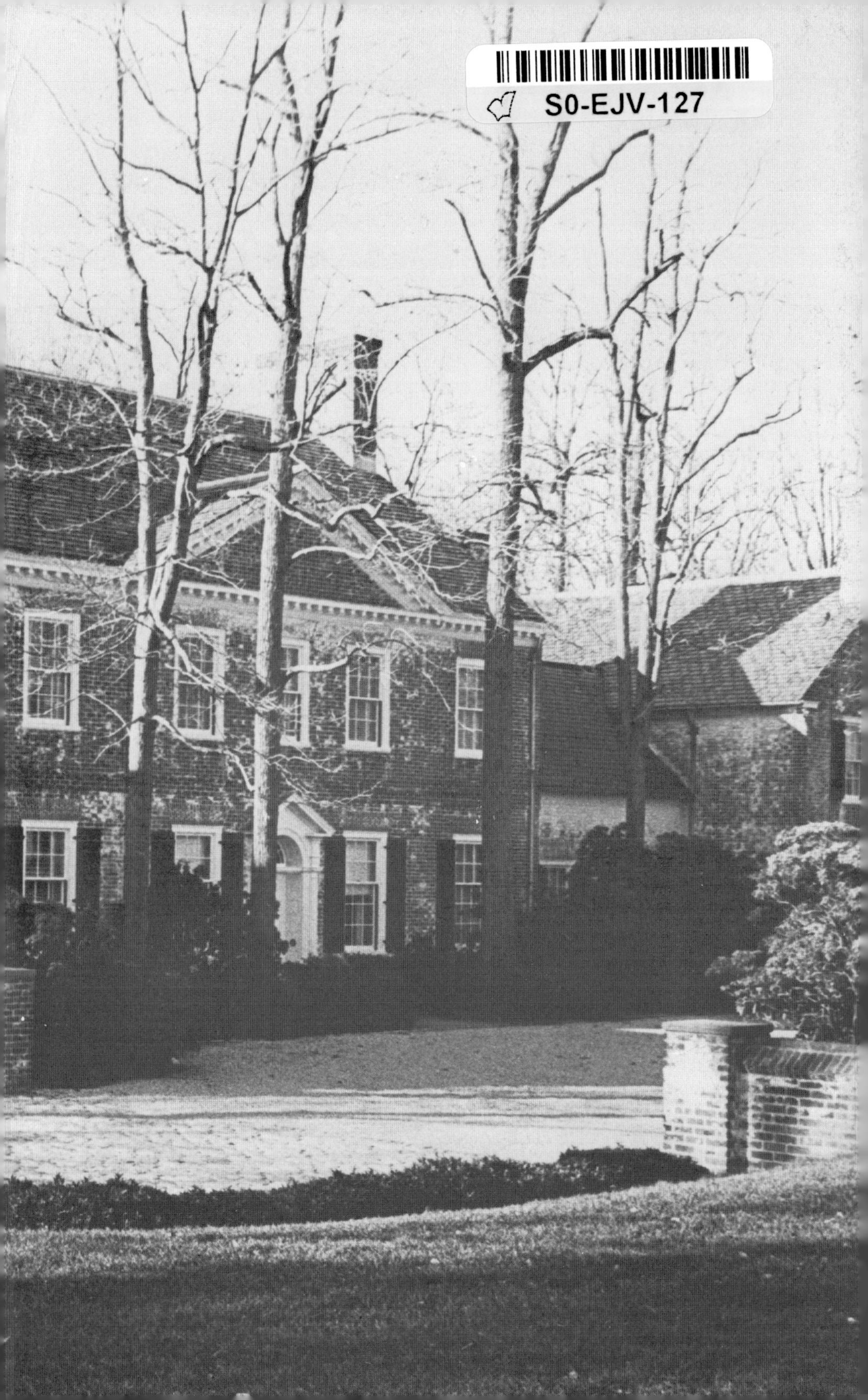

QUANTIFICATION OF OCCUPATIONAL CANCER

First Row: R. Peto; M. Schneiderman; R. Monson, O. Axelson.
Second Row: G. Paddle; J. Cairns, T. Hirayama, J. Peto; S. Darby, D. Berry.
Third Row: M. Sloan; A. Stewart, G. Kneale; O. Wong, S. Austin; W. R. Gaffey.
Fourth Row: A. McMichael; Participants during coffee break; F. Hoerger.

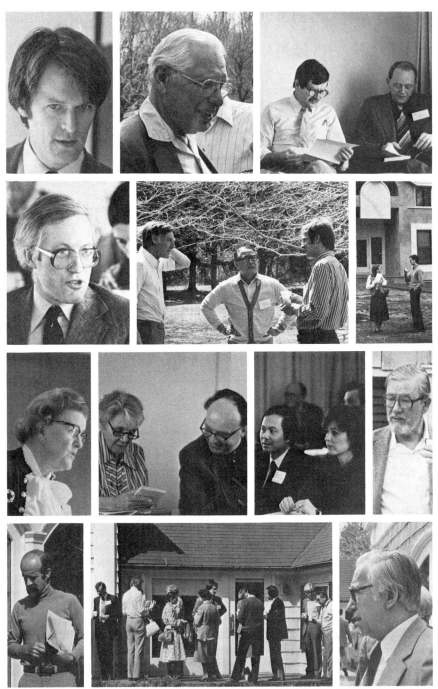

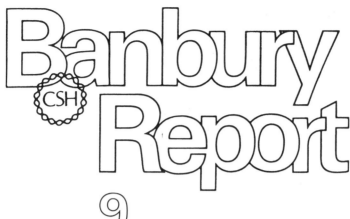

Banbury Report

9

QUANTIFICATION OF OCCUPATIONAL CANCER

Edited by

RICHARD PETO
University of Oxford

MARVIN SCHNEIDERMAN
Clement Associates

COLD SPRING HARBOR LABORATORY
1981

BANBURY REPORT SERIES

Banbury Report 1: Assessing Chemical Mutagens
Banbury Report 2: Mammalian Cell Mutagenesis
Banbury Report 3: A Safe Cigarette?
Banbury Report 4: Cancer Incidence in Defined Populations
Banbury Report 5: Ethylene Dichloride: A Potential Health Risk?
Banbury Report 6: Product Labeling and Health Risks
Banbury Report 7: Gastrointestinal Cancer: Endogenous Factors
Banbury Report 8: Hormones and Breast Cancer

Banbury Report 9
Quantification of Occupational Cancer

Printed in the United States of America

Cover and book design by Emily Harste

Library of Congress Cataloging in Publication Data

Main entry under title:

Quantification of occupational cancer.
(Banbury report; 9)
Includes index.
1. Cancer–Congresses. 2. Occupational diseases–Statistical methods–Congresses. 3. Cancer–Statistical methods–Congresses. 4. Epidemiology–Statistical methods–Congresses. 5. Cancer–Reporting–Congresses. I. Peto, Richard, 1943- . II. Schneiderman, Marvin. III. Series. [DNLM: 1. Neoplasms–Etiology–Congresses. 2. Neoplasms–Occurrence–Congresses. 3. Occupational diseases–Etiology–Congresses. 4. Occupational diseases–Occurrence–Congresses. W3 BA19 v. 9 / QZ 200 013 1981]
RC261.A2Q36 614.5'999 81-10218
ISBN 0-87969-208-1 AACR2

Participants

E. Donald Acheson, MRC Environmental Epidemiology Unit, University of Southampton, England

Michael R. Alderson, Division of Epidemiology, Institute of Cancer Research: Royal Cancer Hospital, Surrey, England

Susan G. Austin, Union Carbide Corporation

Olav Axelson, Department of Occupational Medicine, Medical Informatics and Internal Medicine, Lïnkoping University, Lïnkoping, Sweden

James J. Beaumont, Industrywide Studies Branch, National Institute for Occupational Safety and Health

Gilbert W. Beebe, Clinical Epidemiology Branch, National Cancer Institute, National Institutes of Health

Eula Bingham, University of Cincinnati Medical Center, Institute of Environmental Health

William J. Blot, Environmental Epidemiology Branch, Division of Cancer Cause and Prevention, National Cancer Institute

Patrick Brochard, Service de Pneumologie, Centre Hospitalier Intercommunal, Cedex, France

John Cairns, Harvard School of Public Health

Sarah C. Darby, National Radiological Protection Board, Oxfordshire, England

Devra L. Davis, Environmental Law Institute

Harry B. Demopoulos, Department of Pathology and Coordinated Tumor Registry, New York University Medical Center

Philip E. Enterline, Department of Biostatistics, Graduate School of Public Health, University of Pittsburgh

Samuel S. Epstein, School of Public Health, University of Illinois at the Medical Center

Henry Falk, Chronic Diseases Division, Center for Disease Control

William R. Gaffey, Monsanto Company

Martin J. Gardner, MRC Environmental Epidemiology Unit, University of Southampton, England

Marise S. Gottlieb, Department of Medicine, Tulane University School of Medicine

Takeshi Hirayama, Epidemiology Division, National Cancer Research Institute, Tokyo, Japan

Sheila K. Hoar, Environmental Epidemiology Branch, National Cancer Institute

Fred D. Hoerger, Health and Environmental Sciences, Dow Chemical Company

Bruce W. Karrh, E.I. du Pont de Nemours & Co., Inc.

Myra Karstadt, Environmental Sciences Laboratory, Mount Sinai School of Medicine of The City University of New York

George W. Kneale, Cancer Epidemiology Research Unit, University of Birmingham, England

Marvin Legator, Division of Genetic Toxicology, University of Texas Medical Branch, Galveston

J. Corbett McDonald, TUC Centenary Institute of Occupational Health, London School of Hygiene and Tropical Medicine, England

Victor K. McElheny, Banbury Center, Cold Spring Harbor Laboratory

Anthony J. McMichael, Division of Human Nutrition, Commonwealth Scientific and Industrial Research Organization, Adelaide, South Australia

Jane G. Meikle, Epidemiology and Preventive Medicine Service, Memorial Sloan-Kettering Cancer Center

Samuel Milham, Jr., Epidemiology Section, Washington State Department of Social and Health Services

Richard R. Monson, Department of Epidemiology, Harvard School of Public Health

Norton Nelson, Department of Environmental Medicine, New York University Medical Center

Vaun A. Newill, Medical Department, Exxon Corporation

William J. Nicholson, Environmental Sciences Laboratory, Mount Sinai School of Medicine of The City University of New York

Geoffrey M. Paddle, ICI Central Medical Group, Cheshire, England

Julian Peto, Imperial Cancer Research Fund, Cancer Epidemiology Unit, Oxford, England

Richard Peto, Nuffield Department of Clinical Medicine, Radcliffe Infirmary, University of Oxford, Oxford, England

Edward P. Radford, Center for Environmental Epidemiology, Graduate School of Public Health, University of Pittsburgh

Charles E. Ross, Shell Oil Company

Harry M. Rosenberg, Mortality Statistics Branch, Division of Vital Statistics, National Center for Health Statistics

Sheldon W. Samuels, Industrial Union Department, AFL-CIO

Rodolfo Saracci, Division of Epidemiology and Biostatistics, International Agency for Research on Cancer, Lyon, France

Marvin Schneiderman, Clement Associates, Inc.

Irving J. Selikoff, Environmental Sciences Laboratory, Mount Sinai School of Medicine of The City University of New York

Jack Siemiatycki, Centre de Récherche en Epidémiologie et Médecine Preventie, Institut Armand Frappier, Québec

Michael A. Silverstein, International Union, UAW

Margaret H. Sloan, Occupational Cancer Branch, Division of Resources, Centers, and Community Activities, National Cancer Institute

Martha E. Smith, Vital Statistics and Disease Registries Section, Health Division Statistics Canada, Ottawa

Alice M. Stewart, Cancer Epidemiology Research Unit, Department of Social Medicine, University of Birmingham, England

Joel B. Swartz, School of Public Health, University of Illinois at the Medical Center

Hrafn Tulinius, Icelandic Cancer Registry, Reykjavik, Iceland

Michael D. Utidjian, Union Carbide Corporation

M. Ellen Warshauer, Epidemiology and Preventive Medicine Service, Memorial Sloan-Kettering Cancer Center

James D. Watson, Cold Spring Harbor Laboratory

Richard J. Waxweiler, Industrywide Studies Branch, National Institute for Occupational Safety and Health

Chi Pang Wen, Gulf Oil Corporation

Otto Wong, Biometric Research Institute, Inc.

Preface

The Banbury conference on Quantification of Occupational Cancer, held from 29 March to 2 April 1981, was the ninth in the center's continuing series of small meetings on urgent technical problems of assessing environmental health risks.

The conference explored examples of efforts to trace the influence of substances encountered in the workplace on subsequent illness and death from cancer, and reviewed what is known now about the overall impact of occupation on cancer deaths.

Attacking as it did one of the most difficult and contentious areas of research on environmental health problems, the conference was a kind of climax in the 3-year-old Banbury program. Although the conference was extremely complex to organize, it was conducted with good humor and concentration on facts by the two organizers, Marvin Schneiderman of Clement Associates, Inc., and Richard Peto of the University of Oxford, whom I must thank warmly for all their intense efforts to bring many divergent views together in the same forum. We were lucky, as Dr. James Watson, Director of Cold Spring Harbor Laboratory, said during opening remarks at the conference, to have such "slightly divergent friends" as our organizers.

A crucial reason for starting the Banbury program, as Dr. Watson said, was that the work of Cold Spring Harbor Laboratory, so heavily focused on tumor viruses, and thus on the cancer problem generally, is allied to a growing realization that many carcinogenic substances activate changes in DNA.

Thus it was natural for Cold Spring Harbor Laboratory to stage the 1976 conference on Origins of Human Cancer as part of its continuing series of meetings on cell proliferation. The 1976 meeting, in which I and others at the occupational cancer conference took part, indicated that studies of environmental factors in cancer could throw much light on the agonizingly complex mechanisms of induction of cancer.

The conference on Origins of Human Cancer also indicated that there was need for scientific forums for discussion of environmental health risks that would be somewhat removed from the contentiousness of court rooms and hearing rooms, and would bring together geneticists with specialists in public health, industrial hygiene, and toxicology. The apparent economic costs of environmental regulations were looming larger. There was even the prospect of a backlash against health protection measures in the name of preserving jobs. The factual basis of environmental health risk assessment needed strengthening.

The Banbury series of meetings was not designed to produce a consensus, which, as Dr. Watson notes, is not possible in many difficult cases. The conferences are designed to cover a broad range, including divergent viewpoints. For that reason we seek organizers with different ways of looking at the problems. We strive to have Banbury discussions follow the 50-year tradition of the Cold Spring Harbor Symposia on Quantitative Biology that if people hear something they don't believe, they don't wait very long before questioning it.

The major reason for difficulty in organizing this conference on Quantification of Occupational Cancer rose from the very sharp differences of opinion as to the size of the occupational cancer problem and about what we should do with the answer to the question if we could obtain it.

Despite the difficulties of organization, the conference indicated that previous divergences on this very important topic are narrowing. Everyone realizes that the full dimensions of the problem of occupational cancer cannot be measured yet, and that we need a great deal of attention to what types of research must be encouraged—that is, to better formulating of the questions and lobbying for support to obtain the necessary data (particularly epidemiological data).

I think there may be increasing agreement to the proposition that even if the total proportion of all cancer attributable to occupation turns out to be small, the problem will still have a very high priority for research and action, not only by the private sector but also by governments with responsibility to protect the public health. Even if the total numbers turn out to be small, we are dealing with hundreds or even thousands of separate cancer-risk situations in the workplace, each demanding the best information the scientific community can provide.

With great pleasure, I wish to extend my warmest thanks to all who took part in the conference and production of this volume of proceedings. I must thank particularly my administrative assistant, Beatrice Toliver, and the Banbury editors, Lynda Moran and Judith Cuddihy for their unstinting efforts.

VICTOR K. McELHENY

Foreword

This meeting has been organized to try to help move toward reducing the burden of cancer in industrial countries. We will try to do this, I think, by exploring the science base for efforts to prevent cancer. Our major efforts will be devoted to the tasks of defining better what it is that humans are exposed to that they ought not to be exposed to and suggesting ways to avoid this exposure, without suggesting methods to avoid our industrial society. Like everybody else, I enjoy the fruits of an industrial society. This, as most science meetings, affords us the opportunity to learn a lot about what we do not know. We are fortunate to have here with us some very knowledgeable people.

Industrial health is not an academic problem, although academics are rather deeply involved. Academics are often thought of as thinkers rather than doers. Like so many generalizations, that is partly true. When it comes to taking health-promoting action, there are people who say, "Now," and there are people who say, "Not yet–I need more proof." On the other hand, I read not too long ago a piece that characterized the evidence linking cigarette smoking and cancer as demonstrating that something was "sort of a cause." I wonder if the author is still smoking cigarettes.

I think proof, like beauty, lies in the eyes of the beholder. But people's behavior is related to perceptions of proof, and therefore I think we are going to explore some aspects of proof and I think some aspects of cause.

I don't expect any proof to emerge from this meeting. I do expect that we will hear a great deal of useful information on a limited number of substantive issues. We are going to talk about them as examples of what we know, what we don't know, and how we can get to know better.

I don't expect that we will hear all, or even most, of the things that go into making policy decisions or action decisions with respect to regulation and disease prevention, as very few of the regulators are here. There are suspicions domestically that regulatory decisions in this country for the next several years may be as likely to derive from ideology as from science. There are people who assert that this has always been true, and the only thing that has changed now is not the science, but the ideology.

Those of us who were involved in organizing this meeting have heard a great deal from many people who believe that there are too few participants here from their particular side of the issue, whatever side they may be on, or that the program is unbalanced or biased. I think all the complainers are correct. There are too few people here from all sides, and the program is incomplete. In that sense, I think it must be biased. My only consolation is that having been challenged from all directions, we probably were close to being unbiased in our biases.

In the rapidly changing political climate that we have had here in the United States over the last year or two, while we were trying to put this meeting together, we found it imperative to shift gears on the meeting more than once. Our patient, flexible colleagues and participants deserve substantial thanks for their cooperation in also shifting gears and modifying emphasis along with us. I particularly want to thank those people who responded on very short notice to our needs for better balance.

I also want to thank James Watson for having conceived of the Banbury meetings and for having supported Vic McElheny in his patient, decent, gentlemanly carrying out of all the burdens that organizing and bringing about such a conference like this entail. We have got 4 days here, roughly, in which to get to know each other, to try to talk with each other, to explore what we know and what we don't know, and to point our future behavior toward possible convergences. I think that means improved health.

MARVIN SCHNEIDERMAN

Introduction

The problem is that everyone is exposed to carcinogens. The more we know, the more things seem to be carcinogenic. Everyone is exposed to carcinogens. For example, a year or two ago Sugimura and Nagao (1979) found, using the Ames test, that onions consist of 1 or 2% by net weight of a substance which is highly mutagenic in the Ames test and carcinogenic for animals. It is very difficult to know what to do with such information.

One possible reaction has been to argue that for most carcinogens a 'threshhold' exposure level will exist, below which there is absolute safety, and then by some obscure logical process to believe that we hardly need worry at all about present-day levels of exposure to occupational carcinogens. But, the more that is understood about the mechanisms of carcinogenesis (at least by the more potent chemical carcinogens), the less plausible 'thresholds' become (Crump et al. 1976). We should, in practice, assume that for nearly all occupational carcinogens, there will be hazards associated even with low levels of exposure. It would be exceptional to find occupational carcinogens where there is real safety, although the risks will obviously be lower with lower doses.

An opposite attitude is to ignore differences in dose and to treat all exposure as being equally terrible. But, that is completely impractical: for many agents, complete avoidance of exposure is not possible.

If we are to avoid extreme absurdities such as these, the sensible thing to aim for is some kind of quantitative perspective, which is the purpose of this book. This may in practice ensure that we do at least control the larger risks and thus have some important impact on disease. It really does matter whether you are killing 0.1%, 1%, 10%, or whatever percentage that you are killing by some particular agent. I will try to use an example of this point that for the moment is fairly neutral.

We have reasonably good information about tobacco carcinogenesis, and it is quite clear from this evidence that tobacco accounts for about 30% of all cancer deaths in America, and a rather similar proportion in Britain, and that alcohol accounts for about 3% of all cancer deaths in America, and perhaps also in Britain. The difference matters. Because tobacco is 30% and alcohol is 3%, the prevention of smoking is a much, much more important public health objective, at least in terms of prevention of premature death, than the prevention of drinking. It means that a 10% reduction in exposure to tobacco could confer benefits which are as great as the abolition of alcohol, the complete abolition of all use of alcohol, and it would be considerably easier to achieve as a public health objective.

I cite these numbers for three reasons. First, I want to note that the total due to alcohol and tobacco is 31%. It is not 33%, it is 31%, for cancers of the mouth, larynx, pharynx, and esophagus are caused both by tobacco and by alcohol. There are situations where one individual case of cancer has had two causes, tobacco and alcohol, in the sense that avoidance of either cause would have resulted in avoidance of the cancer. So, if one says 30% of all cancer deaths are caused by tobacco, that is not to say that they do not also have other causes, as we will, of course, be hearing at this conference in the asbestos context.

The second point that I wanted to make is that percentages matter. If we are trying to do something about public health, then we had better really understand the difference between 30% and 3%. Otherwise, we may be much less effective then we might be at preventing premature death.

The last point that is quite interesting is that, although there has been conclusive evidence for more than a quarter of a century of roughly the sort of scale of death that tobacco causes, both in cancer and in chronic obstructive lung disease, and probably in vascular disease as well, it is interesting that the industry and spokesmen for the industry, still do not accept this. There can never be, really, clearer proof that we now have with tobacco. Yet the industry concerned will not accept in public that it is causing these deaths. I think that this will be true of many other industries which are found to cause deaths.

I doubt whether there are any others which cause death on anything like the scale that the tobacco manufacturers do. But when an industry is found to cause substantial numbers of deaths, with a few exceptions within widely diversified industries (as opposed to single-product industries, such as asbestos) there will be deliberate attempts to mislead government and the public as to what the evidence is. Even if certain individuals in such industries want to be humane and want to work in some kind of way towards the general good, and they are effective at doing so, then they will find themselves rendered impotent or fired, because it is not in the commerical interests of an industry to have its products advertised as causing this, that, and the other kind of disease. At present, the tobacco industry is the most blatant example of this. Even knowing what they are doing, knowing the effects that they already have, they are deliberately trying to generate new markets in the third world, selling high-tar cigarettes–much too high to sell any longer in the U.S. or in Britain. Thus, one has to discover the causes of deaths, and then actually do something about them legislatively, because little will happen by the goodness of human nature.

If our aim is a quantitative perspective on cancer in general and on occupational cancer in particular, then there are two things that we need to do. The first, I suppose, will appear rather more sterile than the second, but I think that both are necessary.

We do have to examine previous quantitative assertions that still are maintained. If somebody in the past has made some quantitative assertion and it has disappeared–it is no longer quoted, it is no longer part of the general political process–then, whether or not it was nonsense, we can forget it. But if there are quantitative assertions that have been made and that are still maintained, and if what we want is a quantitative perspective, then we have to examine those assertions.

The two things that seem to me outstanding in this respect are (1) the OSHA document of 1978, the one which generated the statement that 23-38% of all cancers are, or will in the future be due to occupational exposure, and (2) the assertion that whether there is good evidence for a generalized increase in cancer at the moment over and above the effects of tobacco.

My opinion based on my reading of the data, is that both suggestions are demonstrably false. Other people have different opinions, but I do think we have to go into both questions. We cannot skate over them. The difference between the beliefs associated with both of these and what I consider to be the truth is as extreme as the 3%/30% difference between the quantitative effects of alcohol and of tobacco. Either I am wrong or the people who are making these assertions are wrong. These are not assertions that have been made once and have sunk into oblivion, they are assertions that continue to have a considerable influence on the public debate, both in Britain and in America, as many probably know.

The much more enjoyable, interesting, and constructive side to the conference which is reported on in this book is the discussion of what sorts of new evidence to seek. There are many ways in which one can seek new sorts of evidence. One that I particularly urge is that there should be a really large national case-control study of lung cancer that monitors occupational factors and which monitors tobacco usage. It would have a variety of purposes. It would, particularly, give direct information about the present hazards of various occupational cancers, or at least those occupational cancers which we know how to ask about. It would give information, of course, only about the present, but could not give information about the future. Nothing that we can really do now can exclude the possibility that there is a disaster looming in the future as a result of the vast increases in chemical production that have taken place recently. Equally, I think nothing at present can really refute the sort of Pangloss approach, which says that things are getting better and that they will continue to get better and nothing bad is going to happen.

The argument as to what will happen in the future is one in which opinions differ legitimately. The argument as to what is happening in the present is one in which the evidence is not complete but is quite substantial, and it should be easy to agree on what sorts of evidence to seek and then find it.

I don't propose the case-control study as being the only thing that would be of interest. But I do hope that the question of whether such a case-control study really would help solve very much will be considered and criticized.

In this introduction I should mention that Richard Doll and I were asked to prepare a critique of other people's estimates of what percentage of cancer was due to which causes and to prepare our own estimates with which these could be contrasted (Doll and Peto 1981; Peto, this volume). It was our major activity for 18 months to try to make sense of these numbers, and to see what we can say, what we cannot say, and where it is reasonable to be definite and where one cannot yet be definite. The result is a reasonably carefully written report from us to the Office of Technology Assessment on these issues. That document really defines what I think.

In this book it is my hope that we will deal with what is the rather sterile question of past estimates and then try to approach constructively the questions of where we should go from here and what should we ask for.

REFERENCES

Crump, K.S., D.G. Hoel, C.H. Langley, and R. Peto. 1976. Fundamental carcinogenic processes and their implications for low-dose risk assessment. *Cancer Res.* **36**:2973.

Doll, R. and R. Peto. 1981. The causes of cancer: Quantitative estimates of avoidable risks of cancer in the United States today. *J. Natl. Cancer Inst.* **66**:1191.

Sugimura, T. and M. Nagao. 1979. Mutagenic factors in cooked foods. *CRC Crit. Rev. Toxicol.* **6**:189.

RICHARD PETO

Contents

SESSION 1: Asbestos and Other Mineral Fibers

Constraints in Estimating Occupational Contributions to Current Cancer Mortality in the United States

IRVING J. SELIKOFF
Environmental Sciences Laboratory
Mount Sinai School of Medicine
of The City University of New York
New York, New York 10029

There is presently a valid debate concerning how much current cancer is associated with occupational causes. It is likely that there will be no easy resolution because the background for these discussions in many ways reflects the paucity of data needed for definitive judgment. These deficits do not reflect the inadequacies of investigators or evaluators; rather, they are structural and derive from the relatively recent emergence of both the question and the research. A variety of difficulties has been identified, and among the more important ones are:

1. Current estimates generally are based upon what is known so far concerning agents that have caused, are causing, and will cause cancer in man (Althouse et al. 1979) (Table 1). These estimates include those circumstances in which reliable epidemiological data are available. Comparatively few agents have warranted such acceptance, but it is uncertain that benzidine, nickel, asbestos, *bis*(chloromethyl)ether, vinyl chloride, arsenic, β-naphthylamine, and their few brethren form a complete list and that the next decade will not augment what is presently known.
2. There is continuing reluctance to accept, for estimates of potential human cancer risk, animal carcinogens. Even when human exposure occurs, the absence of epidemiological confirmation continues these agents in one or another "suspect" category, and current estimates concerning occupational cancer risk therefore do not include the possibility that these agents are associated with cancer among workers. Laboratory observations concerning mutagenesis are regarded in very much the same way (European Chemical Industry Ecology and Toxicology Centre 1980).
3. Latency has many ramifications, many of which are critically important. Thus, recently introduced agents (1950-1970) may not have had the chance to demonstrate whether or not they will be associated with occupational cancer. For those occupational carcinogens already identified, we often know only the short-term effects, in quantitative terms (Selikoff et al. 1980).

Table 1
IARC Carcinogens for Humans

	Probably carcinogenic	
Carcinogenic for humans	high degree of evidence	lower degree of evidence
4-Aminobiphenyl	aflatoxins	acrylonitrile
Arsenic and certain arsenic compounds	cadmium and certain cadmium compounds	amitrole (aminotriazole)
Asbestos	chlorambucil	auramine
Auramine manufacture	cyclophosphamide	beryllium and certain beryllium compounds
Benzene	nickel and certain nickel compounds	carbon tetrachloride
Benzidine	tris(1-aziridinyl)phosphine sulfide (thio-TEPA)	dimethylcarbamoyl chloride
N,N-bis(2-chloroethyl)-2-naphthylamine (chlornaphazine)		dimethylsulfate
Bis(chloromethyl)ether and technical-grade chloromethyl ether		ethylene oxide
Chromium and certain chromium compounds		iron dextran
Diethylstilbestrol		oxymetholone
Underground hematite mining		phenacetin
Manufacture of isopropyl alcohol by the strong acid process		polychlorinated biphenyls
Melphalan		
Mustard gas		
2-Naphthylamine		
Nickel refining		
Soot, tar, and mineral oils		
Vinyl chloride		

Data from Althouse et al. (1979).

By definition, first reports intend to reflect initial evaluation of experiences. Vinyl chloride is one such example. It has been stated that the first polymerization plant in the United States started production in 1938. The industry remained quite small, with few workers, until the 1950s and 1960s, when expansion proceeded at the rate of approximately 10% per annum. Reports of angiosarcoma of the liver in workers, beginning in 1974, were of individuals who had begun work, on the average, less than 20 years before. Data are not available concerning what the incidence might be 25, 30, or 40 or more years from onset of exposure.

4. The occurrence of "signal" neoplasms has been effective, in epidemiological terms, in identifying human cancer risks with a variety of agents. Sinus cancer with nickel smelting, mesothelioma with asbestos, and vinyl chloride angiosarcoma are good examples. Nevertheless, consideration of such agents only in relation to knowledge of unique associations with otherwise uncommon neoplasms omits the possibility of a much wider, and quantitatively more important, spectrum of associated cancer. With nickel, for example, cancer of the lung takes far more lives among nickel smelter workers than sinus cancer (Sunderman 1978). The same is true among asbestos workers at this time in relation to mesothelioma. It is unfortunate that we do not yet have long-term, large-scale epidemiological investigations of cohorts of vinyl chloride-exposed workers to tell us whether the spectrum of neoplasms observed in experimental animals exposed to vinyl chloride (Maltoni and Lefemine 1974) will also occur in human populations.
5. In the case of populations exposed to known (or suspect) carcinogens, even for those agents that have been identified, there is often only fragmentary information concerning the number of people exposed 1930-1970. For current exposures, we have often depended upon the National Occupational Health Survey I (NOHS I) data, based upon a survey that was not designed for this particular purpose and with many constraints, weaknesses, and deficits. It was pressed into service for population estimates in the absence of other information.
6. It is difficult to make dose-disease-response estimates in the absence of exposure measurements in past years. In the nature of things, measurements were not made when currently suspect or acknowledged agents were introduced originally. With asbestos, for example, we suffer the difficulty of estimating dose-disease-response relationships in the absence of dust measurements in the 1940s, 1950s, and 1960s.
7. Initial data suggest that interaction among agents may significantly alter cancer risk of an occupational carcinogen. Asbestos and smoking and uranium and smoking are examples. Yet, there are only fragmentary data so far to allow evaluation in most circumstances of the potential for multiple factor interaction. Accordingly, we generally continue to regard each agent as if it were the only one to which a worker were exposed.

8. At least in the United States, there is considerable mobility in employment during a worker's lifetime with opportunity for multiple sequential or concomitant exposures to potential carcinogenic agents. This factor of lifetime occupational exposures has been studied only uncommonly in most populations.
9. There are diagnostic and categorization uncertainties. Attempts are made to utilize "signal" neoplasms as indices of the total neoplastic burden associated with specific agents. There are difficulties with this approach, however. At least until experience with such otherwise unusual neoplasms becomes widely known and diagnostic criteria set, there is serious risk of misdiagnosis; this has been the case with mesothelioma and angiosarcoma. The former has also suffered from inadequate opportunity for categorization in the International Classification of Diseases (ICD), 6th to 8th revisions and, unhappily, in the current 9th revision as well. Even in well-established neoplasms, opportunities for inaccurate categorizations exist (Selikoff and Seidman 1981) and comparisons among populations are often insecure (Percy and Dolman 1978).

   Estimates based upon "diagnosed mesothelioma" in the files of pathology departments (especially from the 1960s and 1970s) or on death certificates in vital statistics records inevitably are subject to important underdiagnosis. Projections of total neoplastic risk derived from the use of these yardsticks are inappropriate. Histological review of all diffuse pleural and peritoneal neoplasms would be more effective, but this has not been done often. It is not the practice, for example, even in the Surveillance, Epidemiology, and End Results (SEER) program.
10. There have been secular changes in industrial agents and processes. Estimates vary as to the number of new chemicals introduced into industrial use each year, but it is at least several hundred. It is not yet wide practice to undertake preliminary laboratory investigation of potential carcinogenicity and, of course, epidemiological data cannot be expected. Recommendations have been made concerning examination of structural similarities to known carcinogens. This may prove useful, but has not yet found wide acceptance.
11. In making quantitative projections for future estimates, it should be appreciated that current occupational cancer experience reflects exposures decades ago. Current exposures are often quite different, generally much less intense, and better controlled. Projections concerning future risk need take this into account.
12. We know very little about intrauterine exposures. Thalidomide and diethylstilbestrol have sensitized us to this possibility, however, and the demonstration of transplacental angiosarcoma by Maltoni and Lefemine (1974) has provided experimental data bearing on the matter.
13. The germinal papers of Wagner et al. (1960) and Newhouse and Thompson

(1965) have established the important principle of environmental cancer from occupational sources. Quantitation has been slow in coming, although opportunity exists for such estimates (Selikoff 1977; Anderson et al. 1979). Nevertheless, by and large, this problem has not been investigated for most agents. If Hirayama's data concerning lung cancer rates among nonsmoking wives of smoking husbands are confirmed (Hirayama 1981), the problem of low-level household contact disease will be further sharpened.

CASE STUDY: ASBESTOS-ASSOCIATED NEOPLASMS

It may be instructive to examine how these constraints operated in evaluation of cancer risk associated with occupational exposure to asbestos. Case reports of lung cancer in asbestos workers were recorded in 1935 (Gloyne 1935; Lynch and Smith 1935), and collections of such cases subsequently appeared. It remained for Doll, however, in a classic paper published in 1955, to establish clearly, on a population basis, the association of occupational exposure to asbestos and lung cancer (Doll 1955). This investigation properly is considered a landmark in studies of asbestos cancer (Selikoff 1975).

Doll studied the mortality experience of 113 men who worked for at least 20 years in a "scheduled area" in an asbestos products factory, during the period 1922-1953. Altogether, there were 39 deaths, with 15.4 expected. Based upon rates for England and Wales, 0.8 deaths of lung cancer were anticipated; 11 were observed. Doll stated, "From the data it can be concluded that lung cancer was a specific industrial hazard of certain asbestos workers . . . among men employed for 20 or more years. . . ."

This conclusion was entirely appropriate. Yet, when it is examined closely, one can appreciate how the constraints inherent in the research opportunities available to Doll limited a fuller characterization of the problem.

"Lung Cancer"

All that could be said from the data obtained in the study was that bronchogenic carcinoma was increased significantly. In retrospect, even with hindsight, one could not expect that the panoply of other asbestos-associated neoplasms could have been seen in excess in 39 deaths among 113 people.

Although mesothelioma had been reported in an asbestos worker in 1953 (Weiss. 1953), the strength of the association between asbestos exposure and mesothelioma was not well established until 1960, with Wagner's report from the northwest Cape Province (Wagner et al. 1960). Doll did note that one of the 11 cases of respiratory cancer was an endothelioma of the pleura, but this was insufficient to warrant further special notice. Too, other neoplasms were present in some excess (2.3 expected, 4 observed) but with such limited experience, one could not hope to evaluate the significant excess occurrence

Table 2
Deaths among 17,800 Asbestos Insulation Workers in the United States and Canada, January 1, 1967 - December 31, 1976

Underlying cause of death	Expected[a]	Observed BE[b]	Observed DC[c]	Ratio O/E BE	Ratio O/E DC
Total deaths, all causes	1658.9	2271	2271	1.37	1.37
Total cancer, all sites	319.7	995	922	3.11	2.88
Cancer of lung	105.6	486	429	4.60	4.06
Pleural mesothelioma	**[d]	63	25	–	–
Peritoneal mesothelioma	**	112	24	–	–
Mesothelioma, n.o.s.	**	0	55	–	–
Cancer of esophagus	7.1	18	18	2.53	2.53
Cancer of stomach	14.2	22	18	1.54	1.26
Cancer of colon-rectum	38.1	59	58	1.55	1.52
Cancer of larynx	4.7	11	9	2.34	1.91
Cancer of pharynx, buccal	10.1	21	16	2.08	1.59
Cancer of kidney	8.1	19	18	2.36	2.23
All other cancer	131.8	184	252	1.40	1.91
Noninfectious pulmonary diseases, total	59.0	212	188	3.59	3.19
Asbestosis	**	168	78	–	–
All other causes	1280.2	1064	1161	0.83	0.91

Data from Selikoff et al. (1979).
Number of men, 17,800; man-years of observation, 166,853.
[a]Expected deaths are based upon white male, age-specific U.S. death rates of the U.S. National Center for Health Statistics, 1967-1976.
[b]Best evidence. Number of deaths categorized after review of best available information (autopsy, surgical, clinical).
[c]Number of deaths as recorded from death certificate information only.
[d]Rates are not available, but these have been rare causes of death in the general population.

of neoplasms that were later found to be associated with asbestos exposure. Opportunity to identify excess risk of cancer of the esophagus, colon-rectum, stomach, oropharynx, larynx, and kidney, simply were not available in this initial investigation even though later studies of much larger populations demonstrated the important risk of these neoplasms (Selikoff et al. 1979) (Table 2).

"Was"

The asbestos industry regulations of 1931, which were scheduled for implementation in 1933, were considered to have been effective in controlling hazardous asbestos exposure, although subsequent information indicated that this was not necessarily the case (Lancet 1976). Also, at the time there was little information concerning cancer risk that might be associated with less intense exposures than that which obtained in "scheduled areas." Therefore, all that could be said in 1955 was what had happened in the past. We now know that later exposures in the same plant were, unfortunately, also associated with risk (Peto et al. 1977).

"Specific Industrial Hazard"

The workers whose experiences were studied by Doll were employed in an asbestos products manufacturing factory that originally had been selected for investigation of the disease potential of asbestos (Merewether and Price 1930). The selection had been made for a very good industrial hygiene reason. It was known that asbestos was used in a variety of circumstances. It was considered difficult to evaluate the unique disease potential of the dust in industrial circumstances where other agents (cement, silica, etc.) might be present, as in the construction industry. It was deemed more reasonable to seek an employment setting where the effects of the agent would not be obscured or modified by the presence of other noxious materials. Doll had no way of knowing whether other asbestos-exposed workers, not studied by him, might also have such risk and his statement reflects prudent acceptance of limits inherent in the study. However, it soon became known that users of the manufactured products also were at serious risk (Selikoff et al. 1964) and that it was exposure to asbestos that was associated with risk rather than the exact industrial occupational category of "asbestos products manufacture." Unfortunately, it is likely that for each worker manufacturing asbestos products, there are over 100 exposed during their use (Nicholson, this volume).

"Certain Asbestos Workers"

Doll limited his conclusions to observations of workers studied by him. Comment could not have been made concerning risk other than among these "certain workers." Prediction would have been difficult concerning risk among shipyard workers, brake-repair workers, family contacts, construction workers, residents close by some asbestos facilities, and others.

"Employed 20 or More Years"

In the circumstances that obtained in his study, Doll noted that ". . . the labour involved in searching out the individual records of men employed for shorter periods would be disproportionately great. . . ." Thus, there were not available to him data concerning experiences of workers with shorter exposures—1 month,

Table 3
Age-standardized Lung Cancer Death Rates for Cigarette Smoking and (or) Occupational Exposure to Asbestos Dust Compared with No Smoking and No Occupational Exposure to Asbestos Dust

Group	Exposure to asbestos	History cigarette smoking?	Death rate	Mortality difference	Mortality ratio
Control	no	no	11.3	0.0	1.00
Asbestos workers	yes	no	58.4	+47.1	5.17
Control	no	yes	122.6	+111.3	10.85
Asbestos workers	yes	yes	601.6	+590.3	53.24

Data from Hammond et al. (1979).

Age-standardized lung cancer death rates are rates per 100,000 man-years standardized for age on the distribution of the man-years of all the asbestos workers. Number of lung cancer deaths based on death certificate information.

1 year, 10 years—but followed for equally long periods of duration from onset of such exposure. Yet, we now know that such exposure may be associated with very substantial risk (Seidman et al. 1979). The importance of this is emphasized by our knowledge that there are comparatively few asbestos-exposed workers who have been exposed for 20 or more years, in contrast to the very much larger number exposed for shorter periods.

Other Factors

The terms of Doll's study did not admit the investigation of the health experience of family contacts of asbestos workers or other forms of environmental cancer risk, nor was there opportunity for the investigation of multiple-factor interaction between asbestos exposure and cigarette smoking. The importance of the latter (Selikoff et al. 1968; Hammond et al. 1979) can be appreciated immediately on examination of Table 3, which provides data concerning the relative risk of individuals exposed to cigarette smoke or asbestos or to both.

Doll's was the earliest cohort study of a group of asbestos workers. It was necessarily truncated and at the time of publication recorded, as noted, only 39 deaths among the 113 people in the cohort. Subsequent experiences have shown that the total long-term findings among such groups of workers may give a much more complete analysis of their cancer experience. We studied, for example, a cohort of asbestos workers established on January 1, 1943, until January 1, 1977 (Selikoff et al. 1979). Among the 632 men being observed, 478 deaths had occurred (Table 4). While lung cancer was found to be the most significant neoplastic cause of death, there was also a significant number of deaths of

Table 4
Expected and Observed Deaths among 632 New York-New Jersey Asbestos Insulation Workers, January 1, 1943-December 31, 1976

Underlying cause of death	Expected[a]	Observed
Total deaths, all causes	328.9	478
Total cancer, all sites	57.0	210
Cancer of lung	13.3	93
Pleural mesothelioma	**[b]	11
Peritoneal mesothelioma	**	27
Cancer of esophagus	1.4	1
Cancer of stomach	5.4	19
Cancer of colon-rectum	8.3	23
Cancer of larynx, pharynx, buccal cavity	2.8	6
Cancer of kidney	1.3	2
All other cancer	24.5	28
Noninfectious pulmonary diseases, total	9.3	45
Asbestosis	**	41
All other causes	262.6	223

Data from Selikoff et al. (1979). Man-years of observation, 13,925.

[a]Expected deaths are based upon white male, age-specific U.S. death rates of the U.S. National Center for Health Statistics, 1949-1976. Rates for specific causes of death for 1943-1948 were extrapolated from rates for 1949-1955.

[b]Rates are not available, but these have been rare causes of death in the general population

pleural and peritoneal mesothelioma, as well as of gastrointestinal and other cancers.

COMMENT

If asbestos first had been introduced in 1940 and Doll had investigated the experiences of workers in a plant of this new industry in 1965 or 1970, we might now be pointing to an equally excellent study establishing lung cancer as a risk of workers heavily exposed in this plant. But we would know little or nothing about the full spectrum of asbestos neoplastic risk, the very large number of people who had been exposed, the augmentation of that risk by concomitant cigarette smoking, the problem of environmental cancer with asbestos, the importance of "bystander" exposure in shipyards, and hazards associated with the use of asbestos products, and we might conclude that asbestos could account for very little of the cancer burden in the United States.

REFERENCES

Althouse, R., L. Tomatis, J. Huff, and J. Wilbourn. 1979. Evaluation of the carcinogenic risk of chemicals to humans: Chemicals and industrial processes associated with cancer in humans. *IARC Sc. Publ.* **1-20** (Suppl. 1):1.

Anderson, H.A., R. Lilis, S.M. Daum, and I.J. Selikoff. 1979. Asbestosis among household contacts of asbestos factory workers. *Ann. N.Y. Acad. Sci.* **330**:387.

Doll, R. 1955. Mortality from lung cancer in asbestos workers. *Br. J. Ind. Med.* **12**:81.

European Chemical Industry Ecology and Toxicology Centre. 1980. *A contribution to the strategy for the identification and control of occupational carcinogens.* Monograph No. 2. Brussels, Belgium.

Gloyne, S.R. 1935. Two cases of squamous carcinoma of the lung occurring in asbestosis. *Tubercle* **17**:5.

Hammond, E.C., I.J. Selikoff, and H. Seidman. 1979. Asbestos exposure, cigarette smoking and death rates. *Ann. N.Y. Acad. Sci.* **330**:473.

Hirayama, T. 1981. Non-smoking wives of heavy smokers have a higher risk of lung cancer: A study from Japan. *Br. Med. J.* **282**:183.

Lancet. 1976. Asbestos in the air. *Lancet* **1**:944.

Lynch, K.M. and W.A. Smith. 1935. Pulmonary asbestosis. V. A report of a bronchial carcinoma and epithelial metaplasia. *Am. J. Cancer* **36**:567.

Maltoni, C. and G. Lefemine. 1974. Carcinogenicity bioassays of vinyl chloride. 1. Research plan and early results. *Environ. Res.* **7**:387.

Merewether, E.R.A. and C.V. Price. 1930. Report on effects of asbestos dust on the lungs and dust suppression in the asbestos industry. Part I. Occurrence of pulmonary fibrosis and other pulmonary affections in asbestos workers. Part II. Processes giving rise to dust and methods for its suppression. Her Majesty's Stationary Office, London.

Newhouse, M.L. and H. Thompson. 1965. Mesothelioma of pleura and peritoneum following exposure to asbestos in the London area. *Br. J. Ind. Med.* **22**:261.

Percy, C. and A. Dolman. 1978. Comparison of the coding of death certificates related to cancer in seven countries. *Public Health Rep.* **93**:335.

Peto, J., R. Doll, S.V. Howard, L.J. Kinlen, and H.C. Lewinsohn. 1977. A mortality study among workers in an English asbestos factory. *Br. J. Ind. Med.* **34**:169.

Seidman, H., I.J. Selikoff, and E.C. Hammond. 1979. Short-term asbestos work exposure and long-term observation. *Ann. N.Y. Acad. Sci.* **330**:61.

Selikoff, I.J. 1975. Recent perspectives in occupational cancer. *Ambio* **IV**: 14.

______. 1977. Perspectives in the investigation of health hazards in the chemical industry. *Ecotoxicology and Environmental Safety* **1**:387.

Selikoff, I.J. and H. Seidman. 1981. Cancer of the pancreas among asbestos insulation workers. *Cancer* **47**:1469.

Selikoff, I.J., J. Churg, and E.C. Hammond. 1964. Asbestos exposure and neoplasia. *J. Am. Med. Assoc.* **188**:22.

Selikoff, I.J., E.C. Hammond, and J. Churg. 1968. Asbestos exposure, smoking and neoplasia. *J. Am. Med. Assoc.* **204**:106.

Selikoff, I.J., E.C. Hammond, and H. Seidman. 1979. Mortality experience of insulation workers in the United States and Canada. *Ann. N.Y. Acad. Sci.* **330**:91.

———. 1980. Latency of asbestos disease among insulation workers in the United States and Canada. *Cancer* **46**:2736.

Sunderman, F.W., Jr. 1978. Carcinogenic effects of metals. *Fed. Proc.* **37**:40.

Wagner, J.C., C.A. Sleggs, and P. Marchand. 1960. Diffuse pleural mesothelioma and asbestos exposure in the North Western Cape Province. *Br. J. Ind. Med.* **17**:260.

Weiss, A. 1953. Pleurakrebs bei lungenasbestose in vivo morphologisch gesichert. *Medizinische* **1**:93.

COMMENTS

ENTERLINE: I have always wanted to ask you, Irving [Selikoff], about the Paterson, New Jersey, workers who were employed during World War II. Who was available to be employed at that period of time? Were these people deferred, or were they people who couldn't get into the military?

SELIKOFF: It varied. Until 1943, they were basically very young people who were waiting to go into the service. They were new to the work force, they were unskilled, and they often worked only for a month or two. During the period 1943-1944, people who were too old to go into the service, or were otherwise not easily available for service, were found more frequently.

Therefore, it was quite a mixed group. In fact, Herb Seidman and Cuyler Hammond have found this fascinating, because we now have two groups that were exposed at the same time, to the same agent, in the same city, making the same product, with the same machinery—one group old at first exposure and one young at first exposure. There are some interesting differences between the two groups.

R. PETO: In both of the studies you presented, you described one-quarter of the excess cancer as mesothelioma; you had both best estimates and death certificates. There must have been some likelihood of a mesothelioma being picked up because of your interest in these data. If there had been no particular follow-up of these people, what proportion of that excess cancer do you think would have been certified as mesothelioma?

SELIKOFF: That is a good point. We thought, too, that our interest was going to result in a better diagnostic yield among these people than would have occurred in a group in which there was no interest. It didn't turn out that way, and we didn't help very much.

Margaret Sloan, who is here with us from the National Cancer Institute, is now reviewing these 175 cases, plus another 125 or so, and it's extraordinary how infrequently the right diagnosis gets on the death certificate, even when the pathologist has noted it correctly. Very often, an intern, rather than the doctor treating the patient, signs the death certificate. The pathologist doesn't sign, but very often the pathologist is much more accurate than the death certificate.

I would say, in answer to your question, Richard [Peto], that if we weren't there, it would have been slightly less well done then it was.

R. PETO: Might it be a factor of 2?

SLOAN: Not quite that much.

SELIKOFF: I don't understand why that is, but we will report how accurate the pathologist was compared with the clinician. Very often, the diagnosis during life may be cancer of the pancreas or abdominal neoplasm. When the person dies, the pathology report from the autopsy is not available for 2 or 3 weeks and "cancer of the pancreas" goes on the death certificate. Because the death certificate is necessary for burial, it is prepared within 24 hours. As a result, the pathologist's acumen is not recorded on the death certificate.

R. PETO: In areas where there is specific registration of cancer, such as the Third National Cancer Survey (TNCS), do they seek pathological information where possible? Would their data be reasonably accurate?

SELIKOFF: No, we looked into that. In general, there has been some difficulty in even translating correct hospital diagnoses to the death certificate among cases in the TNCS—only 65% were accurately categorized, even with regard to site of neoplasm, and this percentage was even smaller with less common neoplasms (Percy et al. 1981).

We took our cases in the areas in which a SEER program exists. Unfortunately, they were few in number; but there were a number of difficulties in that small number. The reason is that in the SEER program there is verification of the spelling of the patient's name, the Social Security number, the name of the hospital, and the date of death, but not of the pathological diagnosis. They do not review pathologist's slides.

The SEER program in a registry area includes all the cancer deaths in that area, including those from death certificates, private laboratories, small hospitals, and large hospitals. Therefore, the pathological diagnoses may be varied in quality, yet all must be included and none are reviewed pathologically. I understand that the SEER program is now considering the possibility of pathological review.

RADFORD: I note in your analysis of smoking in relation to asbestos that in 1967 there were no cases among the nonsmokers, only cases in the smokers. By 1976, the relative risk was the same for both smokers and nonsmokers. If the cohort is carried forward another 10 years, would you predict that the relative risk for nonsmokers will be substantially higher than for smokers, even though the absolute risk may be lower for the nonsmokers, perhaps because of competing risks? In other words, the very long latent period for the nonsmokers may be hiding that fact that the nonsmokers are developing almost as much cancer per person-year at risk as the smokers. We've observed this longer period of latency in the miners that have been exposed to radon daughters.

SELIKOFF: This is a very interesting thought that you have presented; that is, we may have a longer period of latency with nonsmokers. I don't know; we'll have to look at that.

But remember also that these were two different cohorts. In the first small cohort in New York, we only had 87 nonsmokers; we expected fewer than 0.2 deaths and none occurred. In the second group, we had over 2000 nonsmokers, so it was not too surprising to see a few cases. It may be a problem of sample size, rather than the second possibility of a longer period of latency.

BLOT: What part, if any, of the rise in the incidence of mesothelioma in the United States do you think might be due to changing diagnostic practices?

SELIKOFF: Until the mid-1970s, there was not a wide appreciation of mesothelioma. But that has changed now, and we have seen a higher proportion of correct diagnoses as time goes on. I suspect that diagnoses will become increasingly better. For example, the College of American Pathologists has been teaching a good deal about mesothelioma and the Armed Forces Institute of Pathology has developed sets of slides and teaching materials for mesothelioma. Many pathologists are now much more experienced than they were 5 or 6 years ago.

However, even in the best of hands, there is still a residual 10% insecurity. Dr. Churg and Dr. Suzuki in our laboratory are unable to say one way or another that "this is or is not mesothelioma" in 10% of cases. We classify these cases as "disseminated carcinomatosis, primary site unknown." Thus, we may be underestimating the true incidence of mesothelioma, but that's the best we can do at present.

Getting back to the latency factor, Bill [Blot], you had two studies on the eastern seaboard—one on the eastern coast of Florida and one in the Newport News-Tidewater area of Virginia. You had excess lung cancer but no mesotheliomas in the Florida area, where they began shipbuilding only during World War II. On the other hand, you had many mesotheliomas in the Tidewater area, which has been an old shipbuilding area.

So it may be that the duration from onset of exposure factor is determining whether or not pathologists in an area are or are not seeing and diagnosing mesothelioma. Your two studies in Florida and Newport News were very effective in teaching us the importance of latency in the comparative frequency of lung cancer and mesothelioma.

SIEMIATYCKI: At a purely methodological level, would you agree that, because of the difficulties that come from the latent period problem, case-control studies might be a more effective way, on the one hand, to discover risks and, on the other hand, to quantify them?

SELIKOFF: Yes and no. They may be a good way to identify risk but not necessarily to quantify it. I do not think there is much competition between prospective cohort studies and case-control studies in quantifying risk methodologically.

References

Percy, C., E. Staneck, and L. Gloeckler. 1981. Accuracy of cancer death cerrificates and its effect on cancer mortality statistics. *Am. J. Publ. Health* **71**:242.

Proportion of Cancer Due to Exposure to Asbestos

PHILIP E. ENTERLINE
Department of Biostatistics
Graduate School of Public Health
University of Pittsburgh
Pittsburgh, Pennsylvania 15261

If the current level of cancer mortality continues, nearly 50 million persons alive today in the United States will die of cancer. This prediction could be modified by the discovery of better methods of treatment or by altering known cancer-causing exposure patterns. Because resources are finite, it is important to allocate these so as to achieve greatest impact on the cancer problem. For this reason, it would be useful to know the proportion of cancer due to various environmental agents. This kind of effort has been greatly stimulated by a widely quoted document, sometimes referred to as the "estimates" document, that concludes that 13-18% of all cancer is caused by a single substance–asbestos (Bridbord et al. 1978). There has been disagreement with this estimate (Higginson et al. 1980; Peto 1980a; Hogan and Hoel 1981).

CURRENT APPROACHES

One approach to the question of how much cancer is caused by asbestos is to find a disease clearly caused by asbestos exposure and then from epidemiologic investigations calculate the ratio of this disease to all cancer caused by asbestos. Higginson, for example, has noted that there are about 1000 annual mesotheliomas in the United States, and that in a long-term mortality study of heavily exposed asbestos workers, for every one mesothelioma there were about 1.5 bronchogenic cancers related to asbestos (Higginson et al. 1980). From this he estimated the total annual incidence of asbestos-caused bronchogenic cancer in the United States to be about 1500. This makes up 2% of the approximately 70,000 such deaths each year. Higginson's report leads to an estimate of 4000 asbestos-caused cancers in the United States each year (including mesotheliomas) or 1% of the total 400,000 cancer deaths that occur annually.

Another approach is to estimate the number of asbestos-exposed workers and, based on epidemiologic studies of subsets of this or other populations, predict the proportion and numbers of these asbestos-exposed workers who will develop cancer as the result of asbestos exposure. This is the approach used by the group that produced the estimates document. In that study, it was estimated that 4 million workers alive today have had a heavy asbestos exposure like asbestos workers, and based on data from a study of asbestos insulators, it was calculated that 1.6 million or 40% of these are expected to die of asbestos-related cancers. It was estimated, in addition, that 1.5-3.5 million workers have had lesser exposures and 400,000-700,000 of these will die of asbestos-related cancers. Thus, over the next 30-35 years, the expected number of cancer deaths associated with asbestos is between 58,000 and 75,000 per year, or 13-18% of the 400,000-450,000 cancer deaths that occur each year.

Hogan and Hoel (1981) have used essentially the same approach followed in the estimates document but with different results. They estimated that 7-8 million workers potentially were exposed to asbestos during the years 1940-1967, of which 50% are alive today. Of these, 15% were exposed heavily and will have cancer mortality rates like asbestos insulators, whereas the remainder will have 12.5-25% of this cancer risk. On this basis, they estimate that future excess cancer deaths due to asbestos exposure will contribute 3% of all cancer deaths (range 1.4-4.4%).

HEAVILY EXPOSED WORKERS

In thinking about the problem of asbestos-caused cancer, it helps to consider the magnitude of another health problem related to asbestos, that is, asbestosis. Asbestosis was seen in asbestos workers long before cancer, and, in fact, it was the high frequency of coexisting asbestosis and lung cancer that led to the conclusion that asbestos was a cause of lung cancer. In the past, many felt that asbestosis was a prerequisite for asbestos lung cancer and that prevention of asbestosis would also prevent lung cancer (Eckardt 1959). It is partly for this reason that the present threshold limit value (TLV) for asbestos is based on preventing asbestosis rather than lung cancer. Moreover, many feel that only very heavy asbestos exposure is likely to lead to an asbestosis death and that the presence of asbestosis at death is important because it indicates the heavy exposure needed to produce asbestos lung cancer (Wagner 1965).

Table 1 shows asbestosis deaths observed in the United States during the period 1950-1977 by year, sex, and race. Clearly the trend is upward until 1972, when numbers of deaths seem to have leveled off. It is important to note that all asbestosis deaths observed in epidemiologic studies conducted in the United States are included in the numbers shown in Table 1. It is possible for each study, then, to see how its asbestosis deaths related to the U.S. total and thus estimate the size of the population that produces all asbestosis deaths in the entire United States.

One estimate can be made from a study we conducted in the early 1960s. In that study, we identified 21,755 male white workers from 35 of the larger U.S. asbestos products plants (Standard Industrial Classification [SIC] 3292)

Table 1
Deaths from Asbestosis, United States 1950-1977 by Sex and Race

		White		Other	
Year	Total	male	female	male	female
1950	8	6	1	1	–
1951	9	9	–	–	–
1952	14	12	2	–	–
1953	12	9	–	1	2
1954	8	7	1	–	–
1955	11	10	1	–	–
1956	20	16	3	1	–
1957	21	17	1	3	–
1958	14	12	1	–	1
1959	18	17	1	–	–
1960	21	19	–	2	–
1961	22	17	4	1	–
1962	18	10	–	7	1
1963	31	23	3	4	1
1964	24	21	2	1	–
1965	22	18	2	2	–
1966	29	26	3	–	–
1967	36	32	3	1	–
1968	29	25	3	1	–
1969	34	29	3	2	–
1970	26	21	1	4	–
1971	33	26	3	4	–
1972	58	54	2	2	–
1973	42	40	–	2	–
1974	35	30	3	2	–
1975	45	42	2	1	–
1976	54	46	1	7	–
1977	55	49	1	5	–

where we can be fairly certain exposures were high (Enterline and Kendrick 1967). These workers had all been employed sometime during the years 1948-1951. During the years 1950-1963 at ages under 65, there were 44 deaths from asbestosis. (Only deaths at ages under 65 were examined in this study.) During the same period, it can be seen from Table 1 that for the entire United States the number of deaths from asbestosis at all ages among white males was 184. Tabulations of asbestosis deaths by age are available for the years 1962-1977. During that period, 52% of all asbestos deaths were at ages under 65. From this it can be estimated that there were 96 deaths from asbestosis at ages under 65 during the years 1950-1963. Thus, this population of 21,755 workers produced 45.8% of the asbestosis deaths that occurred in the United States among white males at ages under 65 during the years 1950-1963. From this it can easily be calculated that the total number of white males producing asbestosis deaths at ages under 65 (exposed like asbestos products workers) must have been equivalent to 47,465. Because the ratio of all deaths in Table 1 to white male deaths is 1.23 for the years 1950-1963, this suggests a total population of 58,381 producing asbestosis. In another study, of 1075 retired male asbestos products workers from a single asbestos company at ages 65 and over, we observed 17 asbestosis deaths during the period 1950-1973 (Henderson and Enterline 1979). During the same period in the entire United States it can be calculated from Table 1 that there were 515 male deaths due to asbestosis of which an estimated 48% or 248 were at ages 65 and over. Thus, the total population at ages 65 and over producing asbestosis deaths must have been 15,183. Again adjusting to the total population, this becomes 17,054. The total at all ages, therefore, must have been 75,314.

Another estimate can be made from a large study by Selikoff and his coworkers of 17,800 male asbestos insulators from the United States and Canada (Selikoff et al. 1980). These workers were observed for deaths over the years 1967-1976 and 78 deaths were coded from death certificates as due to asbestosis. The number of Canadian workers was not reported, but perhaps it was about 10%, so that we can estimate asbestosis deaths among U.S. asbestos insulators at about 70. Table 1 shows that during the same period in the entire U.S. there were 371 male deaths from asbestosis. Thus, from these data we can estimate that during the years 1967-1976 these asbestos insulators produced 18.9% of all male asbestos deaths. The total U.S. male population producing asbestosis deaths (exposed like asbestos insulators) was, therefore, equivalent to 84,906. This is somewhat higher than the estimate made on the basis of asbestos products workers, but as it relates to a later period (1967-1976), it may reflect the presence of a larger heavily exposed population. These two study populations produced over half of all the concurrent asbestosis deaths in the United States and point clearly to the importance of asbestos insulators and asbestos products workers in estimating heavily exposed populations. That asbestos insulators and asbestos products workers are the primary source of asbestosis deaths is confirmed by individual case reports, which almost entirely represent occupations of asbestos insulator and asbestos products worker (McVittie 1965).

Actual numbers of asbestos insulators and asbestos products workers are published regularly by the U.S. government. Table 2 shows the number of workers employed by asbestos products companies in the United States (SIC 3292) for the years 1947-1976, the membership of the International Association of Heat and Frost Insulators and Asbestos Workers, and asbestos and insulation workers reported in each decennial U.S. census. The number of insulators increased steadily during the period 1950-1976 from around 15,000 to 25,000.

Table 2
Numbers of Asbestos Products Workers and Asbestos Insulators, 1947-76

Year	Workers employed by asbestos products companies (SIC 3292)[a]	Annual average membership in asbestos workers union[b]	Asbestos and insulation workers in U.S. Census[c]
1947	21,600		
1948			
1949			
1950			15,500
1951		6,000	
1952			
1953	22,200		
1954	22,000	9,000	
1955	23,700	10,000	
1956	22,800	10,000	
1957	22,900	13,700	
1958	21,300	13,700	
1959	22,800	10,000	
1960	22,400	10,000	20,000
1961	21,700	12,000	
1962	21,800	12,000	
1963	19,500	14,000	
1964	20,400	14,000	
1965	21,000	12,500	
1966	22,700	12,500	
1967	21,300		
1968	21,500		
1969	22,200	17,000	
1970	18,900	17,000	25,700
1971	18,900	18,800	
1972	21,000	18,800	
1973	21,300	18,300	
1974	21,000	18,300	
1975	17,300		
1976	16,600		

[a]Data from Bureau of the Census and Department of Commerce (1952-55, 1957-59, 1962-64, 1968-69, 1972-73, 1975-77, 1979).

[b]Data from Bureau of Labor Statistics and Department of Labor (1953, 1955, 1957, 1959, 1962, 1964, 1966, 1968, 1972, 1974, 1977).

[c]Bureau of the Census and Department of Commerce (1964, 1973).

On the other hand, the number of workers employed by asbestos products producers stayed at around 20,000 during the 1950s and 1960s but dropped rather sharply in the 1970s. (In our 1967 study we identified 12,707 white males working in the first quarter of 1948, so our cohort apparently contained over half of all workers employed by asbestos products companies in 1948.) The period of interest is the period prior to 1970, because after that time increased awareness of the health hazards associated with asbestos probably greatly decreased the cancer risk.

In addition to workers in asbestos products industries (SIC 3292), there are workers making asbestos paper included in a larger category, "Building paper and building board mills" (SIC 2611), and asbestos-exposed workers in a category, "Steam and other packing, and pipe and boiler covering" (SIC 3293). A 1976 study by Weston et al. places the total employment in primary asbestos products industries at 37,539, of which an estimated 22,670 are exposed to asbestos.

How many asbestos products workers and asbestos insulators employed during the period 1940-1970 are alive now in 1981? From data in Table 2, it appears that on average during the period 1947-1970 there might have been about 40,000 such workers in the United States. Our experience in carrying out historical prospective studies of working populations is that over a 30-year period the number of different workers with a year or more work experience is about 3 times the average daily worker census. Thus, I would estimate that an average census of 40,000 asbestos products workers and asbestos insulators over the period 1940-1970 represents 120,000 different workers with a year or more work experience. Of course, all these workers would not be alive today. Assuming a death rate of 1% per year, somewhat higher than the U.S. death rate but similar to the annual death rate observed in the study of 17,800 asbestos insulators, and a midpoint of 1955, we would expect about 85% or about 100,000 to be alive in 1970 and, if no new heavily exposed workers have been added since that time, somewhat less in 1981–say about 90,000. These estimates are somewhat higher than those made on the basis of asbestosis deaths, but indicate that certainly less than 100,000 workers and former workers are alive today who had exposures to asbestos–like asbestos insulators and asbestos products workers.

I would estimate that as of 1981 there are between 70,000 and 90,000 persons alive in the United States who have had heavy asbestos exposure–mostly present and former asbestos insulators and asbestos products workers.[1] This is very low in contrast to estimates made by others, but is in line with an estimate of 20,000 "high risk" workers in the United Kingdom, where the population is about a quarter as large as the U.S. population (Smither 1979).

[1] I had earlier estimated somewhere between 43,000 and 1.7 million heavily exposed workers alive in 1967, with a best guess of 250,000 (Hogan and Hoel 1981). The reason for the best guess of 250,000 was that at that time death certificate data on the number of deaths among the 17,800 asbestos insulators had not been reported and I assumed that death certificates showed far fewer than 78 asbestosis deaths.

Assuming a best estimate of 80,000 heavily exposed or high-risk workers alive in 1981, how many of these will die of asbestos lung cancer? As we have actual epidemiologic data on both asbestos products workers and asbestos insulators, this is not difficult to estimate. If data from the cohort of 17,500 asbestos insulators is used to predict, it appears that after 20 years from first exposure 22% will die of asbestos lung cancer (Selikoff et al. 1980).[2] If data from cohorts of asbestos products workers were used, this percentage would be somewhat lower. Among retired asbestos products workers from the Johns Manville Corporation, about 14% died of asbestos lung cancer, while in a study of workers from a British asbestos textile plant 15% died from asbestos lung cancer (Peto et al. 1977; Henderson and Enterline 1979). If we can assume 20% is a good overall estimate for the entire cohort, then the number of asbestos lung cancers that will appear in this group of 80,000 is 16,000. If this cohort lives just 30 more years, asbestos lung cancer deaths will occur at a rate of 530 per year.

LESS THAN HEAVILY EXPOSED WORKERS

It was Hueper's view that heavy exposure to asbestos dust produced asbestosis, whereas lower levels permitted lung cancer to develop (Hueper 1955). He was undoubtedly right, and the cancer problem is not confined to heavily exposed workers, but rather includes those more lightly exposed. Therefore, there is a population of exposed workers that does not experience many asbestosis deaths, but which does have an increased cancer risk. Populations most frequently mentioned are shipyard workers, construction workers, and automotive brake mechanics.

World War II Shipyard Workers

Hogan and Hoel (1981) have estimated that during World War II there were 4.3-5.4 million shipyard workers exposed to asbestos and that perhaps 50% of these or about 2.5 million are alive today. The only data that appear to apply to the probable lung cancer excess in these shipyard workers are those published by Blot et al. (1978, 1980). In two case-control studies involving interviews of lung cancer cases and a matched control group, relative risks (RR) for lung cancer among World War II shipyard workers of 1.6 and 1.7 were calculated.

In view of the fact that World War II shipyard and employment must have been fairly brief and, for occupations other than asbestos insulators, exposure

[2] This is calculated as:

$$\text{Percent excess} = \frac{\text{observed lung cancer} - \text{expected lung cancer}}{\text{expected deaths from all causes}}$$

levels must have been relatively low, these risks are surprisingly high. From labor turnover rates, it appears that the average duration of employment in the shipyard was about a year (Selikoff et al. 1979b). Moreover, shipyards only operated at high employment levels for 2 or 3 years. Under these conditions, the entire cohort would have had to be exposed to very high levels of asbestos to produce RR of 1.6 and 1.7.[3] As Blot et al. (1978) point out, however, the comparison of occupational histories between cases and controls may have been affected by a lower interview response rate among controls and by publicity surrounding the issue of asbestos and cancer. The second point needs emphasis in light of a report by Najarian and Colton (1978) of a fivefold excess in leukemia among shipyard workers exposed to ionizing radiation based on a similar kind of case-control study. Subsequently, they discovered that reports of occupational histories by next of kin for decedents were biased by the knowledge that radiation and leukemia were related (Colton 1979). This was confirmed by a recent historical prospective study which shows no excess in leukemia among radiation exposed workers in the same shipyard (Rinsky et al. 1981). More direct evidence that brief casual exposure in World War II shipyards probably caused little lung cancer excess comes from a recent study of shipyard workers in Hawaii that shows essentially no excess in lung cancer in those followed 15-24 years and exposed to asbestos for less than 10 years (Kolonel et al. 1980). This study also indicates that about 40% of shipyard workers have no asbestos exposure at all. To apply a 1.6-1.7 RR to this large cohort of former shipyard workers seems inappropriate.

One way to predict lung cancer deaths among the cohort of 2.5 million former World War II shipyard workers alive today is by extrapolation from the several studies of asbestos insulators and asbestos products workers. To do this, some estimate of the actual exposure levels is needed.

The time-weighted asbestos exposure for insulation workers has been estimated at 4-12 f/cc (Nicholson 1976). What might the exposure of other exposed shipyard workers have been? There are no published data for shipyard workers to answer this. However, an informed guess is that during World War II for those workers actually exposed to asbestos, fiber counts were probably around 2 f/cc (J. Thorton, pers. comm.). (Current [1979] fiber counts in one shipyard ranges from .08 to .66 [G. Matanoski, pers. comm.].) From the study by Kolonel et al. (1980), we can estimate that about 60% or 1.5 million of the 2.5 million World War II shipyard workers actually were exposed to asbestos. For these 1.5 million workers alive today with a year's exposure at 2 f/cc nearly 50 years ago, we can estimate future asbestos lung cancer incidence by extrapolation from asbestos insulation workers data.

[3] On the basis of a 22% lung cancer excess observed among asbestos insulators where exposure apparently averaged 25 years at 8 f/cc it can be estimated that a 2.5% excess (RR = 1.4) after 1 year's exposure would require continuous exposure at around 22 f/cc.

From data on asbestos products workers and asbestos miners, it appears that the dose-response relationship is linear (McDonald et al. 1974; Henderson and Enterline 1979). Moreover a time-weighted measure of exposure seems appropriate because intensity and duration appear to make roughly equal contributions to lung cancer incidence (Enterline et al. 1973; McDonald et al. 1974).

If for asbestos insulators the exposure averaged 8 f/cc (4-12 f/cc) on a continuous basis and produced a 22% excess in mortality for lung cancer after about 25 years of exposure, we can easily calculate the excess for a single year's exposure at 2 f/cc. The total exposure for asbestos insulators needed to produce a 22% excess in mortality due to asbestos lung cancer can be calculated as (8) (25) = 200 fiber years. For shipyard workers, on the other hand, exposure would have been (2) (1) = 2 fiber years. Therefore, we can calculate that the percent cancer excess in the 1.5 million World War II shipyard workers will be 2/200 or 1/100 of the lung cancer excess in asbestos insulators, or a .22% excess. Applied to the 1.5 million workers alive today, this suggests 3300 will die of asbestos lung cancer. If these workers live just 20 more years, this is about 165 excess deaths per year.

Post-World War II Shipyard Workers

A much more important population consists of workers who continued employment in shipyards after World War II or were hired after World War II, because their exposure lasted a considerable period of time. Shipyard employment is reported to have been around 200,000 since 1945 (Selikoff et al. 1979a). Assuming labor turnover as in the industrial cohorts we have studied, this would produce about 600,000 different workers with a year or more work experience.[4] With a mortality rate at 1% per year, we would expect 528,000 of these to be alive in 1970 and about 475,000 to be alive today. Based on the Kolonel study (1980), we can estimate that 285,000 of these were exposed to asbestos.

There have been several epidemiologic studies dealing with long-term shipyard workers. Three of these show a clear lung cancer excess like the Blot et al. studies (1978, 1980) (Puntoni et al. 1979; Kolonel et al. 1980; Gottlieb and Stedman 1980), one an intermediate excess (Milham 1976), and two essentially no excess (Lumley 1976; Beaumont and Weiss 1980). These offer little consistent guidance for estimating a lung cancer excess. However, an informed guess as to post-World War II continuous fiber levels is around 1 f/cc for those exposed, so we can estimate the lung cancer excess as for World War II shipyard workers (J. Thorton, pers. comm.).

[4] This is consistent with a count made by G. Matanoski (pers. comm.). As part of a study on the health effects of low-level radiation, she has estimated that there have been nearly 500,000 workers employed at shipyards now employing about 120,000 workers.

Assuming continuous exposure was at 1 f/cc for 25 years and projecting from the experience of asbestos insulators, we would expect the excess in lung cancer to be 25/200 or 1/8 the excess in asbestos insulators. Thus, of the 285,000 workers alive today, 2.7% or 7695 would be expected to die of asbestos lung cancer. Over the next 30 years, this would average 256 deaths per year. This estimate of excess lung cancer yields a RR of 1.4, which is a rough average of RRs actually reported for long-term shipyard workers.

Auto Mechanics and Garage Workers

Auto mechanics and garage workers are frequently mentioned as an asbestos-exposed population. This population has been estimated at about 900,000 continuously exposed to asbestos (Weston et al. 1976). Since World War II, this number has probably grown considerably and might have averaged around 750,000 over the period 1940-1970. Again, using experience from industrial epidemiologic studies, we might estimate that there were 2.2 million workers exposed for a year or more. At a death rate of 1% per year, 1.9 million would have been alive in 1970 and about 1.7 million alive today.

Studies indicate that the asbestos fiber concentrations to which auto mechanics and garage workers are exposed continuously are around .3 f/cc, well below that for shipyard workers (Hickish and Knight 1970). Probably the most applicable epidemiologic studies for estimating the effects of this kind of exposure comes from asbestos products workers. One study provides estimates of actual fiber exposure (Peto et al. 1977). In that study the lung cancer excess was 15% and historic fiber concentrations were around 12 f/cc.[5] Exposure was about 25 years duration. Extrapolating from that experience permits an estimate of a (.3)(25)/(25)(12) = 7.5/300 or (.025)(15) = .375% lung cancer excess. Applied to a population of 1.7 million, this suggests 6375 asbestos lung cancer deaths over the next 30 years or 212 deaths per year.

Secondary Asbestos Products

Weston (et al.) estimate that there are 240,000 employees in manufacturing operations using asbestos products and whose exposure is fairly high. From their data, it appears that exposure of these workers is around 2 f/cc. Considering this group of industries during the period 1940-1970 and a mortality rate of 1% per year, there are probably about 540,000 workers and former workers alive in 1981. If historic fiber counts were double the counts available when Weston made its survey (4 f/cc), workers had an average of 25 years employment, if the experience in the primary asbestos industries applies,

[5] Substantially higher exposure estimates appear in a paper just made available but which the author feels must be regarded as provisional (Peto 1980b).

then we can estimate that 5% of this population, or 27,000, will die of asbestos lung cancer. This is 900 deaths per year over the next 30 years.

All Other Workers

Finally, what about all other potentially exposed workers in the United States? This must include construction workers, other workers using asbestos at their jobs, plus workers employed very briefly ($<$ 1 year). A few of these might be in jobs with heavy but unrecognized exposure. The 1973 NIOSH Occupational Hazards Survey identified 1.6 million workers in the United States potentially exposed to asbestos, of which 430,000 were in construction and 648,000 were in manufacturing. We have thus far dealt only with 40,000 heavily exposed, 240,000 secondary asbestos products workers, 200,000 shipyard workers, and 900,000 auto mechanics and garage workers. It is not entirely clear how these groups relate to the 1.6 million workers identified by the Occupational Hazards Survey. Many garage workers and auto mechanics appear to have been omitted. If so, there must be over 1 million workers with potential exposures, many from the construction industry, that still need to be accounted for. I would estimate this represents 3.5 million persons alive today. Considering occasional exposures and brief exposures as well as some longer or heavy exposures, I would estimate an exposure equivalent to .3 f/cc for 25 years–like garage workers and auto mechanics. Projecting as before from the experience of asbestos products workers yields an estimate lung cancer excess of 7.5/300 or (.025)(.15) = .375%. Applied to a population of 3.5 million, this yields an estimate of 13,140 asbestos lung cancer deaths or 438 deaths per year over the next 30 years.

Table 3 summarizes the results of these calculations with regard to asbestos lung cancer. To this I added other cancers resulting from asbestos exposure under the assumption that for every two asbestos lung cancers there is one other cancer. I also added one-third of the approximately 1000 mesotheliomas that occur in the United States each year on the grounds that at least two-thirds are due to exposures other than occupational exposures to asbestos (McDonald and McDonald 1980). The total 4084 extra annual cancer occupational asbestos deaths is about 1% of all cancer deaths in the United States.

Finally, deaths due to nonoccupational exposures to asbestos have been added. Asbestos lung cancer is estimated under the assumption that background is 1.5 ng/m^3 or .00006 f/cc (Nicholson 1978). Predicting from asbestos products workers, but assuming continuous exposure rather than 8 hours per day, 5 days per week, and assuming 70 years exposure suggests 28 asbestos lung cancer deaths per year for the entire United States:

$$\frac{(.00006)\,(70)}{(300)\,(.24)} \times .15 \times \frac{225{,}000{,}000}{70} = 28. \qquad (1)$$

Table 3
Estimated Cancer Deaths Which Will Be Caused by Asbestos Exposure over the Next 20-30 Years

Exposure group and cause of death	Number with exposures alive today	Equivalent exposure level (f/cc)	Number of deaths per year
Occupational Exposure			
Asbestos Lung Cancer			
Insulation and primary asbestos products workers	80,000	8-12	530
Secondary asbestos products workers	540,000	4	900
World War II shipyard workers	1,500,000	2	165
Post-World War II shipyard workers	285,000	1	256
Auto mechanics and garage workers	1,700,000	.3	212
All other exposed workers	3,500,000	.3	438
Total	7,605,000		2501
Other asbestos cancers	–		1250
Mesotheliomas caused by occupational exposure to asbestos	–		333
Total extra cancer deaths per year			4084
Nonoccupational exposure			
Asbestos lung cancer	225,000,000		28
Mesothelioma	225,000,000		333

I have added an estimate of mesotheliomas produced by nonoccupational exposure under the assumption that two-thirds of all mesotheliomas are due to asbestos and the rest due to something else (McDonald and McDonald 1980).

DISCUSSION

From available information, it appears that about 1% of all cancer is due to asbestos exposure. This means that elimination of all asbestos from our environment would have an imperceptible effect on the cancer problem. It would ultimately have a great effect on asbetosis and mesothelioma deaths, but these are relatively unimportant as causes of death.

We can pinpoint some populations at high risk of cancer as the result of asbestos exposure and some special effort might be made here. Asbestos products workers and asbestos insulators exposed mostly before adequate controls were put in place for their protection are clearly high-risk populations. The identities of most of the workers are known either to the asbestos workers union or to the government. Efforts to prevent disease in this population would be an important public service to them, although an almost meaningless effort in terms of the overall cancer problem confronting us. Perhaps there are other such populations. I would be concerned about workers using asbestos products in the secondary asbestos products industry. For example, workers making asbestos gloves from asbestos textile. These are usually small, highly competitive operations and dust control efforts may sometimes be inadequate.

It would be satisfying to believe that a single substance within our ability to control is responsible for a large part of an otherwise mysterious problem. Unfortunately, this is not often the case. The role of asbestos in our overall cancer problem has been greatly exaggerated. One reason may be that we are becoming accustomed to exaggeration in dealing with environmental hazards in the belief that this somehow protects people, and is in the public interest. This may be true in initially drawing attention to a situation, but in the long run exaggeration is foolish because it leads to a wasteful effort and diverts resources from more fruitful areas. Moreover, falsely designating populations at high risk involves other human costs and is clearly not in the public interest.

REFERENCES

Beaumont, J.J. and N.E. Weiss. 1980. Mortality of welders, shipfitters, and other metal trades workers in Boilermakers Local No. 104, AFL-CIO. *Am. J. Epidemiol.* **112**:775.

Blot, W.J., L.E. Morris, R. Stroube, I. Tagnon, and J.F. Fraumeni. 1980. Lung and laryngeal cancers in relation to shipyard employment in coastal Virginia. *J. Natl. Cancer Inst.* **65**:571.

Blot, W.J., J.M. Harrington, A. Toledo, R. Hoover, C.W. Heath, Jr., and J.F. Fraumeni. 1978. Lung cancer after employment in shipyards during World War II. *New Engl. J. Med.* **299**:620.

Bridbord, K., P. Decoufle, J.F. Fraumeni, D.G. Hoel, R.N. Hoover, D.P. Rall, U. Saffiotti, M.A. Schneiderman, and A.C. Upton. 1978. "Estimates of the fraction of cancer in the United States related to occupational factors." Prepared by: National Cancer Institute, National Institute of Environmental Health Sciences, National Institute for Occupational Safety and Health, September 15.

Colton, T. 1979. Presentation before Society for Epidemiologic Research, June 13.

Eckardt, R.E. 1959. Industrial Carcinogens. In *Modern monographs in industrial medicine* (ed. A.J. Lanza and R.H. Orr), p. 99. Grune & Stratton, New York.

Enterline, P.E. and M.A. Kendrick. 1967. Asbestos-dust exposures at various levels and mortality. *Arch. Environ. Health.* **15**:181.

Enterline, P.E., P. Decoufle, and V. Henderson. 1973. Respiratory cancer in relation to occupational exposures among retired asbestos workers. *Br. J. Ind. Med.* **30**:1.

Gottlieb, M.S. and R.B. Stedman. 1979. Lung cancer in shipbuilding and related industries in Louisiana. *South. Med. J.* **72**:1099.

Henderson, V. and P.E. Enterline. 1979. Asbestos exposure: Factors associated with excess cancer and respiratory disease mortality. *Health Hazards of Asbestos Exposure* (eds. I.J. Selikoff and E.C. Hammond), vol. 330, p. 117. New York Academy of Sciences, New York.

Hueper, W.C. 1955. *A quest into the environmental causes of cancer of the lung.* Public Health Service Monograph No. 36, PHS Pub. No. 152. U.S. Public Health Service.

Hickish, D.E. and K.L. Knight. 1970. Exposure to asbestos during brake maintenance. *Ann. Occup. Hyg.* **13**:17.

Higginson, J., J.C. Bahar, J. Clemmesen, H. Demopoulos, L. Garfinkel, T. Hirayama, and D. Schottenfeld. 1980. Proportion of cancers due to occupations. *Prev. Med.* **9**:180.

Hogan, M.D. and D.G. Hoel. 1981. Estimated cancer risk associated with occupational asbestos exposure. *Risk Analysis* (in press).

Kolonel, L.N., T. Hirohata, B.V. Chapell, F.V. Viola, and D.E. Harris. 1980. Cancer mortality in a cohort of naval shipyard workers in Hawaii: Early findings. *J. Natl. Cancer Inst.* **64**:739.

Lumley, K.P.S. 1976. A proportional study of cancer registrations of dockyard workers. *Br. J. Ind. Med.* **33**:108.

McDonald, A.D. and J.C. McDonald. 1980. Malignant mesothelioma in North America. *Cancer* **46**:1650.

McDonald, J.C., A.D. McDonald, G.W. Gibbs, J. Siemiatycki and C.E. Rossiter. 1971. Mortality in the chrysotile asbestos mines and mills of Quebec. *Arch. Environ. Health* **22**:677.

McDonald, J.C., M.R. Becklake, G.W. Graham, A.D. McDonald, and C.E. Rossiter. 1974. The health of chrysotile asbestos mine and mill workers of Quebec. *Arch. Environ. Health.* **28**:61.

McVittie, J.C. 1965. Asbestosis in Great Britain. *Ann. N.Y. Acad. Sci.* **132**:128.

Milham, S. 1976. *Occupational mortality in Washington State, 1950-71.* Vols. I, II, III. National Institute of Occupational Safety and Health Research Report.

Nicholson, W.J. 1976. Case study 1: Asbestos–the TLV approach. In *Occupational carcinogenesis* (ed. U. Saffiotti and J.K. Wagoner), vol. 271, p. 152. New York Academy of Sciences, New York.

_____. 1978. "Control of sprayed asbestos surfaces in school buildings: A feasibility study." Report to the National Institute of Environmental Health Sciences, June 15.

Najarian, T. and T. Colton. 1978. Mortality from leukemia and cancer in shipyard nuclear workers. *Lancet* i:1018.

Peto, R. 1980a. Distorting the epidemiology of cancer: The need for a more balanced overview. *Nature* **284**:297.

Peto, J. 1980b. Lung cancer mortality in relation to measured dust levels in an asbestos textile factory. In *Biological effects of mineral fibers* (ed. J.C. Wagner), vol. ii, p. 829. IARC, Lyon.

Peto, J., R. Doll, S.V. Howard, L.J. Kinlen, and H.C. Lewinsohn. 1977. A mortality study among workers in an English asbestos factory. *Br. J. Ind. Med.* **34**:169.

Puntoni, R., M. Vercelli, F. Merlo, F. Valerio, and L. Santi. 1979. Mortality among shipyard workers in Genoa, Italy. *Health Hazards of Asbestos Exposure.* (ed. I.J. Selikoff and E.C. Hammond), vol. 330, p. 353. New York Academy of Sciences, New York.

Rinsky, R.A., R.D. Zumwalde, R.J. Waxweiler, W.E. Murray, Jr., P.J. Bierbaum, P.J. Landrigan, M. Terpilak, and C. Cox. 1981. Cancer mortality at a naval nuclear shipyard. *Lancet* i:231.

Selikoff, I.J., E.C. Hammond, and H. Seidman. 1979a. Mortality experience of insulation workers in the United States and Canada, 1943-1976. In *Health hazards of asbestos exposure.* (ed. I.J. Selikoff and E.C. Hammond), vol. 330, p. 91. New York Academy of Sciences, New York.

Selikoff, I.J., R. Lilis and W.J. Nicholson. 1979b. Asbestos disease in United States shipyards. In *Health hazards of asbestos exposure.* (ed. I.J. Selikoff and E.C. Hammond), vol. 330, p. 295. New York Academy of Sciences, New York.

Selikoff, I.J., E.C. Hammond, and H. Seidman. 1980. Latency of asbestos disease among insulation workers in the United States and Canada. *Cancer* **46**:2736.

Smither, W.J. 1979. Surveillance of high-risk groups–a survey of asbestos workers: The present position in the United Kingdom. *Ann. N.Y. Acad. Sci.* **330**:525.

Wagner, J.C. 1965. The sequelae of exposure to asbestos dust. *Ann. N.Y. Acad. Sci.* **132**:691.

Weston, R.F., A.R. Daly, A.J. Zupko, and J.L. Hebb. 1976. "Technological feasibility and economic impact of OSHA proposed revision to the asbestos standard." Prepared for Asbestos Information Association of North America, Washington, D.C.

COMMENTS:

ACHESON: What dose-response relationship did you use to make your calculations? Were you dealing with f/cc?

ENTERLINE: Right, and I assumed a straight-line extrapolation to zero. For example, using Irving's [Selikoff] data, the estimate is that insulators on average are exposed to 4-12 f/cc—an average of 8 f/cc.

NICHOLSON: It would probably have been 10-15 f/cc in the early years.

ENTERLINE: I am using 8 f/cc because that seems to be what is published. If 8 f/cc produces a RR of something like 4-5, then you could easily calculate what 2 f/cc would produce. It is just a simple extrapolation. I think that most data support a straight-line relationship between asbestos and lung cancer.

ACHESON: There have been conversions. In World War II nobody was dealing with f/cc.

ENTERLINE: That's correct. Data I used must have been converted from particles to fibers at some point in time.

J. PETO: How were these estimates derived? There are obviously a lot of complex assumptions that can't be tested, but they finish up with more or less the right number of mesotheliomas, don't they? There's a reasonably steady relationship between excess lung cancer and mesothelioma. It seems from the conversation following Irving's talk that there is general agreement that the majority of mesotheliomas are being recorded in cancer registries. Everyone seems to agree that there are approximately 1000 mesotheliomas occurring annually. In some ways, the most reliable way of getting an estimate is to multiply that factor by 3 or 4 for lung cancer, and you arrive at 4000 lung cancers and 1000 mesotheliomas, which is more or less the answer you got.

ENTERLINE: Right. I was surprised when this happened.

DAVIS: I have a few comments on some methodological problems. I wonder if you would agree to differentiate between exposure and dose. It is important to try to reconstruct exposure historically, using the best available estimates of an industrial hygienist. I think recent studies of indoor air pollution and personal monitoring systems that have been developed suggest that, even within a room of this size—given the differences in metabolism, respiration rate, and the like—people can be exposed to conditions with very different doses being taken in. I would suggest that we could think about exposure as being material potentially available for uptake and dose being what is taken up. It is important to differentiate between those two, even though it is usual to be able to try to reconstruct potential past exposure.

Further with respect to your critique of Bill Blot's work, while it is of course to be preferred that we continue to follow the classic Doll model in the case-control studies, it makes it difficult to criticize a case-control study by a noncase-control study. I might call your attention to the fact that I have recently learned from Herbert Sauer that mortality data from the years 1959-1961 seem to be missing for certain key Virginia counties, such as Portsmouth and Newport News. These are the areas of the country with one of the longest traditions of shipbuilding and asbestos work. And so it would suggest, at least, that we still have a lot of missing pieces with respect to using aggregate county-type data in discussing mesothelioma.

McDONALD: Did you make a distinction between men and women?

ENTERLINE: No, I didn't. I just took the total population producing the asbestosis cases. Some of the asbestosis cases are women, some are black, some are white, some are young, some are old. I didn't make any distinction. In effect I assumed that the ratio of asbestosis deaths to lung cancer deaths is the same for men and women, black and white, and so forth.

McDONALD: You didn't have a final figure of the proportion of excess deaths that were male or female.

ENTERLINE: No, I didn't.

BLOT: Just a couple of comments about the shipyard statements. It could very well be that the RRs at 1.6 or so that we found are high. But the one advantage we did have is that we had direct observations on patients with lung cancer, and we didn't have to rely on extrapolations.

There are a couple of other pieces of evidence to indicate that the risk is somewhere close to that order. I think the data that you mentioned from Hawaii—the Kolonel cohort study of Pearl Harbor shipyard workers—indicates a RR figure in the same ballpark. It was a cohort study of several thousand shipyard workers who had been employed from the 1950s onward. Information about wartime exposures was unknown. The overall RR for lung cancer in the total cohort was something like 1.1 or 1.2, which is not very high. But when they restricted the cohort to those who had been followed at least 20 years, which, by definition in their study, means that these workers had to have been employed in the early 1950s and were probably more likely to have also been employed during the war, then they came up with a RR estimate of 1.7.

In the negative study of the Portsmouth nuclear shipyard workers, there may be a similar phenomenon. The overall RR for lung cancer was something like 1.06 or 1.07, which wasn't high. But again, that was a cohort followed up mainly for interest in radiation exposures. Many employees at that yard began work only in the 1950s or later. Furthermore many of the person-years of observation occurred in either the late 1950s or the early 1960s. From what we know about latent periods for lung cancer and for mesothelioma, this may be too early to pick up an increase in the overall RR for lung cancer.

In fact, if you look at some of the lung cancer data broken down by time periods that are given in the detailed report that NIOSH prepared, there is some excess in lung cancer, with risks of 1.2 or 1.3 in the late 1960s and early 1970s.

Although we didn't have a direct estimate of cancer risk among the total cohort of World War II shipyard workers, it is quite conceivable that the overall risk of lung cancer to this large group of people who did work during the war, even though they did work for only a few years, could very well be 40-50% or so. If that is the case, then the numbers of lung cancers resulting today would be a bit higher, perhaps quite a bit higher than you predicted.

ENTERLINE: Well, this needs to be made clear. The Hawaiian study may be correct for long-term shipyard workers, but I don't think it should be applied to short-term World War II shipyard workers. If you believe, as I do, that it is a time-weighted measure that gives you the response, it must be recognized that there was only a very short time period involved in the dose for World War II shipyard workers.

BLOT: It could be that intense, short-term exposures could carry the same effect as long-term, less intense ones.

Cancer among Shipyard Workers

WILLIAM J. BLOT AND JOSEPH F. FRAUMENI, JR.
Environmental Epidemiology Branch
National Cancer Institute
Bethesda, Maryland 20205

In the 1960s, case reports of pleural mesothelioma in several European shipbuilding centers suggested an asbestos hazard among shipyard workers. Large numbers of this ordinarily rare cancer have been recorded since then, and lung cancer has been documented as an occupational disease among shipyard employees. This presentation summarizes the results of a series of case-control studies in the United States that have evaluated the risk of respiratory cancer among shipyard workers and discusses some of the research questions that remain. The combined data from these studies provide relatively stable risk estimates which may be useful in assessing the contribution of occupational determinants to human cancer.

THE SHIPBUILDING INDUSTRY IN THE UNITED STATES

Ship construction and repair has been a major industry in western nations throughout most of the 20th century. In the United States, large seagoing vessels have been constructed and repaired in areas along the Atlantic, Gulf, and Pacific coasts as well as some inland centers. The U.S. shipbuilding industry was only of moderate size until World War II, when it underwent massive expansion and became the largest single manufacturing industry in the country. In 1941 there were 8 Navy and 24 private shipyards with facilities to build 2000-ton vessels. By the end of the war, there were 99 additional yards. Construction was completed on over 5000 new merchant ships and 1500 combatant vessels; in over 60,000 instances during 1942-1945, these and other ships were repaired or converted (Fassett 1948).

Figure 1 shows estimates of the number of persons employed in U.S. shipyards during the period 1915-1965. The total peaked at about 1.7 million persons in late 1943. In comparison, the World War I maximum employment was about 475,000, whereas less than 100,000 worked in shipyards during the 1920s and 1930s; employment was somewhat over 200,000 from 1950 onwards. About 90% of the World War II workforce in shipyards was male, but the age

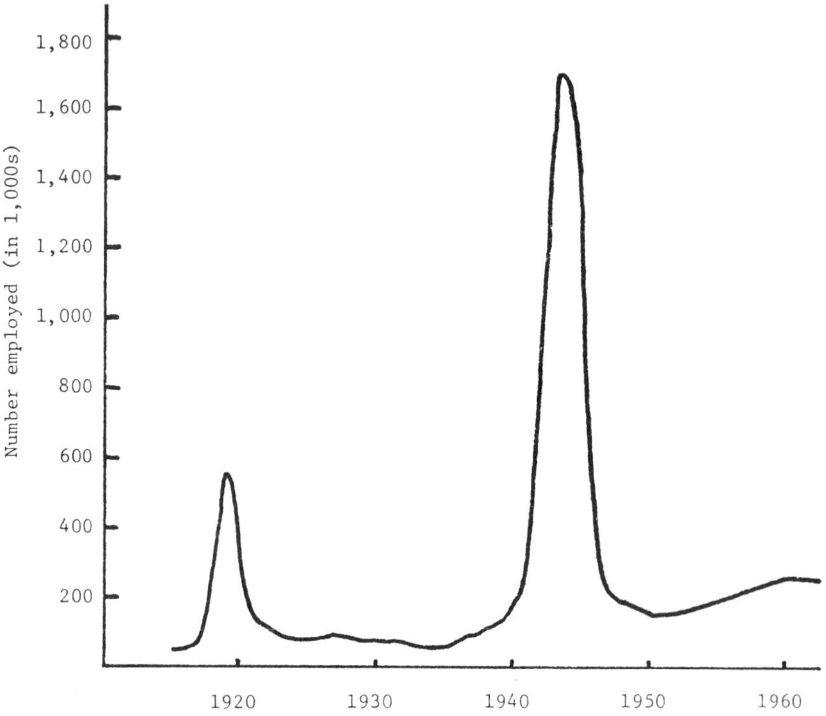

Figure 1
Numbers Employed in the U.S. Ship Construction and Repair Industry, 1915-1965. (Data from Bureau of Labor Statistics 1945; Fasset 1948; Bureau of Census 1960.)

and race distribution is uncertain. It seems likely, however, that the newly hired workers during the war were mainly white and generally younger than those more experienced shipbuilders employed before and after the war (estimated median age, 40 years). Turnover among shipyard workers was high during the wartime escalation, with separations running 5-10% per month (Bureau of Labor Statistics 1945). Because the percentage that left the work force but later returned is unknown, it is difficult to determine precisely the number of individuals ever employed in the industry during the war. Selikoff et al. (1979) estimated 4.5 million. This is probably a reliable figure, but under the assumption that only a very small fraction of newly hired workers were former employees, the estimated total would be even higher and may approach 6 million. It is the enormous size of the shipbuilding industry that makes it worthy of special attention when efforts are made to quantify the extent of occupational cancer.

Very limited data are available on exposure to particular carcinogens among individual shipyard workers. However, classification of jobs held can provide useful information. The largest single group within U.S. shipyards in

1943 was welders (15%), followed by shipfitters (11%), machinists (8%), pipefitters (7%), electricians (7%), carpenters (6%), and laborers (6%). Only 0.2% were pipecoverers (Bureau of Labor Statistics 1945). This group had especially high exposure to asbestos dust, as shown by an environmental survey in 1945 of pipecovering operations in two Navy and two private shipyards (Fleischer et al. 1946). The recognition that asbestos exposures were widespread throughout the shipyards came in the 1970s when pleural and parenchymal X-ray changes characteristic of asbestos disease were observed among long-term shipyard workers of virtually all trades, not just those directly handling asbestos products (Polakoff et al. 1979; Selikoff et al. 1979; Felton 1980). In addition to asbestos, the wartime shipbuilding construction effort required large expenditures for various other materials. Indeed, about 60% of nonlabor shipbuilding costs were for machinery and structural iron and steel, with foundries on the premises of the larger yards.

THE MESOTHELIOMA OUTBREAK

In 1964 a British series of 17 patients with mesothelioma was reported in Liverpool; 5 had worked in the ship-repair industry (Owen 1964). Other cases subsequently were identified among shipyard workers of Plymouth (Harries 1968) and Barrow-in-Furness (Edge 1979) in Great Britain; Walcheren Island (Stumphius 1971), St. Nazaire-Nantes (deLajartre and deLajartre 1979), and Genoa (Puntoni et al. 1976) in continental Europe; and recently, Seattle (Hinds 1978) and Norfolk-Newport News (Tagnon et al. 1980) in the United States. It is noteworthy that in each report nearly all the mesotheliomas were pleural (259 of the 269 mesotheliomas that specified the site of origin) compared with the predominance of peritoneal tumors reported among insulation and asbestos factory workers (Selikoff 1977; Newhouse and Berry 1979).

There is little doubt that occupational asbestos exposure induced these cancers. There are several research questions, however, concerning the amount of exposure sufficient to cause mesothelioma and the carcinogenic potential of different types of asbestos fibers. Both issues have been difficult to evaluate because of the rarity of the tumors—and consequently small numbers of cases in any single study—and because of uncertainties concerning individual exposures. In each series, however, mesotheliomas occurred among workers in several shipyard jobs where asbestos materials would not be handled ordinarily and thus exposure was likely to be indirect and comparatively light. In many instances, the duration of employment was only a few years. For other settings also, mesotheliomas have been reported following incidental and apparently low exposure to asbestos (Greenberg and Davies 1974). Nevertheless, the risk of mesothelioma among shipyard workers, and other occupational groups exposed to asbestos (Newhouse and Berry 1979), is greater among those with higher exposures. A dose-response gradient is suggested by the higher incidence in laggers, who experienced more intense exposures than other dockyard trades in Devonport (Sheers and Coles 1980); by the increasing prevalence of mesothelioma with higher estimated asbestos exposure in Walcheren Island (Stumphius 1979); and by the higher risks among pipecoverers and pipefitters than other shipyard workers in Tidewater, Virginia (Tagnon et al. 1980). Furthermore, in Virginia, the mesotheliomas in the shipyard industry arose mainly among long-term employees, with lower risks among persons employed for limited periods, usually during World War II. Finally, an examination of asbestos-fiber content in lung tissue in patients and controls in Merseyside, England, revealed that the risk of mesothelioma rose with increasing body burden (Whitwell et al. 1977). Thus, the measurable evidence indicates that the risk of mesothelioma is proportionate to the amount of asbestos exposure, but the data are not sufficient to delineate adequately the shape of the dose-response curve. It is not possible from these data to distinguish a linear from a probit or other mathematical model that might predict a proportionately smaller response at low doses. Furthermore, the data are not sufficient to determine whether short-term intense exposure carries a higher, or lower, risk than long-term, lighter exposure.

Which asbestos fibers are responsible for mesothelioma in the shipyards? Chrysotile is generally a major component in ship fireproofing and insulation. However, exposures generally are mixed, as other fiber types, particularly amosite in the United States and crocidolite in Europe, have also been used extensively in the industry. Separating the effects of the different fibers is difficult, but there are bits of evidence that suggest a major role for chrysotile. First, examination of lung tissue from autopsies of mesothelioma patients in Great Britain revealed that the chrysotile fibers were shorter and finer than crocidolite or amosite, perhaps enhancing their deposition on the pleural lining (Pooley and Clark 1979). Also, lung and pleural tissue from mesothelioma patients in shipyard regions in the Netherlands and in France contained mixed fiber types, but more often chrysotile than crocidolite (deLajartre and deLajartre 1979; Stumphius 1979). Second, the pleural origin of most mesotheliomas seen in shipyard workers corresponds to the pattern described in Canadian chrysotile miners believed to be lightly exposed or unexposed to other fiber types (McDonald et al. 1980), although amphiboles were detected in the lungs of some miners who developed asbestosis (Pooley 1976). Thus, inhaled asbestos fibers of all types seem capable of inducing mesothelioma in humans. Among shipyard workers, chrysotile, which some investigators suspect is the least potent carcinogen among the asbestos fibers (International Agency for Research on Cancer 1977), may actively account for a large percentage of pleural mesotheliomas.

The shipyard mesotheliomas resemble mesotheliomas in other settings regarding the long duration between initial exposure and clinical onset, with the latent period averaging nearly 40 years and few cases developing within 20 years of first employment. As indicated by J. Peto (this volume), elevated risks

Table 1
RR of Lung Cancer Associated with Shipbuilding Employment along the Atlantic Coast

Location	Years cases diagnosed	Total sample	Percent employed in shipyards	RR[a]
Coastal Georgia	1970-1976	1057	21	1.6
Jacksonville, Florida	1976-1978	789	22	1.4
Tidewater, Virginia	1976	641	33	1.5
Bath, Maine	1974-1978	64	67	1.7

[a]Adjusted for cigarette smoking.

of mesothelioma should continue into the 1990s among the large cohort of men employed in shipbuilding during the 1940s, with perhaps 10,000 deaths from this tumor occurring in the United States as a legacy of their wartime shipyard exposures.

LUNG CANCER AS A SHIPYARD DISEASE

Whereas a few cases of a rare disease such as mesothelioma may arouse suspicion of an occupational hazard, clustering of a more common disease such as lung cancer may not be detected so easily. Thus, although lung cancer was linked to asbestos exposure in the 1950s (Doll 1955) and accounted for nearly 20% of the deaths among asbestos insulation workers in the 1960s (Selikoff 1977), it was not until the late 1970s that excess risks were documented among shipyard workers. Today there is considerable evidence from case-control and cohort studies that the risk of lung cancer is increased by a factor of less than 2 among men employed in shipyards during World War II. Asbestos has been incriminated, although other agents in the shipyard environment may have contributed to this risk (Cowles 1978).

Case-control studies of lung cancer have been conducted by the National Cancer Institute in 4 areas along the Atlantic coast where the shipbuilding industry has been prominent. In each survey, the cancer patients and controls (or their next of kin) matched for age, sex, race, source of ascertainment (e.g., hospital, death certificate), and vital status were interviewed for information on occupational and smoking histories. In all areas there were elevated risks associated with prior work in area shipyards, particularly during World War II (Table 1) (Blot et al. 1978, 1980, 1981). The percentage of the cases identified in the 1970s that had worked in the industry varied from 21% in Georgia, where major shipyards operated during the war and closed shortly thereafter, to a high of 67% in Bath, Maine, site of the oldest continuing shipyard in the United States. About one-third of the cases in coastal Virginia worked in the

Table 2
RR of Lung Cancer According to Cigarette Smoking and Shipyard Employment

	Employment in shipyards	
Cigarette smoking status	no	yes
Nonsmoker	1.0	2.2
Former smoker	3.7	3.0
Light (.5 pack/day)	4.8	5.2
Moderate (.5-1.5 packs/day)	7.2	10.2
Heavy (2+ packs/day)	10.3	21.7

All risks relative to noncigarette smokers never employed in shipbuilding. Data from 4 Atlantic coast case-control surveys.

shipbuilding industry, currently the area's largest single employer with about 30,000 workers, somewhat less than one-half of the 1943 total. The risk of lung cancer in Virginia was elevated among those who had worked in the shipyards during World War II, but not among those first employed after 1950. Combining data from over 2500 interviews in the 4 areas, the relative risk (RR) of lung cancer associated with ever-employment in shipbuilding, adjusted for cigarette smoking, was 1.44 with relatively tight 95% confidence limits of 1.17-1.78 ($p < .001$). The RR of lung cancer for workers employed during World War II but not thereafter was also 1.4, with the temporary work averaging about 3 years.

In the combined data set, the increased risk of lung cancer among shipyard workers was seen in nearly all cigarette smoking categories (Table 2). There was a twofold increased risk among nonsmokers, but the largest absolute excess occurred among heavy smokers. A synergistic relation with smoking is characteristic of asbestos-induced lung cancer (Saracci 1977). However, only in the Florida study were asbestos exposures reported more often among cases than controls. It may be that workers were unaware of asbestos exposure in the past, or that next of kin had incomplete knowledge. The shipyard jobs of the cases did not tend to differ from those of the controls, but airborne asbestos dusts apparently were widespread throughout the yards during the heightened wartime activity.

That asbestos is primarily responsible for the lung cancer excess is also suggested by a cohort study of workers employed in the early 1950s at the Pearl Harbor Naval Shipyard in Hawaii (Kolonel et al. 1980). There was a 70% increase in lung cancer deaths among men whose particular jobs suggested exposure to asbestos, but no excess risk for the remainder of the workforce. Further evidence comes from the radiologic detection of pleural plaques suggesting asbestotic change among several workers in Barrow-in-Furness within a few years of lung cancer diagnosis (Edge 1979). It is not possible, however, to exclude the influence of carcinogens other than asbestos in shipyards. An evaluation of mortality patterns among welders of a boilermakers union in Seattle, Washington, who were primarily engaged in shipyard work, revealed a 69% excess of lung cancer beginning 20 or more years after first employment (Beaumont and Weiss 1980). It was suggested that by-products of welding may have been partly responsible for the excess risk.

The precise contribution of asbestos to shipyard lung cancer will remain clouded because of the uncertainties in the actual exposures of individual workers. Epidemiologic surveys of shipyard workers first employed after asbestos controls were instituted in the 1970s may help clarify the issue, but only in another 10 years or longer. Although in mesothelioma the lung tissue has shown higher asbestos fiber content than controls, the results in lung cancer have not been as clear-cut (Whitwell et al. 1977). Although lung cancer in asbestos insulation workers tends to arise more often in the lower lobes, the excess risk appears to affect all histologic types (Selikoff et al. 1977), in contrast to the predeliction for small cell anaplastic carcinoma following occupational exposures to agents such as radon and *bis*(chloromethyl)ether (Lundin et al. 1971; Pasternack et al. 1977). Limited data were available on the histology of lung cancers among shipyard workers in the United States, and no cell type pecularities were seen.

It has been shown that the risk of lung cancer among asbestos workers increases with the duration and intensity of exposure (Henderson and Enterline 1979; Newhouse and Berry 1979). It is noteworthy then that the excess risk of lung cancer among shipyard workers in Georgia, where yards operated only during World War II, was of the same magnitude as in Virginia, where the industry was established before the war and continues to prosper today Furthermore, in Virginia, there was no major difference in risk between those who worked temporarily during the war years and those who spent their careers in shipyard work. These findings do not necessarily argue against a dose-response relation, but they may reflect the latency period for asbestos-related cancer. That is, shipyard exposures during the 1940s seem largely responsible for the excess lung cancers detected in the 1970s, with later and perhaps earlier employment not measurably affecting the risk in recent years.

OTHER CANCERS IN SHIPYARD WORKERS

Cancers outside of the respiratory system have not been reported in excess among shipyard workers, but sufficiently large studies to detect small increases, such as those on the order of 50% or so, have not been completed. A report of excess leukemia among Portsmouth, New Hampshire, shipyard workers handling nuclear materials introduced in the late 1950s (Najarian and Colton 1978) was not confirmed by a recent cohort study of nuclear workers at that yard (Rinsky et al. 1981).

CONCLUSION

During World War II, the shipbuilding industry in the United States was huge, with 4.5 million or more workers employed for limited periods during the 1940s. As a consequence of asbestos exposures, mesotheliomas of the pleura now occur excessively in this cohort and will possibly continue to be seen into the 1990s because of the long latency period. The major health effect of wartime shipyard employment is lung cancer. At the rates prevailing in the United States, with about 20% of all deaths in males attributable to cancer and one-third of these from lung cancer, about 300,000 of the total cohort would be expected to die from lung cancer. If the 40% excess risk observed among east coast shipyard workers in the 1970s holds in general, then another 120,000 deaths from this cancer may occur as a result of wartime exposures.

REFERENCES

Beaumont, J.J. and N.E. Weiss. 1980. Mortality of welders, shipfitters, and other metal trades workers in Boilermakers Local No. 104, AFL-CIO. *Am. J. Epidemiol.* **112**:775.

Blot, W.J., L.E. Morris, R. Stroube, I. Tagnon and J.F. Fraumeni, Jr. 1980. Lung and laryngeal cancers in relation to shipyard employment in coastal Virginia. *J. Natl. Cancer Inst.* **65**:571.

Blot, W.J., J.M. Harrington, A. Toledo, R. Hoover, C.W. Heath, and J.F. Fraumeni, Jr. 1978. Lung cancer after employment in shipyards during World War II. *N. Engl. J. Med.* **299**:620.

Blot, W.J., J.E. Davies, L.E. Morris, C.W. Nordwall, E. Buiatti, A. Ng, and J.F. Fraumeni, Jr. 1981. Occupation and the high risk of lung cancer in northeast Florida. *Cancer* (in press).

Bureau of Census. 1963. Census of population 1960. U.S. Government Printing Office, Washington, D.C.

Bureau of Labor Statistics. 1945. *Wartime employment, production, and conditions of work in shipyards,* Bull. No. 824. Washington, D.C.

Cowles, S.R. 1978. Cancer in the workplace. Percivall Pott to the present. *Mil. Med.* **143**:395.

deLajartre, M. and A.Y. deLajartre. 1979. Mesothelioma on the coast of Brittany, France. *Ann. N.Y. Acad. Sci.* **330**:323.

Doll, R. 1955. Mortality from lung cancer in asbestos workers. *Br. J. Ind. Med.* **12**:81.

Edge, J.R. 1979. Incidence of bronchial carcinoma in shipyard workers with pleural plaques. *Ann. N.Y. Acad. Sci.* **330**:289.

Fasset, F.G., Jr. 1948. *The shipbuilding business in the United States of America,* vol. 1. Society of Naval Architects and Marine Engineers, New York.

Felton, J.S., E.N. Sargent, and J.S. Gordenson. 1980. Radiographic changes following asbestos exposures experience with 7500 workers. *J. Occup. Med.* **22**:15.

Fleischer, W.E., F.J. Viles, R.L. Gade, and P. Drinker. 1946. A health survey of pipe-covering operations in constructing naval vessels. *J. Ind. Hyg. Toxicol.* **28**:9.

Greenberg, M. and L. Davies. 1974. Mesothelioma register 1967-68. *Br. J. Med.* **31**:91.

Harries, P.G. 1968. Asbestos hazards in naval dockyards. *Ann. Occup. Hyg.* **11**:135.

Henderson, V.L. and P.E. Enterline. 1979. Asbestos exposure: Factors associated with excess cancer and respiratory disease mortality. *Ann. NY Acad. Sci.* **330**:117.

Hinds, M.W. 1978. Mesothelioma in shipyard workers. *West J. Med.* **128**:169.

International Agency for Research on Cancer (IARC). Asbestos. *IARC Monogr.* **14**.

Kolonel, L.N., T. Hirohata, B.V. Chappell, F.V. Viola, and D.E. Harris. 1980. Cancer mortality in a cohort of naval shipyard workers in Hawaii: early findings. *J. Natl. Cancer Inst.* **64**:739.

Lundin, F.E., Jr., V.E. Archer, and J.K. Wagoner. 1971. Radon daughter exposure and respiratory cancer. NIOSH and NIEHS Joint Monograph 1. NTIS, Springfield, Va.

McDonald, J.C., F.D. Liddell, G.W. Gibbs, G.E. Eyssen, and A.D. McDonald. 1980. Dust exposure and mortality in chrysotile mining, 1910-1975. *Brit. J. Ind. Med.* **37**:11.

Najarian, T. and T. Colton. 1978. Mortality from leukemia and cancer in shipyard nuclear workers. *Lancet* i:1018.

Newhouse, M.L. and G. Berry. 1979. Patterns of mortality in asbestos factory workers in London. *Ann. N.Y. Acad. Sci.* **330**:53.

Owen, W.G. 1964. Diffuse mesothelioma and exposure to asbestos dust in the Merseyside area. *Br. Med. J.* **2**:214.

Pasternack, B.S., R.E. Shore, R.E. Albert. 1977. Occupational exposure to chloromethyl ethers. *J. Occup. Med.* **19**:741.

Polakoff, P.L., B.R. Horn, and D.R. Scherer. 1979. Prevalence of radiographic abnormalities among northern California shipyard workers. *Ann. N.Y. Acad. Sci.* **330**:333.

Pooley, F.D. 1976. An examination of the fibrous mineral content of asbestos lung tissue from the Canadian chrysotile mining industry. *Environ. Res.* **12**:281.

Pooley, F.D. and N. Clark. 1979. Fiber dimensions and aspect ratio of crocidolite, chrysotile, and amosite particles detected in lung tissue specimens. *Ann. N.Y. Acad. Sci.* **310**:711.

Puntoni, R., F. Valerio, and L. Santi. 1976. Il mesotelioma pleurico fra i lavoratori del porto di Genova. *Tumori* **62**:205.

Rinsky, R.A., R.D. Zumwalde, R.J. Waxweiler, W.E. Murray, Jr., P.J. Bierbaum, P.J. Landrigan, M. Terpilak, and C. Cox. 1981. Cancer mortality at a naval nuclear shipyard. *Lancet* i:231.

Saracci, R. 1977. Asbestos and lung cancer: An analysis of the epidemiological evidence on the asbestos-smoking interaction. *Int. J. Cancer* **20**:123.

Selikoff, I.J. 1977. Cancer risk of asbestos exposure. *Cold Spring Harbor Conf. Cell Proliferation* **4**:1765.

Selikoff, I.J., R. Lilis, and W.J. Nicholson. 1979. Asbestos disease in United States shipyards. *Ann. N.Y. Acad. Sci.* **330**:295.

Sheers, G. and R.M. Coles. 1980. Mesothelioma risks in a naval dockyard. *Arch. Environ. Health* **35**:276.

Stumphius, J. 1971. Epidemiology of mesothelioma on Watcheren Island. *Br. J. Ind. Med.* **28**:59.

______. Mesothelioma incidence in a Dutch shipyard. *Ann. N.Y. Acad. Sci.* **330**:311.

Tagnon, I., W.J. Blot, R.B. Stroube, N.E. Day, L.E. Morris, B.B. Peace, and J.F. Fraumeni, Jr. 1980. Mesothelioma associated with the shipbuilding industry in coastal Virginia. *Cancer Res.* **40**:3875.

Whitwell, F., J. Scott, and M. Grimshaw. 1977. Relationship between occupations and asbestos fiber content of the lungs of patients with pleural mesothelioma, lung cancer, and other diseases. *Thorax* **32**:377.

COMMENTS

KARSTADT: You and others have reported on the experience of the male shipyard workers in the U.S. during World War II. A significant number of women were also employed. Could you report on any data about women?

BLOT: No, I can't. In the beginning war years, females made up 5% of the work force. By 1945 it increased to an overall 10%. We didn't look at women in our case-control studies mainly because of the small numbers. But, to answer your question: I believe that Johns Hopkins University is conducting a cohort study of over 250,000 people who worked at seven U.S. shipyards. They are looking at radiation risks, primarily among people working in the 1950s and 1960s when radiation materials were introduced. For some of the cohorts, they are tracing and identifying people, including women, who worked during the war.

J. PETO: The question of chrysotile causing mesothelioma is too large a subject to discuss now. Nobody has a very firm opinion about it, but there is a considerable distribution of probability assignment in the industry and it is a very important question in England particularly, because the exposure there is predominantly chrysotile. I suppose that is increasingly true in the States now as well.

BLOT: I mentioned the possible carcinogenic potential of chrysotile in particular because chrysotile is generally regarded as less hazardous. But there are a few bits of information that indicate that we may be writing it off too soon.

J. PETO: I always maintained that, but nobody ever agreed with me.

BEEBE: Why do you think you don't see much higher risks in certain occupations? I don't quite understand why it should seem that the exposure was so homogeneous throughout.

BLOT: We do for mesothelioma. The cases tend to cluster in those jobs where the exposure is the most intense. But there wasn't much of that for lung cancer. I am not sure what the reason is. It may have to do with the interaction of cigarette smoking and asbestos, or it could be that it takes less of an exposure to induce a lung cancer because of the contribution of cigarette smoke, whereas it requires a more intense exposure to induce a mesothelioma, as the asbestos has to act entirely on its own.

ENTERLINE: I wanted to ask two questions about the way you determine occupations. One: Do you think that the bias that was in the study by Najarian and Colton (1978) in which people tended to associate the leukemias with radiation exposure, could be present? Two: I have never seen the actual occupation on the death certificates. What happens when you look at the death certificate occupation like Marise Gottlieb did?

BLOT: In answer to the first question, I think there is probably not much room for error in a person telling you the fact that he worked in a shipyard. It is unlikely that someone would fabricate that, although it is possible. The information tends to break down when you get into the details of precisely what the person did or what materials he was handling. They often didn't know.

As far as the second question is concerned, it depends where you do the study. We preceded the interview study in Georgia with a death certificate search and found that out of 1700 people—half lung cancer and half controls deaths—essentially none had listed shipyard work as their usual occupation in the 1960s and 1970s because the yards closed shortly after World War II. It was only when we went back and got an occupational history that we found that something like over 20% of these people who were dying of lung cancer had, in fact, worked in the yards.

ENTERLINE: But in Newport News, would you have picked up the shipyard workers with lung cancer by just using death certificate occupation?

BLOT: I don't know, because we didn't do it. In Newport News there would be the potential for a monitoring of death certificate information on occupation since the industry has continued.

ENTERLINE: I think it would be good to check.

McDONALD: I don't want to get into the fiber type controversy but there was a point you mentioned about body burden of chrysotile and amphiboles that worried me. One has to do well-controlled studies of body burdens; I mentioned this because in both the British and the American case-controlled studies, the chrysotile levels seem much higher than the amphibole levels in both cases and controls, whereas the difference in level was in the amphiboles.

SIEMIATYCKI: Did you interview the proxies of cases and the controls themselves?

BLOT: No. Almost all these studies were matched according to what we call the vital status. If the case was deceased, we attempted to interview a next of kin of the control.

R. PETO: There is a disagreement as to how much of the excess lung cancer that you have seen is genuinely ascribable to asbestos. Could this be resolved if you look at the mesothelioma data in corresponding areas? If you assume that the amount of lung cancer caused in the shipyards is about three or four times the amount of mesothelioma caused in the shipyards, would you get something like your 1.5 risk, or would you get something substantially lower? I know your studies don't address this directly, but you must have data on this.

BLOT: The projected lung cancer risk would be much higher than 1.5 in Virginia, but it would be much less in Georgia and Florida. These studies are not strictly comparable, however, because the shipbuilding industry has been in operation since the early 1900s in Virginia but only during World War II in the other two states. Another problem is that the factor of 3 or 4 is a guess. It is an extrapolation from other sources of data. Perhaps the shipyard setting is different.

NICHOLSON: You also have the diagnostic problem, in that you were using mesothelioma to pick it out.

References

Najarian, T. and T. Colton. 1978. Mortality from leukemia and cancer in shipyard nuclear workers. *Lancet* i:1018.

Trends in Mesothelioma Incidence in the United States and the Forecast Epidemic Due to Asbestos Exposure During World War II

JULIAN PETO
Imperial Cancer Research Fund
Cancer Epidemiology Unit
Oxford OXI 30G England

BRIAN E. HENDERSON AND MALCOLM C. PIKE
Department of Family and Preventive Medicine
University of Southern California
Los Angeles, California 90033

The incidence of mesothelioma in those not exposed to asbestos is of the order of one per million per annum; however, among men heavily exposed to asbestos, the risk may be increased by a factor of 1000 or more. About 1000 cases are now diagnosed each year in the United States, and it has been suggested that increasing asbestos exposure, particularly in shipyards and other industries that flourished during World War II, may result in very much higher rates in the near future. We have tried to produce more formal estimates of the pattern of past exposure and the likely evolution of future incidence by combining incidence patterns observed in industrial cohorts with the results of a survey of cases diagnosed in Los Angeles County in which age and year of first exposure to asbestos were ascertained. Our results suggest that the extent of shipyard and other wartime exposure has been grossly exaggerated, although the effects of more recent exposure may be greater than is generally appreciated. In particular, it seems that the total number of mesotheliomas caused by shipyard exposure during World War II is likely to be about 5000, almost half of which have already occurred.

Projections of future numbers are based on classification of the population into cohorts first exposed to asbestos at different ages in each period. These subgroups are not observed directly, however, and our results do not provide estimates of risk that can be applied usefully to identifiable individuals. A formal account of this unusual method of analysis is given in the Appendix of this paper but the results are presented in a less formal but hopefully more comprehensible form within the text.

THE AGE AND TIME DEPENDENCE OF MESOTHELIOMA CAUSED BY ASBESTOS EXPOSURE

The proportion of mesotheliomas in asbestos workers that are peritoneal in origin varies widely under different conditions. Among North American insulation workers who have been exposed to amosite, a high proportion are peritoneal, but the majority of mesotheliomas are pleural among miners and factory workers exposed only to chrysotile or crocidolite. For both practical and theoretical purposes, however, the two sites can be amalgamated. Both diseases are quickly fatal, and the incidence of cases caused by asbestos exposure for both appears to be approximately proportional to the 3.5th power of time since first exposure, irrespective of age at first exposure, duration of exposure, or fiber type (Peto et al. 1981). North American insulation workers provide the only substantial data on incidence beyond 40 years after first exposure, but other cohorts followed up for shorter periods conform to the same incidence pattern (Peto et al. 1981). Therefore, we have assumed that incidence will continue to increase as (time since first exposure)$^{3.5}$ indefinitely in the following analyses, but deaths occurring after age 80 are ignored in the resulting predictions of future mesothelioma incidence. Projection beyond this age would entail extrapolation beyond the range of observation in any existing cohort and probably could not be tested, as misdiagnosis is common in extreme old age.

THE RELATIONSHIP BETWEEN CURRENT AND FUTURE MESOTHELIOMA INCIDENCE

Table 1 shows the numbers of cases that would be expected to occur in successive quinquennia up to age 80 among equal cohorts of men first exposed at various ages. The median ages at first exposure (18½, 23½, 28½, etc.) have been chosen so that each entry in Table 1 corresponds to a conventional age group and period of first exposure in our survey (see Table 2 below). Thus, for example, men first exposed at age 23½ in mid-1942 (the middle of the 1940-1944 period) would have been aged 55-59 in 1974-1978. Apart from an arbitrary multiplying factor, the figures in Table 1 are the product of (time since first exposure)$^{3.5}$ and the appropriate life-table for men in the United States. They are based on two assumptions: (1) that mesothelioma incidence continues to rise as (time since first exposure)$^{3.5}$ up to age 80, and (2) that overall age-specific mortality in exposed workers is similar to that of other men of the same age in the United States. Therefore, predictions of the future rate of increase based on these figures might be somewhat exaggerated, as mortality in heavily exposed asbestos workers is higher than in the general population. The proportion surviving may fall progressively below the survival curve based on national mortality figures, and there would then be proportionately fewer mesotheliomas in the future.

The last row in Table 1, giving the cumulative risk of developing mesothelioma by age 80, illustrates the enormous effect of age at first exposure. A man first exposed below age 20 suffers more than 10 times the risk of a man aged over 40, for example, and the assumed distribution of age at first exposure may substantially affect predictions of future risk.

Table 1
Predicted Numbers of Mesotheliomas That Would Occur among a Given Number of Men in Each Quinquennium Following First Exposre to Asbestos at a Fixed Level, by Age at First Exposure

	Age first exposed							
	16-20	21-25	26-30	31-35	36-40	41-45	46-50	51-55
	Median age first exposed							
	18½	23½	28½	33½	38½	43½	48½	53½
Age at diagnosis	Predicted numbers of mesotheliomas							
25-29	.04							
30-34	.17	.04						
35-39	.48	.17	.04					
40-44	1.07	.47	.16	.04				
45-49	2.02	1.05	.47	.16	.03			
50-54	*3.40*	1.97	1.02	.46	.16	.03		
55-59	5.19	*3.24*	1.87	.97	.43	.15	.03	
60-64	7.22	4.77	*2.98*	1.72	.90	.40	.14	.03
65-69	9.12	6.31	4.17	*2.60*	1.51	.79	.36	.13
70-74	10.32	7.40	5.12	3.39	*2.12*	1.23	.65	.30
75-79	10.15	7.50	5.39	3.73	2.47	*1.55*	.91	.49
Total below age 80	49.18	32.92	21.22	13.07	7.62	4.15	2.09	0.95

Figures corresponding to cases occurring in 1974-1978 in men first exposed in 1942 are italicized.

MESOTHELIOMA INCIDENCE IN LOS ANGELES COUNTY AND IN THE UNITED STATES

The case or a close relative was interviewed in 87% (101/116) of male and 81% (25/31) of female pleural or peritoneal mesotheliomas diagnosed in Los Angeles County in 1974-1978, a period in which ascertainment probably was very close to complete. Exposure to asbestos was reported for 69 of the men for whom an interview was obtained; 22 reported no exposure, and in the remaining 10 it could not be determined if exposure had occurred. The 69 men with recorded asbestos exposure are tabulated according to age at first exposure and year of first exposure in Table 2. The 18 men first exposed in shipyards during World War II (1939-1945) are shown separately, both because the effects of such exposure are of particular interest and because they appear to have been rather older at first exposure than other men. The remaining 51 exposed men include only four shipyard workers.

Table 2
69 Male Mesotheliomas with Dated Asbestos Exposure Diagnosed in Los Angeles County in 1974-1978

Year first exposed	Age at first exposure to asbestos							
	16-20	21-25	26-30	31-35	36-40	41-45	over 45	Total
1915-1919	1	0						1
1920-1924	3	0	1					4
1925-1929	2	1	2	0				5
1930-1934	0	0	1	1	0			2
1935-1939	3	1	4	1	0	0		9
1940-1944	1	3	1	1	2	0	0	8
1945-1949	1	4	0	2	2	3	1	13
1950-1954	1	0	1	2	0	0	0	4
1955-1959	0	1	1	0	1	0	0	3
1960-1964	0	0	0	0	0	1	0	1
1965-1969	0	0	0	0	0	0	1	1
Total except WW II shipyard	12	10	11	7	5	4	2	51
1939-1945 (WW II shipyard)	1	2	2	4	3	4	2	18

Cases originating in World War II shipyard exposure are not included in the upper part of the table.

The incidence of mesothelioma in Los Angeles County in 1974-1978 was similar in both sexes to that observed in eight Surveillance, Epidemiology, and End Results Program (SEER) cancer registries between 1970 and 1976, except perhaps in the older age groups, where rates were rather higher among men and lower among women (Table 3). Based on these average rates, Hinds (1978) has estimated that approximately 900 cases were occurring each year in the United States between 1970 and 1976, of which almost 700 were in men. It appears that incidence was still rising during this period, however, and we shall assume that a total of 4000 male cases (800 per annum) were diagnosed in the United States between 1974 and 1978 as a basis for projections of national incidence.

Among the 91 men in our survey for whom adequate histories were obtained, 20% (18/91) were World War II shipyard workers, 56% (51/91) were first exposed to asbestos in other environments, and 24% (22/91) had never been exposed to asbestos. If this pattern is typical of the whole United States, approximately 800 World War II shipyard workers (20% of 4000), 2240 men with other asbestos exposure (56% of 4000), and 960 unexposed men (24% of 4000) developed mesothelioma between 1974 and 1978.

Table 3
Mesothelioma Incidence per Million per year in the United States in 1970-1976, and in Los Angeles in 1974-1978

	Male		Female	
Age	United States[a]	Los Angeles	United States[a]	Los Angeles
10-19	0.0 (0)[b]	0.0 (0)	0.2 (1)	0.0 (0)
20-29	0.7 (3)	0.4 (1)	0.2 (1)	0.0 (0)
30-39	3.2 (9)	0.0 (0)	1.2 (4)	2.9 (6)
40-49	7.0 (22)	4.6 (10)	1.6 (5)	0.9 (2)
50-59	12.3 (33)	12.1 (22)	2.6 (10)	4.6 (9)
60-69	29.9 (54)	36.3 (41)	7.8 (15)	4.3 (6)
70-79	34.7 (45)	54.9 (42)	10.9 (19)	5.9 (8)

[a]Data from Hinds (1978).
[b]Number of cases in parentheses.

FUTURE INCIDENCE DUE TO SHIPYARD EXPOSURE DURING WORLD WAR II

A high proportion of men employed in shipyards during World War II were aged 35 or more at first exposure, as younger men were often on active service. We have drawn a small random sample of former employees at the Long Beach Naval Dockyard, and within this sample 68% (17/25) of men first employed during World War II were aged 35 or more when they joined the dockyard; the youngest of the 10 who worked there for more than 3 years was aged 33. The effects of such an age distribution, with 70% of men aged over 35 at first exposure and 10% aged 25 or under, are shown in the left half of Table 4. The corresponding numbers of mesotheliomas expected in successive periods, both overall and in each age cohort, are expressed as a percentage of the number of cases diagnosed in the period 1974-1978. These figures were calculated by averaging adjacent cohorts in Table 1. Thus, for example, the predicted number in each period for men aged 25 or less is the sum of the numbers shown in Table 1 for men aged 16-20 and those aged 21-25 at first exposure multiplied by 0.10, the proportion of men aged 25 or under; for men aged 26-35 the calculation is based on the sum for ages 26-30 and 31-35, and so on. Men aged over 55 at first exposure are ignored, as their risk is negligible. The figures are standardized to sum to 100 for the period 1974-1978.

Table 4 also shows the corresponding total numbers of cases in World War II shipyard workers in the United States, assuming 800 in the period 1974-1978. The predicted total number, past and future, is 5280, of which about half have already occurred. To assess the effect of the assumed age distribution, the calculation is repeated in the right half of Table 4 for a population in which equal numbers of men were first exposed at each age from 16 to 45.

Table 4
Two Age Distributions at First Exposure to Asbestos in 1942 and Corresponding War II Shipyard Workers Assuming 800 Cases in 1974-1978.

	Age at first exposure					
	16-25	26-35	36-45	46-55	Total	
	Proportion of men					
	.10	.20	.35	.35	1.00	
Year of diagnosis	Predicted numbers of mesotheliomas					WW II shipyard workers
1949-1953	0	1	1	1	3	24
1954-1958	1	2	4	3	10	80
1959-1963	3	6	9	8	26	208
1964-1968	7	13	19	13	52	416
1969-1973	13	23	31	10	77	616
1974-1978	22	36	42	–	100	800
1979-1983	33	49	28	–	110	880
1984-1988	44	58	–	–	102	816
1989-1993	54	35	–	–	89	712
1994-1998	58	–	–	–	58	464
1999-2003	33	–	–	–	33	264
Total up to age 80:					660	5280

The older distribution (left side of the table) may be more representative of the war-
seems more characteristic of other industries. All figures except the World War II shipyard

Surprisingly, the predicted total number is increased by only 25%, to 6624. Therefore, it appears that the only critical assumption underlying these projections is that about 20% of currently diagnosed male cases are due to World War II shipyard exposure. There are certainly areas in which this is not true, notably Tidewater, Virginia, where 77% of mesotheliomas had been shipyard workers, and almost 40% were first exposed during World War II (Tagnon et al. 1980). In this area, however, the incidence of mesothelioma was approximately four times the national rate among white males, due to the extraordinarily high level of shipyard employment. Thus, we are inclined to believe that Los Angeles is more typical of the national average. The total number of mesotheliomas diagnosed among World War II shipyard workers is unlikely to exceed 7000, and could be considerably less.

FUTURE INCIDENCE DUE TO ASBESTOS EXPOSURE OTHER THAN IN WORLD WAR II SHIPYARDS

The figures in Table 1 give estimates of past and future numbers of cases in relation to the number currently occurring in each birth cohort according to age

Predictions of Total Numbers of Mesotheliomas in Successive Periods in World

	Age at first exposure					
	16-25	26-35	36-45	46-55	Total	
	Proportion of men					
	.25	.25	.25	.25	1.00	
Year of diagnosis	Predicted numbers of mesotheliomas					WW II shipyard workers
1949-1953	1	1	0	0	2	16
1954-1958	2	2	2	2	8	64
1959-1963	6	6	5	4	21	168
1964-1968	13	13	11	7	44	352
1969-1973	25	23	17	6	71	568
1974-1978	42	35	23	–	100	800
1979-1983	63	48	16	–	127	1016
1984-1988	85	56	–	–	141	1128
1989-1993	104	34	–	–	138	1104
1994-1998	112	–	–	–	112	896
1999-2003	64	–	–	–	64	512
Total up to age 80:					828	6624

time recruitment pattern in shipyards. The right side of the (uniform) age distribution workers columns are expressed as percentages of the 1974-1978 total.

at first exposure, but they also can be interpreted as estimates of the distribution of the numbers that would have been expected to occur in 1974-1978 for each cell in Table 2 if equal numbers of men at each age up to 45 had been first exposed under uniform conditions in each quinquennium since 1915. The figures in Table 1 are rearranged in this way in Table 5, together with the observed numbers of cases other than World War II shipyard workers from Table 2. The standardization constant used in calculating the numbers in Table 1 was chosen to make their sum equal the observed number, 20, among nonshipyard workers first exposed at age 45 or below since 1945. They can thus be interpreted as the numbers that would be expected subject to the exposure conditions of post-War recruits. The ratios of observed to expected in each row of Table 5 provide estimates of the relative "levels of exposure" of men first exposed at ages 16-20, 21-25, 26-30, 31-35, 36-40, and 41-45 in each period, while differences between the total ratios for different periods (right-hand column in Table 5) indicate secular changes in exposure. (Level of exposure is formally defined in the Appendix. It depends on asbestos dust level and duration of subsequent exposure as well as on the number of men first exposed in each age range and period.)

Table 5
Male Mesotheliomas with Recorded Asbestos Exposure Diagnosed in Los Angeles County in 1974-1978

Year first exposed	Age at first exposure to asbestos												Total	
	16-20		21-25		26-30		31-35		36-40		41-45			
	O[a]	E[b]	O	E	O	E	O	E	O	E	O	E	O	E
1915-1919	1	10.2	0[c]										1	10.2
1920-1924	3	10.3	0	7.5	1[c]								3	17.8
1925-1929	2	9.1	1	7.4	2	5.4	0[c]						5	21.9
1930-1934	0	7.2	0	6.3	1	5.1	1	3.7	0[c]				2	22.4
1935-1939	3	5.2	1	4.8	4	4.2	1	3.4	0	2.5	0[c]		9	20.0
1940-1944	1	3.4	3	3.2	1	3.0	1	2.6	2	2.1	0	1.6	8	15.9
1945-1949	1	2.0	4	2.0	0	1.9	2	1.7	2	1.5	3	1.2	12	10.3
1950-1954	1	1.1	0	1.1	1	1.0	2	1.0	0	0.9	0	0.8	4	5.8
1955-1959	0	0.5	1	0.5	1	0.5	0	0.5	1	0.4	0	0.4	3	2.7
1960-1964	0	0.2	0	0.2	0	0.2	0	0.2	0	0.2	1	0.2	1	1.0
1965-1969	0	<0.1	0	<0.1	0	<0.1	0	<0.1	0	<0.1	0	<0.1	0	0.2
Total 1945-1969	2	3.8	5	3.7	2	3.6	4	3.4	3	3.0	4	2.6	20	20.0

Cases first exposed after age 45 are omitted.
[a]O = Observed (see text for explanation).
[b]E = Expected from Table 1 (see text for explanation).
[c]Men with the median ages and year of first exposure corresponding to these cells would be aged over 80 during the survey period [1974-78]. The one observed case is omitted from the total in the right-hand column.

Separate predictions of past and future numbers of cases could in principle be calculated for each cell in Table 5 (see Appendix of this paper), but as the observed distribution of cases more or less conforms to the pattern of expected numbers for each age range up to age 45 in each period of first exposure since 1945, it seems more sensible merely to observe that our data suggest a fairly uniform distribution of age at first exposure (or, more correctly, level of exposure at each age) over this period and show no evidence of any change in extent of exposure since 1945. A reasonable prediction of future numbers of cases originating in exposure in each period since 1945 thus can be calculated directly from the pattern shown in the right half of Table 4, which corresponds to a uniform initial age distribution. If conditions have not altered since 1945, the same number of cases will arise in men first exposed in each successive quinquennium, possibly up to 1960-1964 or even later. The ratios of observed to expected in Table 5 are very much lower than unity before 1945, however, indicating considerably lower exposure than in 1945 or later. The ratio of observed to expected for all periods of first exposure from 1915 to 1934 is 11/72.3, or 15%, and 17/35.9, or 47%, for 1935-1944. There are too few cases to provide separate estimates for each age and period, and we have assumed that cases caused by first exposure in each 5-year period from 1915 to 1944 will also follow the pattern shown in the right half of Table 4, and that the total for each 5-year period from 1915-1919 to 1930-1934 will be 15% of the total for 1945-1949 or later, and 47% for 1935-1939 and 1940-1944. The calculation is shown in Table 6. The predicted numbers are standardized to give a total in 1974-1978 of 2240 due to asbestos exposure other than in World War II shipyards, and thus represent the overall numbers for the whole United States.

OVERALL INCIDENCE

The projection in the left half of Table 4 for World War II shipyard exposure, the right-hand column of Table 6 for other exposure, and a constant incidence of 960 cases per quinquennium unrelated to asbestos exposure, give the overall projections of total numbers of cases shown in Table 7. [If the age-specific incidence of unexposed cases remains constant, the annual number will in fact rise, as the average age of the U.S. population is still increasing. This effect has been ignored.] The least reliable aspect of these predictions is the suggestion that the eventual number of mesotheliomas in men first exposed in 1960-1964, and perhaps even 1965-1969, may be as high as for 1945-1949. Only eight cases in our survey were first exposed between 1950 and 1964, and our projections for 1950 onwards could be too high or too low by a factor of 2. The pattern of exposure levels (ratios of observed:expected in Table 5) suggested by our data, increasing from 15% before 1935 to 100% by 1945 and subsequently remaining at about this level until 1965 or later, corresponds reasonably close to total U.S. asbestos consumption, however (Fig. 1, shown on page 63), and industrial exposure was probably not controlled effectively in many areas until about 10 years ago.

Table 6
Projections of Past and Future Numbers of Male Mesotheliomas in the United States due to Asbestos Exposure, Excluding World War II Shipyard Workers

	Assumed "level of exposure"										
	0.15	0.15	0.15	0.15	0.47	0.47	1.00	1.00	1.00	1.00	
	Period first exposed										
Year of diagnosis	1915-1919	1920-1924	1925-1929	1930-1934	1935-1939	1940-1944	1945-1949	1950-1954	1955-1959	1960-1964	Total
1924-1928	2										2
1929-1933	8	2									10
1934-1938	22	8	2								32
1939-1943	46	22	8	2							78
1944-1948	75	46	22	8	7						158

1949-1953	105	75	46	22	26	7					281
1954-1958	134	105	75	46	69	26	14				469
1959-1963	149	134	105	75	145	69	56	14			747
1964-1968	145	149	134	105	234	145	148	56	14		1130
1969-1973	118	145	149	134	330	234	309	148	56	14	1637
1974-1978	67	118	145	149	419	330	499	309	148	56	2240
1979-1983		67	118	145	466	419	703	499	309	148	2874
1984-1988			67	118	456	466	892	703	499	309	3510
1989-1993				67	370	456	991	892	703	499	3978
1994-1998					211	370	970	991	892	703	4137
1999-2003						211	787	970	991	892	3851
2004-2008							450	787	970	991	3198
2009-2013								450	787	970	2207
2014-2018									450	787	1237
2019-2023										450	450
Total	871	871	871	871	2733	2733	5819	5819	5819	5819	32,226

The figures are standardized to give a total of 2240 cases in 1974-1978.

Table 7
Overall Projections of Numbers of Mesotheliomas Diagnosed in the United States in Successive Periods in Men First Exposed to Asbestos before 1965, or Unexposed

	World War II shipyards	Other asbestos exposure	Unexposed	Total
1924-1928		2	960	962
1929-1933		10	960	970
1934-1938		32	960	992
1939-1943		78	960	1038
1944-1948		158	960	1118
1949-1953	24	281	960	1265
1954-1958	80	469	960	1509
1959-1963	208	747	960	1915
1964-1968	416	1130	960	2506
1969-1973	616	1637	960	3213
1974-1978	800	2240	960	4000
1979-1983	880	2874	960	4714
1984-1988	816	3510	960	5286
1989-1993	712	3978	960	5650
1994-1998	464	4137	960	5561
1999-2003	264	3851	960	5075
2004-2008		3198	960	4158
2009-2013		2207	960	3167
2014-2018		1237	960	2197
2019-2023		450	960	1410
1924-2023	5,280	32,226	19,200	56,706

THE ETIOLOGY AND AGE DISTRIBUTION OF INCIDENTAL CASES

The multistage model of carcinogenesis provides a qualitative, and sometimes quantitative, explanation for a variety of observations on spontaneous and induced cancer rates in both animals and humans, and of cellular transformation rates in various in vitro systems. In its simplest form, such a model predicts that exposure to an initiator (a carcinogen effecting the first change in a multi-stage process) is likely to increase cancer incidence in approximate proportion to some power of time since first exposure, irrespective of age at first exposure, and that the incidence of spontaneous tumors of the same type will be proportional to age raised to the same power. An example of such relationships is provided by lung cancer rates in smokers and nonsmokers. Lung cancer incidence appears to be approximately proportional to the 4th or 5th power of duration of smoking among continuing cigarette smokers, irrespective of age,

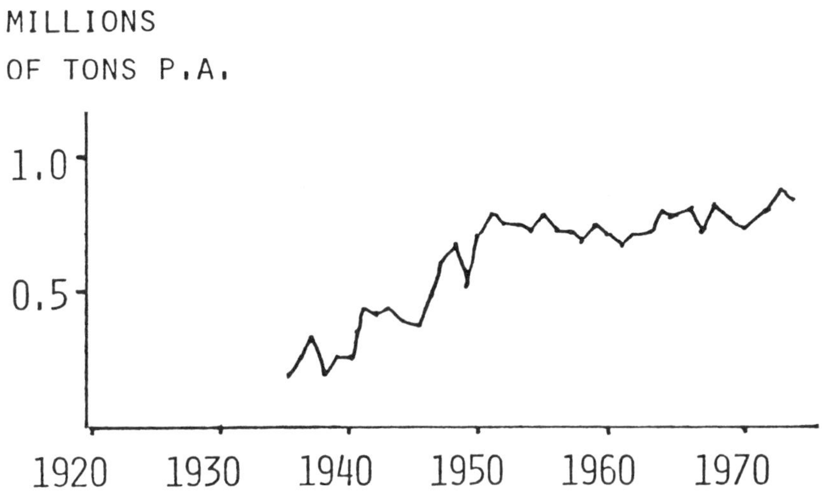

Figure 1
Total U.S. asbestos consumption

and to more or less the same power of age in nonsmokers (Doll 1978). This suggests: (1) that smoking increases the frequency of the first of an ordered (or at least partially ordered) sequence of changes involved in the transformation of a normal cell to malignancy, and (2) that the rates at which these cellular changes occur are not strongly age dependent.

The close analogy between these observations and the incidence pattern of asbestos-induced mesothelioma, for which incidence is proportional to (time since first exposure)$^{3.5}$, suggests that the incidence in individuals who have not been exposed to asbestos might be expected to rise as (age)$^{3.5}$. That this is approximately so is shown in Table 8, where the age distribution of the 22 male and 19 female cases in our survey who were reported as unexposed is compared with the distribution that would have been expected if incidence were proportional to (age)$^{3.5}$.

The assumption that cases reporting no asbestos exposure are really spontaneous, and will therefore persist at the current level, is supported by the similar incidence in men (22 cases) and women (19 cases), although they could be due to ambient asbestos exposure, which presumably would affect the sexes equally. A more banal explanation is that many are not mesotheliomas at all. Preliminary results of a pathological review of our material suggest that the diagnosis will be revised in a significantly higher proportion of "unexposed" cases than of those with a history of asbestos exposure. Their inclusion in future projections, and the suggestion that such cases follow the age-incidence curve that might be expected by analogy with lung cancer rates in smokers and nonsmokers, must therefore be regarded as provisional.

Table 8
Age Distribution of Unexposed Mesothelioma Cases Diagnosed in Los Angeles County, 1974-1978, and Population in Thousands

	Age								
	20-	30-	40-	50-	60-	70-	80-	90-94	Total
Men									
number	1	0	3	3	8	5	2	0	22
Los Angeles population	540	423	435	365	226	112	38	3	2142
Women									
number	0	3	2	5	6	1	1	1	19
Los Angeles population	575	418	458	394	280	185	76	8	2394
Both sexes									
number	1	3	5	8	14	6	3	1	41
Los Angeles population	1115	841	893	759	506	297	114	11	4536
expected	0.8	1.9	4.7	8.1	9.7	9.4	5.6	0.7	41.0

Expected numbers are based on the assumption that incidence is proportional to $age^{3.5}$.

DISCUSSION

The accuracy of our predictions relating to particular periods, notably the effects of World War II shipyard exposure, depends on the assumption that Los Angeles is typical of the rest of the United States. The method appears to be surprisingly robust even against substantial variation in the assumed distribution of age at first exposure, however, and as we have standardized our predictions to correspond to current national rates, any underestimation of numbers originating in a particular period or industry is at least partially compensated by a corresponding overestimate elsewhere. The overall prediction, at least for the effects of first exposure before 1950, is unlikely to be much in error. Our estimate of 5280 mesotheliomas due to World War II shipyard exposure, together with less than 3000 due to other exposure during World War II, is less than 3% of the lowest estimate of future numbers due to past asbestos exposure in the estimates paper of Bridbord et al. (1978). This report predicted that previous asbestos exposure, principally during World War II, would eventually cause at least 280,000 mesothelioma deaths, but the calculations were not presented in sufficient detail for the effects of World War II and later exposure to be separated.

The predictions relating to first exposure after 1945 are necessarily speculative, but they are of some value, if only to indicate that although there is a growing epidemic of asbestos-related disease, the incidence may never much exceed the current rate, and is unlikely to double. A national study conducted and analyzed along the lines of this paper is evidently needed. Such a survey would provide more precise estimates of the effects of exposure in various periods, particularly between 1950 and 1965 where our data are most sparse, and definitive data on shipyard workers.

It is difficult to know what adjustment, if any, should be made to allow for misdiagnosis. In our view, the disease is usually diagnosed in asbestos workers, but it may never be possible to establish the true incidence. We have not discussed the incidence due to asbestos exposure among women. Twenty-one percent of the cases diagnosed in Los Angeles County were women, but the majority had had no known exposure (19/25 interviewed). Three had been exposed at work (one only 3 years before the disease was diagnosed), two had been married to asbestos workers, and one reported childhood exposure. It is not yet possible to distinguish a secular increase in incidence among women from the effects of improving diagnosis in the United States, but in England the female rate has not increased much since 1967, while the reported incidence in men has doubled (Acheson and Gardner 1979). Thus, it seems unlikely that the incidence among women will ever much exceed the current relatively low level, although the possibility remains that substantial numbers of women were first exposed since 1950.

The lifelong risk of mesothelioma following asbestos exposure is very low among men first exposed after age 40, but for lung cancer the relative risk, and hence the lifelong risk, does not change markedly with age at first exposure (Peto 1979; Seidman et al. 1979). The overall excess of lung cancer among men who have been exposed industrially to asbestos has in most studies been of the order of three times the number of mesotheliomas (McDonald and McDonald, this volume), but this ratio may be higher among World War II employees, many of whom were considerably older at first exposure than most earlier or later recruits. If our predictions of approximately 5000 mesotheliomas in men first exposed in shipyards and 3000 for other industries in World War II are correct, the excess number of lung cancers could exceed 30,000. The "mesothelioma epidemic" is the most obvious manifestation of World War II exposure, as the disease is normally so rare, but it may be a relatively minor component of the resulting morbidity and mortality.

The predicted number of mesotheliomas caused by asbestos in men first exposed in the U.S. at any time before 1965 shown in Table 7 is about 37,500, and a corresponding excess of lung cancer of about three times this figure implies a total of about 150,000 cancer deaths, most of which have yet to occur. The extent of wartime asbestos exposure may have been exaggerated, but the effects of later exposure, which are only beginning to be seen, may prove considerably greater than has been generally realized.

REFERENCES

Acheson, E.D. and M.J. Gardner. 1979. The ill effects of asbestos on health. In *Asbestos, vol. 2: Final report of the Advisory Committee on Asbestos.* Her Majesty's Stationery Office, London.

Bridbord, K., P. Decoufle, J.F. Fraumeni, D.G. Hoel, R.N. Hoover, D.P. Rall, U. Saffiotti, M.A. Schneiderman, and A.C. Upton. 1978. "Estimates of the fraction of cancer in the United States related to occupational factors." National Cancer Institute, National Institute of Environmental Health Sciences, and National Institute for Occupational Safety and Health, Bethesda, Maryland, September 15.

Doll, R. 1978. An epidemiological perspective of the biology of cancer. *Cancer Res.* **38**:3573.

Hinds, M.W. 1978. Mesothelioma in the United States. *J. Occup. Med.* **20**: 469.

Peto, J. 1979. Dose-response relationships for asbestos-related disease: implications for hygiene standards. II. Mortality. *Ann. N.Y. Acad. Sci.* **330**:195.

Peto, J., H. Seidman, and I.J. Selikoff. 1981. Mesothelioma incidence among asbestos workers: implications for models of carcinogenesis and risk assessment calculations. *Br. J. Cancer* (in press).

Seidman, H., I.J. Selikoff, and E.C. Hammond. 1979. Short-term asbestos work exposure and long-term observation. *Ann. N.Y. Acad. Sci.* **330**:61.

Tagnon, I., W.J. Blot, R.B. Stroube, N.E. Day, L.E. Morris, B.B. Peace, and J.F.

Fraumeni, Jr. 1980. Mesothelioma associated with the shipbuilding industry in coastal Virginia. *Cancer Res.* **40**:3875.

APPENDIX

The excess cancer incidence caused by a specific pattern of carcinogenic exposure will in general increase with increasing dose, but the time-dependence is usually independent of dose. In other words, for some functions D and f

$$\text{incidence} = D(d) \cdot f(a,t) \tag{1}$$

at age a following a specified pattern of exposure at dose d starting at age t. (This equation cannot, in general, be applied to a group of individuals who have suffered different patterns of exposure. For example, a smoker who increased his consumption steadily from 10-20 cigarettes per day over 10 years and then stopped smoking has suffered double the dose of one who increased from 5-10 cigarettes per day over the same period and then stopped, but his dose cannot be compared directly with that of a continuing smoker, whose incidence will follow a quite different time course.) For industrial carcinogens, usually it is not possible to obtain accurate enough data on either dose or incidence to establish the form of D, the dose dependence. For the purposes of the present analysis, however, we shall define D as the "effective dose," thereby guaranteeing linearity, and write (1) as

$$\text{incidence} = D \cdot f(a,t). \tag{2}$$

This formulation, in which dose-response is by definition linear, greatly simplifies the analysis. Exposure levels are poorly measured and vary widely, but for a specific pattern of exposure the overall incidence in a cohort of individuals who were first exposed at the same time and age can also be described by equation (2), the constant factor D now denoting the average "effective dose" of the cohort. (The selective loss of the most heavily exposed individuals would in fact progressively reduce D, the average exposure of the survivors. This relatively minor effect is ignored.)

National Incidence

Ignoring those who have never been exposed to asbestos, the general population can be divided into cohorts on the basis of age at first exposure and period of first exposure to asbestos. Thus C_{ij} denotes the cohort first exposed in year i at age j. The function f specifying the time and age dependence of the resulting cancer incidence would for many carcinogens depend strongly on whether exposure was brief or continuous, and the proportions suffering various patterns of exposure might vary considerably between cohorts. For asbestos-induced mesothelioma, however, incidence appears to rise approximately as (time since first exposure)$^{3.5}$ irrespective of age, fiber type, or exposure pattern. Denoting the average "effective dose" of cohort C_{ij} by D_{ij}, the incidence I_{ij} at age a in cohort C_{ij} will be approximately

$$I_{ij}(a) = D_{ij} \cdot (a - j)^{3.5}. \tag{3}$$

The expected number of cases $e_{ij}(a)$ occurring in unit time at age a in cohort C_{ij} will be approximately

$$e_{ij}(a) = n_{ij} \cdot D_{ij} \cdot (a - j)^{3.5} \cdot p(a)/p(j), \tag{4}$$

where $p(a)$ is the probability of surviving to age a, and n_{ij} is the number of people first exposed in year i at age j—that is, the initial size of cohort C_{ij}. The life-table p should in principle also be suffixed by i,j to take account of secular changes in national mortality and the higher mortality of those who have been exposed; but to simplify the analysis we shall ignore these effects and replace p by the life-table based on current national mortality rates. Therefore, our predictions will be somewhat inflated if, as seems likely, an appreciable proportion of mesotheliomas occur among men whose exposure was high enough to reduce life expectancy significantly.

Definition of "Level of Exposure"

Finally, equation (4) can be simplified further by combining n_{ij} and D_{ij}. It may be difficult and pointless to attempt to estimate the numbers n_{ij} who were first exposed to an agent such as asbestos at a particular age and period, as there will be great heterogeneity of exposure levels within each cohort, and the results could not be used to provide meaningful estimates of individual risk. For the purpose of analyzing the evolution of national cancer incidence, however, the product $N_{ij} = n_{ij} \cdot D_{ij}$, the average "level of exposure" of the population resulting from first exposure at age j in year i, is equally useful and more convenient. Equation (4) thus can be written

$$e_{ij}(a) = N_{ij} \cdot (a - j)^{3.5} \cdot p(a)/p(j). \tag{5}$$

To simplify the notation, it has been assumed that analysis is based on single years of age, age at first exposure, year of first exposure, and period of observation of incident cases. In practice, it is more convenient to use quinquennial divisions, a, i, and j denoting quinquennial midpoints. In particular, $e_{ij}(a_s)$ denotes the expected number of cases diagnosed in the study period (1974-1978) aged between a_s - 2½ and a_s + 2½ years among men first exposed in the quinquennia of age and period centered at age j and year i respectively. (Note that if the year i_s is the midpoint of the survey period, $a_s = j + i_s - i$ for cohort C_{ij}.) Approximating $p(a)$ by the life-table based on current national death-rates, this formula provides a basis for estimating N_{ij}, and hence the numbers of cases in each past and future quinquennium from the present rate of occurrence in cohort C_{ij}. Moreover, the average "levels of exposure" N_{ij} of different cohorts provide a useful indication of the relative degree of overall exposure in different periods, although they do not enable us to distinguish periods in which a few individuals were heavily exposed from those in which a larger number suffered moderate exposure.

The expected numbers $e_{ij}(a_s)$ are estimated by interviewing a sample of cases to determine age and period of first exposure. A random sample of controls should, in principle, also be interviewed and the "attributable fraction" of cases estimated in the usual way in each cohort. This adjustment, which would slightly reduce the proportion of cases attributed to asbestos exposure, has not been attempted. We have simply assumed that all cases with recorded exposure were caused by asbestos and have classified the remainder as "incidental," although some, or even all, such "incidental" cases may be due to ambient asbestos or unrecorded acute exposure.

Standard Errors of Predicted Future Incidence

The most severe limitation is the inaccuracy of predictions resulting from recent exposure. This is an inevitable consequence of the time distribution of industrial cancers, which are usually rare until 20 or more years after first exposure to a carcinogen. Thus, for example, less than 1% of the total number of mesotheliomas that eventually will occur in a cohort of men first exposed to asbestos in the age range 21-25 will be diagnosed before age 40. The diagnosis of a single case in 1980 of a man born in 1942 who was first exposed in 1965 would (in expectation) imply that about 150 further cases will occur in his birth cohort, but the 95% confidence interval of this predicted number would be (4-840). In practice, of course, reasonably smooth trends over time and age will be observed and outliers can be ignored; but it is difficult to assign confidence intervals either within any particular cohort or overall.

COMMENTS

SLOAN: I would like to ask how great the effort was to be sure that mesothelioma cases that did not seem to be associated with asbestos really were such.

J. PETO: A simple multi-stage model would predict the same age distribution if these cases were caused by ambient asbestos. If there is a background exposure to asbestos, then exposure starts at age zero. So $(\text{age})^{3.5}$ is the same as $(\text{time since first exposure})^{3.5}$. You would get exactly the same pattern, whether it is a natural disease without cause or whether it is caused by ambient asbestos. The unexposed cases are significantly younger than the exposed cases, as they are for lung cancer in nonsmokers compared with smokers, these differences in age distribution must be interpreted cautiously.

RADFORD: In the case of lung cancer induced by radon daughters, it appears that your model does not work. Mesothelioma is a disease that apparently does not require a promoter or other factors such as host factors, which may be important in the onset of the disease. At least one may postulate this concept.

In the case of lung cancer, on the other hand, we find that miners exposed at older ages show a rapid increase in excess risk, whereas miners that are exposed at younger ages have a long period before they develop it.

J. PETO: Exactly the same thing seems to happen with asbestos and lung cancer. It hasn't been published, but this is something that Irving Selikoff is now looking into. The pattern of relative risk (RR) is such that if you are exposed at a younger age, the RR seems to rise slowly for some time. If you are exposed at an older age, it seems to go up more sharply, but more or less to the same eventual level.

RADFORD: So the model you described would not apply?

J. PETO: Not for lung cancers due to asbestos or radiation. Radiation and asbestos appear to behave in an almost identical manner in relation to causing lung cancer. They interact with smoking, probably, and both produce this sort of pattern.

RADFORD: Radiation doesn't interact with smoking according to the only lifetime follow-up studies we have.

J. PETO: I thought there was evidence that it did in uranium miners.

RADFORD: It is an artefact of follow-up time. The progression that I asked Irving [Selikoff] about this morning can be shown. In other words, if follow up is only to 25 years, you get a multiplicative effect. But if you carry it out to 45 years, as we have in Swedish miners, the RR is much higher in the nonsmokers than in the smokers, although the absolute risk is somewhat higher for the smokers.

SCHNEIDERMAN: Does this imply that the effect of smoking is to just shorten the latent period?

RADFORD: Yes. When the radiation dose rate is high, the initiating step becomes rate limiting for the onset of cancer.

MILHAM: In Phil Enterline's analysis of copper smelter workers with heavy arsenic exposure, he saw the same smoking and lung cancer relationship that Dr. Radford was talking about, in that either there was no synergistic effect or, indeed, the nonsmokers per given arsenic exposure seemed to have higher lung cancer rates.

ENTERLINE: Actually, the absolute excess was higher in the smokers, but RR was higher in the nonsmokers.

DAVIS: Let me address the issue of the apparent shorter latency if the age of exposure is later. If I understand this correctly, Julian, it would seem to me very important to look at male and female differences in terms of the immune system, to study whether women who would be exposed later would have a similar shorter latency or perhaps a longer one for mesothelioma.

J. PETO: The incidence pattern depends on age of exposure for lung cancer, but not for mesothelioma. Incidentally, I don't think that latency is a very useful concept in cancer epidemiology. You don't usually see any cases within 10 years of first exposure because the risk is so low, and you don't see many beyond 60 years because most people don't live long enough. Latency is a secondary effect of the incidence pattern and the duration of follow-up and effects of age at exposure or sex should be examined by looking directly at the pattern of incidence.

McMICHAEL: I want to raise again this question of whether we can glean useful information by looking at the data for women. Of course, often there aren't sufficient numbers in the usual type of study carried out by a single epidemiological research unit; or the exposure levels for women workers may be lower than for men.

J. PETO: Molly Newhouse's studies included men and women, and the incidence rates were very much the same in the two sexes with comparable exposure. I suspect that lung cancer rates in men and women who have smoked the same amount all their lives are similar.

McMICHAEL: Yes, but I am not concerned here with any innate biological differences in the way the sexes may respond to certain exposures. In the large case-control study that NCI has done recently of bladder cancers, they were able to assemble a sufficient number of persons that otherwise had lower background risk—that is, women nonsmokers. In that sort of situation, we may be able to tease out some of the subtleties in the etiology of the cancer that can't be teased out in the males that are being heavily exposed and have a confused, complex lifetime exposure in the occupational setting and the personal behavioral setting.

I am just suggesting that methodologically, wherever possible, we ought to gather as much data as we can from minorities with apparently low-risk-factor backgrounds, because they provide some research opportunities that aren't there in the majority group.

Mesothelioma as an Index of Asbestos Impact

J. CORBETT McDONALD
TUC Centenary Institute of Occupational Health
London School of Hygiene and Tropical Medicine
London, WC1E 7HT, England

and

ALISON D. McDONALD
Department of Epidemiology
St. Mary's Hospital Medical School
London, W2 1PG, England

A few attempts have been made to assess the contribution made by asbestos to overall cancer mortality by applying estimated numbers of persons exposed under various circumstances to risks derived from epidemiological surveys on working groups (see Lancet 1978). This approach is difficult and unreliable because it depends heavily on two very poorly defined sets of information: (1) the frequency, nature, and intensity of exposure in the entire population many years ago and, (2) the scanty quantitative data available on exposure-response. In fact, the attempts made to date have not dealt deeply with either of these aspects.

This paper will explore a different approach, depending on two sets of data that we believe may be more reliable and easy to use and that, moreover, could be improved fairly readily. The first requirement is information on the incidence in the population of fatal malignant mesothelial tumors (mesothelioma); the second is information on the ratio in relevant circumstances of deaths attributable to asbestos exposure caused by mesothelioma on the one hand and other malignant diseases on the other. We believe that the incidence of mesothelioma is measurable (without great difficulty) and that fairly good estimates already exist. These tumors are relatively rare, rapidly fatal, and strongly (though not invariably) related to asbestos exposure. Although very few of the 30 or so cohort studies of asbestos workers contain any quantitative information on exposure (apart from duration), most give a useful indication of the ratio of mesothelioma to other malignancies under various circumstances.

This paper is exploratory. We have used only data that are readily available and no statistical sophistication whatever. We have focused on the "recent present" in North America (United States and Canada) and have deliberately avoided the more complex issues of trends in time and major geographical variations. If our approach is acceptable, it should be possible to improve both the quality of the statistical base and the methods of analysis.

INCIDENCE OF MESOTHELIOMA IN NORTH AMERICA

Information on mortality from these tumors in North America can be obtained from three data sets: (1) the Third National Cancer Survey (TNCS) (Cutler and Young 1975), (2) population-based cancer registries from the SEER Program in five states (Connecticut, Hawaii, Iowa, New Mexico, and Utah) and five city areas (Atlanta, Detroit, New Orleans, San Francisco-Oakland, and Seattle) (Biometry Branch, NCI, unpubl.), and (3) our own efforts at complete ascertainment of fatal cases through pathologists in Canada (1960-1975) and in the United States (1972) (McDonald and McDonald 1980). It is clear from these sources that, in the 1970s, the incidence was two to three times greater in males than in females, much higher in some areas than in others, and steadily rising over the period in males but less certainly in females. Allowing for these variations, we believe that the three sets of data, as summarized in Table 1, are not incompatible.

Starting with our own data, for example, all three characteristics listed above are evident. We have presented reasons (McDonald and McDonald 1977) for thinking that the true rate of mesothelioma in the United States was probably about 50% higher than that obtained through pathologists. From the latter source, we estimated that in 1972 the incidence per 10^6 population in Canada was 2.3 for men and 1.3 for women and, in the United States, 1.9 and 0.6 (McDonald and McDonald 1980). After correction for the 50% under-ascertainment, the rates for the United States would become about 2.9 and 0.9. These figures may be compared with 3.6 and 1.9 from TNCS. However, the TNCS figures (like our own) include only malignant mesotheliomas and not suspicious cases or tumors of uncertain malignancy. Inclusion of the latter brings the TNCS rates to 5.1 and 2.0. The rates for these same categories of mesothelioma obtained from tumor registries in the five states and five city areas about 5 years later (1973-1978) were appreciably higher in males ($8.8/10^6$) and somewhat higher for females ($2.6/10^6$). It is impossible to say how representative these rates are because they include four major ports and naval shipyards. For the present purpose, however, we are inclined to conclude that reasonable estimates of mesothelioma incidence for North America in the mid-1970s should be higher than those of the TNCS, say about $8.0/10^6$ for males and about $2.5/10^6$ for females.

MESOTHELIOMA AND OTHER ASBESTOS CANCERS

In this exercise, we shall consider only the relationship between mesothelioma and respiratory and digestive cancers, i.e., of the trachea, bronchus, and lung

Table 1
Incidence per 10^6 Population per Annum of Fatal and Cancer Registry Cases of Mesothelioma in North America in the 1970s

Cases	Source	1970-1972	1975
	Males		
Fatal cases			
Canada	McDonald and McDonald (1980)	2.3	3.0
United States	McDonald and McDonald (1980)	2.9	
	TNCS	3.6	
Cancer registry cases			
United States	TNCS	3.4	
Cancer registry cases, including 'suspicious' and 'malignancy unspecified'			
United States	TCNS	5.1	
	SEER program		8.8
	Females		
Fatal cases			
Canada	McDonald and McDonald (1980)	1.3	1.0
United States	McDonald and McDonald (1980)	0.9	
	TNCS	1.9	
Cancer registry cases			
United States	TNCS	1.8	
Cancer registry cases, including 'suspicious' and 'malignancy unspecified'			
United States	TNCS	2.0	
	SEER program		2.6

(ICD 162-164) and gastrointestinal tract and digestive organs (ICD 150-159). Some other cancers, of the larynx for example, may be caused by asbestos, but they are not sufficiently important numerically to affect the issue. Table 2 summarizes the essential findings from all cohort studies of asbestos workers of which we are aware. They vary considerably in size, in nature, intensity, and duration of exposure and in the types of asbestos fiber used. In males, the ratios between deaths from mesothelioma and excess deaths from lung cancer (observed minus expected [0 - E]) range from 0.3 to 18.5. Generally speaking, however, the extremes were from surveys in which the numbers of mesotheliomas or excess lung cancers were very small. Most ratios (excluding the three highest and three lowest) were in the range of 1.0 to 5.2 (median 2.4). The gradient in ratios showed some association with asbestos fiber type–higher in the absence of amphiboles and lower in their presence.

Table 2
Ratios of Fatal Mesotheliomas to Excess Mortality from Respiratory and

		Reference	Country[a]	Cohort traced	Deaths	Mesoth-elioma
						Males
Mining and milling						
	Chrysotile	McDonald et al. (1980)	A	9,850	3,291	10
		Nicholson et al. (1979)	A	544	178	1
		Rubino et al. (1979)	I	933	332	0[b]
	Anthophyllite	Meurman et al. (1974)	F	1,041	248	0
	Talc	Kleinfeld et al. (1967b)	A	220	91	2
		Brown et al. (1979)	A	382	74	1
	Crocidolite	Hobbs et al. (1980)	Aus	4,960	181	16
Manufacture						
	Chrysotile	Elwood and Cochrane (1964)	B	1,024	46	1
		Weiss (1977)	A	264	66	0
		Dement et al. (1981)	A	746	191	1
	Crocidolite	McDonald and McDonald (1978)	A	93	43	8
	Amosite	Seidman et al. (1979)	A	820	528	14
	Mixed	Newhouse and Berry (1979)	B	2,887	545	46
		Newhouse et al. (1981)	B	8,804	1,640	8
		Peto et al. (1977)	B	796	293	9
		Henderson and Enterline (1979)	A	1,075	781	4
		Robinson et al. (1979)	A	2,666	912	13
		Hughes and Weill (1980)	A	5,645	601	0[b]
		Mancuso and Coulter (1963)	A	1,266	175	4
Insulation						
	Mixed	Kleinfeld et al. (1967a)	A	152	46	4
		Selikoff et al. (1979)	A	632	478	38
		Selikoff et al. (1979)	A	17,800	2,271	175
		Elmes and Simpson (1977)	B	162	122	13
		Newhouse and Berry (1979)	B	1,368	83	10
Shipyards						
	Mixed	Rossiter et al. (1980)	B	6,076	1,042	28
		Kolonel et al. (1980)	A	4,779	385	3[d]
						Females
Manufacture						
	Crocidolite	Jones et al. (1980)	B	578	166	17
		McDonald and McDonald (1978)	A	83	13	2
	Mixed	Peto et al. (1977)	B	284	24	1
		Newhouse and Berry (1979)	B	783	200	21
		Newhouse et al. (1981)	B	4,219	346	2
		Robinson et al. (1979)	A	544	128	4
		Mancuso and Coulter (1963)	A	229	20	1

[a]A = America, Aus = Australia, B = Britain, F = Finland, I = Italy.
[b]One possible case (Rubino et al. 1979); 2 cases not meeting criteria (Hughes and Weill 1980).
[c]Estimated from proportional mortality data.
[d]Three cases after end of follow up; expected figure based on nonexposed cohort.
[e]Not applicable.
[f]Not stated.
[g]def. = Deficient.

Digestive Cancers in Cohort Studies of Asbestos-exposed Workers

Respiratory (162-4)				Digestive (150-9)			
O	E	O − E	O − E / Mesothelioma	O	E	O − E	O − E / Mesothelioma
230	184.0	46.0	4.6	276	272.4	3.6	0.4
28	11.0	17.0	17.0	10	9.5	0.5	0.5
10	10.4	0	na[e]	19	19.3	0	na
21	12.6	8.4	na	7	8	def.[g]	na
9	2.3[c]	6.7	3.4	6	1.5[c]	4.5	2.3
8	2.8	5.2	5.2	3	3.0	0	na
38	22.6	5.4	0.3	ns[f]			
6	3.0	3.0	3.0	ns			
8	8.6	def.	na	2	2.0	0	na
26	7.5	18.5	18.5	9	7.1	1.9	1.9
8	4.0[c]	4.0	0.5	1	2.0[c]	def.	na
83	22.8	60.2	4.3	ns			
103	43.2	59.8	1.3	40	34.0	6.0	0.1
143	139.5	3.5	0.4	103	107.2	def.	
49	22.9	26.1	2.9	ns			
63	23.3	39.7	9.9	55	39.9	15.1	3.7
49	36.1	12.9	1.0	50	41.4	8.6	0.7
49	49.1	0	na	25	50.1	def.	
15	5.5	9.5	2.4	12	7.0	5.0	1.3
10	1.4[c]	8.6	2.2	7	2.7[c]	4.3	1.1
93	13.3	79.7	2.1	ns			
429	105.6	381.4	2.2	122	84.1	37.9	0.2
35	5.0	30.0	2.3	ns			
21	5.6	15.4	2.5	3	4.3	def.	na
88	100.7	def.	na	73	83.3	def.	na
35	23.5[d]	11.5	3.8	ns	ns	def.	na
12	3.8	8.2	0.5	10	20.3	def.	na
0	0[c]	def.	na	1	0[c]	1.0	0.5
2	0.9	1.1	1.1	ns			
27	3.2	23.8	1.1	3	4.3	def.	na
6	11.3	def.	na	29	27.4	1.6	0.8
14	1.7	12.3	3.2	8	6.0	2.0	0.5
4	0.2	3.8	3.8	2	1.0	1.0	1.0

Data relating to the digestive cancers in males were quite scanty, less detailed, and more difficult to interpret. Most surveys showed little or no increase over expectation, and generally the ratios of excess deaths from this cause to those from mesothelioma were unstable because of small numbers. Perhaps the more useful ratios were those from the two largest cohorts, 0.22 for insulation workers (Selikoff et al. 1979) and 0.36 for Quebec chrysotile workers (McDonald et al. 1980). However, the overall range for the ten values available was from 0.1 to 3.7 (median 0.9).

For females, even data on lung cancer are extremely sparse and are obtained mainly from cohorts exposed to crocidolite or to mixtures of which crocidolite was an important component. The observed ratios ranged from 0.5 to 3.8 (median 1.1).

MESOTHELIOMA AND ASBESTOS EXPOSURE

Given the estimated incidence of mesothelioma (derived from Table 1) and the ratios of mesothelioma to excess deaths from other forms of cancer in asbestos workers (derived from Table 2), two further points deserve consideration: (1) the proportion of deaths from mesothelioma in the mid-1970s attributable to asbestos exposure, and (2) the distribution of occupations (and other forms of asbestos exposure) responsible for the attributable cases.

So far as we are aware, our own surveys in Canada and the United States represent the only effort made to address either question directly. In a recent paper (McDonald and McDonald 1980), we summarized the findings from case-referent surveys in Canada (1960-1972) and in the United States (1972). For the present purpose, we shall use only the 183 male case-referent pairs for both Canada and the United States in 1972 (not shown separately in the published paper). In these pairs, 118 (64.5%) of the cases and 45 (24.6%) of the referents had been employed 10 or more years before death in an occupation that entailed exposure to asbestos and in which an excess of cases over referents was observed. On the assumption that the 183 cases were representative of "all cases" in that year in North America, that referents were typical of the general population in terms of exposure, and the true relative risk was the same as the estimated value, our statistical colleague, Dr. David Oakes (pers. comm.), calculated that the proportion of the cases that would be prevented by removing the occupational exposure to asbestos would be 53%. Taking into account the possible errors in the data and uncertainty about the three basic assumptions, we believe that the true proportion in 1972 might be as high as about 70%, and somewhat higher, about 75%, in 1975. No corresponding estimate for 1972 could be made from observations on the 56 female case-referent pairs. In only one female case and no referent was a history of occupational exposure to asbestos obtained; however, one additional female case and no referent had been exposed at home to the dusty clothing of an asbestos worker. Clearly, only a small proportion (less than 10%) of female cases was attributable to occupational asbestos exposure directly or indirectly.

The same data source provides an indication of the proportions of "attributable mesotheliomas" associated with various types of work and this throws some light on the appropriate ratios to apply in estimating the accompanying excess of other cancers (respiratory and digestive). The results indicated that some 90% of male cases probably were caused by exposure to insulation materials in heating, construction, and shipyard trades, for which a ratio to other cancers of about 2.5 seems appropriate; the remainder had worked in a variety of jobs in production or manufacture, with a wider and somewhat higher range of ratios. We conclude that a ratio of 3.3 based on median values (2.4 for respiratory cancers plus 0.9 for digestive) adequately represents existing knowledge and has the virtue of simplicity.

SYNTHESIS

The midyear population of North America in 1975 was 236 million (115 million males and 121 million females); in that year malignant (and benign) neoplasms were registered as the cause of death in 219,000 males and 181,000 females. From the data presented above, our best estimate is that in 1975 there were about 920 deaths from mesothelioma in North America in men and about 300 in women. If we were to assume that all male cases were caused by occupational exposure to asbestos, application of a ratio of 3.3 would yield a further 3040 deaths from other asbestos-related cancers. However, the resultant total—3960—would require adjustment to allow for the proportion of mesotheliomas in the general population caused by asbestos (best estimate, 75% in men) and for any modification considered necessary in the ratio to other cancers. These principles underlie the calculations presented in Table 3, where our best estimate for the contribution of asbestos to total cancer mortality in males is seen to be 1.4% with a range of 0.5% to 2.9%, depending on the assumptions. On the same basis, the contribution of asbestos to female cancer mortality must be lower by an order of magnitude, but we are reluctant to make any specific estimate on the limited data available.

CONCLUSION

If our approach has any validity, it is clear that the estimate produced depends heavily on the population incidence of mesothelioma. The proportion of these tumors due to occupational exposure is probably increasing, must be less than 100%, is unlikely to be less than 50%. Equally, the ratio to other asbestos-related cancers surely must lie between about 1 and 5. However, selection of the correct ratio(s) presents difficulties because it depends both on the distribution of industrial exposures and the types of asbestos fiber used. The

Table 3
Estimated Proportion of All Cancer Deaths in American Males in 1975 Attributable to Occupational Asbestos Exposure under Various Assumptions

Estimate	Annual incidence of mesothelioma per 10^6 population (cases)	Proportion of mesotheliomas attributable to asbestos	Ratio of mesotheliomas to excess mortality from respiratory and digestive cancers	Proportion of male cancer deaths attributable to asbestos
Lowest	5.0 (575)	50%	2.5	0.5%
Low		50%	3.0	0.8%
Best	**8.0** (920)	**75%**	**3.3**	**1.4%**
High		100%	3.5	1.9%
Highest	11.0 (1265)	100%	4.0	2.9%

considerable need to monitor the impact of potent environmental carcinogens calls for systematic programs of ascertainment and registration for such readily identifiable indicators as malignant mesothelioma. Possible methods have been discussed elsewhere (McDonald 1979).

REFERENCES

Brown, D.P., J.M. Dement, and J. K. Wagoner. 1979. Mortality patterns among miners and millers occupationally exposed to asbestiform talc. In *Dusts and disease* (ed. R. Lemon and J.M. Dement), p. 317. Pathotox, Park Forest, Illinois.

Cutler, S.J. and J.L. Young (ed.). 1975. *Third National Cancer Survey: Incidence data.* DHEW. Publication No. (NIH) 75-787. National Cancer Institute, Bethesda.

Dement, J.M., R.L. Harris, M.J. Symons, and C. Shy. 1981. Estimates of dose-response for respiratory cancer among chrysotile asbestos textile workers. In *Inhaled particles V* (ed. H. Walton). (In press)

Elmes, P.C. and M.J.C. Simpson. 1977. Insulation workers in Belfast. A further study of mortality due to asbestos exposure (1940-75). *Br. J. Ind. Med.* **34**:174.

Elwood, P.C. and A.L. Cochrane. 1964. A follow-up study of workers from an asbestos factory. *Br. J. Ind. Med.* **21**:304.

Henderson, V.L. and P.E. Enterline. 1979. Asbestos exposure: Factors associated with excess cancer and respiratory disease mortality. *Ann. N.Y. Acad. Sci.* **330**:117.

Hobbs, M.S.T., S.D. Woodward, B. Murphy, A.W. Musk, and J.E. Elder. 1980. The incidence of pneumoconiosis, mesothelioma and other respiratory cancer in men engaged in mining and milling crocidolite in Western Australia. *IARC Sci. Publ.* **30**:615.

Hughes, J. and H. Weill. 1980. Lung cancer risk associated with manufacture of asbestos-cement products. *IARC Sci. Publ.* **30**:627.

Jones, J.S.P., P.G. Smith, F.D. Pooley, G. Berry, G.W. Sawle, B.K. Wignell, R.J. Madeley, and A. Aggarwal. 1980. The consequences of exposure to asbestos dust in a war-time gas mask factory. *IARC Sci. Publ.* **30**:637.

Kleinfeld, M., J. Messite, and O. Kooyman. 1967a. Mortality experience in a group of asbestos workers. *Arch. Environ. Health* **15**:177.

Kleinfeld, M., J. Messite, O. Kooyman, and M.H. Zaki. 1967b. Mortality amongst talc miners and millers in New York State. *Arch. Environ. Health* **14**:663.

Kolonel, L.N., T. Hirohata, B.V. Chappell, F.V. Viola, and D.E. Harris. 1980. Cancer mortality in a cohort of naval shipyard workers in Hawaii: Early findings. *J. Natl. Cancer Inst.* **64**:739.

Lancet. 1978. What proportion of cancers are related to occupation? *Lancet* **ii**: 1238.

Mancuso, T.F. and E.J. Coulter. 1963. Methodology in industrial health studies. *Arch. Environ. Health* **6**:210.

McDonald, A.D. 1979. Mesothelioma registries in identifying asbestos hazards. *Ann. N.Y. Acad. Sci.* **330**:441.

McDonald, A.D. and J.C. McDonald. 1978. Mesothelioma after crocidolite exposure during gas mask manufacture. *Environ. Res.* **17**:340.

______. 1980. Malignant mesothelioma in North America. *Cancer* **46**:1650.

McDonald, J.C. and A.D. McDonald. 1977. Epidemiology of mesothelioma from estimated incidence. *Prev. Med.* **6**:446.

McDonald, J.C., F.D.K. Liddell, G.W. Gibbs, G.E. Eyssen, and A.D. McDonald. 1980. Dust exposure and mortality in chrysotile mining, 1910-75. *Br. J. Ind. Med.* **37**:11.

Meurman, L.O., R. Kiviluoto, and M. Hakama. 1974. Mortality and morbidity among the working population of anthophyllite asbestos miners in Finland. *Br. J. Ind. Med.* **31**:105.

Newhouse, M.L. and G. Berry. 1979. Patterns of mortality in asbestos factory workers in London. *Ann. N.Y. Acad. Sci.* **330**:53.

Newhouse, M.L., G. Berry, and J.W. Skidmore. 1981. A mortality study of workers manufacturing friction materials with chrysotile asbestos. In *Inhaled particles V* (ed. H. Walton). (In press)

Nicholson, W.J., I.J. Selikoff, H. Seidman, R. Lilis, and P. Formby. 1979. Long-term mortality experience of chrysotile miners and millers in Thetford Mines, Quebec. *Ann. N.Y. Acad. Sci.* **330**:11.

Peto, J., R. Doll, S.V. Howard, L.J. Kinlen, and H.C. Lewinsohn. 1977. A mortality study among workers in an English asbestos factory. *Br. J. Ind. Med.* **34**:169.

Robinson, C., R. Lemen, and J.K. Wagoner. 1979. Mortality patterns 1940-1975 among workers employed in an asbestos textile friction and packing products manufacturing facility. In *Dusts and diseases* (ed. R. Lemen and J.M. Dement), p. 131. Pathotox, Park Forest, Illinois.

Rossiter, C.E. and R.M. Coles. 1980. H.M. Dockyard Devonport: 1947 mortality study. *IARC Sci. Publ.* **30**:713.

Rubino, G.F., G. Piolatto, M.L. Newhouse, G. Scansetti, G.A. Aresini, and R. Murray. 1979. Mortality of chrysotile asbestos miners at the Balangero Mine, Northern Italy. *Br. J. Ind. Med.* **36**:187.

Seidman, H., I.J. Selikoff, and E.C. Hammond. 1979. Short-term asbestos work exposure and long-term observation. *Ann. N.Y. Acad. Sci.* **330**:61.

Selikoff, I.J., E.C. Hammond, and H. Seidman. 1979. Mortality experience of insulation workers in the United States and Canada, 1943-1976. *Ann. N.Y. Acad. Sci.* **330**:91.

Weiss, W. 1977. Mortality of a cohort exposed to chrysotile asbestos. *J. Occup. Med.* **19**:737.

COMMENTS

GARDNER: In discussing the ratio of excess lung cancer deaths to mesothelioma deaths in the various studies you did not mention cigarette smoking. It seems probable that because of the different relationships of the two diseases to smoking habits, the ratio would be expected to vary between different surveys.

McDONALD: I am sure it does. Ours is a sort of a de facto approach. We are simply saying, given the smoking habits of these cohorts and given the mesotheliomas in the populations, this is our estimate of the cancer excess. Yes,–it does ignore it.

McMICHAEL: You commented on the apparently inconsistent or varied picture with respect to digestive tract cancers. I have just done some very quick arithmetic on it. If you subdivide the industry into two categories: insulation workers and "others," you find that for "others" the observed is 740 and the expected is about 741. If you look at the insulation workers the observed is 132 and the expected is 91, implying a RR perhaps of about 1.4.

I think that suggests that we should be looking for critical differences in associated non-occupational exposures between subgroups of workers or maybe at differences in cigarette smoking, or differences in dietary patterns related to ethnicity or subcultural profiles.

McDONALD: I would add that the Quebec group fared well. They were very heavily exposed to asbestos in the chrysotile mines and they do not have a very high excess mortality from respiratory causes, nevertheless, they do have an excess mortality from digestive causes. One of the mysteries was that, whereas the respiratory causes have a linear relationship to exposure, the digestive ones simply don't. They are all over the place.

ENTERLINE: It is interesting to note that our estimates come very close although we used different approaches. My estimate is approximately 4,000 per year. Out of the 4,000 deaths, approximately 2,000 cancer deaths were males who were occupationally exposed. The worst category seems to be that of male shipyard workers.

SCHNEIDERMAN: In 1978 the SEER program reported that the cancer death rate for males was 12.2. That is more than a 10% increase per year. The increase occurred in the registries from Hawaii, Seattle, San Francisco, and Connecticut, all coastal areas. There were no increases evident in New

Mexico, Utah, Detroit, and Iowa, which I think is really quite consistent with what we expect in terms of exposure.

McDONALD: I certainly wouldn't want the Canadian trend to be taken too literally. But it does emphasize that the annual rate of increase is substantial, and that fits in with Julian Peto's 'epidemic.'

SCHNEIDERMAN: The increases appeared to have occurred in places where there was occupational exposure.

J. PETO: Regarding the ratio of mesothelioma to excess lung cancer, any reasonable model would suppose that what is determined by asbestos is the *absolute* risk of mesothelioma but only the RR for lung cancer, since the effect interacts with smoking. It is the RR rather than the absolute excess that we should analyze. In women, for example, you would expect to see roughly equal numbers of asbestos-induced mesotheliomas and lung cancer, because at the moment their lung cancer rate is so much lower. But the RR for lung cancer might be the same.

The other point I wanted to make in relation to these extremes is that I don't think the extremes are as large as you suggest. If you take certain specific instances–in Hobbs, for example there was a division on nonBritish migrant workers and others. The nonBritish migrant workers had ridiculous results–20 mesothelionas and approximately 13 lung cancers, compared to ten expected, and a total number of deaths which was half the expected number of total deaths in the nonBritish migrant workers. Those numbers are off. They are inappropriate expected numbers perhaps because there is very poor follow-up because they are migrants.

I think that you can consistently review the studies and suppose there is obviously some variation–some outside causes pertinent to mesotheliomas and other types are not.

But the variation in the ratio is not large. I think a factor of 2 between the RR for lung cancer and the absolute mesotheliona incidence would be the sort of variation that you would see between the extremes, if you allow for those sort of technical errors and sample effects.

BEAUMONT: I wonder if these medians aren't a little bit high, because if the study does not observe mesotheliomas or if there is a deficit of respiratory cancer or digestive cancer, then no ratio is calculated and therefore it was not entered into the median.

McDONALD: I did also calculate the average, which did not count deficiencies as deficiencies, but simply as zero. The averages came out very close to the median–slightly lower, actually.

SIEMIATYCKI: The area around the Quebec asbestos mines is an area where the general population appears to be highly exposed to asbestos and has been for many years.

First of all, have measurements of ambient asbestos exposure been made in these areas? If so, how do they compare to occupational exposures?

The second question: Are there mesotheliomas in the general population in these areas? Do they appear among young people who have started exposure at age 0?

McDONALD: The first point is that ambient levels have been measured, and they are still relatively high. They used to be very high indeed, in the 2 to 5 fiber level in Thetford Mines.

The second point concerns mesotheliomas in the general population. We did not find any cases in our studies of the general population which were not either directly or indirectly occupationally exposed. There were some cases in the families of miners. Some of these cases were exposed as children and these individuals developed mesotheliomas with early onset, as you might expect.

Cancer from Occupational Asbestos Exposure Projections 1980–2000

WILLIAM J. NICHOLSON, GEORGE PERKEL, AND IRVING J. SELIKOFF
Environmental Sciences Laboratory
Mount Sinai School of Medicine
of the City University of New York
New York, New York 10029

HERBERT SEIDMAN
Department of Epidemiology and Statistics
American Cancer Society
New York, New York 10017

In recent years, considerable data have accumulated that allow estimates to be made of the cancer mortality associated with past exposure to asbestos. These include new information on the dose- and time-dependence of asbestos-related cancers in various occupational circumstances, an increased awareness of the various trades in which possible asbestos exposure has occurred in past years, as well as information on the absolute and relative exposures of these different occupational groups. Although the relevant data are less complete than desirable, they are sufficient to allow estimates of future asbestos-related mortality to be made. These may be useful in directing priorities for appropriate surveillance and possible interventive activities that might be undertaken.

THE DOSE- AND TIME-DEPENDENCE OF ASBESTOS-RELATED CANCERS

The spectrum of malignant disease that occurs from asbestos exposure is best seen in data from the mortality study of Selikoff et al. (1979) on 17,800 insulation workers. This information is shown in Table 1 in which the number of deaths, by cause, over a 10-year period, is tabulated along with those expected from national rates. Causes of death are characterized both according to those listed on the certificates of death (DC) and according to the best evidence (BE) available from a review of autopsy protocols, medical records, and pathological or surgical specimens. The agreement is relatively good for most causes of death but considerable differences exist for mesothelioma and asbestosis. Because deaths from these causes are rare in the absence of asbestos exposure, their misdiagnosis has little effect upon general population rates. However, as they are common causes of death among asbestos-exposed workers, their misdiagnosis can affect seriously a determination of asbestos mortality. Thus,

Table 1
Deaths Among 17,800 Asbestos Insulation Workers in the United States and Canada, January 1, 1967-December 31, 1976

Underlying cause of death	Expected[a]	Observed (BE)[b]	Observed (DC)[c]	Ratio o/e (BE)	Ratio o/e (DC)
Total deaths, all causes	1658.9	2271	2271	1.37	1.37
Total cancer, all sites	319.7	995	922	3.11	2.88
Cancer of lung	105.6	486	429	4.60	4.06
Pleural mesothelioma	†[d]	63	25	–	–
Peritoneal mesothelioma	†	112	24	–	–
Mesothelioma, n.o.s.	†	0	55	–	–
Cancer of esophagus	7.1	18	18	2.53	2.53
Cancer of stomach	14.2	22	18	1.54	1.26
Cancer of colon-rectum	38.1	59	58	1.55	1.52
Cancer of larynx	4.7	11	9	2.34	1.91
Cancer of pharynx, buccal	10.1	21	16	2.08	1.59
Cancer of kidney	8.1	19	18	2.36	2.23
All other cancer	131.8	184	252	1.40	1.91
Noninfectious pulmonary diseases, total	59.0	212	188	3.59	3.19
Asbestosis	†	168	78	–	–
All other causes	1280.2	1064	1161	0.83	0.91

Data from Selikoff et al. (1979). Number of men = 17,800. Man-years of observation = 166,853.

[a]Expected deaths are based upon white male age-specific U.S. death rates of the U.S. National Center for Health Studies, 1967-1976.

[b]Best evidence. Number of deaths categorized after review of best available information (autopsy, surgical, clinical).

[c]Number of deaths as recorded from death certificate information only.

[d]Rates are not available, but these have been rare causes of death in the general population.

the "best evidence" mortality will be used for the estimate of the asbestos-related cancers. However, as we will attribute all excess cancer among insulators to their asbestos exposure (see below), the overall results will not differ greatly from those using certificate of death diagnosis. Lower rates of death at one site (as mesothelioma) will be balanced by higher rates at another (as pancreas).

In addition to mesothelioma and cancer of the lung, cancer of the stomach, colon, rectum, esophagus, larynx, pharynx and buccal cavity, and kidney each are elevated significantly compared with rates expected for these sites in the general population. (This group will be referred to subsequently as "asbestos-related" malignancies.) Opportunity for fiber contact with the epithelial surfaces of the lung and gastrointestinal tract clearly is evident. Exposure to the mesothelial tissue and kidney can occur as fibers readily penetrate lung membranes and can lodge in the mesothelium or be transported by body fluids to the kidney. Similarly, fiber dissemination occurs to other extrapulmonary organs, such as brain, liver, spleen, etc. (Langer 1974). Although excesses at these other sites are not of significance for an individual malignancy, the category "all other cancers" is elevated at a high level of significance ($p < 0.0001$) and we will attribute these excess malignancies to asbestos exposure as well. Their contribution accounts for less than 8% of the total excess cancer.

The time course of the asbestos-related mortality from lung cancer is shown in Figure 1 according to age of observation for individuals exposed initially from ages 15 through 24 and from 25 through 34. As can be seen, the two curves of relative risk (RR), according to age, rise with the same slope and are separated by approximately 10 years. This suggests that the RR of developing lung cancer is independent of age and of the preexisting risk at the time of exposure. In contrast, had one plotted the added risk of cancer,

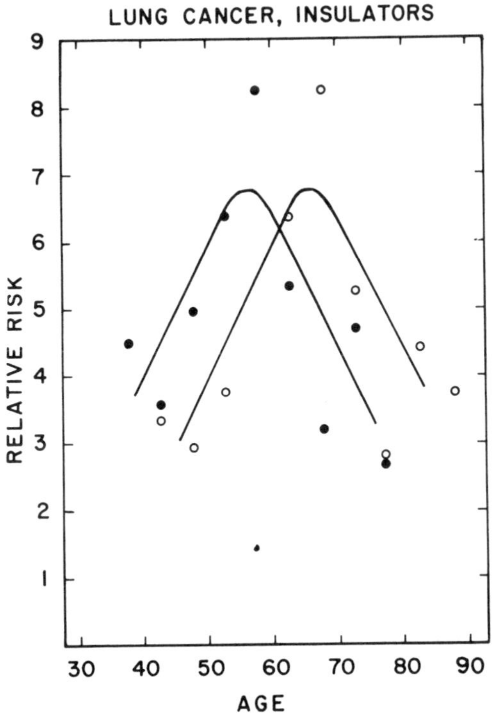

Figure 1
The ratio of observed to expected deaths from lung cancer among insulation workmen according to age of observation and age at onset of employment. Age at onset (•) 15-24 years; (○) 25-34 years.

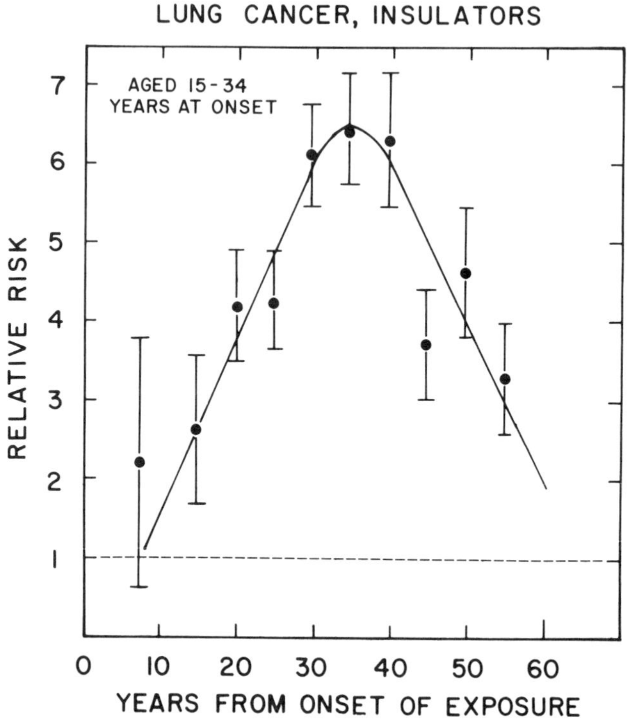

Figure 2
The ratio of observed to expected deaths from lung cancer among insulation workmen (aged 15-34 years at onset) according to time from onset of employment.

the slope for groups first exposed at older ages would have been two to four times as great as for those exposed at younger ages. If one combines these data and plots them according to time from onset of exposure, the curve of Figure 2 is obtained. A linear increase with time from onset of exposure is seen for 35 to 40 years. After 40 years, the RR falls significantly, rather than remaining constant as might be expected after cessation of exposure. The decrease is not the result of the elimination of smokers from the population under observation, as a similar rise and fall occurs for those individuals who were smokers in 1967. Selection processes, such as differing exposure patterns or differing individual biological susceptibilities may play a role, but the exact nature of the effect is not understood. It is, however, a general phenomenon seen in many mortality studies.

The early portion of the curve of Figure 2 is remarkable in two aspects. First, it shows a linear increase in the RR of lung cancer according to time from onset of exposure. This suggests that the dose of asbestos received in a given period of time increases the risk of cancer by an amount that is proportional to that which existed in the absence of exposure. This increased RR is proportional to the dose of inhaled asbestos, which in turn is proportional to the time worked. This results in the linear rise in Figure 2. However, the linear rise can occur only if the increased RR that is created by a given dose of asbestos continues to multiply the background risk for several decades (at least until age 60), even though the background risk will increase by 10- or 20-fold in 30 years. Second, the extrapolated line through the observed data points crosses the line of RR equal to one (that expected in an unexposed population) very close to the onset of exposure. At most, the line might be adjusted so that it passes through the RR of one line at a time from onset of exposure of about 10 years. (Note that we are plotting the RR of death. Irreversible malignancy would occur several years earlier, as usually 1 or 2 years elapse between identification of lung cancer and death and it is likely that a malignant growth was present, unseen, for at least 1 or 2 years before becoming clinically evident.) This means that an increased RR appropriate to a given exposure is achieved very shortly after the exposure takes place. However, if there is a low risk in the absence of asbestos exposure, the cancers that will arise from that increased RR may not be seen for many years or even decades until the background risk becomes significantly greater.

The same two points–(1) that the effect of an external exposure to asbestos is to multiply the preexisting risk of cancer in the exposed population and (2) that the multiplied risk becomes manifest in a relatively short time–can also be seen in the mortality from lung cancer in a study of Seidman et al. (1979). Figure 3 depicts the time course of the mortality for lung cancer of a group exposed for short periods of time beginning 5 years after onset of exposure. As 77% were employed for less than 2 years, exposure largely ceased prior to the follow-up period. As can be seen, there is a rise to a significantly elevated RR that occurs within 10 years, and then that increased RR remains constant throughout the observation period of the study. Furthermore, the RR from a specific exposure is independent of the age at which the exposure began. This is seen in Table 2 where the RR of death for lung cancer for individuals exposed for less than and greater than 9 months is listed according to the age at entrance into a 10-year observation period. Within a given age category, the RR is similar in different decades of observation, as we saw before in Figure 3 with the overall data. However, the RR also is independent of the age decade at entry into a 10-year observation period. (See lines labelled "All" in each exposure category.) There is some reduction in the oldest groups. This can be attributed to the same effects manifest at older ages in insulators or to relatively fewer cigarette smokers that might be present in the 50-59 year observation groups because of selective mortality.

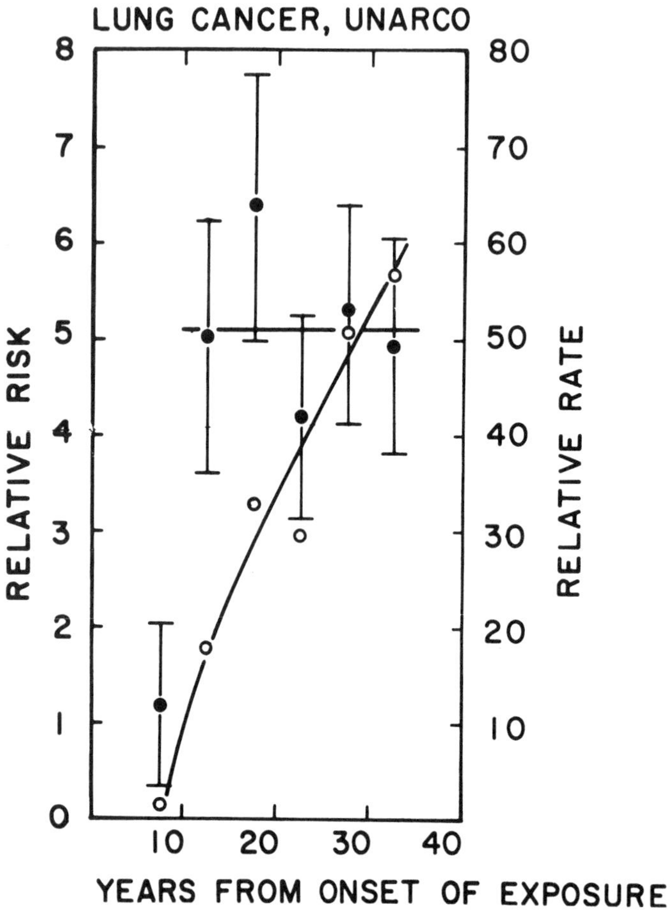

Figure 3
The ratio of observed to expected deaths from lung cancer and the relative lung cancer mortality rates among asbestos insulation production employees according to time from onset of employment. (•) Risk; (○) Rate.

In the calculation of asbestos-related cancer, the time course of non-mesothelial tumors will be treated as follows: The increase in the RR of lung cancer will begin 7.5 years after onset of exposure and increase linearly, following the line of Figure 2, for the number of years a specified group is employed. At termination of employment, the RR will remain constant until 40 years from onset of exposure, after which it will linearly decrease to 1 over the subsequent 3 decades. The magnitude of the increase will be equal to that of Figure 2 for insulators and factory employees. The rate of increase for other groups will be proportional to their estimated exposure relative to that of insulators. (See below.) The same time course will be used for all other non-mesothelial cancer with the magnitude of the increase in insulators being adjusted by the observed

Table 2
Relative Risk of Lung Cancer During 10-year Intervals at Different Times from Onset of Exposure

Years from onset of exposure	Age at start of period		
	30-39	40-49	50-59
	Lower exposure (< 9 months)		
5	0.00 [0.35][a]	3.75 (2)[b]	0.00 [3.04]
15	6.85 (1)	4.27 (3)	2.91 (4)
25	-	2.73 (2)	4.03 (6)
All	3.71 (1)	3.52 (7)	2.58 (10)
	Higher exposure (> 9 months)		
5	0.00 [0.66]	11.94 (4)	9.93 (8)
15	19.07 (2)	11.45 (5)	5.62 (5)
25	-	13.13 (6)	7.41 (8)
All	11.12 (2)	12.32 (15)	7.48 (21)

Data from Seidman et al. (1979)

[a]No cases seen. Number of cases expected on the basis of the average relative risk in the overall exposure category.

[b]Number of cases given in parentheses.

frequency of these tumors compared to that expected and that of other groups by their estimated exposure relative to insulators.

The treatment of the time course of mesothelioma differs from that of lung cancer and other malignancies in that there is no background rate in the absence of asbestos exposure to which to compare the asbestos-related risk. Thus, it is necessary to utilize absolute risks of death. Figure 4 shows the risk of death of mesothelioma according to age for individuals exposed first between ages 15 and 24 and between ages 25 and 34 as in Figure 1. As can be seen, these data, although somewhat uncertain because of small numbers, roughly parallel one another by 10 years as did the increased RR for lung cancers. Thus, the absolute risk of death from mesothelioma appears to be directly related to onset of exposure and is independent of the age at which the exposure occurs. The risk of death from mesothelioma among the insulation workers is plotted according to time from onset of exposure on the right side of Figure 4. It increases about 45 or 50 years from onset of exposure and then appears to fall. Whether the decrease is real or simply the result of misdiagnosis of the disease in individuals age 70 and older is not certain. The relationship of Figure 4 will be used for the risk of mesothelioma among insulation workers employed 25 or more years. After 45 years from onset of exposure, it will be considered to remain constant at 1.2 per 100 person-years. For other exposed groups, the risks will be reduced by the relative exposure of the group compared to insulators and by the fraction of 25 years that a population is exposed.

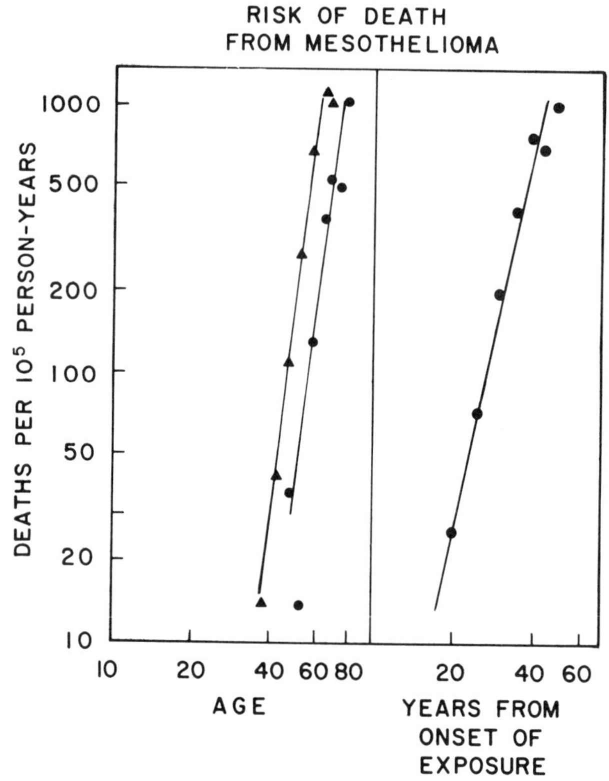

Figure 4
The death rates for mesothelioma among insulation workmen according to age of observation and age at onset of employment, and according to time since onset of employment. (▲) Age at onset < 25 years; (●) > 25 years.

LINEARITY OF DOSE-RESPONSE RELATIONSHIPS

Four recent studies have demonstrated that the risk of lung cancer increases linearly with dose over a fairly wide range of exposures (Liddell et al. 1977; Henderson and Enterline 1979; Seidman et al. 1979; Dement et al. 1981). Unfortunately, they are not directly comparable. For three, the measure of dose was the exposure to asbestos and other dusts in terms of millions of particles per cubic foot (mppcf) times the duration of exposure. This exposure categorization is highly dependent upon the proportion of nonfibrous material in the aerosol being considered. Some relationships between particle counts and fiber concentrations in fibers longer than 5 μm/ml (f/ml) have been provided in the literature, but these are tenuous at best, based as they are upon a limited number of observations. Further, the study of Henderson and Enterline (1979) was limited to retirees of a major asbestos products manufacturer in the United States. As was seen in Figure 2, observations of exposed groups begun late in life can differ considerably from those in which follow up starts at younger years (as, for example, at age 40-45, 20 years after onset of employment). In the fourth study, that of Seidman et al. (1979), exposure characterization involved the use of data from plants other than that in which the mortality experience occurred. An analysis of some of the differences of the slopes of the dose-response functions obtained in these studies has been made elsewhere (Nicholson 1981a). For the purposes of this discussion, the important aspect is the shape of the curve with increasing amounts of asbestos inhaled.

In the analysis which follows, it is not necessary that one fully understand the reasons for the differences in the slopes of dose-response relationships in mining and various manufacturing operations as the RRs in different industries will be based largely upon the observed mortality experience in those industries or upon a comparison of the number of cases of mesothelioma or excess lung cancers in different work activities. In this subsequent comparison, however, we will utilize a linear dose-response relationship to adjust for different periods of employment. Although the evidence of linearity is strong for lung cancer, we will assume that it also obtains for mesothelioma and other malignancies. The evidence for this is more limited, but an analysis of the risks of mesothelioma according to time of employment in the study of Seidman et al. (1979) would suggest that it is true for that tumor as well.

POPULATION AT RISK

Asbestos exposure occurs in a wide variety of industrial pursuits, from mining and milling, through primary and secondary manufacturing, to utilization of asbestos-containing products by a wide variety of workmen. In addition to those directly using asbestos products in the course of their employment, many other individuals may be exposed by virtue of work in jobs requiring that they be near the installation or repair of asbestos-containing materials. This occurs, to a great extent, in the construction and shipbuilding industry and has led to documentation of widespread disease potential from asbestos exposure in these industries (Harries 1976; Selikoff et al. 1981). Estimates on the number of individuals potentially exposed in various occupations and industries are listed in Table 3. The data come largely from Bureau of Labor Statistics (1979) estimates of work populations and new employees in various industries in different periods of time. A detailed report of the estimates is published elsewhere (Perkel 1981).

For the primary asbestos industry (Standard Industrial Classification [SIC] code 3292), all hourly employees were considered at risk. For some of the secondary manufacturing industries, such as heating equipment (SIC 3433), fabricated plateworks (SIC 3443), and industrial furnaces and ovens (SIC 3567),

Table 3
Population Potentially Exposed to Asbestos. Selected Occupations and Industries, 1940-1979

Industry or occupation	Employed 1940	New entrants[a] 1940-1949	1950-1959	1960-1969	1970-1979
Primary and secondary manufacturing	33	57	33	32	33
Insulation work	18	23	35	28	35
Shipbuilding and repair (except insulation)	150	4525	154	162	151
Construction trades (except insulation)	426	652	530	681	721
Railroad engine repair	69	103	12	0	0
Utility services	44	71	37	37	41
Stationary engineers and firemen	295	354	194	171	159
Chemical plant and refinery maintenance	113	118	61	57	59
Automobile maintenance	531	641	374	436	605
Marine engine room personnel (except U.S. Navy)	34	58[b]	22	19	13
Totals	1713	6602	1452	1623	1817
Overall total			13,207[c]		

Data from Perkel (1981).
[a]Numbers given are in thousands.
[b]Excludes World War II personnel.
[c]9,200,000 are estimated to be alive on Jan. 1, 1980.

only half the individuals employed in those industries were considered to have possible asbestos exposure; for electric housewares and fans (SIC 3634), it was estimated that 10% of production and maintenance employees had potential exposure. The shipbuilding and repair industry was a major source of asbestos exposure and the finding of widespread exposure among individuals employed in all crafts in this industry leads us to attribute significant asbestos exposure to all shipyard employees (Selikoff et al. 1981). The number of employees in Naval and civilian yards during World War II was obtained from data of the U.S. Navy (J. K. Nunneley, pers. comm.) and publications of the Bureau of Labor Statistics (1945, 1979). Corresponding widespread potential for asbestos exposure also occurs among maintenance personnel in chemical processing plants and petroleum refineries where the installation, removal, and repair of insulation on high-temperature equipment leads to exposures of many in maintenance crafts. This has been demonstrated by the finding of a significant percentage of X-ray abnormalities among various nonproduction crafts in such operations (Lilis et al. 1979, 1980). Thus, we have included, as a group potentially at risk from asbestos disease, all maintenance employees in chemical plants and refineries as well as those employed in the maintenance of buildings, including the heating facilities therein.

The opportunity for asbestos-exposure among various construction trades is also significant. This industry alone accounts for an estimated 70-80% of the total U.S. consumption of asbestos fiber. Direct exposure to asbestos occurred among individuals engaged in the installation of asbestos cement sheets and pipes; asbestos-filled roofing materials; dry-wall installation, replacement, and removal; insulation of pipes, turbines, heating units, and electrical power-generating equipment; application and sanding of spackle; and during numerous plumbing and pipefitting activities. Second, in high-rise construction, the spraying of asbestos-containing fireproofing material led to widespread contamination of building sites with virtually all employed thereon exposed to considerable concentrations of asbestos, particularly during the years 1958 through 1972 (Reitze et al. 1972). Additional possible exposures date back to the mid-1930s from the use of such spray material for acoustic purposes. For the population estimates of Table 3, we have considered that all painters, pipefitters, and plumbers would have had potential exposure to asbestos and that, among the remaining construction crafts, 20% would have had exposure, except during the years 1958 through 1972. During those years it is estimated that 50% of the construction craftsmen would have had potential exposure. All engine room personnel in the merchant marine and all auto mechanics engaging in brake repair were considered to have potential exposure. Railroad repair shop workers were included during the period steam engines were repaired.

The numbers in Table 3 are necessarily uncertain. This comes from our lack of knowledge of the numbers of individuals with actual asbestos exposure in any given trade and to uncertainties of the number of new employees entering the work force in each decade. These uncertainties, however, will have only a limited impact on the eventual number of asbestos cancers estimated to occur in these industries. This occurs because, for an industry where the population at risk and the exposure are not well known, the RR for the population in Table 3 will be determined by the ratios of mesotheliomas observed in the industry to those seen in manufacturing, insulation work, and shipbuilding, where the populations exposed and the mortality risks are better known. Thus, an overestimate of the number of individuals at risk in Table 3 would lead to the adoption of a lower relative exposure index. Similarly, uncertainties in the turnover rates within a given industry are relatively unimportant compared to the total person-years at risk. A high turnover with more individuals at risk would lead to the use of a shorter period of exposure.

Table 4
Employed Population Potentially Exposed to Asbestos in Selected Occupations and Industries, 1950-1975

	Number employed[a]					
Industry or occupation	1950	1955	1960	1965	1970	1975
Primary and secondary manufacturing	60	62	63	66	68	68
Insulation work	40	42	42	44	47	49
Shipbuilding and repair (except insulation)	132	187	190	191	194	196
Construction trades (except insulation)	741	893	1102	1215	1341	1029
Railroad engine repair	71	56	0	0	0	0
Utility services	62	65	65	64	69	74
Stationary engineers and firemen	311	348	385	289	291	293
Chemical plant and refinery maintenance	93	100	94	93	103	100
Automobile maintenance	599	653	682	791	837	1102
Marine engine room personnel (except U.S. Navy)	37	37	34	35	31	22

Data from Bureau of Labor Statistics (1979).
[a]Numbers given in thousands.

Table 4 provides information on the average number of employees in each of 4 decades for the same industries and trades of Table 3. The average period of employment for individuals hired during a given decade will be calculated from the ratio of the average work force to the number of new entrants per year. The age distribution of new manufacturing employees in 1960 (Table 5) will be used to calculate age-related mortality of new entrants into a trade or industry. This distribution also was found in new hires during 1974 at a major northeast U.S. shipyard (E. Christian, pers. comm.).

RELATIVE RISK BY INDUSTRY

To calculate the asbestos-related cancer mortality in a given industry or occupation, it is necessary to have an absolute or relative measure of exposure for the employee groups listed in Table 3. Inasmuch as we are utilizing data for insulation workers for the dose- and time-dependence of asbestos cancer for all other trades, all asbestos-related risks will be relative to the RR of insulators. These RRs will be determined by three indices. One is the directly measured mortality data, especially that of mesothelioma or lung cancer, in an industry or

Table 5
Age Distribution of Employees Hired During 1965 but Not Working January 1, 1965

Age	Number[a]	Percent in age interval	Percent of shipyard workers in age interval[b]
18-19	892	15.1	17.8
20-24	1614	27.3	31.6
25-34	1431	24.3	27.6
35-44	861	14.6	12.0
45-54	588	10.0	6.1
55-64	361	6.1	2.9
65+	146	2.5	0.0

Data from Bureau of Labor Statistics (1965).
[a]Numbers given in thousands.
[b]Based on 478 new hires during 1974. Data from Christian (pers. comm.).

trade. A second index is directly measured average concentrations of asbestos that can be attributable to the work activity. The third index is the prevalence of X-ray abnormalities after long-term employment in an industry. Here we will assume that the percentage of X-ray abnormalities attributable to an exposure circumstance after 20 years of employment will be proportional to the total dose of asbestos inhaled by the workers in that industry. Where the percentage of abnormal X-rays approaches 100% the RRs will be determined using the percentages of X-rays having a category 2 or greater parenchymal abnormality on the ILO U/C scale. These direct and indirect measures are shown in Table 6 along with the sources of the various data.

For industries in which none of the above indices are available or for which the data are very uncertain, RR estimates will be made from the numbers of mesotheliomas identified among individuals in different asbestos exposure circumstances. These data will utilize the nationwide survey of mesothelioma in 1972 and 1973 by McDonald and McDonald (1980). The numbers from this series are shown in Table 7. The RRs, by industry, estimated from all of the above data are listed in Table 8. For the years 1972-1979, the RRs for manufacturing, insulation work, shipbuilding, and utility employment were reduced to 0.1 and those of the other industries (except automobile maintenance) to 0.05 to reflect the adoption of control measures. Further, exposures subsequent to 1979 were not considered.

CALCULATION OF ASBESTOS-RELATED MORTALITY

As discussed previously, for those trades in which workers have possible asbestos exposure, estimates were made of the number of employees potentially at risk,

Table 6
Indices of Relative Asbestos Exposure in Selected Occupations and Industries

Industry or occupation	Estimated average fiber concentrations	Relative risk of lung cancer	Percentage of deaths from mesothelioma	Applicable employment period	Percentage of parenchymal abnormalities 1+	2+	Percentage of pleural abnormalities	Applicable employment period
Primary and secondary manufacturing	20-40	2.8[a]-6.1	2.6[b]-9.1[a]	1-20+ years				
Insulation work	15[a]	4.8[c]	8.7	20+ years	85[d]	42[d]	56[e]	20+ years
Shipbuilding and repair		1.6[f]		2-3 years	86[g]	17[g]	54[g]	20+ years
Chemical plant and refinery maintenance		1.5[h]		15 years (estimated)	33[i]	3[i]	44[i]	20+ years
Automotive maintenance	0.1-0.3[j]							
Marine engine room personnel							16-20[k]	15 years (estimated)

[a]Nicholson (1981)
[b]Seidman et al. (1979)
[c]Selikoff et al. (1979)
[d]Selikoff et al. (1965)
[e]Selikoff (1965)
[f]Blot et al. (1978)
[g]Selikoff et al. (1981)
[h]Hanis et al. (1979)
[i]Lilis et al. (1980)
[j]Nicholson (1979)
[k]Jones (1980)

Table 7
The Numbers of Mesotheliomas by Work Activity in North America (1960-72, Canada; 1972, United States)

Occupation or industry	Number of cases
Primary and secondary manufacturing	21
Insulation work	27
Shipbuilding and repair (except insulation)	21-49[a]
Construction trades (except insulation)	45
Railroad engine repair	5
Utility services	
Stationary engineers and firemen	13+
Chemical plant and refinery maintenance	3
Automobile maintenance	11
"Heating Trades"	59[b]

Data from McDonald and McDonald (1980).
[a]Highest number includes some insulators.
[b]Includes many individuals who would be assigned to other categories, such as stationary engineers and firemen (furnace repair), shipyard employment (welders, steamfitters), utilities (plumbing, heating, boiler work), and manufacturing (boilermakers).

Table 8
The Relative Risk of Asbestos Cancer from 25 years of Employment in Selected Occupations and Industries

Occupation or industry	Relative risk
Primary manufacturing	1
Secondary manufacturing	0.5
Insulation work	1
Shipbuilding and repair (except insulation)	0.5
Construction trades[a] (except insulation)	0.15-0.25[b]
Railroad engine repair	0.2
Utility services	0.3
Stationary engineers and firemen	0.15
Chemical plant and refinery maintenance	0.15
Automobile maintenance	0.02
Marine engine room personnel (except U.S. Navy)	0.1

[a]See text for percentage of construction population considered at risk.
[b]Risk for years 1958-1972 when the use of sprayed asbestos-fireproofing was common.

the relative exposure of those workers compared to insulators, the average employment time of an individual entering a particular trade or industry, and the age distribution of new hires in the various trades or industries. The asbestos-related cancer mortality was calculated as follows. For those employees entering a trade subsequent to 1940, the above data were utilized to obtain the age and calendar year distribution of men in 5-year periods of time. For each quinquennium at entry, the appropriate age- and calendar year-specific rates were applied to calculate the excess non-mesothelial cancer mortality, the risk of death from mesothelioma, and the total mortality expected according to U.S. rates for each quinquennium until the year 2000 (assuming 1975-1979 rates to apply to 2000). This was done for each quinquennium of entry and the calculated numbers summed for each calendar quinquennium. For those employed in 1940, the appropriate age distribution for an industry or trade in 1940 was used. It was assumed that onset of asbestos exposure occurred at age 22.5. The excess non-mesothelial cancer mortality was calculated using the time dependence displayed in Figure 2 with the assumption that the first manifestation of risk from a given exposure takes place 7.5 years from its occurrence and increases linearly until 7.5 years after cessation of exposure. The risks of death from mesothelioma were calculated using the data of Figure 4, adjusted for each industrial group, with the risk assumed to be constant after 45 years from first exposure.

The results of such calculations are shown in Tables 9 and 10, which list the average annual number of mesotheliomas and total excess cancer attributable

Table 9
The Projected Annual Deaths from Asbestos-related Mesotheliomas in Selected Occupations and Industries, 1977-1997

Industry or occupation	Number of deaths per year				
	1977	1982	1987	1992	1997
Primary and secondary manufacturing	176	247	319	340	319
Insulation work	64	92	128	153	171
Shipbuilding and repair (except insulation)	450	664	906	895	797
Construction trades (except insulation)	330	470	679	891	1011
Railroad engine repair	39	48	55	52	39
Utility services	70	95	123	133	124
Stationary engineers and firemen	141	214	293	330	323
Chemical plant and refinery maintenance	48	69	93	103	99
Automobile maintenance	75	95	115	120	112
Marine engine room personnel (except U.S. Navy)	19	23	27	28	26
Totals	1412	2017	2738	3045	3021

to asbestos exposure in each quinquennium from 1970 through 2000. As can be seen, the dominant factors in the asbestos-related disease are the shipbuilding and construction industries. Industries directly involved in the manufacturing of asbestos products or with the application of insulation material contribute a significantly smaller proportion to the current asbestos disease and that to be expected for the next 2 decades.

It is instructive to look at a display of the number of mesotheliomas and asbestos-related cancers in the shipbuilding industry from the years 1940 through 2000. These data are displayed in Figures 5 and 6 for the populations first employed prior to 1940, during World War II, and subsequent to 1945. As can be seen, the relative importance of the wartime and postwar exposures are roughly equal, even though a considerably greater number of individuals were employed in World War II. This, of course, comes about because of the relatively short periods of work for the wartime group. Further, while the exposures in the construction industry are more uncertain, the important disease experience is also ahead of us in that industry, largely because of the extensive use of asbestos in spray fireproofing materials. A measure of the overall future disease experience can be seen in Figure 7 which depicts the projected annual mesothelioma deaths from 1940 to the year 2000. Although the estimates of the total number of cases are uncertain, the data on the time course of the cancers that will occur are relatively good. They suggest that of all the mesotheliomas that are to occur between the years 1940 and 2000, only 32% have occurred to date (1981).

Table 10
The Projected Annual Deaths from all Asbestos-related Cancer in Selected Occupations and Industries, 1977-1997

	Number of deaths per year				
Industry or occupation	1977	1982	1987	1992	1997
Primary and secondary manufacturing	885	991	1072	1028	952
Insulation work	374	455	527	549	537
Shipbuilding and repair (except insulation)	2267	2747	2890	2659	2159
Construction trades (except insulation)	1912	2423	2909	3150	3123
Railroad engine repair	165	179	177	151	115
Utility services	324	375	407	398	355
Stationary engineers and firemen	725	881	985	992	1004
Chemical plant and refinery maintenance	238	285	310	309	277
Automobile maintenance	308	353	378	363	324
Marine engine room personnel (except U.S. Navy)	74	85	94	93	85
Totals	7142	8774	9749	9692	8931

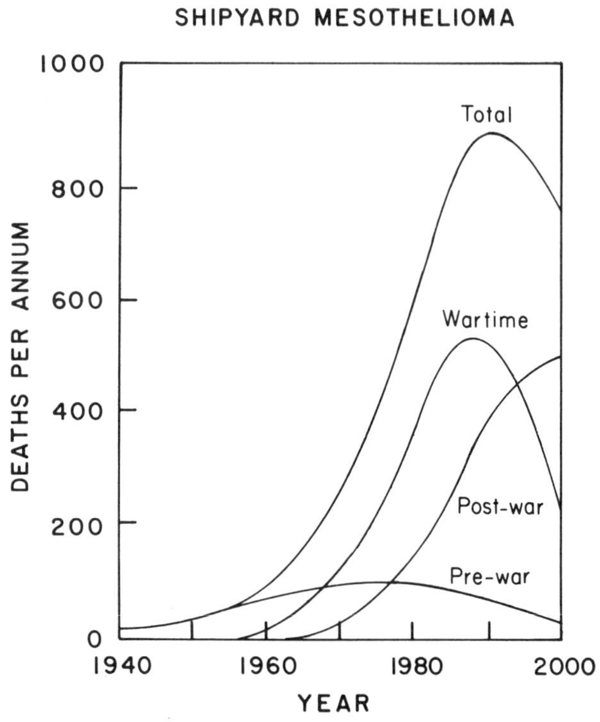

Figure 5
The estimated and projected numbers of mesothelioma deaths per annum from past asbestos exposure from 1940 through 1999 among three groups of shipyard employees (those employed in 1940 or earlier, those employed during World War II, and those employed subsequent to World War II).

The number of mesotheliomas estimated by this procedure is approximately 40% greater than those that would be estimated to occur nationwide using data of the Surveillance, Epidemiology, and End Results (SEER) program. In this comparison, however, it should be noted that the information used for the estimate of asbestos-related cancers in this work relied upon data that identified asbestos malignancy using all medical evidence available and after a review of all surgical or pathological material available. The SEER program, on the other hand, used records-based reports with no review of pathological material. Further, although it represented the shipbuilding industry well, the ten SEER areas underrepresent industrial areas and metropolitan regions that would have had significant construction activities 30 or more years ago. Thus, it is not unexpected that actual U.S. rates may exceed those estimated from the SEER program.

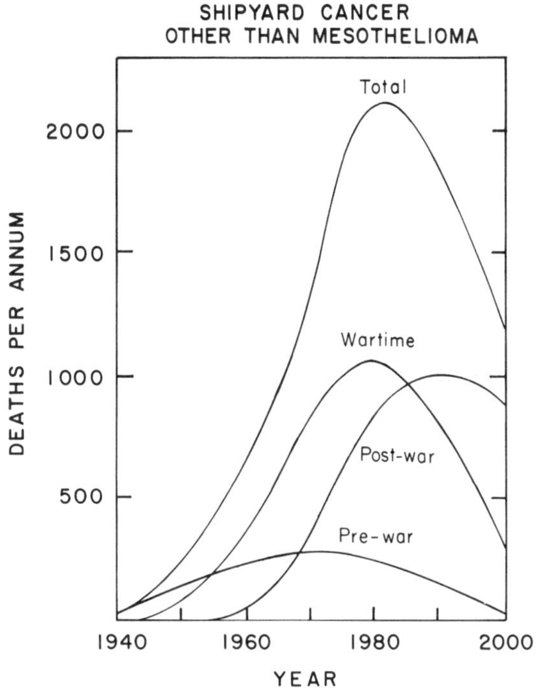

Figure 6
The estimated and projected numbers of excess asbestos-related cancers per annum from 1940 through 1999 among three groups of shipyard employees (those employed in 1940 or earlier, those employed during World War II, and those employed subsequent to World War II).

Some previous estimates of asbestos-related mortality exceed these discussed here. In the Department of Health, Education and Welfare (Bridbord et al. 1978) estimate, recognition was taken of the large number of individuals potentially exposed to asbestos, their estimate being 8-11 million compared to ours of 13.2 million. However, their estimates of the number of "heavily exposed individuals" was subjective and no explicit adjustment was made for the periods of time different groups of individuals were employed in asbestos exposure circumstances. The estimates by Hogan and Hoel (1981) placed great emphasis upon possible effects from the shipbuilding industry. They, too, subjectively estimated the number of "heavily exposed individuals" in this trade and did not account explicitly for variations in employment time and may have overestimated the asbestos-related mortality. However, their estimates of the effect of other industries neglected large numbers of individuals with

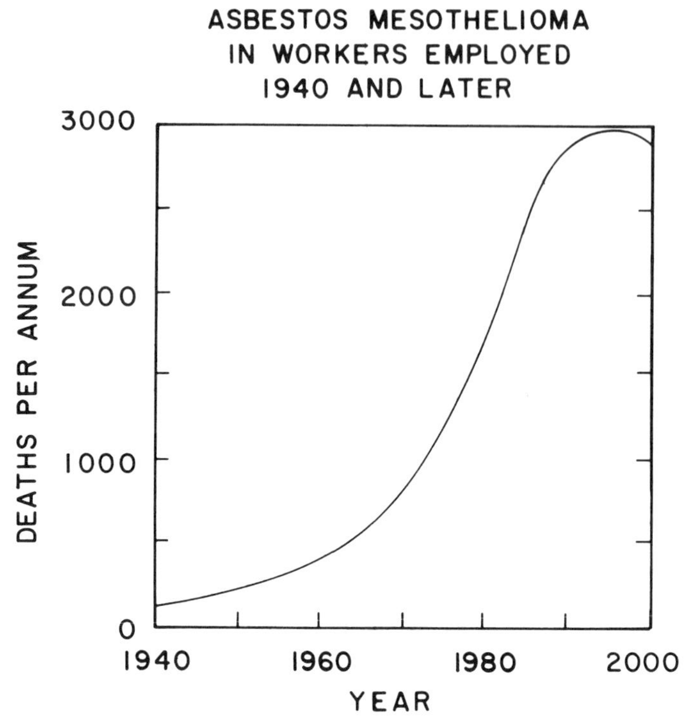

Figure 7
The estimated and projected numbers of mesotheliomas per annum from 1940 through 1999 from occupational asbestos exposure.

potential exposure. Thus, their estimates for other than shipbuilding would appear to understate the asbestos disease potential (Nicholson 1981b).

SUMMARY AND CONCLUSIONS

Estimates have been made of the number of cancers that are projected to result from past exposures to asbestos in a variety of occupations and industries. Only those potentially exposed by virtue of their employment have been considered. Additional deaths will result from exposure through family contacts (household contamination), from environmental exposures, from exposure during consumer use of asbestos products, and from exposure while in the Armed Forces, particularly in engine rooms of naval ships. No estimates have been made of deaths resulting from asbestosis. These estimates indicate that:

1. From 1940 through 1979, 13,200,000 individuals had significant potential asbestos exposure at work. As of January 1, 1980, 9,200,000 are estimated to be alive.

2. Approximately, 8500 asbestos-related excess cancer deaths are currently occurring on an annual basis. This will rise to approximately 10,000 annually by the year 1990.
3. Thereafter, the mortality rate from past exposures will decrease, but still remain significant for another three decades (2000-2030).

These projections are from past exposures to asbestos. Over 1,000,000 tons of friable asbestos material are in place in buildings, ships, factories, refineries, power plants, and other facilities. The maintenance, repair, and eventual demolition of these facilities provide opportunities for continued significant exposures. If such work is not properly done, or asbestos is otherwise used with inadequate controls, the burden of disease and death from past exposures will be increased by the environmental exposures of the future.

REFERENCES

Blot, W.J., J.M. Harrington, A. Toledo, R. Hoover, C.W. Heath, Jr., and J.F. Fraumeni, Jr. 1978. Lung cancer after employment in shipyards during World War II. *New Eng. J. Med.* **299**:620.

Bridbord, K., P. Decoufle, J.F. Fraumeni, Jr., D.G. Hoel, R.N. Hoover, D.P. Rall, U. Saffiotti, M.A. Schneiderman, and A.C. Upton. 1978. "Estimates of the fraction of cancer in the United States related to occupational factors." National Cancer Institute, National Institute of Environmental Health Sciences, and National Institute for Occupational Safety and Health, September 15.

Bureau of Labor Statistics. 1945. *Wartime employment, production, and conditions of work in shipyards.* BLS Bulletin 824. Government Printing Office, Washington, D.C.

———. 1965. Occupational mobility of employed workers. Special Labor Force Rept. 84. Government Printing Office, Washington, D.C.

———. 1979. *Employment and earnings, United States, 1909-1978.* BLS Bulletin 1312-11. Government Printing Office, Washington, D.C.

Dement, J.M., R.L. Harris, Jr., M.D. Symons, and C. Shy. 1981. Estimates of dose-response for respiratory cancer among chrysotile asbestos textile workers. In *Fifth Int. Conf. on Inhaled Particles.* Cardiff, Wales. (In press)

Hanis, N.M., K.M. Stavraky, and J.L. Fowler. 1979. Cancer mortality in oil refinery workers. *J. Occ. Med.* **21**:167.

Harries, P.G. 1976. Experience with asbestos disease and its control in Great Britain's naval dockyards. *Environ. Res.* **11**:261.

Henderson, V.L. and P.E. Enterline. 1979. Asbestos exposure: Factors associated with excess cancer and respiratory disease mortality. *Ann. N.Y. Acad. Sci.* **330**:117.

Hogan, M.D. and D.G. Hoel. 1981. Estimated risk associated with occupational asbestos exposure. *Risk Analysis* **1**.

Jones, R.N. 1980. Shipboard asbestos exposure. Hearings before the Subcommittee on Coast Guard and Navigation, U.S. House Committee on Merchant Marine and Fisheries, Serial No. 96-41. Washington, D.C.

Langer, A.M. 1974. Inorganic particles in human tissues and their association with neoplastic disease. *Environ. Health Perspect.* **9**:229.

Liddell, F.D.K., J.C. McDonald, and D.C. Thomas. 1977. Methods of cohort analysis: Appraised by application to asbestos mining. *J. R. Stat. Soc. A* **140**:649.

Lilis, R., S. Daum, H. Anderson, M. Sirota, G. Andrews, and I.J. Selikoff. 1979. Asbestos disease in maintenance workers of the chemical industry. *Ann. N.Y. Acad. Sci.* **330**:127.

Lilis, R., S. Daum, H. Anderson, G. Andrews, and I.J. Selikoff. 1980. Asbestosis among maintenance workers in the chemical industry and oil refinery workers. In *Biological effects of mineral fibres,* p. 795. International Agency for Research on Cancer, Lyon.

McDonald, A.C. and J.C. McDonald. 1980. Malignant mesothelioma in North America. *Cancer* **46**:1650.

Nicholson, W.J. 1979. Asbestos exposure estimates among garage maintenance workers. Report to the National Institute for Occupational Safety and Health, Contract 210-77-0119.

______. 1981a. Dose-response relationships for asbestos and inorganic fibers. In *Arbete och Hälsa.* No. 17, p. 1. Arbetarskyddsstryrelsen, Solna, Sweden.

______. 1981b. Comment: The role of occupation in the production of cancer. *Risk Analysis* **1**:77.

Perkel, G. 1981. "Occupational exposure to asbestos: Population at risk, 1940-1979." Report to the Department of Labor, Contract No. J-9-M-8-0165.

Reitze, W.B., W.J. Nicholson, D.A. Holaday, and I.J. Selikoff. 1972. Application of sprayed inorganic fiber containing asbestos: occupational health hazards. *Am. Ind. Hyg. Assoc. J.* **33**:179.

Seidman, H., I.J. Selikoff, and E.C. Hammond. 1979. Short-term asbestos work exposure and long-term observation. *Ann. N.Y. Acad. Sci.* **330**:61.

Selikoff, I.J. 1965. The occurrence of pleural calcification among asbestos insulation workers. *Ann. N.Y. Acad. Sci.* **132**:351.

Selikoff, I.J., J. Churg, and E.C. Hammond. 1965. The occurrence of asbestosis among insulation workers in the United States. *Ann. N.Y. Acad. Sci.* **132**:139.

Selikoff, I.J., E.C. Hammond, and H. Seidman. 1979. Mortality experience of insulation workers in the United States and Canada. *Ann. N.Y. Acad. Sci.* **330**:91.

Selikoff, I.J., W.J. Nicholson, and R. Lilis. 1981. Hazard of asbestosis with ship repair. *Am. J. Indust. Med.* **1**:9.

COMMENTS

CAIRNS: This morning we have had a lot of estimates by different methods of the total contribution of asbestos to U.S. cancer death rates. It seems to me that there is an amazing congruence in the conclusions. The present estimate lies somewhere between 1 and 2%, but we may expect that the asbestos cancer death rate will increase through various cohort effects and the change in use of asbestos. It might increase to somewhere between 1.5 and 3% of cancer rates. But, it is not clear to me whether this congruence of opinion is due to a sampling error. Is there anyone present who thinks that these estimates are off by a factor of twofold or more?

NICHOLSON: When one does these calculations, as uncertain as they may be, you get a feeling that goes beyond the simple numbers. In shipyards it is not possible to have a much greater contribution than what I estimated. It is uncertain if it would be significantly less, because one finds very high relative risks of death from lung cancer and other asbestos malignancies in shipyard studies. But from the available data, I would be surprised if it were significantly higher. On the other hand, I think that the construction rates might be higher, because the ratios of mesotheliomas among different construction trades indicates considerable risks are present and we have yet to see the full effects of the spraying of asbestos for fireproofing purposes.

The estimate that Phil [Enterline] gave—about half of what I obtained—doesn't attribute as much to the construction industry and to maintenance activities. However we are remarkably close, and our estimates probably represent a reasonable range for these estimates.

ENTERLINE: It seems to me that the areas of disagreement are mostly "don't know" areas. For example, I don't know how to estimate the historic exposure in shipyards, except by talking to people that worked there. You did say this morning there are dust counts available.

NICHOLSON: No, I didn't. There are environmental data only for insulation workers.

ENTERLINE: I think that gets very confused. A lot of people think that is shipyard workers.

NICHOLSON: I think there are fairly reasonable data that indicate the exposure of insulators was about 10-15 f/ml. If your data from Newport News suggesting general environmental exposures of 2-3 f/ml are correct, that implies that the RR of shipyard workers to insulators would be about 0.2 or 0.3. The risk that I used, 0.5, is close to that which Bill [Blot] obtained with his case-control studies, if the average shipyard employment time is 3 or 4 years.

BLOT: That is right—about a 3-year average.

McDONALD: I think these answers apply to male workers. We shouldn't include females at the present time since the ratios are probably a lot lower there.

NICHOLSON: But the number employed in these trades would be relatively few, except in the wartime shipyard group.

R. PETO: I wanted to make a very similar point to John Cairns'. The numbers that different people have attributed are: Enterline, 4000-5000 at present, with no prediction of the future; McDonald, about 3000 at present, with no prediction of the future; Julian Peto, about 3000 at present, predicting that there might be a rise to about 5000 in the future; Blot, 4000 from shipyards alone, plus some from people not in shipyards; and, Bill [Nicholson], you predicted 8000 at present, predicting a rise to 10,000. You indicated that these are perhaps the upper limits to what is reasonable—the 10,000 being at approximately the turn of the century, and Julian's 5000 being at approximately the turn of the century. Although there is a consensus here, there is a marked divergence between what has been presented here and what was reported in the OSHA document. The numbers I am talking about are thousands of cancer deaths per year in the United States due to the asbestos, in males or females together, or males alone (the numbers are really virtually the same), excluding asbestosis.

Now, there is *not* a consensus that this is reasonable, because there is also the figure of 58,000 to 75,000, which is in the OSHA document (Bridbord et al. 1978). This is 13%-18% of all cancer deaths. Marvin [Schneiderman], will you comment on this? Is this a figure you still regard as reasonable?

SCHNEIDERMAN: I am very impressed by the work that has been done and presented here today. I was also impressed with the work that Hogan and Hoel (1981) did, which showed results somewhat like Nicholson's, or perhaps somewhat higher.

I am inclined to believe the original estimates made by Selikoff and reported in the OSHA document, are too high.

References

Bridbord, K., P. Decoufle, J.F. Fraumeni, Jr., D.G. Hoel, R.N. Hoover, D.P. Rall, U. Saffiotti, M.A. Schneiderman, and A.C. Upton. 1978. "Estimates of the fraction of cancer in the United States related to occupational factors." National Cancer Institute, National Institute of Environmental Health Sciences, and National Institute for Occupational Safety and Health, September 15.

Hogan, M.D. and D.G. Hoel. 1981. Estimated risk associated with occupational asbestos exposure. *Risk Analysis* 1:77.

SESSION 2:
Radiation Risks,
Animal Experiments

Exposure to Ionizing Radiation and Cancer Mortality among Workers at the Hanford Plant

SARAH C. DARBY AND JOHN A. REISSLAND
National Radiological Protection Board
Chilton, Didcot, Oxfordshire OX11 0RQ, England

The question of whether or not occupational exposure to ionizing radiation within the maximum permissible limits results in any discernible health damage to those exposed has been an outstanding issue in radiological protection for many years. In 1964, an investigation was initiated in the United States under Dr. Thomas F. Mancuso with the objective of correlating the lifetime health and mortality experience of workers in the atomic energy industry with their occupational radiation exposure. After a feasibility study, the collection of personal, radiation, and mortality data began for employees at selected facilities, including the Hanford Works in Richland, Washington, Mound Laboratories in Miamisburg, Ohio, and the installations at Oak Ridge, Tennessee. This project was viewed as a pilot study with the intention of extending it to include all employees of the former U.S. Atomic Energy Commission and its contractors. It was also planned to extend the study by considering health indices other than mortality, for example, through the use of Social Security Administration (SSA) records of disability. An extensive account of the methodology and some preliminary findings of the early stages of the project have been given by Mancuso et al. (1971).

Great publicity was attracted in 1977 when Dr. Mancuso, in collaboration with Dr. Alice Stewart and Mr. George Kneale, published an analysis of data relating to employees at the Hanford plant, in which it was estimated that 5.8% of the 442 certified deaths from cancer in males were radiation-induced (Mancuso et al. 1977). This paper was presented as a preliminary analysis, and shortly afterwards a reanalysis of a slightly extended data set using a revised methodology was published in which it was again estimated that approximately 5% of the cancer deaths of Hanford workers were radiation-induced (Kneale et al. 1978). Risks were estimated in these papers in the form of doubling doses (i.e., doses of radiation that double the normal risk) and the values given are summarized in Table 1. When these are applied to current U.S. cancer mortality rates, it is clear that they imply a substantially greater risk than the values given by the International Commission on Radiological Protection (ICRP 1977),

Table 1
Doubling Doses for Certain Types of Cancer in Males Estimated from the Hanford Data by Mancuso, Stewart, and Kneale

	Estimated doubling dose (rads)	
Cause of death	from Table 16 of Mancuso et al. (1977)	from Table 10 of Kneale et al. (1978)
Multiple myeloma and myeloid leukemia	0.8	3.6
Cancer of the pancreas	7.4	–
Cancer of the pancreas, stomach, and large intestine	–	15.6
Lung cancer	6.1	13.7
All cancers	12.2	33.7

which estimates that the total risk of fatal cancer is 10^{-4} per rem (10^{-2} per Sv) for workers by extrapolation from data obtained at higher doses. It is also difficult to reconcile an estimated doubling dose of either 0.8 rad or 3.6 rad for multiple myeloma and myeloid leukemia with typical background radiation doses of around 0.1 rad per year.

Although several substantial criticisms of Mancuso et al. (1977) have been published (see Anderson 1978; Hutchison et al. 1979), the present authors wished to be in a position to form a first-hand opinion of this new data base. A copy of the raw data on the Hanford workers was requested from the U.S. Department of Energy, and this was kindly supplied by the Pacific Northwest Laboratories of Battelle. The analysis of these data is now complete and this paper presents the main features of it; a full account will be published shortly (Darby and Reissland 1981).

THE DATA

Basic employment and vital information was received on all individuals with initial employment at the Hanford works prior to 1965. Annual dose histories were available only for white males who remained employed for at least 2 years; but as they received almost all the radiation dose, the analysis has been concentrated on them. The annual dose histories given represent whole-body penetrating radiation and were obtained chiefly from personal dosemeter readings. Additional information available for this group of workers comprised date and place of birth, employment dates at Hanford, date and place of death as revealed by searching the SSA files, and cause of death as given on the death certificate and classified according to the 8th revision of the International

Classification of Diseases (ICD) (World Health Organization 1967). For a few individuals, there was an indication that internal irradiation from radioactive material taken into the body had occurred. However, the authors were informed that there was considerable doubt as to the accuracy of this information, and so, initially, it was ignored in the analysis. Subsequent examination found that the conclusions would not have differed if the actual doses received by these individuals had been somewhat higher than was indicated by their annual dose histories.

COMPARISON OF OBSERVED DEATHS WITH U.S. NATIONAL MORTALITY

To compare the mortality of Hanford workers with that of the U.S. population, calculations were made of the number of person years at risk for white male employees from the second anniversary of the time they started work at Hanford until the cut-off date for the study or their date of death, whichever came first. This procedure is shown schematically for three hypothetical individuals in Figure 1. As death rates vary with age and calendar year, the number of person years at risk grouped by age within each calendar year of the study was multiplied by the corresponding annual death rate in the United States to give the number of deaths expected in that category if national death

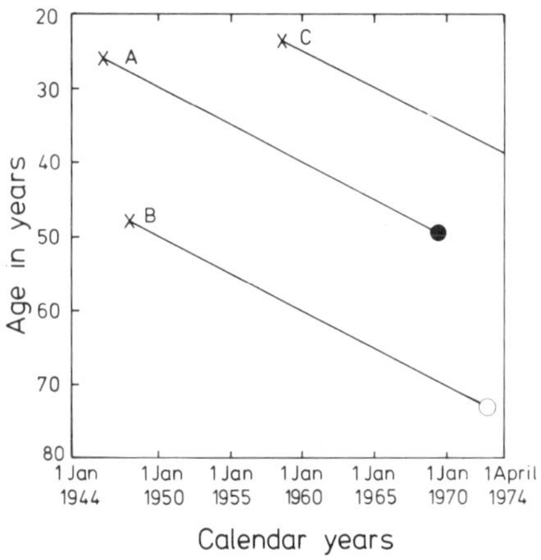

Figure 1

Schematic representation of three hypothetical individuals who, on their second anniversary after starting work at Hanford, contribute to the person years at risk in the study until they either die from cancer (A), die from some other cause such as an accident or heart disease (B), or survive until April 1, 1974, the cut-off date for the study (C). (X) Second anniversary of commencement of employment at Hanford; (–) period during which an individual contributes to the person years at risk; (•) death from cancer; (○) death from some other cause.

Table 2
Observed and Expected Deaths from All Causes in White Males by Length of Time since Starting Employment at Hanford

Length of time since starting employment at Hanford (yr)	Observed deaths from all causes	Expected deaths from all causes	Ratio of observed to expected deaths
2-	71	176.8	.40
5-	231	378.3	.61
10-	345	500.6	.69
15-	475	642.3	.74
20+	967	1146.4	.84

Expected deaths are calculated from U.S. national rates.

rates were applicable to Hanford workers. Observed and expected deaths from all causes, classified according to length of time since starting employment at Hanford, are given in Table 2. It can be seen that the ratio of observed to expected deaths is very low in the years soon after commencement of employment at Hanford and gradually increases. This phenomenon is characteristic of the mortality of employed groups (Fox and Collier 1976), although it is unusual for the ratio of observed to expected deaths to remain substantially below unity 20 years after commencement of employment. This result rules out the possibility that these data contain evidence of excess overall mortality in the Hanford workforce as a whole when compared with national mortality rates. However, because the most obvious explanation for the continuing deficit of observed deaths more than 20 years after commencement of employment is incomplete tracing of deaths, the finding is nevertheless a disturbing one.

INTERNAL COMPARISON OF OBSERVED DEATH RATES

It is difficult to make detailed comparisons between the Hanford data and U.S. national mortality because all the Hanford deaths are coded according to the 8th revision of the ICD, whereas the published national mortality rates for the period prior to 1968 are coded according to the 6th and 7th revisions. In addition, as there is an overall deficit of deaths from all causes in the Hanford data when compared with the national figures, an overall deficit in any individual cause of death might well conceal a concentration of the deaths among individuals with high recorded radiation doses. Therefore, a more detailed internal comparison was carried out in which the observed death rates for specific types of cancer were examined for trends with recorded dose.

Each man's contribution to the person years at risk was allocated among various strata according to the current calendar year, and also his current age and length of time since commencing employment. Inside each stratum, the person years at risk were further subdivided according to each man's recorded radiation history. To allow for uncertainties in the latent period between irradiation and any resulting death from radiation-induced cancer, separate analyses were carried out using various different criteria for calculating radiation dose. The first analysis took each man's radiation dose at any point in time to be equal to his total dose recorded before the end of the calendar year ending 2 years previously (ignoring all radiation in the most recent 2 years). Further analyses then were carried out considering the total recorded dose more than 5 years previously, more than 10 years previously, and between 2 and 10 years previously (ignoring all radiation dose received more than 10 years ago).

For each cause of interest, every observed death was also allocated to the relevant stratum and dose category, and a test for trend in the observed death rates was carried out by means of a test statistic that summarized the information from all strata which could provide any information about a trend in death rates with dose. For further details see Darby and Reissland (1981).

Analyses were carried out for the following reported causes of death:

1. All causes.
2. All solid tumors (ICD, 8th revision, codes 140-199).
3. All solid tumors excluding those known to be associated with smoking (ICD, 8th revision, codes 140-199 with 140-150, 157, 161-163 and 188 removed).
4. All leukemias (ICD, 8th revision, codes 204-207).
5. Acute leukemia (ICD, 8th revision, codes 204.0, 205.0, 206.0, 207.0).
6. Chronic leukemia (ICD, 8th revision, codes 204.1, 205.1, 206.1, 207.1).
7. Leukemia unspecified as to chronic or acute (ICD, 8th revision, codes 204.9, 205.9, 206.9, 207.9).
8. All neoplasms of lymphatic and hematopoietic tissues other than leukemia (ICD, 8th revision, codes 200-203, 208, 209).

Separate analyses were also carried out for all ICD, 8th revision, three-digit categories of neoplasm and all four-digit categories of leukemia for which there were one or more observed deaths.

When deaths from all causes were considered, there was no evidence of a trend towards increased mortality with increasing dose. On the contrary, there was some evidence of a deficit of deaths in the higher dose groups, particularly when the more recent doses were considered. This is illustrated in Table 3 where the observed deaths in each dose category are compared with those expected, assuming that within each stratum the total number of deaths expected is equal to that observed, and that the expected deaths are distributed between the close categories in proportion to the person years at risk. The slight negative trend is

Table 3
Observed and Expected Deaths from All Causes Occurring after 2 Years of Employment by Dose Category

	Total recorded radiation dose in rem between 2 and 10 years previously							
	< 1	1-	5-	10-	15-	20-	25-	30+
Observed deaths	1464	270	48	31	22	10	0	0
Expected deaths	1402.84	306.97	62.25	34.25	26.75	11.49	0.32	0.00

Deaths occurring in individuals over the age of 80 have been excluded, as have deaths belonging to strata where all the person years at risk fell in a single dose category. Expected deaths are calculated by internal comparison.

due to the fact that an individual's total recorded radiation dose is highly correlated with the length of time worked at Hanford. Because it is the healthier men who tend to remain in an industry, there will be a natural tendency for those receiving the larger radiation doses to be selected from the healthier members of the study population. In addition, when considering doses received in the recent past, only those men healthy enough to be working at that time will have received any dose.

Deaths due to solid tumors, whether or not those associated with smoking are excluded, showed a very similar pattern to deaths from all causes. Deaths from leukemia as a whole showed no evidence of a trend with dose, nor did acute, chronic, and unspecified leukemia when considered as three separate groups. In contrast, neoplasms of lymphatic and hematopoietic tissue other than leukemia did show a positive trend with dose when the dose was taken to be that occurring more than 10 years previously. Inspection of the relevant individual three-digit ICD categories revealed that this was entirely accounted for by a very clear trend for multiple myeloma. The observed and expected deaths from multiple myeloma in the individual dose categories are illustrated in Table 4 for total dose received more than 10 years previously. The evidence points to an excess of between two and three deaths among those whose total dose exceeded 5 rem. Similar conclusions emerge when other criteria are used for classifying the dose. For the remaining three- and four-digit ICD categories of neoplasm, there was no evidence of a trend in death rates with dose apart from two exceptions, pancreatic cancer, and renal cancer. Observed and expected deaths from these causes are also shown in Table 4.

The authors' overall interpretation of the results in the individual three- and four-digit ICD categories is that multiple myeloma is the only category for which there is firm evidence of a trend in the observed death rates with increasing radiation dose. The reason for this is that for pancreatic cancer the evidence of a trend was strongest when the more recent doses were considered, which is contrary to expectation for a radiation-induced solid tumor, whereas for renal cancer the evidence of a trend was entirely due to one death in a high-dose category. Therefore, it seems likely that these two findings are spurious and attributable to the large number of significance tests that have been carried out on the data. Conversely, in view of the relatively small numbers of observed deaths and the size of the recorded doses, there are no malignancies for which an association with radiation can be ruled out.

DISCUSSION

At the end of 1973, the Hanford work force was recorded as having received a collective dose of about 60,000 person rem. ICRP risk factors (ICRP 1977) suggest that this eventually will give rise to a total of about six radiation-induced fatal cancers of which about 1.2 will be leukemia. In view of the latent periods involved, not all the extra deaths are likely to have occurred by the end of the period included in this analysis, and therefore one would not expect to be able to detect the influence of radiation on the mortality patterns of the Hanford work force. The present analysis confirmed these expectations, both overall and for leukemia. The finding of excess multiple myeloma among those with high recorded doses comes shortly after excesses have been noted in a number of cohorts of persons exposed to radiation (Cuzick 1981). These include the atomic bomb survivors (Ichimaru et al. 1979), although the risk implied by the Hanford data is somewhat higher. Clearly there is a need for additional data to be collected in this area.

Table 4
Observed and Expected Deaths from Multiple Myeloma, Pancreatic Cancer, and Renal Cancer by Dose Category

	Total recorded dose in rem more than 10 years previously						
	< 1	1-	5-	10-	15-	20-	25+
Multiple myeloma							
Observed deaths	3	0	1	1	0	1	0
Expected deaths	4.53	1.19	0.18	0.05	0.04	0.01	0.00
Pancreatic cancer							
Observed deaths	21	2	0	2	0	0	0
Expected deaths	19.92	4.18	0.51	0.24	0.12	0.03	0.00
Renal cancer							
Observed deaths	8	0	0	1	0	0	0
Expected deaths	7.92	0.93	0.13	0.00	0.00	0.00	0.00

Deaths occurring after 2 years of employment are included except where the death occurred in an individual over the age of 80 or belonged to a stratum where all person years at risk fell in a single dose category. Expected deaths are calculated by internal comparison.

By now there have been many analyses of the mortality of Hanford workers. Two of these (Sanders 1978; Brodsky 1979) are by members of the original Mancuso team. These analyses examine the mortality of Hanford workers in relation to the siblings of radiation workers; Sanders (1978) also compares exposed with nonexposed employees. Neither analysis finds any evidence of harmful effects. Marks et al. (1978) and Gilbert and Marks (1979) have also analyzed the Hanford data, and the present authors' conclusions are very similar to theirs.

The difference between the Mancuso, Stewart, and Kneale conclusions and those reached by ourselves, Gilbert and Marks (1979), and Hutchison et al. (1979) seem largely attributable to methodological differences. The first analysis of Mancuso et al. was limited to considering those known to have died, and initially was carried out with no adjustment for factors, other than radiation, that are known to influence mortality rates. Although there was some discussion of the likely effect of various factors individually, their combined effect was not investigated. In addition, doubling doses were estimated after selecting for each group of cancers the predeath interval for which the contrast between the mean dose of those who have died was maximized when compared with that for all noncancer deaths. It seems clear that such doubling doses will be biased downwards.

The reanalysis by Kneale et al. (1978) employed revised methodology to the extent that several factors thought to be possible sources of bias were now controlled simultaneously, however this included the unusual step of controlling for internal radiation. In spite of doubts about the quality of the data on internal irradiation, almost all those involved also had high external recorded radiation doses; thus, controlling for internal radiation in this way is to some extent controlling for external radiation dose. It seems likely therefore that such a procedure will distort any ensuing estimates of doubling dose. The reanalysis by Kneale et al. (1978) also continued to ignore data on the substantial majority of Hanford workers who survived to the end of the period of analysis, and used the same method for estimating doubling doses as in the previous paper.

REFERENCES

Anderson, T.W. 1978. Radiation exposures of Hanford workers: A critique of the Mancuso, Stewart and Kneale report. *Health Phys.* **35**:743.

Brodsky, A. 1979. A statistical method for testing epidemiological results, as applied to the Hanford worker population. *Health Phys.* **36**:611.

Cuzick, J. 1981. Radiation-induced myelomatosis. *N. Engl. J. Med.* **304**:204.

Darby, S.C. and J.A. Reissland. 1981. Low levels of ionising radiation and cancer—Are we underestimating the risk (with discussion). *J. R. Statist. Soc. A* (in press).

Fox, A.J. and P.F. Collier. 1976. Low mortality rates in industrial cohort studies due to selection for work and survival in the industry. *Br. J. Prev. Soc. Med.* **30**:225.

Gilbert, E.S. and S. Marks. 1979. An analysis of the mortality of workers in a nuclear facility. *Radiat. Res.* **79**:122.

Hutchison, G.B., B. MacMahon, S. Jablon, and C.E. Land. 1979. Review of report by Mancuso, Stewart and Kneale of radiation exposure of Hanford workers. *Health Phys.* **37**:207.

Ichimaru, M., T. Ishimaru, M. Mikami, and M. Matsunaga. 1979. *Multiple myeloma among atomic bomb survivors and controls in Hiroshima and Nagasaki by dose, 1950-1976.* Hiroshima, Radiation Effects Research Foundation, Technical Report No. 9-79.

International Commission on Radiological Protection (ICRP). 1977. Recommendations of the International Commission on Radiological Protection. In *Annals of the ICRP.* Publ. 26. Pergamon Press, Oxford.

Kneale, G.W., A. Stewart, and T. Mancuso. 1978. Reanalysis of data relating to the Hanford study of the cancer risks of radiation workers. *IAEA Proc. Ser.* **1**:387.

Mancuso, T.F., B.S. Sanders, and A. Brodsky. 1971. In *Proceedings 6th Annual Health Physics Society Topical Symposium, Radiation Protection Standards: Quo Vadis, III.* Study of the lifetime health and mortality experience of employees of AEC contractors, part I: Methodology and some preliminary findings limited to mortality of Hanford employees. COO-3428-1.

Mancuso, T.F., A. Stewart, and G. Kneale. 1977. Radiation exposures of Hanford workers dying from cancer and other causes. *Health Phys.* **33**:369.

Marks, S., E.S. Gilbert, and B.D. Breitenstein. 1978. Cancer mortality in Hanford workers. *IAEA Proc. Ser.* **1**:369.

Sanders, B.S. 1978. Low level radiation and cancer deaths. *Health Phys.* **34**:521.

World Health Organization (WHO). 1967. *Manual of the International Statistical Classification of Diseases, Injuries and Causes of Death.* World Health Organization, Geneva.

COMMENTS

GAFFEY: Did you check the background rates for multiple myeloma in Washington State or in the counties around the plant? I wonder whether this excess might not reflect a regional difference from the national average.

DARBY: The background rates for multiple myeloma in the northwest are slightly higher than in the rest of the United States, and this might have some bearing on the interpretation of our comparison of Hanford mortality with U.S. national rates. However, a high background rate for multiple myeloma would not affect the conclusions from our internal comparison, which shows that there is an upwards trend in mortality from multiple myeloma with increasing dose.

RADFORD: I think it is worth pointing out a number of aspects of this. First, does or doesn't it fit the ICRP risk estimates or is it a test of anything? I think it is clear from your presentation that, even if the ICRP mortality data are off by a factor of 2, which I believe they are, we are still not going to see an excess in this time frame.

Second, oddly enough, multiple myeloma has been popping up in these occupational groups that have been exposed to relatively low-dose rates over long periods of time. I refer, for example, to the Windscale workers, who also showed an excess of multiple myeloma. There has been some indication from Gene Matanoski's follow-up on the younger radiologists that multiple myeloma has been one form of cancer that seems to be in excess, whereas leukemia is not.

This is a bizarre observation. Myeloma seems to be coming out for reasons that aren't apparent at all to me. Excess leukemia is not present in these groups, but multiple myeloma may be. I understand that Dr. Matanoski has new data, which I have not seen, so perhaps I won't put too much stress on the radiologists.

ACHESON: Where you have such a small number of observed deaths, it is particularly important that the diagnosis is correct. Can you tell us anything about the diagnosis? In multiple myeloma, the diagnosis is often very contentious.

DARBY: In the data that we have analyzed, the diagnosis is as given on the death certificate. The data were supplied to us in anonymous statistical form by the U.S. Department of Energy, so we have not been able to investigate the accuracy of these diagnoses. However, I understand that the staff of the Pacific Northwest Laboratory are carrying the study on and doing such investigations.

McDONALD: I am a little worried about diagnosis also. I wondered if you happen to know what the actual location of death is for the multiple myeloma patients. I am always interested in pathologists who are fond of certain diagnoses.

DARBY: The only information that we have as to the location of death of the multiple myeloma patients is the state in which the death occurred. Out of the seven multiple myeloma deaths, five, including all three with substantial doses, occurred in Washington State. The remaining two occurred in Maryland and California.

J. PETO: To what form of radiation are these people exposed?

DARBY: Our analysis considers exposure to whole-body penetrating radiation as measured by film badges or thermoluminescent dosemeters. A few workers at the Hanford plant also may have received some additional exposure from inhaled or ingested radionuclides, and when we were supplied with the data we were given an indication of whether there was any evidence of internal contamination in addition to the external dose for each individual. We were also told that this evidence was very uncertain and that is why we have ignored it in our basic analysis. However, after we had finished the analysis, we checked to see if the conclusions would have been different if those individuals about whom there was a possibility of internal contamination had received slightly higher doses than indicated by their external dose. The answer is that within a wide margin the conclusions don't change at all.

R. PETO: I wanted to make a couple of points. First, there was a review paper by Jack Cuzick (1981) in which he reviewed all of the studies of radiation and found that an excess of myelomatosis was found quite consistently in many different studies. Your findings are really typical of many other studies.

Second, in reply to Radford's comment. Surely what we are doing is not trying to really get a direct estimate of the effects of radiation from these data. There are other data that are, perhaps, better suited to that. Rather, we are trying to examine whether the claims of very large effects of irradiation based on these data are justified from these data.

SARACCI: I am not entirely clear why you analyzed the data going backward, in a sense. Your cutoff, if I understand correctly, is exposure 2 years before the death.

DARBY: We calculated a "dose" applicable to every individual at each moment in time for the total period that person was in the study. To allow for uncertainties in the time between irradiation and any resulting radiation-induced death, we carried out several analyses using different criteria for calculating this "dose." For example, in our first analysis, we considered it to be his total recorded radiation dose 2 years previously, so that at the time the man died we would be considering dose up to 2 years previously. Thus, this analysis ignores dose received in the very recent past as it is very unlikely to be a relevant factor in a death occurring so soon afterwards.

WAXWEILER: It appears to me that you are more or less summarily dismissing pancreatic cancer because the effect was longer than the 2-10 years before death. Occasionally, I have seen in other occupational cohorts that there is what you might call autocorrelation over time in the person's job history. They tend to stay in the same types of jobs for a period of time. It may not necessarily mean that there is not an association between radiation and pancreatic cancer.

DARBY: We feel that the observed association between radiation dose and death from pancreatic cancer may well be spurious for two reasons. Firstly, the majority of work on radiation-induced cancer shows rather long latent periods for solid cancers of this type. In these data, the association is actually stronger when the more recent doses are considered as compared with dose received in the distant past. Secondly, specific diagnosis of cancer of the pancreas is rather difficult; it is quite often confused with cancer of the stomach. If one combines the two conditions in these data, the excess disappears.

I should add that we do not interpret these data as providing evidence that radiation does not cause pancreatic cancer. This is one condition that should certainly be looked at in other data sets of this type. It would also be interesting to examine the medical records of those reported on the death certificate as dying from cancer of the pancreas or stomach.

WAXWEILER: You didn't mention the percent lost to follow-up in your cohort study. Was it looked at by dose?

DARBY: The data tape that we received from the Department of Energy contained no indication as to which individuals were lost to follow-up, but the ratio of observed to expected deaths calculated from national mortality rates is still only 0.84 for those who started employment at Hanford over 20 years previously (see Table 2). We feel that this ratio is surprisingly low, and it certainly raises the possibility that the percent lost to follow-up is substantial. We received the data in anonymous statistical form, thus we have not been able to investigate this possibility ourselves, but we understand that the Pacific Northwest Laboratory staff are continuing the study.

MILHAM: Are radiation doses that these men received characterized as low or high dose? By anybody's definition, this population had low-dose radiation. Would you be willing to say from your study results that low-dose radiation can cause cancer in human beings?

DARBY: This study provides strong evidence of an association between exposure to low-dose radiation and death from multiple myeloma. Because it is an observational study, there is no way of establishing from these data alone whether the association is a causal one, especially when one considers the nature of the work carried out at Hanford, which would include exposure to a large number of possible carcinogens. The recent review paper by Cuzick (1981) concludes that there is strong evidence that radiation can cause myelomatosis, but much of this evidence is based on higher doses than are involved here. Clearly, further cohorts of individuals exposed to low-dose radiation need to be studied before any firm conclusions can be drawn as to whether the observed association in these data is a causal one.

References

Cuzick, J. 1981. Radiation-induced myelomatosis. *N. Engl. J. Med.* **304**:204.

Analyses of Hanford Data: Delayed Effects of Small Doses of Radiation Delivered at Slow-Dose Rates

THOMAS F. MANCUSO
University of Pittsburgh School of Public Health
Pittsburgh, Pennsylvania 15261

ALICE M. STEWART AND GEORGE W. KNEALE
Cancer Epidemiology Research Unit
Department of Social Medicine
University of Birmingham
Edgbaston, Birmingham, B15 2TT, England

This presentation describes the work of Mancuso and his associates, who spent more than 10 years assembling Hanford data from work records, social security transactions, and death certificates before reporting the findings that are now in dispute.

THE MANCUSO-STEWART-KNEALE ANALYSES

The general reaction to our 1977 paper in *Health Physics* (Mancuso et al. 1977) (see MSK I, Table 1) began by being, and has remained, one of total disbelief. Yet much of what this report contains might have been deduced from known effects of pregnancy X-rays (Kneale and Stewart 1976a, b) and much since has been confirmed by research workers who were asked, either by the Department of Energy or the General Accounting Office, to check our findings (Hutchinson et al. 1979; General Accounting Office 1981). Furthermore, if the International Commission on Radiological Protection (ICRP) had realized that the trend of noncancer mortality for A-bomb survivors has always been steeper than normal, they would have hesitated before assuming that risk estimates for this population were applicable directly to workers in radiation medicine or the nuclear industry (Fig. 1).

MSK I (Mancuso, Stewart, and Kneale) was concerned with men and women who worked at Hanford after 1943 and died before 1973, and the first finding was that, at two very low-dose levels (one for males and the other for females), the mean cumulative dose was significantly higher for workers whose deaths were ascribed to cancers than for other nonsurvivors. Shortly before

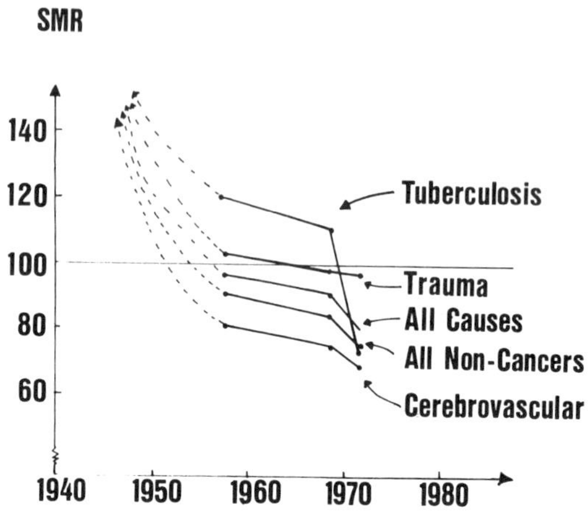

Figure 1
Mortality trends of A-bomb survivors.

this, Milham (1976) had found a high proportion of cancer deaths among the workers whose deaths were reported to the Washington State Health Department and Gilbert (1976) had found that the cancer death rate was dose related. Therefore, it only remained for us to include all certified deaths in a comparative mean dose (CMD) analysis and thus discover which types of cancer were most affected and obtain some provisional estimates of relative risk, cancer latency, and exposure age.

The first test of these estimates was made by ourselves (Kneale et al. 1978) (see MSK II in Table 1) after we had:

1. achieved a separation between workers with zero doses and workers who were not issued film badges;
2. identified a larger sample of deaths (1944-1977);
3. discovered that in relation to Hanford data a CMD analysis had at least four times the power of a conventional standardized mortality ratio (SMR) analysis;
4. found that an independent classification of tissue sensitivity to cancer induction by radiation existed (ICRP 1969) which made it possible to

Table 1
MSK Analyses of Hanford Data

MSK series	Published reports	Data base
I	Mancuso et al. (1977)	1944-1972 deaths
II	Kneale et al. (1978)	1944-1977 deaths
	Stewart et al. (1980)	
III	Kneale et al. (1981)	1944-1977 deaths and 1944-1978 survivors

Table 2
Specifications of A and B Cancers Included in MSK III

Group	Tissue	ICD numbers (8th rev.)	Cases[a] male	Cases[a] female
A cancers				
(sensitive tissues)	pharynx	145-149	10	–
	digestive	150-159	201	19
	respiratory	160-163	215	10
	female breast	174	–	19
	thyroid	193	1	–
	hemopoietic	200-209	76	10
		remainder		
B cancers				
(other tissues)	other sites	140-209	199	28
	other unspecified	195-199	41	3

[a]Excluding cases that were never issued film badges.

work with only two cancer groups, namely, cancers of sensitive and insensitive tissues (so-called A and B cancers, see Table 2);

5. obtained a nonskewed distribution of the film-badge doses by fitting them to a scale of natural logarithms (Fig. 2); and
6. devised a scale of bioassay levels for use in distinguishing between safe and dangerous occupations (Table 3).

The main findings of MSK II have been available since 1978. They include evidence of a radiation effect for cancers in a Mantel-Haenszel analysis of certified causes of death, higher mean cumulative doses for A than B cancers, evidence that the radiation effect for lung cancer was unlikely to be a by-product of smoking habits (Stewart et al. 1980), and signs of underreporting

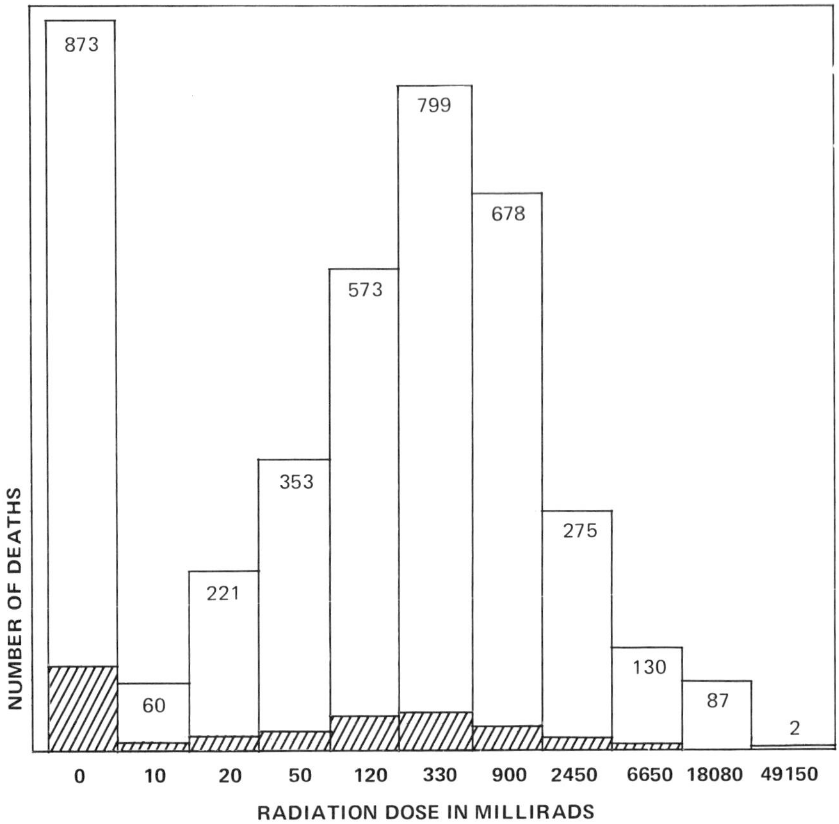

Figure 2
Log distribution of radiation doses. (▨) Females.

Table 3
Specifications of Bioassay Levels

Level	Specifications
1	no testing of urine or blood
2	tested with wholly negative findings
3	tested with false positive findings
4	either false positive findings and a whole-body count or definite evidence of internal radiation[a]

[a]Only 225 male workers were ever suspected of having an internal deposition of plutonium.

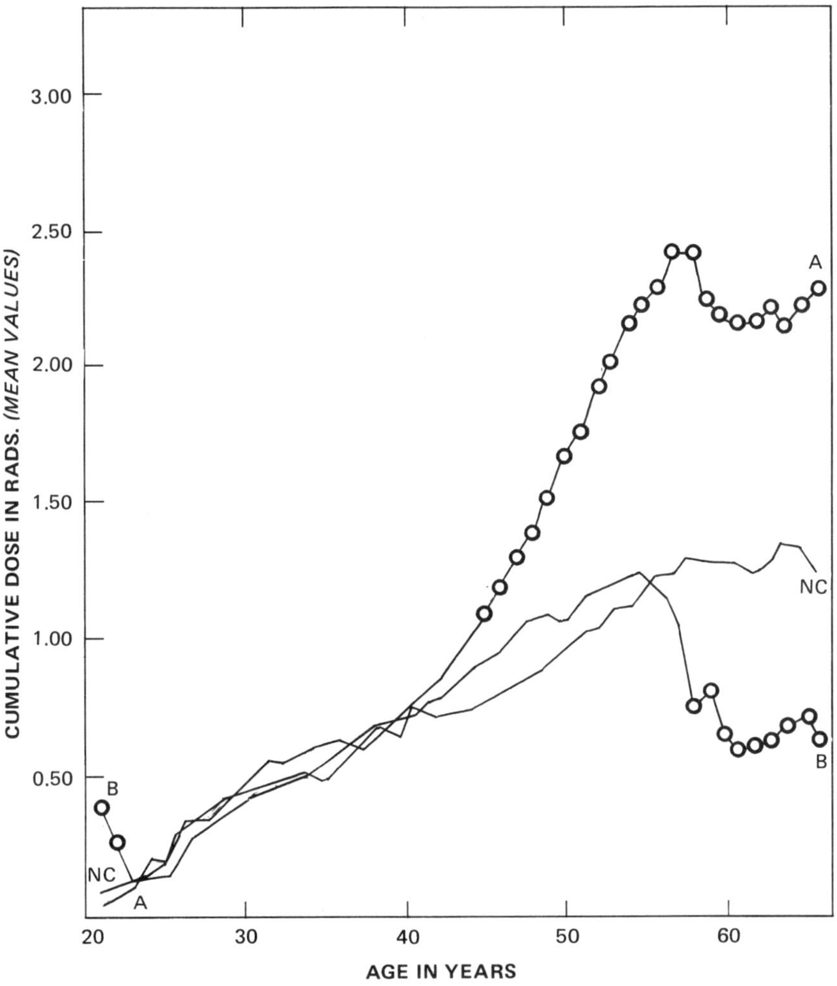

Figure 3
Age trend of cumulative radiation for the groups of male workers. (NC) Noncancers; (A) sensitive cancers; (B) other cancers; (○) any cancer dose that differs by a significant amount from the corresponding dose for noncancers.

of cancers after 56 years of age with more involvement of B than A cancers in the underreporting (Fig. 3).

Nevertheless, there remained two unsolved problems: (1) Even after standardization for sex, dates of birth, and hire, and employment period, the mean cumulative dose was higher for live than dead workers and (2) also higher for noncancer deaths than B cancers (Table 4). The difference between live and

Table 4
Radiation Doses of Live and Dead Workers

Group	All workers	Never monitored	Mean radiation dose in rads
Alive in 1977	29,251	5,486	2.03
1944-1977 deaths			
A cancers	754	193	1.77
B cancers	371	100	0.87
Noncancers	4,472	1,107	1.18
All deaths	5,597	1,400	1.24

dead workers was well known to us, as were the following facts: The first difference (between live and dead workers) was much reduced by having as one of the controlling variables a three-point scale of bioassay levels (Mancuso et al. 1977), and for Hanford workers the risk of dying from natural causes was 25% below the national average (Marks and Gilbert 1978). These findings were suggestive of selective recruitment of workers who combined exceptional health with being born less than 25 years before Hanford began to manufacture plutonium (1944) and obtaining jobs either as production managers or operatives.

A test of this hypothesis required for each occupation a healthy-worker scale (i.e., a scale that measured relative levels of general mortality) as well as a classification of occupations that separated production workers from supporting staff and separated highly paid workers from lowly paid workers. This required a long period of preparation for the following reasons. Although there had been coding of Hanford jobs (according to the 1970 Census classification), there had been little or no supervision of this work, which was error prone, because there was no flagging of production workers in the original records and no clear distinction between these workers and supporting staff in the Census classification. Furthermore, workers often changed their jobs and this made it extremely difficult to be sure that even the most obvious mistakes had been fully corrected. However, after months of screening for punching and coding errors, there finally emerged an occupational classification that had separate positions for production workers and supporting staff at two salary levels (Table 5). A healthy-worker scale, based on all certified deaths, could then be used to show the effects on general mortality of working for 1 year in each of the occupational groups. Thus, we have discovered that, at Hanford, the healthy-worker effect is positively correlated with radiation dose.

Though MSK III is not yet in print (Kneale et al. 1981), the analysis predated the search for errors in the recording of occupations and, therefore, had as the only indication of the work being done by individuals, the four-point

Table 5
Job Specifications of Hanford Workers Related to Dose and Fitness Levels

Job specifications	Mean dose in centirads	Fitness levels index	Fitness levels rank
Producers			
Scientists	14.2	-2.41	1
Technicians	35.1	-1.50	2
Operatives	46.1	-0.17	4
Supporting staff			
Managers	22.0	-0.46	3
Clerical	3.4	+0.56	5
Others	6.2	+0.95	6

Table 6
MSK III Summary Statistics

Controlling factors: usual	Controlling factors: extra	*t* values: All deaths	*t* values: A cancers
Sex and date of birth Date of hire Employment period	nil	-3.59[a]	0.33
	bioassay levels	-0.48	2.47[a]
	job fitness levels	-0.61	1.69
	job fitness levels exposure age latency		2.63[a]

[a]Significant at the 5% level.

scale of bioassay levels in Table 3. Originally, we had intended this measure to be a temporary expedient, but we are now reasonably certain that the bioassay data are reliable, as well as convenient, guides to the dangerousness of work at Hanford. We can say this because in the MSK III test of the null hypothesis (of no radiation effect for cancers of sensitive tissues) the temporary expedient proved to be a better indicator of the healthy worker effect than even the revised occupational classification (Table 6).

The statistical procedures used in MSK III, which are illustrated in Figure 4 and Table 7, were developed from first principles by George Kneale. But essentially the same method had already been developed by Cox for the express purpose of measuring the beneficial effects of drugs in a therapeutic trial (Cox 1972). When the procedures are applied to Hanford data without control for

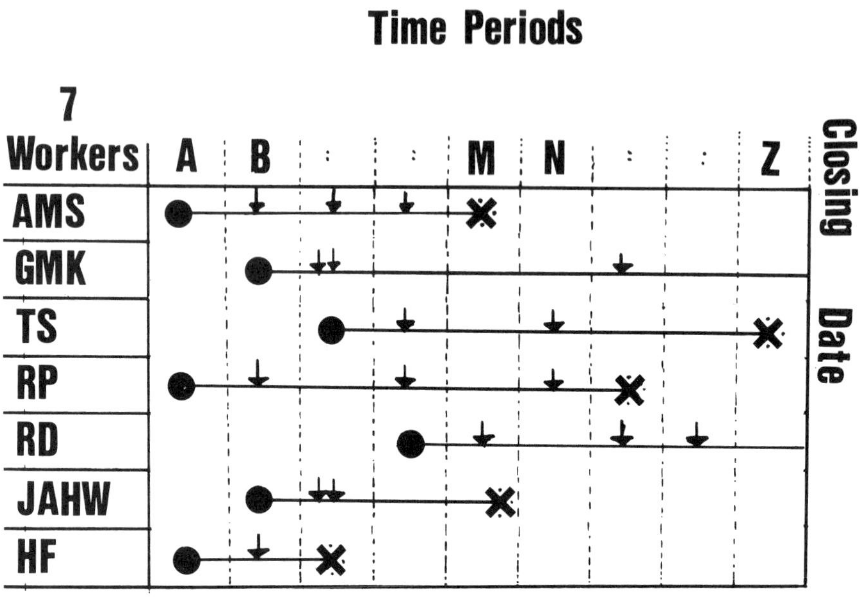

Figure 4
Follow-up of hypothetical study subgroup. (•) Hire; (ẋ·) death; (↓) exposure.

Table 7
Statistics Relating to Hypothetical Study Subgroup Described in Figure 4

		Cumulative exposures by start of period			
Period	Quantity	0	1	2	3
A-L	–	–	–	–	–
M	At risk	1	1	3	1
	Deaths observed	0	0	1	1
	Deaths expected	0.33	0.33	1.0	0.33
N-Z	–	–	–	–	–
Total	Observed	0	1	2	2
	Expected	0.74	1.18	1.83	1.25

bioassay levels or job specifications, literal interpretation of the findings requires the radiation to have unbelievably strong life-saving effects. But with either of these factors as a controlling variable, the method produces definite evidence of a radiation effect for A cancers (Table 6). Therefore we were free to apply

Table 8
Results of Model Testing after Confirming a Radiation Effect

Radiation effects	Maximum likelihood estimate
Dose response (E)	nonlinear, with $E = 0.5$ ($E = 1.0$ rejected at the 1% level)
Doubling dose (D)	$D = 15$ rads with 95%; confidence interval of 2-150 rads
Latency (L)	where L = interval between cancer induction and death $L = 25$ years (type of cancer not specified)
Exposure age (S)	where S = the age increase needed to increase sensitivity to cancer induction by e (the base of natural logarithms); $S = 8$ years ($S = \infty$ rejected at 1% level)

maximum likelihood theory to our data with the results shown in Table 8. According to these results, there is (1) nonlinearity of dose response, with the curve obeying the square root law, (2) a cancer latency effect with an optimal interval of 25 years, and (3) an exposure age effect which implies that a 40-year-old worker is twice as vulnerable (to the cancer induction effects of radiation) as a 32-year-old worker.

An opportunity to test our MSK III estimates has been provided by a follow-up of 1110 women who worked in the radium luminizing industry in World War II and were still alive in 1961 (Baverstock et al. 1981). During the next 16 years, there was a significant excess of deaths from breast cancer (16 observed and 10.2 expected) that was largely the result of women who were under 30 years of age when first exposed, who had an average absorbed dose of 51 rads of gamma radiation, and who died between 1971 and 1977 (high-risk group with 10 observed and 3.05 expected deaths). Therefore, it is possible to calculate the MSK III risk for a typical woman in the high-risk group, i.e., a woman who (1) worked from 1940-1945 and was 26 years of age in 1940, (2) had a mean absorbed dose of 50 rads in equal amounts each year, and (3) died from a breast cancer in 1972 (Table 9). For this hypothetical worker, the actual dose (50 rads) was much higher than the cancer-effective dose (14.6 rads), but even so the extra risk was equal to 98% of the normal risk. Because this estimate of relative risk is much lower than the ratio of observed to expected deaths (3.28), there is no question of the MSK III estimate exaggerating the cancer effect of the gamma radiation, though we are left with the possibility that, in females, the rule of low sensitivity (to cancer induction) between 20 and 30 years of age does not apply to breast tissue.

Other examples of how cancer-effective doses can be derived from actual doses are shown in Tables 10-12. To these we have added two tables that show,

Table 9
Application of Hanford Estimates to Individuals: A Typical Radium Luminizer

Year	Age[a]	Dose in rads actual	Dose in rads transformed	Relative risk
1940	26	8.5	1.7	
1941	27	8.5	2.0	
1942	28	8.5	2.2	
1943	29	8.5	2.5	
1944	30	8.5	2.9	
1945	31	8.5	3.3	
Total		51.0	14.6	1.98

After Baverstock et al. (1981).
[a]Age at death–58 years; cause of death–breast cancer.

Table 10
Application of Hanford Estimates to Individuals: A Process Worker at Hanford

Year	Age[a]	Dose in rads actual	Dose in rads transformed	Relative risk
1960	41	0.9	0.8	
1961	42	2.3	2.3	
1962	43	2.5	2.7	
1963	44	1.5	2.0	
1964	45	2.0	2.3	
1965	46	5.1	6.1	
1966	47	4.4	5.3	
Total		18.7	21.5	2.20

[a]Age at death–53; cause of death–stomach cancer.

Table 11
Application of Hanford Estimates to Individuals: A Process Worker at Windscale

Year	Age[a]	Dose in rads actual	Dose in rads transformed	Relative risk
1951-1955	31-35	32.4	15.4	
1956-1960	36-40	32.9	24.8	
1961-1965	41-45	22.8	29.8	
1966-1970	46-50	21.9	43.3	
1971-1975	51-55	29.5	63.2	
Total		139.6	176.5	4.0

[a]Age at death–56 years; cause of death–pancreatic cancer.

Table 12
Application of Hanford Estimates to Individuals: A Chargehand at Windscale

Year	Age[a]	Dose in rads		Relative risk
		actual	transformed	
1959-1963	38-42	14.3	14.0	
1964-1968	43-47	15.9	27.3	
1969-1973	48-52	22.4	51.9	
1974-1978	53-57	15.4	36.0	
1979	58	1.8	1.8	
Total		69.8	131.0	4.0

[a]Age at death–59 years; cause of death–lung cancer.

first, that cancer mortality in 329 Japanese cities was related to background radiation (Ujeno 1978) (Table 13) and, second, what proportion of A cancers would be caused by a background radiation dose of 0.1 rads per annum if the mortality experiences of Hanford workers have been correctly interpreted in MSK III (Table 14).

Finally, everyone who has had an opportunity to examine Hanford data, including Darby and Reissland (1981), has found evidence of higher doses for noncancer deaths than B cancers. Therefore it should be noted that, in MSK III, inclusion of place of death among the controlling variables and exclusion of two groups of sudden death (myocardial infarction and accidents) left the positive findings for A cancers unchanged and removed the negative findings for B cancers (Kneale et al. 1981). Since writing this paper, we have examined the records relating to primary and secondary causes of death of Hanford workers and thus discovered how the cancers that do not feature in any analysis

Table 13
Cancer Mortality and Background Radiation in 329 Japanese cities

Sex	Background radiation	Cancer mortality[a]
Males	under 60	753
	60-79	839
	80-99	840
	100+	868
Females	under 60	464
	60-79	541
	80-99	554
	100+	567

Data from Ujeno (1978).
[a]Deaths over 40 years in the period 1969-1970.

Table 14
Background Radiation (0.1 rads per annum) and Cancers of Sensitive Tissues

Death age	Cumulative dose: actual	Cumulative dose: transformed	Radiogenic[a] cases (%)
40	4.0	2.6	30
45	4.5	2.8	31
50	5.0	3.3	32
55	5.5	4.2	35
60	6.0	6.8	40
65	6.5	9.9	45
70	7.0	15.0	50

Sensitive tissues include digestive, hemopoetic, respiratory, and breast.
[a]As proportion of all sensitive cancers.

Table 15
Certified and Uncertified Cancers: Age at Death

Age (years)	Cancers: certified (%)	Cancers: uncertified (%)
Under 50	15.3	2.4
50-59	26.1	7.1
60-69	37.3	27.4
70+	21.3	63.1
Number of cases	743	84

Table 16
Certified and Uncertified Cancers: Cancer Sites

Cancers	Certified (%)	Uncertified (%)
Prostate	7.0	22.6
Other B cancers	21.8	15.5
A cancers	71.2	61.9

of Hanford data (because they were not certified causes of death) differ from the certified cases. The uncertified cases were distinctly older than the certified ones (Table 15). They were also biased in favor of prostate cancer and other cancers of insensitive tissues (Table 16) and the commonest cause of death was a cardiovascular disease (Table 17). Therefore, the fact that all investigators have recorded negative findings for B cancers is probably an artefact caused by

Table 17
Certified and Uncertified Cancers: Stated Cause of Death

	Uncertified cancers		Other
D/C diagnosis	prostate (%)	other (%)	deaths
Cardiovascular	73.7	´9.2	65.5
Other causes	26.3	,8	34.5

underreporting of nonfatal cancers whose effects included high blood pressure and other damage to the cardiovascular system.

Other Analyses of Hanford Data

According to Hutchinson et al. (1979) "the excess proportional mortality [of Hanford workers] at doses above 10 rems for cancer of pancreas and multiple myeloma is likely to be explainable in terms of a correlate of dose rather than in terms of radiation." Equally lame conclusions have been drawn by other investigators, but they are probably the result of using methods that were capable of recognizing some but not all the effects of Hanford exposures. For example, critics of our findings have always insisted upon using the International Classification of Diseases (ICD) classification of cancers. This classification makes no concessions to radiosensitivity. Therefore, without reference to the ICRP classification of tissue sensitivity (ICRP 1969), one is left either with groups that are too small to draw firm conclusions or consist of a mixture of sensitive and insensitive cancers. In view of everyone's findings for group-B cancers, this is peculiarly unfortunate.

The idea that Hanford workers are exceptionally healthy is not a new one. However, the possibility of differences between production workers and supporting staff has been overlooked by our critics, as has also the possibility that (because the nuclear industry has only been in existence for 36 years) the long-term consequences of these differences are still in the future. But the main reasons for finding excuses for all findings that smack of a cancer effect from the Hanford exposures can be found in Atomic Bomb Casualty Commission (ABCC) publications relating to A-bomb survivors who were still alive in October 1950.

Both the study population of Hanford workers and the study population of A-bomb survivors are biased in favor of disease-resistant persons. But for Hanford workers, the selection predated the exposures (healthy-worker effect) and for A-bomb survivors it was radiation-induced (survival of the fittest). Therefore, detection of delayed effects of Hanford exposures is much easier than detection of delayed effects of A-bomb radiation. In ABCC data, the selection effects are so strongly correlated with dose levels that a relative risk analysis of 1950-1974 deaths failed to recognize any extra noncancer deaths apart from blood diseases (Beebe et al. 1977). However, there must have been many deaths due to nonstochastic effects of the radiation after, as well as before, 1950 because an SMR analysis of 1950-1972 deaths (Moriyama and Kato 1973) disclosed the significant differences between A-bomb survivors and other Japanese citizens (which are here depicted in Fig. 1).

SUMMARY

Following the discovery of relatively high doses for Hanford workers who subsequently died from cancer, Mancuso, Stewart, and Kneale first established a connection between this finding and tissues that are sensitive to cancer induction by radiation and then used the method of regression models in life tables to show (1) that for cancers of these tissues there was nonlinearity of dose-response (with the curve obeying the square root law), (2) that the cancer risk increased progressively with adult age (doubling of the risk every 8 years), (3) that the commonest interval between induction and death was 25 years, and (4) that for a man aged 40 years the doubling dose was 15 rads (with a 95% confidence interval of 2-150 rads).

ACKNOWLEDGMENTS

The latest analysis of Hanford data was financed by the Environmental Policy Institute, 317 Pennsylvania Avenue, SE, Washington D.C. 20003. Earlier analyses and the cost of data collection were supported by the Division of Biology and Medicine, and Division of Occupational Safety of the former Atomic Energy Commission, AEC Contract No. AT (30-1)-3394 and No. C11-AT(11-1)-3428, and ERDA Contract No. E(11-1)-3428.

REFERENCES

Baverstock, K.F., D. Papworth, and J. Vennart. 1981. Risks of radiation at low dose rates. *Lancet* i:430.

Beebe, G.W., H. Kato, and C.E. Land. 1977. *Mortality experience of atomic bomb survivors 1950-74. Life span study report 8.* RERF TR 1-77. U.S. National Academy of Sciences, Washington D.C.

Cox, D.R. 1972. Regression models and life-tables. *J. Roy. Stat. Soc. B34* 2:187.

Darby, S.C. and J.A. Reissland. 1981. Low levels of ionising radiation and cancer–Are we underestimating the risk? *J. Roy. Stat. Soc.* (in press).

General Accounting Office (GAO). 1981. *Problems in assessing the cancer risks of low-level ionizing radiation exposure.* General Accounting Office, Gaithersburg, Maryland.

Gilbert, E.S. 1976. *Proportional mortality analysis of Hanford deaths–Progress report.* Battelle Memorial Institute, Pacific Northwest Laboratory, Richland, Washington.

Hutchinson, G.B., B. MacMahon, S. Jablon, and C.E. Land. 1979. Review of report by Mancuso, Stewart & Kneale of radiation exposure of Hanford workers. *Health Phys.* **37**:207.

International Commission on Radiological Protection (ICRP). 1969. Radiosensitivity and spatial distribution of dose. In *Annals of the ICRP.* Publ. 14. Pergamon Press, Oxford.

Kneale, G.W. and A.M. Stewart. 1976a. M-H analysis of Oxford data. I. Independent effects of several birth factors including fetal irradiation. *J. Natl. Cancer Inst.* **56**:879.

_____. 1976b. M-H analysis of Oxford data. II. Independent effects of fetal irradiation subfactors. *J. Natl. Cancer Inst.* **57**:1009.

Kneale, G.W., T.F. Mancuso, and A.M. Stewart. 1981. Hanford radiation studies III: A cohort study of the cancer risks from radiation to workers at Hanford (1944 to 1977 deaths) by the method of regression models in life-tables. *Br. J. Ind. Med.* **38**:156.

_____. 1978. Re-analysis of data relating to the Hanford study of the cancer risks of radiation workers. *IAEA Proc. Ser.* **1**:387.

Kneale, G.W., A.M. Stewart, and T.F. Mancuso. 1979. Radiation exposures of Hanford workers dying from cancer and other causes. *Health Phys.* **36**:87.

Mancuso, T., A. Stewart, and G. Kneale. 1977. Radiation exposures of Hanford workers dying from cancer and other causes. *Health Phys.* **33**:364.

_____. 1976. *Radiation exposures of Hanford workers dying from various causes.* Paper presented at 10th Mid-Year Topical Symposium of the Health Physics Society. Proceedings of Saratoga Springs, October 1976, p. 204. Rensselaer Polytechnic Institute, Troy, New York.

Marks, S. and E.S. Gilbert. 1978. Cancer mortality in Hanford workers. *IAEA Proc.*, Ser. **1**:369.

Milham, S. 1976. *Occupational mortality in Washington state 1950-71.* HEW Publ. no. (NIOSH 76-175).

Moriyama, I.M. and H. Kato. 1973. *Mortality experience of A-bomb survivors 1970-72, 1950-72. Atomic Bomb Casualty Commission life span study report 7*, Japanese National Institute of Health. RERF TR 15-73.

Stewart, A.M., G.W. Kneale, and T.F. Mancuso. 1980. Hanford IIB. The Hanford data—A reply to recent criticisms. *Ambio* **9**:66.

Ujeno, Y. 1978. Carcinogenic hazard from natural background radiation in Japan. *J. Radiat. Res.* **19**:205.

APPENDIX: EXACT ESTIMATES OF JOB-ASSOCIATED HEALTH RISKS

Let cohorts be indexed by g and let age be indexed by a, so that P_{ag} = probability of dying at age a in cohort g. Let workers be indexed by i; let d_i = 1 if worker i is dead, 0 otherwise. Let jobs be indexed by k and j; let N_{ika} = total number of years (not necessarily consecutive) for which worker i

has held job k by time he has reached age a. Let r_k = health index of job k be so defined that if

$$S_{ia} \ (= \sum_k N_{ika} r_k) \tag{1}$$

is cumulative health index score of worker i by age a, then corrected probability of dying (taking into account special risks of jobs and also any special healthy-worker effects due to selective recruitment) is given by

$$P_{ag}\exp(S_{ia}) / [1 + P_{ag}\exp(S_{ia}) - P_{ag}], \tag{2}$$

or in other words S_{ia} is the change in the logit of the probability of dying. Then it can be shown by Cox's method of regression models in life tables that if the r_k are all small compared with 1, the maximum likelihood estimates of the r_k satisfy the equation

$$\sum_k V_{kj} r_k = Y_j \tag{3}$$

where

$$V_{kj} = \sum_i [\sum_{a=1}^{A_i} N_{ika} N_{ija} P_{aG_i} (1 - P_{aG_i})] \tag{4}$$

and

$$Y_j = \sum_i [N_{ijA_i} d_i - \sum_{a=1}^{A_i} N_{ija} P_{aG_i}] \tag{5}$$

and A_i = final age of worker i and G_i = cohort of worker i.

Because of the complexity of the calculations to obtain the matrix V and the necessity to invert it, these exact estimates of health risks can only be obtained if there are fewer than about 20 jobs in the whole classification of jobs. On the other hand, the approximate method can deal with several thousand jobs at once.

COMMENTS

NICHOLSON: One thing that bears upon the former presentation as well as yours is the method of follow-up. If you rely on Social Security, there may be deaths occurring, particularly before 1967, that were unknown to the system. This might have a greater effect on workers with short employment periods than other workers and thus give rise to what was seen by Darby as a healthy-worker effect of a significant magnitude throughout the exposed group. Can you make a comment about how it might affect what you would do? And would it also be greater for women than for men?

STEWART: I think the point about the healthy-worker effect is that it would be important if we had compared Hanford workers with an outside population as was done by Darby.

NICHOLSON: But how about "lost to follow-up."

STEWART: This too is unimportant for a survey that relies upon internal comparisons. Nevertheless, it is true that there are two subgroups of unidentified deaths not identified.

R. PETO: Your standardization procedures included a factor that changed with time, i.e., the bioassay factor, but this is not permissible in a life-table analysis. In a proper life-table analysis standardized for the monitoring of individuals, an individual whose monitoring status changes at a certain point in time should contribute to all contingency tables relating to previous times and as a monitored individual to all subsequent tables. One person's category is not fixed, but variable in time, and the only way to avoid bias is to take this variation into account in your analysis. You cannot categorize people by what may happen to them in the future or serious biases may be engendered.

STEWART: We had this difficulty pointed out to us before. The best sensitive index is something like the final stage of this thing because you are going to be at risk for a time before you actually show positive results in a testing. But this point has been taken, and of course doesn't apply to the job classification. Those are just your man-years in the job. I believe George can explain this to you in detail.[1]

[1] Following private discussion between G. Kneale and R. Peto, they jointly wrote the following statement: Because the various groups analyzing the Hanford data now have adopted statistical methods which in principle resemble each other, their conclusions should ultimately converge, if they apply their methods to the same set of data.

George Kneale has recently been working with a set of data including all deaths up to mid-1977, while Sarah Darby has been working with a set of data that include only deaths up to mid-1974. Moreover, Kneale has standardized for a detailed measure of job category (see below) before estimating the role of radiation, while Darby has not. Both Kneale and Darby agree that the relationship of myelomatosis to dose is highly significant statistically. Unless this finding is due to some other cause of myeloma in the chemical manipulation of the various components of the nuclear fuel cycle, it indicates that some of the cases of myeloma are radiogenic, a conclusion supported by the recent Cuzick (1981) article.

Moreover, although the suggestive excess of "A-cancers" other than myeloma found in Kneale's most recent analysis is not statistically significant, this does not imply that none of these cases of "A-cancers" were radiogenic. For example, one or two of the pancreatic cancers among men exposed to more than 10 rems might well have been radiogenic. (After standardization by a Cox-type model for calendar year of death, sex, age at hire, length of continuous employment, and job fitness by indices which, in contrast with those used by Stewart and Kneale previously (1981) varied with time, and depended logistically on job hazard the t-value for the "A-cancers," including myelomatosis, was +1.8, indicating somewhat more cases among irradiated workers; the t-value for the "B-cancers" was −2.7; the t-value for the aggregate of all A or B cancers was approximately zero.)

It would be particularly desirable, in the interests of resolving the previous divergence of interpretations, for the National Radiological Protection Board to be willing to analyze exactly the same data that Stewart and Kneale have studied, rather than to continue to obtain their data from different sources.

J. PETO: Did you standardize for the period since first employed or not?

STEWART: Yes, also for sex, date of hire, and either bioassay level or general mortality rating (fitness rating).

KNEALE: I should make it clear that the diagram relating to seven people was supposed to be one of the 480 cohorts. Also note that the Cox methodology is just a minor generalization of your own log-rank tests for testing differences between drugs in clinical trials. The only difference is that workers have radiation exposures through their employment years and patients usually have only short treatment periods. There might be a spread of about 5 years for each subset.

R. PETO: Apart from your bioassay standardization, your analysis seems to be virtually the same as that of Sarah Darby. Why are the findings so different?

STEWART: Did you notice that she was working with 400 deaths from the years 1944-1972 and we with 1100 deaths from the years 1944-1977?

WAXWEILER: Were all your comparisons among monitored workers?

STEWART: Yes, monitored for external radiation, that is.

WAXWEILER: I think this is an important point to make, because what we found in the Portsmouth nuclear shipyard was that there was an ultrahealthy-worker effect. There was a double selection. First, there was a selection to get into the shipyard and, second, selection to become a monitored worker.

STEWART: We think that is happening in Hanford.

MILHAM: I now have all deaths through 1979 in Hanford workers who died in Washington State. The pancreatic cancer excess is still there. There has been no change over time in the RR. There is the same ratio of observed to expected now as men dying, say, between 1950 and 1960. For men dying between ages 45 to 49 of bowel cancer, there are six deaths observed to one expected. I don't know what that means yet.

As you well know, a lot of men worked at Hanford who aren't in your file. J. A. Jones, the construction group, had fairly heavy radiation exposures and these people are not in the data set. I wish they were.

ACHESON: Could I ask for clarification about cases of cancer that were not the cause of death? Are we talking about registered cases on a cancer register or are we talking about cancers in part 2 of the death certificate?

STEWART: Part 2.

ENTERLINE: I would like to make an observation that Hanford is one of the few studies that I know of where two research teams are studying the same population almost totally independently of each other—separate clearance with Social Security, separate procuring of death certificates, and so on.

My question is related to hidden prostatic cancers. Were you implying that if they had been coded as cancer, there would have been a dose effect?

STEWART: I can't say that for certain.

ENTERLINE: Would you be able to do so eventually?

STEWART: Yes.

BLOT: The interesting aspect of Dr. Darby's presentation was the excess of myeloma, which I think is intriguing in view of the Windscale findings and in view of the recent evidence from Japan that myeloma is indeed a high-dose radiation effect.

You mentioned that you are dealing with something like 1100 deaths, whereas Dr. Darby had 400 deaths. So you obviously must have a much bigger cohort. If you take Dr. Darby's finding as a hypothesis, i.e., that myeloma is increased, can you use the additional information you have, whether it is in terms of follow-up or whatever it is that causes more deaths, to test that hypothesis in this particular data set?

In other words, can you use part of this large data set to test an hypothesis generated by another part?

STEWART: It isn't true that all data collecting processes were different. They were in fact the same but I don't know exactly what was or was not included on the tape sent to Darby by the DOE.

ENTERLINE: You never matched the two tapes?

STEWART: Well, not in detail, but they must be much the same. All the dose data come from the same source (Hanford) and all the death benefit claims come from the same source (Social Security).

DARBY: I'd like to comment on this presentation. The paper presented by Dr. Stewart at this meeting discusses the third analysis of mortality in the Hanford work force that has been carried out by MSK. In their first analysis, based on deaths that occurred between 1944 and 1972, MSK reported that fatal malignancies were induced in radiosensitive tissues with a much higher frequency per unit radiation dose than was accepted generally. It was also estimated that 6% of all cancers and 1% of all certified deaths among Hanford workers were radiation-induced, and doubling doses were given for some tumors that would be less than cumulative background exposure for most workers. The authors rightly asserted that these estimates differed from the recommendations of the ICRP by an order of magnitude. MSK's second analysis was based on deaths that occurred between 1944 and 1977, and it was reported that approximately 5% of the cancer deaths of Hanford workers were radiation-induced. Somewhat higher doubling doses were quoted in this analysis than previously, although they still differed from the ICRP estimates by an order of magnitude, and a RR for all cancers of 1.26 was estimated for those with doses of 5.11 rads or more. The third MSK analysis is also based on mortality between 1944 and 1977, but the conclusions reached in it differ somewhat from those reached in the previous analyses. This latest analysis finds no evidence of radiation-related effects when deaths from all causes are considered together, and it makes no claim to find excesses when deaths from all types of cancer are taken as a single group; any excesses are found to be confined to a particular group of cancers.

The methodology used in this latest analysis also differs from that used in the previous two in that available information on members of the work force who survived to the end of the follow-up period is taken into account together with information on those who have died. This methodology is actually very similar to that used by ourselves (Darby and Reissland, in this volume) and others (Gilbert and Marks 1979, 1980), despite initial appearances to the contrary due to the differing nomenclature and somewhat unusual presentation used by the MSK team. The change in methodological approach allows for more detailed comparison among the various analyses and their corresponding conclusions. Thus, there now seems to be a general consensus of opinion that there is no evidence of radiation-related excesses when considering either mortality from all causes or from all cancers when taken as a single group.

There are however, still important differences between the conclusions reached in the third MSK analysis and other analyses of the Hanford data. These are due chiefly to the different controlling factors used. The extreme sensitivity of analyses of this type of data to the controlling factors is well illustrated in Table 6 of Mancuso et al. (this volume). Here it can be seen that there is only evidence of an excess of type A cancers when either bioassay level or a combination of job fitness levels, exposure age, and latency are included among the controlling factors. The various bioassay levels are specified in Table 3 of Mancuso et al. (this volume) and represent levels of monitoring for internal contamination. On general grounds, it seems likely that those who are more thoroughly monitored for internal contamination are likely to be those who work in contaminated areas of the plant and consequently are likely to be exposed to higher levels of external radiation. Hence, it is to be expected that there is a strong correlation between the bioassay level and external radiation dose. This expectation is confirmed in Table 2 of Kneale et al. (1981). Thus, the inclusion of bioassay level as a controlling factor is to a large extent controlling for radiation dose because those at bioassay level 4 (which includes almost everyone in the highest external dose categories) are not then compared with those at bioassay level 1 (which includes the majority of those in the lowest external dose category). The implications of including such a variable as a controlling factor are unclear as it potentially obscures a large part of the relevant information. An additional difficulty is that each worker is classified right from the start of his employment by the highest level of bioassay that he will ever reach, rather than progressing through the bioassay levels changing at the appropriate dates (see Kneale et al. 1981 for details). By comparing the results given in Table 7 of Mancuso et al. (this volume) with the results given in Kneale et al. (1981), it seems clear that bioassay level has been included as a controlling factor throughout the model-fitting procedure used in this latest paper and thus casts doubt upon many of its conclusions.

The original justification for using bioassay level as a controlling factor given in Stewart et al. (1980) was that it distinguished between safe and dangerous occupations, and in Kneale et al. (1981) it was claimed that switching from using bioassay levels to a job hazard index would have made very little difference to the results. Table 6 of Mancuso et al. (this volume) indicates that this claim was not entirely justified because the inclusion of job fitness instead of bioassay levels as a controlling factor now gives a test statistic for A cancers that is not significant at the 5% level, and it is only when exposure age and latency are also included as controlling factors that the test statistic for A cancers again becomes significant. Clearly job fitness, latency, and exposure age are potentially useful factors to control for in an analysis of this type. It would be interesting to see the full details of how the job fitness index has been constructed and also how exposure age and latency were taken into account. Unfortunately these details have not been given in their paper. Obviously, it is unacceptable to continue to add further controlling factors until a significant result is achieved. Therefore, before accepting the significant result in the bottom line of Table 6 it is particularly important to know how the decision to include these extra factors was reached.

References

Cuzick, J. 1981. Radiation-induced myelomatosis. *N. Engl. J. Med.* **304**:204.

Gilbert, E.S. and S. Marks. 1979. An analysis of the mortality of workers in a nuclear facility. *Radiat. Res.* **79**:122.

———. 1980. An updated analysis of mortality of workers in a nuclear facility. *Radiat. Res.* **83**:740.

Kneale, G.W., T.F. Mancuso, and A.M. Stewart. 1981. Hanford radiation study III: A cohort study of the cancer risks from radiation to workers at Hanford (1944-77) deaths by the method of regression models in life-tables. *Br. J. Ind. Med.* (in press).

Stewart, A.M., G.W. Kneale, and T. Mancuso. 1980. The Hanford data—a reply to recent criticisms. *Ambio* **9**:66.

Radon Daughters in the Induction of Lung Cancer in Underground Miners

EDWARD P. RADFORD
Center for Environmental Epidemiology
Graduate School of Public Health
University of Pittsburgh
Pittsburgh, Pennsylvania 15261

Work in underground mines was the first occupation found to be associated with lung cancer (Arnstein 1913), but recognition of the relationship of this cancer to radioactivity in the mines was not achieved until some years later (Uhlig 1921). As in the case of many occupational cancers, resistance to identification of the causative agent was encountered (Lorenz 1944). Hueper reports that in 1948, when he attempted to establish a register of uranium ore miners and millers on the Colorado Plateau for an epidemiological study of the lung cancer hazard, government officials claimed that "scientists recommending such fact-finding epidemiologic procedures in Colorado were displaying 'bad scientific judgment' and deserved to be dismissed from the government service. They insisted, moreover, that any mentioning of the extensive experiences made since 1879 on occupational lung cancer hazards in Saxon and Bohemian radioactive mines in Schneeberg and Joachimsthal at medical conferences be suppressed as not being in the 'public interest' " (Hueper 1966).

Although the climate for epidemiologic investigation of occupational cancers has improved somewhat since that time, even in the case of exposure to a bronchial carcinogen as well established as radon daughters, epidemiologic investigations still are not properly supported nor prosecuted. For example, the Ontario uranium miners constitute a group unsurpassed in terms of opportunities to elucidate some of the important issues still outstanding concerning the epidemiology of bronchial cancer induced in miners by radon daughters: Air measurements have been carried out since the mines opened, radon daughter concentrations range from low to high, the number of miners at risk is over 15,000, and Canadian officials already have been alerted to this problem by the "epidemic" of lung cancer cases in the St. Lawrence, Newfoundland, fluorspar miners (deVilliers et al. 1971). Yet, the only report of lung cancer experience in these miners, published 5 years ago (Ham 1976), is so incomplete epidemiologically that only limited conclusions concerning factors associated with risk can be drawn; it is impossible to derive quantitative risk estimates from the evidence presented, and the role of smoking, which surely could be studied in these miners, remains unevaluated. I cite this example because it is another case in which the agency responsible for regulation of occupational carcinogens also assumes the responsibility for epidemiologic studies of the problem. Moreover, many industry or governmental groups are often quick to say that evidence linking a particular agent to excess cancer risk in workers exposed to it is incomplete, while at the same time ignoring opportunities to set in motion studies of exposed workers under their jurisdiction that could resolve the outstanding questions.

EPIDEMIOLOGY OF LUNG CANCER IN MINERS

In the case of radon daughters, we are fortunate to have at least four mining populations that have had sufficient epidemiologic follow-up to permit assessment of dose-response relationships and quantitative expression of risk. In one of these, the historical prospective study of Swedish iron miners that I have been carrying out in collaboration with Dr. K.G.S. Renard and which is summarized briefly within, we have nearly a lifetime follow-up. Such lifetime follow-up is essential to good definition of total cancer risk when exposures are to low doses, the latent period to onset of cancer is long, and when other factors potentially involved in cancer expression may affect the latent period, such as cigarette smoking in the case of bronchial cancer.

The four mining populations are: 4146 U.S. uranium miners identified in 1950 as a result of Dr. Hueper's efforts cited above and studied prospectively since with data to 1974 (BEIR III 1980); 1118 Newfoundland fluorspar miners first identified as at high risk of lung cancer in 1959 and studied for the period 1949-1971 (BEIR III 1980); 2433 Czechoslovakian uranium miners from the Joachimsthal area studied from 1949 to 1975 (Kunz et al. 1979); and 1290 Swedish iron miners whose mortality experience has been evaluated from 1951 to 1976 (E.P. Radford and K.G.S. Renard, unpubl.). In addition to these four groups, a lung cancer excess has been reported in other underground miners exposed to radon daughters: British iron miners (Boyd et al. 1970), Ontario uranium miners (Ham 1976), and Swedish zinc miners (Axelson and Sundell 1978), but these studies do not permit adequate evaluation of dose-response relationships in quantitative terms. Nevertheless, they are important because they show that whenever mining populations exposed to even modest elevations of radon daughters have been studied, an excess risk of lung cancer has been found, even though mining conditions and the types of minerals mined vary enormously. This last fact indicates that the exposure factors common to these mining groups are the presence of elevated levels of radon daughters and nonspecific dusts and, of course, cigarette smoking.

Underground mining per se, however, does not necessarily carry a significant excess risk of lung cancer. Coal miners have only a slightly increased lung cancer rate (Crofton 1969; Rockette 1977); exposure to mineral dusts or diesel fumes occurs in coal mining, but levels of radon in coal mines have been found to be low (Lucas and Gabrysh 1966; Duggan et al. 1970). It is reasonable to conclude that other factors in mine atmospheres play at most a minor role in lung cancer induction compared to radon daughters.

In three of the four more detailed studies listed above, exposure to radon daughters has had to be determined retrospectively, a problem common to many studies of occupationally related cancers and a source of uncertainty in dose estimates. In one, however, the study of Czechoslovakian uranium miners, dose measurements of radon and later radon daughters have been made extensively in the mines for most of the period of study. In this case, there was a coefficient of variation of ±30% in individual cumulative doses, but probably much less uncertainty in the aggregated data for all miners. Thus, if we accept the Czechoslovakian data as having relatively good dosimetry and if the quantitative risk coefficients obtained in the other miner groups check closely with the Czechoslovakian data, then the cumulative dose estimates in the other studies are given additional support.

The dose rates in these four studies differ considerably. The U.S. uranium miners were exposed to very high concentrations of radon daughters prior to 1960, and have correspondingly high cumulative exposures (mean 1180 WLM[1]). The Czechoslovakian uranium miners and the Newfoundland fluorspar miners were exposed at about 10-100 WLM/year and have accumulated on average about 200-300 WLM. The Swedish iron miners accumulated on average about 5 WLM per year and have total doses of only about 90 WLM. The most recent evaluations of the relevant alpha dose to the bronchial epithelium give values of 0.3-0.8 rad per WLM (Harley and Pasternack 1972; Jacobi 1976). Thus, the average dose to the epithelium in these mining populations has ranged from about 50-500 rad, but within each study there is a wide range of doses observed.

U.S. Uranium Miners

The U.S. uranium miners followed to 1974 have shown no excess of lung cancers in the lowest dose range (0-119 WLM), but an absolute risk of lung cancer of about 8 cases/(10^6 person years • WLM) for doses up to 600 WLM, and lower risk/WLM for higher doses. In other words the dose-response curve is curvilinear downward, as would be expected for alpha radiation exposures to these higher levels. When the data for those exposed to less than 360 WLM are combined, the absolute risk in this dose range is 6 excess lung cancers/(10^6 person

[1]Working level month, a measure of cumulative exposure to radon daughters. One working level (WL) is defined as an air concentration of radon daughters giving rise to 1.3×10^5 Mev per liter of alpha radiation energy from daughter decay. One working level month (WLM) represents exposure to one WL for 170 hours, the average number of hours worked per month.

years · WLM) for person-years more than 10 years after mining began (little or no excess was found for this interval).

Early follow-up of this group found that nearly all cancers occurred in cigarette smokers, but more recently cases among the nonsmokers are starting to appear. In the smoking miners, the latent period to death from lung cancer has been relatively short, whereas for nonsmokers, it is longer–generally well after 20 years. For this reason, the risk in relation to smoking status is not yet defined in these men, and will not be until the follow-up is closer to the lifetime of the workers.

Newfoundland Fluorspar Miners

In the Newfoundland fluorspar miners, 65 deaths (27% of all deaths) from lung cancer were reported up to 1971, with only 6 among surface workers. For underground miners with more than 840 WLM cumulative dose, 19 of 26 deaths (73%) were from lung cancer, a finding reminiscent of the Joachimsthal miners several decades earlier, about half of whom died of lung cancer. The excess risk of lung cancer was dose-related. Generally, these miners were heavy smokers, yet the latent periods were longer between start of mining and death than for the U.S. miners, perhaps because of the lower dose rate from radon daughters present in these mines. The absolute risk observed for miners studied from 1949 to 1971 (excluding the first 10 yr from start of mining) is 17.7 excess lung cancer deaths/(10^6 person years · WLM), or three times as high as was found in the U.S. uranium miners.

Czechoslovakian Uranium Miners

The Czechoslovakian uranium miners have now been followed to 1975, a mean follow-up of 25 years. Kunz et al. (1979) have given a dose-response curve which is clearly curvilinear downward at doses above 300 WLM. When a straight line is fitted to the data up to 300 WLM and the first 10 years of experience are deleted, the result is an absolute risk estimate of 21-24 excess cases/(10^6 person-year · WLM), the range depending on the fraction of exposure years that should be omitted because they were within 5 years of death and thus did not contribute to cancer induction. The authors have shown that the risk per unit dose at low doses was lower when the dose was delivered over a short period (5.6 yr) than when it was delivered over a longer period (10-14 yr); in other words the lower the dose rate, the greater the risk per unit dose. (This effect of dose protraction has also been observed for bone cancer in experimental animals and man exposed to the alpha-emitter, ^{224}Ra.) This dose rate effect may account for the lower risk among the U.S. uranium miners exposed at high dose rates; neither smoking experience nor the age distribution can account for the difference observed in risk between the U.S. uranium miners and the other two groups.

Swedish Iron Miners

The study of Swedish iron miners is now nearing completion, and I shall summarize a few of the highlights. This group of miners has offered an unusual opportunity to study several aspects of the lung cancer-radon daughter problem: Unusually complete work records, low levels of exposure to radon daughters, and age-specific smoking histories obtained on a large sample of active and retired miners. The study population has been 1435 men born between 1880 and 1919, and known to be alive on January 1, 1920. The main analysis of mortality has been made from January 1, 1951 to December 31, 1976, with 1290 men alive January 1, 1951.

After 10 years from beginning mining, 50 deaths from lung cancer were observed (one death occurred less than 10 yr); of these 50 cases, 32 were in current or recent (<5 yr) smokers, and 18 never smoked or had given up smoking 18 or more years previously. Swedish national data have been used for calculating expected cases. A survey of smoking and its outcomes on a population of 55,000 Swedish citizens begun in 1963 by the Karolinska Institute of Hygiene has allowed us to determine expected rates for both smoking and nonsmoking miners.

On the minimum assumption that the miners smoked the same as the Swedish sample, the expected cases were 2.00 for nonsmokers and 12.60 for smokers, thus the relative risk (RR) was 18/2.00 = 9.00 for non-smokers and 32/12.60 = 2.54 for smokers. Absolute risk values were 16.0 cases/(10^6 person-years · WLM) for nonsmokers, and 18.5 cases/(10^6 person-years · WLM) for smokers. If we correct for the difference in proportion of smokers and the amount smoked between the miners and the Swedish sample, the observed/expected values are 18/1.67 = 10.78 for nonsmokers and 32/8.41 = 3.81 for smokers. In this case the absolute risk is 16.3/(10^6 person-years · WLM) for nonsmokers, and 22.3 cases/(10^6 person-years · WLM) for smokers.

Although the exposure dose-rate to radon daughters was lower and the follow-up longer in these Swedish miners than in the Newfoundland or Czechoslovakian miners, the results of the three studies are very close in terms of risk estimates. Of interest is the long latent period to death in these Swedish miners. An excess of lung cancer was not evident until about 25 years after the start of mining, and the mean latent period was 40 years, with little effect of smoking observed.

It is evident from the Swedish data that in this study smoking and radiation-induced effects are nearly additive. Note that these cohorts have been studied for nearly their lifetime. I believe that previous assertions of a multiplicative effect of smoking and radon daughter exposures arise as an artefact of incomplete follow-up in men exposed to high dose rates. I suspect that a similar phenomenon will be found to apply to asbestos and other respiratory carcinogens.

COMPARISON OF RISK ESTIMATES AMONG THE FOUR STUDIES

Table 1 summarizes the results of the estimates of risk per 10^6 person-years per WLM for the four studies cited above, with an approximate result obtained from the case-control study of Swedish zinc miners by Axelson and Sundell (1978). The concordance of results from the Czechoslovakian uranium miners, the Newfoundland fluorspar miners, and the Swedish iron miners is striking. This concordance lends considerable support to the dose estimates made in the latter two studies, as mentioned above. Moreover, the fact that these three studies with different follow-up periods agree as well as they do suggests that the absolute risk estimates are not likely to change with further follow-up. Results from the Swedish zinc miners are in reasonable agreement with the other studies, but the estimate of risk is less certain in this group; this small study with very long follow-up is, however, in accord with the results in the Swedish iron miners with regard to the similarity of absolute risk in smokers and nonsmokers.

The findings in the U.S. uranium miners stand out as anomalous. Either the retrospective dose calculations have been overestimates, or the effect of a higher dose rate is substantial in reducing the risk. Possibly both factors may be important in explaining the discrepancy in risk determined for this group. If the Ontario uranium miners eventually are studied adequately, these problems can be resolved.

In the Czechoslovakian, Newfoundland, and Ontario miners, an effect of age at start of mining has been demonstrated. That is, those men who have begun mining at older ages, over 35 or 40, have shown a significantly higher (2-4 times) risk of lung cancer than those whose exposure began at younger ages. This effect may also be a result of incomplete follow-up. We know that the radon-daughter induced cancers follow the rate of lung cancer observed normally by age, and the RR model appears to hold for age as a variable, even though not for smoking. For this reason, we would anticipate that any exposed population would show a steadily increasing excess number of lung cancers with age until competing risks reduced the population size. On this basis, for studies with only 20-30 years of follow-up, those who began mining at young ages are not yet in the age range where the high risk would be expected. It is significant that we have found no evidence of this effect of age at start of mining among the Swedish iron miners who have been studied on average for about 45 years since the start of mining; the absolute risk per WLM is the same for those who began mining before age 30 as for those who began later.

Table 1
Summary of Risk Estimates for Lung Cancer Induced by Radon Daughters among Mining Populations

Mining population	Time period	Reference	Excess cases per 10^6 person-years per WLM	Remarks
U.S. uranium miners ($N = 3366$)	1950-1974	BEIR III (1980)	6	exposed to high doses and dose rates; cases in nonsmokers now appearing
Czechoslovakian uranium miners ($N = 2433$)	1950-1975	Kunz et al. (1979)	21	70% smokers; markedly higher rate for those started after age 40
Newfoundland fluorspar miners ($N = 1118$)	1949-1971	BEIR III (1980)	18	high proportion of heavy smokers
Swedish zinc miners ($N \sim 150$)	1956-1970	Axelson and Sundell (1978)	~ 30	very long follow-up; nonsmokers and smokers have equivalent risk
Swedish iron miners ($N = 1290$)	1951-1976	E. P. Radford and K. G. St. Clair Renard (unpubl. results)	20	nearly lifetime follow-up; RR in nonsmokers high
			22[a]	smokers
			16	nonsmokers

[a]Smoking characteristics of miners used to correct expected rates derived from Swedish national data for mortality and smoking.

CANCER TYPE OBSERVED

For the U.S. and Czechoslovakian uranium miners, the principal types of cancers observed in excess have been epidermoid and small cell or oat cell cancers, with some excess of adenocarcinomas as well (Archer et al. 1974; Horáček et al. 1976). The proportion of excess cancers of these three types has been found to be independent of dose. Epidermoid and small cell cancers also predominated in the Swedish iron miners, and somewhat surprisingly the proportion of small cell undifferentiated cancers was independent of smoking status. Wright and Couves (1977), studying 29 Newfoundland fluorspar miners by sputum cytology, found that almost all (26 of 29) samples showed squamous cell carcinomas, an observation supporting the view that the degree of dedifferentation of these cancers may be merely a function of the stage of progression of the disease, with observations at autopsy more likely to reflect the highly anaplastic oat cell carcinomas because the cancer is more advanced at that time.

It is now evident that a significant risk of lung cancer exists from exposure to doses close to the current occupational exposure standard. The control of radon daughters in underground mines will be difficult, especially if exposure limits are reduced, as it appears they probably will have to be. In my opinion, this is a type of occupational cancer that will prove to be unusually troublesome to control in the coming years.

REFERENCES

Archer, V.E., G. Saccomanno, and J.H. Jones. 1974. Frequency of different histologic types of bronchogenic carcinoma as related to radiation exposure. *Cancer* **34**:2056.

Arnstein, A. 1913. Uber des sogenannten "Schneeberger Lungenkrebses." *Verh. d. Dtsch. Pathol. Ges.* **16**:332.

Axelson, O. and L. Sundell. 1978. Mining, lung cancer and smoking. *Scand. J. Environ. Health* **4**:46.

BEIR III. 1980. *Report of the Advisory Committee on the Biological Effects of Ionizing Radiation. The effects on populations of exposures to low levels of ionizing radiation.* National Academy of Sciences, Washington, D.C.

Boyd, J.T., R. Doll, J.S. Faulds, and J.P. Leiper. 1970. Lung cancers in iron ore (haematite) miners. *Br. J. Ind. Med.* **26**:97.

Crofton, E.C. 1969. A study of lung cancer and bronchitis mortality in relation to coal-mining in Scotland. *Br. J. Prev. Soc. Med.* **23**:141.

deVilliers, A.J., J.P. Windish, F. de N. Brent, B. Hollywood, C. Walsh, J.W. Fisher, and W.D. Parsons. 1971. Mortality experience of the community and of the fluorspar mining employees at St. Lawrence, Newfoundland. *Occup. Health Rev.* **22**:1.

Duggan, M.J., P.J. Soilleux, J.C. Strong, and D.M. Howell. 1970. The exposure of United Kingdom miners to radon. *Br. J. Ind. Med.* **27**:106.

Ham, J.M. 1976. *Report of the Royal Commission on the Health and Safety of Workers in Mines.* Ministry of the Attorney General, Province of Ontario, Toronto, Canada.

Harley, N.H. and B.S. Pasternack. 1972. Alpha absorption measurements applied to lung dose from radon daughters. *Health Phys.* **23**:771.

Horáček, J., V. Plaček, and J. Ševc. 1976. Histologic types of bronchogenic cancer in relation to different conditions of radiation exposure. *Cancer* **40**:832.

Hueper, W.C. 1966. Occupational and environmental cancers of the respiratory system. *Recent Results in Cancer Research,* p. 138. Springer-Verlag, New York.

Jacobi, W. 1976. "Interpretation of measurements in uranium mines: Dose evaluation and biomedical aspects." Proceedings of the NEA Specialist Meeting, Elliott Lake, Canada.

Kunz, E. J. Ševc, F. Plaček, and H. Horáček. 1979. Lung cancer in man in relation to different time distribution of radiation exposure. *Health Phys.* **36**:699.

Lorenz, E. 1944. Radioactivity and lung cancer: Critical review of lung cancer in miners of Schneeberg and Joachimsthal. *J. Natl. Cancer Inst.* **5**:1.

Lucas, H.F. and A.F. Gabrysh. 1966. *Radon in coal mines.* Argonne National Laboratory Report 7220.

Rockette, H. 1977. Cause specific mortality of coal miners. *J. Occup. Med.* **19**:795.

Uhlig, M. 1921. Uber den Schneeberger Lungenkrebs. *Virchows Arch. fur Pathol. Anat.* **230**:76.

Wright, E.S. and C.M. Couves. 1977. Radiation-induced carcinoma of the lung—the St. Lawrence tragedy. *J. Thorac. Cardiovasc. Surg.* **74**:495.

COMMENTS

RADFORD: I will draw a graph on the board, more to provoke discussion than anything else. Here is what I think the story is comparing smokers and nonsmokers. This is the difference in latent period, or time to tumor, I suppose is a better term, between smokers and nonsmokers. If you plot the mean difference against dose rate, the results are as follows:

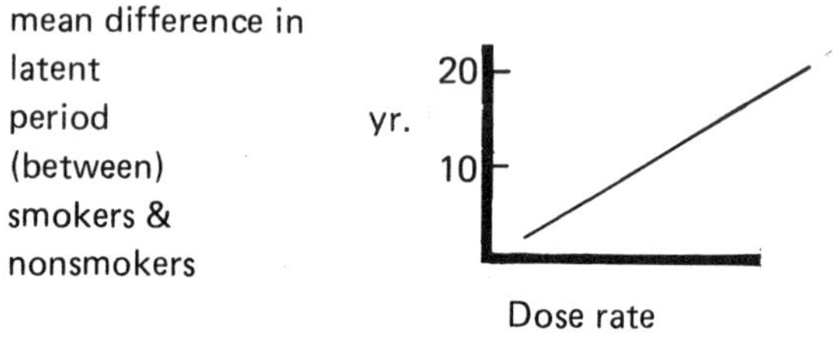

I will leave it at that.

AXELSON: Another mining community in Sweden has shown that the accumulated number of lung cancers over 3-year subperiods from 1957 to 1980 is higher after 1960. Practically no lung cancers before 1959-60. We suspect that this is an effect of a change in ventilation, because the water flows underground. So, it was an invention in the forties and fifties to take down the air through old shafts and heat it a little from the ground, and then bring it to the workplaces which led to the build-up of radon daughters in the mine air. What is shown here in terms of lung cancer is probably the effect of this changed ventilation. We made the air better from the viewpoint of dust and so on, but worse with regard to radon daughters.

This just affects a few cases. There are 50 cases now, and six of those were never smokers. Lung cancer has rarely been found in the municipality outside of the miner population.

RADFORD: In other words, this epidemic is almost entirely accounted for by the deaths in the miners.

AXELSON: In total, lung cancer among miners is less than 0.5% of the total lung cancer in Sweden. It is really a small contribution to lung cancer in general, but a big contribution in the mining community.

CAIRNS: I vaguely remember in the back of my mind somebody having once suggested that the high cancer rates seen in the colder parts of the United States might be partly due to accumulation of radon inside houses, particularly ones built out of stone or brick. Is there any substance to this idea?

RADFORD: That is a very apt question. It is not occupational cancer, but it is of considerable concern, especially to the Swedish Government. Olav Axelson has done a case-control study showing the comparison of lung cancer in individuals living in brick and stone houses to those in frame houses and found a positive effect. I was just in Sweden a couple of weeks ago, and they have a special problem because they have uranium-bearing shales that are quite close to the surface. A lot of towns and houses have been built on them, and quite high radon levels are found in houses.

As you know, the U.S. government is looking into this matter. It has been found that so-called technologically enhanced release of radon is occurring quite widely in both natural gas and in artesian well waters. You can get a fairly good release of radon in the shower if you happen to have water that is fairly high in dissolved radon.

There are big problems in Butte, Montana, because it is built over mines which are now worked out. Radon is seeping up through the ground and getting into the houses. There are phosphate mine tailings in Florida and uranium mine tailings used for buildings, with high radon found in these buildings. An ongoing study is being done in a Pennsylvania town which has uranium mine tailings from an old radium separation plant, where they imported the uranium and left it around.

I stress the data on the Swedish miners because it is a very widespread problem. This is about the lowest dose range that anyone has found evidence of a quantitative nature of the risk. Olav has the data from the houses, and I know there are other studies going on in Sweden on this problem.

BLOT: Is there a general North-South difference in the amount of radon found in homes?

RADFORD: I doubt it very much. It is a question of the uranium or radium content of the soil in which the house is built. Second, it is a question of the amount of air changes in the house, because with more insulation of homes, radon levels go up. You would expect that people living in the south would have lower levels, except now many people in the South keep air conditioners running and I don't know what that does to the radon. Maybe somebody else does.

In central Florida, there are a lot of houses that are very high in radon because they were built on slabs from phosphate mine tailings high in radium.

BEAUMONT: Using the attributable rate, you showed a strong dose response with the various mining populations. I wonder if you would have seen the same dose response if you had used a RR plot, because the low-dose categories are based on younger person-years and therefore have a lower background rate, and just the opposite with high-dose person-years.

RADFORD: In other words, you are saying that because of the contribution of background radon exposure, you might find a problem. Well, you could in the Swedish miner data, because exposures were in the low-dose range. You might expect that background would contribute at most, 10 WLM in ranges up to 300 WLM, almost negligible.

It happens that in the section of Sweden studied, the miners generally lived in frame houses, and it is not the part of Sweden that has these uranium-bearing ores, so it is very likely that the background contribution of radon is relatively low.

BEAUMONT: I was referring to the background of lung cancer in the general population.

RADFORD: Well, we have used standard methods to correct for that. In other words, these are all age-specific, year-specific adjusted.

BEAUMONT: Are the categories age adjusted to each other?

RADFORD: There really isn't much difference , because it is mostly a function of duration not the concentration of work underground.

ENTERLINE: The longer the duration, the older the people are going to be and the higher the dose. If you do an absolute difference, you get a quite different answer than if you did a relative difference, because the young people will have low death rates. An absolute difference would result in high RR. Old people with high death rates, result in the same absolute difference for a low RR.

RADFORD: I see.

ENTERLINE: You get a very different picture if you do RR.

RADFORD: Well, we will do it.

R. PETO: Did you get fairly constant RRs in your population?

RADFORD: Yes.

R. PETO: I was worried that you were plotting risk of cancer against cumulative dose. Cumulative dose is roughly proportional to age. If you plot cancer risk against age, we know that you get a relationship. What you are plotting is a mixture of a real effect of radiation and just the fact that cancer gets common in old age. I wish you would do something like dose rate over the previous 20 years or some measure which is not correlated with age. You really need to present all your analyses because until you do you are merely demonstrating that there is a relationship between cancer and age.

RADFORD: I sense that that is the same point made earlier. Knowing this cohort as well as I do, I suspect it is unimportant, because miners began mining at different ages and don't necessarily have a direct correlation of duration of exposure with age. Obviously it plays a role. The duration of exposure underground varied substantially among the miners, so I wouldn't want to take any bets. But I agree that confounding age and exposure duration ought to be taken into account in the analysis. It will be done.

The IARC Monograph Program On the Evaluation of the Carcinogenic Risk of Chemicals to Humans as a Contribution to the Identification of Occupational Carcinogens

RODOLFO SARACCI
Division of Epidemiology and Biostatistics
International Agency for Research on Cancer
Lyon, France

This presentation is an overall sketch of the IARC monograph program which Lorenzo Tomatis initiated, shaped, and supervised on the evaluation of the carcinogenic risk of chemicals to humans. Some participants here today have first-hand knowledge of this program because they have worked hard in Lyon by participating in one or more of its sessions to make it effective.

THE MONOGRAPH PROGRAM

The program started in 1971 and represents an approach to try to identify chemical carcinogens in a systematic way through literature searches and evaluation. It was born in response to requests to the World Health Organization to provide a list of recognized chemical carcinogens. The philosophy with which the program was started was, in fact, antagonist to that implicit in most requests, namely to provide just a list in which chemicals would have been quickly and nicely rated as "strong carcinogens," "mild carcinogens," and so on. On the contrary, the basic philosophy that was adopted after preparatory discussion meetings with scientists from a number of countries recognized that such a list could, perhaps, be the end product of a systematic program of in depth evaluations carried out individually for each chemical, starting with those for which an assessment of carcinogenicity was likely to present less difficulty. A second feature of the program philosophy, reflecting the state of knowledge of the early 1970s, was to limit the evaluation to the strictly qualitative aspect, namely to try to reply, as unequivocally as possible, to the key question, "Is this compound carcinogenic or not?" Attempts at quantitative assessment deliberately were set aside.

The program operates in the following manner. Compounds are selected for carcinogenicity evaluation mainly on two grounds: (1) human exposure to the compound is known to occur and (2) there is some suspicion (derived from human data, animal data, or other laboratory data) that the chemical may be carcinogenic.

It is apparent that the selection is highly "biased," and one cannot in any way compare the group of compounds hitherto evaluated (over 500) to a random sample of all chemicals (e.g., those listed in Chemical Abstracts). Instead, the group represents a purposively selected series of compounds. The evaluation process for each compound begins with an extensive bibliographic search, followed by the preparation of a series of draft documents covering chemical and physical data, production, use, occurrence and analysis, carcinogenicity studies in animals, other relevant biological data including toxicological data and mutagenicity data, and, finally, case reports and epidemiological data.

These documents constitute the raw material on which an international Working Group of scientists from a variety of fields (chemistry, experimental and human pathology, mutagenesis, toxicology, epidemiology, etc.) works for 6-7 days with the twin purposes of achieving a final version of the documents (which form the monograph body) and of expressing an evaluation on what the animal evidence and the human evidence described in the documents means in terms of carcinogenicity. On average, three Working Groups per year are convened in Lyon, each composed of scientists particularly acquainted with the compounds to be examined and evaluated. The evaluative judgment was, in the early years of the program, performed separately under two sections headed respectively "Animal data" and "Human data."

THE PRESENT EVALUATION CRITERIA

When I joined the IARC in 1976 and began to participate in the program meetings as an epidemiologist, it was difficult for me to make up my mind about the human data knowing that I had to ignore completely the animal data evaluation written one line above. This difficulty (which, judging from how the discussions developed within the Working Groups, was often shared by other participants) stemmed from the fact that because the human data evaluation was the final section it was bound to end up as a global evaluation (albeit not explicitly designed and acknowledged as such) rather than an evaluation strictly limited to the human evidence.

This difficulty prompted, along with other considerations aimed at improving the program, the introduction of the following changes.

1. The section now headed "Summary of the data reported and evaluated" was divided into three subsections–"Experimental data," "Human data," and "Evaluation," the latter now encompassing in three successive and brief paragraphs the experimental data evaluation, the human data evaluation,

and a combined, overall evaluation of carcinogenic risk to humans that takes into account the animal evidence. This arrangement has the advantage that a separate and independent assessment of the animal and human evidence is more easily and freely achievable by scientists who know that in any case there is a place for a final paragraph expressing a judgment that tries to integrate informally all the available evidence and its bearing to the risk in man.

2. If a quantitation is not made, at least a categorization of a sort is made not of "potency" of carcinogens or of dose-responses but of "degrees of evidence." In the first phase of the program, evaluations were expressed in an entirely narrative form, without any attempt at formally rating the strength of the evidence on which the evaluation was based. It is easy to see, going through volumes 1-16 of the monographs, that there are variations from one Working Group to another in the way that the evaluations were conceived and written up. This was natural and had to be expected, as, on the other hand, it was natural to seek to reduce the variation after some experience had been gained.

These changes were adopted by an ad hoc Working Group specially convened in October 1977 to review the criteria for the assessment of the carcinogenic risk of chemicals to humans and have been maintained ever since. Two other ad hoc Working Groups were convened subsequently to bring the evaluations for the compounds examined in the previous years in line with the new criteria. The results of their work are summarized in the Supplement No. 1 to the IARC Monograph Series (September 1979), which covers the 442 compounds included in volumes 1-20 of the monographs.

The following series of tables outlines the categorization of the evidence of carcinogenicity, in animals, in humans, and in the final (combined) judgment, as well as some results of the application of this categorization as presented in Supplement No. 1.

Table 1 indicates the criteria specifying the degrees of evidence of carcinogenicity in animals (for completeness there are, in fact, two extra categories not included in the table, namely "Negative evidence" and "No data"). The categorization of the evidence–and this applies to the animal as well as to the human evidence–is, of course, contingent on the time of the evaluation and may change as new data are accrued. It is also apparent that the strength of evidence is an altogether different concept than the "strength" or "potency" of a carcinogen (however defined). However, the two properties may happen to be related to the extent that a compound that is very active may be relatively easy to detect and the evidence concerning its carcinogenicity may reach more easily the level of "sufficient."

Table 2 indicates the criteria specifying the degrees of evidence of carcinogenicity in humans, and Table 3 shows the definition of the three degrees of evidence to be used in the final combined evaluation.

Table 1
Degrees of Evidence for Carcinogenicity from Experimental Animal Studies

1. *Sufficient evidence* of carcinogenicity indicates that there is an increased incidence of malignant tumors: (a) in multiple species or strains, or (b) in multiple experiments (preferably with different routes of administration or using different dose levels), or (c) to an unusual degree with regard to incidence, site or type of tumor, or age at onset. Additional evidence may be provided by data concerning dose-response effects, as well as information on mutagenicity or chemical structure.
2. *Limited evidence* of carcinogenicity means that the data suggest a carcinogenic effect but are limited because: (a) the studies involve a single species, strain, or experiment; or (b) the experiments are restricted by inadequate dosage levels, inadequate duration of exposure to the agent, inadequate period of follow-up, poor survival, too few animals, or inadequate reporting; or (c) the neoplasms produced often occur spontaneously or are difficult to classify as malignant by histological criteria alone (e.g., lung and liver tumors in mice).
3. *Inadequate evidence* indicates that because of major qualitative or quantitative limitations, the studies cannot be interpreted as showing either the presence or absence of a carcinogenic effect.

Table 2
Degrees of Evidence for Carcinogenicity from Human Studies

1. *Sufficient evidence* of carcinogenicity indicates a causal association between exposure and human cancer.
2. *Limited evidence* of carcinogenicity indicates a possible carcinogenic effect in humans, although the data are not sufficient to demonstrate a causal association.
3. *Inadequate evidence* of carcinogenicity indicates that the data are qualitatively or quantitatively insufficient to allow any conclusion regarding carcinogenicity for humans.

THE CATEGORIZATION OF THE CHEMICALS

Results of the application of these criteria and definitions are presented in Tables 4-6. Of these, Table 4 shows the 18 compounds or industrial processes classified as carcinogenic in humans; with the exception of 3 drugs, the human exposure to the other 15 is largely or exclusively occupational.

As one easily can see, no element of true quantification in the sense we are discussing at this meeting is present in the monograph program. Quantitative data, when available, are summarized in the body of the monograph and are taken into account in the discussion that leads to the evaluation, but this is

Table 3
Evaluation of the Carcinogenic Risk to Humans

Group 1
The chemical, group of chemicals, or industrial process is carcinogenic for humans. This category was used only when there was *sufficient evidence* to support a causal association between the exposure and cancer.

Group 2
The chemical or group of chemicals is probably carcinogenic for humans. This category includes chemicals for which the evidence of human carcinogenicity is almost "sufficient" as well as chemicals for which it is only suggestive. To reflect this range, this category has been divided into higher (group A) or lower (group B) degrees of evidence. The data from experimental animal studies played an important role in assigning chemicals to category 2, and particularly for those in group B.

Group 3
The chemical or group of chemicals cannot be classified as to its carcinogenicity for humans.

Table 4
The Following 18 Chemicals, Groups of Chemicals, and Industrial Processes Are Carcinogenic for Humans (Group 1)

1. 4-Aminobiphenyl
2. Arsenic and certain arsenic compounds
3. Asbestos
4. Manufacture of auramine
5. Benzene
6. Benzidine
7. *N,N-bis*(2-chloroethyl)-2-naphthyl-amine (chlornaphazine)
8. *Bis*(chloromethyl)ether and technical-grade chloromethyl methyl ether
9. Chromium and certain chromium compounds
10. Diethylstilbestrol
11. Underground hematite mining
12. Manufacture of isopropyl alcohol by the strong acid process
13. Melphalan
14. Mustard gas
15. 2-Naphthylamine
16. Nickel refining
17. Soots, tars, and mineral oils
18. Vinyl chloride

formulated essentially as a judgment on the presence or absence of carcinogenicity and not in terms of grades of carcinogenic activity of a compound.

Table 5
Chemicals or Groups of Chemicals which Are Probably Carcinogenic for Humans

Subgroup A–higher degree of human evidence
1. Aflatoxins
2. Cadmium and certain cadmium compounds
3. Chlorambucil
4. Cyclophosphamide
5. Nickel and certain nickel compounds
6. Tris (1-aziridinyl) phosphine sulphide (thiotepa)

Subgroup B–lower degree of human evidence
1. Acrylonitrile
2. Amitrole (aminotriazole)
3. Auramine
4. Beryllium and certain beryllium compounds
5. Carbon tetrachloride
6. Dimethyl carbamoyl chloride
7. Dimethyl sulfate
8. Ethylene oxide
9. Iron dextran complex
10. Oxymetholone
11. Phenacetin
12. Polychlorinated biphenyls

Table 6
The Following 18 Chemicals and Groups of Chemicals Could Not Be Classified as to Their Carcinogenicity for Humans (Group 3)

1. Chloramphenicol
2. Chlordane/heptachlor
3. Chloroprene
4. Dichlorodiphenyltrichloroethane (DDT)
5. Dieldrin
6. Epichlorohydrin
7. Hematite
8. Hexachlorocyclohexane (technical-grade HCH/lindane)
9. Isoniazid
10. Isopropyl oils
11. Lead and certain lead compounds
12. Phenobarbitone
13. *N*-Phenyl-2-naphthylamine
14. Phenytoin
15. Reserpine
16. Styrene
17. Trichloroethylene
18. Tris(aziridinyl)-1-*para*-benzoquinone (triaziquone)

THE QUANTIFICATION ISSUE

Two considerations bearing on quantification need to be made. First, an exploration of the feasibility of including quantitative aspects into the evaluation will be carried out soon for some chemicals (by the Working Group convened for October of this year). Of course, this does not ensure necessarily that the attempt will be successful and that the present form of the evaluation will be changed as a result. Second, another element of a quantitative nature arises rather naturally when facing, as one often does within the monograph program, animal data along with human data on carcinogenicity. What can one say about the quantitative correlation between human data and animal data? In my opinion at least three points can be made:

1. It is impracticable to draw a complete conventional two-by-two table (with frequencies of animal carcinogenicity test positivity and negativity in the two rows and frequencies of human data positivity and negativity in the two columns) to derive correct formal estimates of the specificity, sensitivity, and predictive value of animal data (tests) in respect to human data as the yardstick. The main, although not the sole, reason for this is that one simply does not have reliable figures to fill in the "specificity" column, i.e., the one that ought to include the frequencies with which compounds clearly shown negative for carcinogenicity in humans are positive or negative in animal experiments.
2. Of 13 individual chemicals (the 18 in Table 4 minus the 5 industrial processes) that have been classified as carcinogenic for humans, only 2, arsenic and benzene, are not positive in animal experiments (notably for benzene, the evidence is inadequate rather than negative). Thus, 11 out of 13 are positive in animal experiments, pointing towards a high sensitivity of animal long-term tests in detecting human carcinogens.
3. Of the 442 compounds in volumes 1-20, there is sufficient evidence of carcinogenicity in experimental animals for 142 (32%) of them, while published human data of any type (case reports or epidemiological studies) are available for only 60 compounds (14%, i.e., the 54 listed in Tables 4-6, plus 6 with limited human data that could not be reviewed by the ad hoc Working Group due to time limitations). One may wonder why human evidence (positive or negative) in published form exists for only a low proportion of compounds. Several reasons may be invoked legitimately, including: too short a period from onset of use of certain compounds to make an epidemiological study worthwhile; great difficulty in identifying sizable populations with sufficiently well-defined exposure to individual chemicals and without concurrent exposure to many other agents; difficulty in obtaining access to the relevant information (on exposures, on causes of death) due, for example, to confidentiality reasons or pretexts; shortage of qualified epidemiologists willing to carry out such types of studies.

Be this as it may, the problem remains scientific as well as practical (i.e., in public health terms)—for about one-third of the 442 compounds having "sufficient evidence" of carcinogenicity in animals, there is known human exposure (occupational in a large number of the cases) and, at the same time, no human data are available about carcinogenicity. For these compounds, the following sentence is now appended to the statement of "sufficient evidence" of carcinogenicity in animals: "In the absence of adequate data on humans it is reasonable, for practical purposes, to regard the chemical as if it presented a carcinogenic risk to humans."

This qualifying sentence obviously is not a scientific solution to the problem, nor is it a recommendation (which would fall outside the province of the monograph program). Because we are confronted with an unsolved problem, it is intended as an interpretative aid for the reader and user of the monographs who tries to work out, comparatively for the different compounds, the exact meaning and implications of the Working Groups' evaluations.

COMMENTS

SCHNEIDERMAN: The paper that Dr. Saracci referred to will be presented by Myra Karstadt (this volume) as a follow-up to this. She will ask the questions "What has been done with these compounds? Are the industries and people who are using them gathering any data? And, what have they learned?"

ROSS: I would like to find out about your isopropyl oil category. After some recent work done by Lynch and others (Lynch et al. 1979) and Dr. Enterline (1980) for Shell over the past several years, we are looking at the chemical compound diisopropyl sulfate as possibly being the high-acid concentration intermediate product that might be the chemical of interest. I think that the words "isopropyl oils" is probably too loose of a term and passé.

SARACCI: This is supplemental information that you are really providing. It would show how one can go down from the overall indication to something more specific. I would be grateful if you could provide that information.

ENTERLINE: I'm not clear about the 60 compounds listed in Category 1.

SARACCI: Sixty out of 442 were classified: 18 in Category 1, 18 in Category 2, and 18 in Category 3. This adds up to 54. We deliberately lost six in the classification because of time limitation at the Working Group Session.

RADFORD: What about the reference you made to the 142?

SARACCI: They are another group. There is sufficient evidence of carcinogenicity for the 142 in animals, but not in humans.

RADFORD: Do any of the 142 end up in Categories 1, 2, or 3?

SARACCI: Only very few end up there. There is human evidence for about a dozen compounds. All the others of this group of 142 stay outside the classification and compose a group by themselves.

SCHNEIDERMAN: Which volume of the monograph series has this breakdown of the 18, 18, 18?

SARACCI: It is in Supplement No. 1 (IARC 1979).

RADFORD: I think you can safely remove hematite from your list and just list the radon daughters. The quantitative risk obtained in our study of the iron mines is very similar to that for the fluorspar mines. It correlates with the radon, but it doesn't correlate with the mineral at all.

SARACCI: No. But the animal evidence on iron oxide is also one of the few which is flatly negative.

SIEMIATYCKI: Rodolfo, I think the 14% for which there is *any* type of human evidence is a very optimistic statistic. In fact, the denominator can be tens of thousands. Those 442 are strongly biased to those for which there is something suspect in the data.

SARACCI: Yes. They are biased in that. They are selected according to several criteria. There is a suspicion of carcinogenicity, that may come from animals or man. But the other is that there is evidence of human exposure. So, speaking on those two criteria, it is strongly biased in the sense of enriching heavily the proportion of compounds for which there is any information in man. In short, I agree with you that the real denominator is much larger.

SIEMIATYCKI: Could you comment on the absence of a "non-carcinogenic" category in your classification?

SARACCI: In fact, in Supplement 1 (IARC 1979), Table 3 lists all 442 compounds. You can find that only for iron oxide is the category "negative." This was used only for the evidence in experimental animals and seems to be the exception which confirms the general tendency of the Working Groups to use the "negative" category with prudence. Before committing ourselves to a proven negative, we require a good deal of negative evidence.

DAVIS: Of the 442 substances examined there were enough data for 142 to be evaluated as animal carcinogens. It is my understanding in absence of human data, that the policy recommendation is that for practical purposes an animal carcinogen should be regarded as if it were a human carcinogen. This coincides with the NCI policy elaborated by U.S. Government last year.

There are probably a little bit more than 70,000 substances in commercial production. Approximately 50,000 of these are on the inventory under our TSCA law. The others are pesticides, drugs, cosmetics, and other agents.

With respect to Group 3, are chlordane-heptachlor and aldrin-dieldrin both on that list?

SARACCI: No, there is only limited evidence (not sufficient evidence) for these compounds in experimental animals.

DAVIS: In the United States, the Carcinogen Assessment Group at the Environmental Protection Agency has evaluated animal evidence on chlordane-heptachlor under the Federal Insecticide, Fungicide and Rodenticide Act, and has determined that they should be treated—again this is policy—as human carcinogens. They decided that the animal data are such that they are animal carcinogens.

I understand that in the U.K. they are not regarded as animal carcinogens. Is there anyone here who could enlighten us on that? How would you go about deciding how to remove a compound from Group 3 and place it into Group 1 or 2?

SARACCI: The only way of putting it out of Group 3 and into Group 2 is reevaluating the evidence which is usually done—within the IARC program—when new data become available. The fact that the judgments expressed by different groups of scientists don't coincide means that the evidence is indeed not that strong.

HOERGER: What would you forecast as the rate at which you will handle the study of additional compounds in the next 2-5 years?

SARACCI: It would be more or less the same rate, unless the program is expanded substantially. We are running into compounds for which we have less and less hard data. Of course, we also take into account evidence from short-term studies—but this is considered a very different level of evidence. The required hard evidence is the long-term carcinogenicity and the human data.

R. PETO: I would like to draw your attention to Section 4.2 of our recent paper (Doll and Peto 1981) which takes a more pessimistic view of the ability of the laboratory experiments to pick out the important causes of human cancer.

CAIRNS: This idea of defining something as a potential human hazard because it is carcinogenic in animals is going to run into great difficulty with dietary components like flavonoids. In terms of benzo[*a*] pyrene equivalents, the flavonoid quercetin may be the main mutagen that we are exposed to. Must the Federal Government now declare that the onion is a human carcinogen, because it is rich in quercetin, which is highly mutagenic and has been reported to be carcinogenic in animals?

WATSON: But it doesn't say that an onion is a carcinogen.

R. PETO: There is a paper by Pamucku et al. (1980) that reports on this.

References

Doll, R. and R. Peto. 1981. The causes of cancer: Quantitative estimation of avoidable risks of cancer in the United States today. *J. Natl. Cancer Inst.* **66**:1091.

Enterline, P.E. 1980. Cancer in men manufacturing alcohol. Report to the Shell Oil Company.

Lynch, L., N.M. Hanis, M.G. Bird, K.L. Murray, and L.P. Walsh. 1979. An association of upper respiratory cancer with exposure to diethyl sulfate. *J. Occup. Med.* **21**:333.

Pamucku, A.M., S. Yalciner, J. F. Hatcher, and G.T. Bryan. 1980. Quercetin, a rat intestinal and bladder carcinogen present in bracken fern (*Pteridium aquilinum*) *Cancer Res.* **40**:3468.

IARC. 1979. Chemicals and industrial processes associated with cancer in humans. *IARC Monogr. Eval. Carcinog. Risk Chem. Hum.* **1-20** (Suppl. 1).

A Strategy for the Identification of Carcinogens in a Large, Complex Chemical Company

GEOFFREY M. PADDLE
ICI Central Medical Group
Wilmslow, Cheshire, SK9 1QB England

The estimation of the influence on the incidence of cancer of such factors as the environment, or all chemicals, is essentially an epidemiological problem. The occupational and health records maintained by industry can help to resolve the problem, but their quality is such that studies based upon them are almost always subjected to damning criticism. The advantages that toxicology has in the assessment of individual compounds, particularly novel ones, can be discounted in this more general debate. It is a debate in which it is more constructive to promote the virtues of the epidemiological approach than to denigrate it for its inability to match the rigor of laboratory experiments. It is, therefore, a debate in which industrial records can play an important role.

The penchant of epidemiologists for the generation of hypotheses rather than the testing of them has been criticized elsewhere (Paddle 1980). Much of the concern about carcinogens in the environment is due to the multitude of hypotheses that have been put forward but remain unverified. This situation is, itself, due to the widely held view that hypotheses can only be tested in well-conducted cohort studies. Any other form of study is considered capable only of leading to a recommendation that an appropriate cohort study should be done. Industry has not the resources to respond to every such recommendation for each chemical compound that comes under suspicion. Besides which, the design would often have to fall well short of the ideal.

Industry can however adopt an alternative strategy with the dual objectives of displaying readily available information for specific compounds and of identifying carcinogens in the workplace by the careful scrutiny of clusters of cases. This strategy relies upon techniques other than cohort studies, and will, therefore, be discounted by peer review for as long as these techniques are regarded as inferior. The aim of this presentation is to show that, when the strengths and weaknesses of occupational records are taken into account, this strategy is a better option than a succession of cohort studies.

THE INDUSTRIAL CONTEXT

Imperial Chemical Industries Limited (ICI) was formed in 1926 by the amalgamation of four companies, two of which were established in the 1870s. Today ICI is an international organization and among the largest chemical companies in the world. Its range of products is very broad, as can be judged from the names of its divisions in the United Kingdom—agricultural, explosives, fibers, mond (e.g., general chemicals, alkali, lime, and salt), organics (e.g., dyestuffs), paints, petrochemicals and plastics, pharmaceuticals, and plant protection. The plants and offices are spread widely geographically, being located in areas with very disparate health statistics. The multiplicity of chemical compounds handled is illustrated by the presence of 20,000 compounds in its computerized Process Chemical Register and over 50,000 compounds in its Chemical Compound Centre's directory of research chemicals. The U.K. ICI workforce has varied in size with the growth of new business areas and the decline of others. At its peak, it numbered over 100,000, of whom roughly 55% were male weekly staff, 30% were male monthly staff, 10% were female monthly staff, and 5% were female weekly staff. The turnover rate, a key epidemiological figure, has averaged about 10% per annum, concentrated largely among those with short service and those reaching retirement age.

The need to record information for purely epidemiological purposes was not formally recognized until a working party on epidemiology and biostatistics set up by the Medical Policy Group reported in 1973. Prior to the creation of the systems recommended by this team, epidemiological information had to be extracted from records that were held for other purposes. Fortunately the company has always adopted a progressive attitude to the maintenance of personnel records, the provision of medical care, and the introduction, and extension, of pension rights. The minimum retention periods for these records were not mutually consistent, and were insufficient for cohort studies of suspect carcinogens, but in many locations data for much longer than the minimum periods have been kept.

A computerized system for medical and occupational records, known as MORAS, was implemented in 1976. Many of the concepts incorporated in this system were based on Pell (1968). The system consists of a personnel file, the process chemical register, and health data, which are limited to mortality and internally diagnosed absence records for periods of 28 calendar days or more. The death records since 1976 have been supplemented by those for the period 1970-1975 and a separate file has been created from less authentic data for the period 1950-1969. As the personnel and compound files are linked by location codes, the system can be used to construct cohort studies automatically. Alternatively, the details of studies set up by conventional methods can be held for routine updating. The advantages of such systems are now accepted widely in the chemical and other industries, and they will undoubtedly influence the progress of epidemiology in the 1990s. More extravagant claims that the computerization of detailed health records and occupational hygiene data will permit the precise estimation of dose-response curves must be treated with reservation, until some practical examples are available for comment.

ALTERNATIVE COURSES OF ACTION

It would not be appropriate for industry to maintain such comprehensive and expensive records simply to be able to react to accusations about the carcinogenicity of chemicals. Ott (1977) describes a variety of ways in which the records can be analyzed in other than a purely reactive fashion. His recommendation that the occupational records for all decedents from certain areas should be codified for computerized retrieval is particularly relevant, and has been adopted in one division of ICI. On the other hand, most attempts to analyze the information in a constructive manner are plagued by the certainty that a host of false positives will result. A suitable strategy for the efficient use of the data should allow for a division of effort between the provision of prompt, reliable information about specific, suspect compounds, and a rational attempt to detect any carcinogens that are discernible by statistical methods. The draft Interagency Regulatory Liaison Group guidelines on epidemiological research have not met with universal approval. Though they may be too superficial for very detailed, highly specialized studies, it has proved to be helpful to adopt them in forming a strategy for industrial effort. In particular, they highlight the need for specific objectives. The objective which industry has been encouraged to direct attention to is: (1) Is compound X related to diagnosis Y among employees Z? The question addressed in this paper is whether the set of such hypotheses for all suspect combinations (X, Y, Z) can be replaced adequately by the single hypothesis: (2) Is any compound X related to any diagnosis Y among any employees Z? The possibility that it can becomes less remote when the available information is assessed objectively.

PREFERRED STRATEGY

At present, by far the most informative set of data available in industry is the death records for pensioners and employees. ICI (United Kingdom) has over 10,000 of these for the period 1970-1978 with authentic diagnoses and over 18,500 for 1950-1969 with less reliable diagnoses. It must make sense to analyze these to extract any information that they may contain about carcinogens in the workplace. The approach has been to calculate age-adjusted proportionate mortality ratios (PMRs) for the company vs the population of England and Wales, and similar tables for each division versus the remainder of the company. The tables are presented as in Table 1 with the diagnostic groups

Table 1
Ranked PMRs for Selected Causes (age-adjusted), All Age Groups

Cause of death	ICI			England and Wales—
	observed deaths	expected deaths	PMR	observed deaths
083 Accidental poisoning, other unspecified solids and liquids	0.12	0.00	48200	1
047 Disease of eye	0.12	0.03	399	7
046 Disease of nerves and peripheral ganglia	0.37	0.12	306	28
020 Malignant neoplasms of other and unspecified respiratory organs	1.87	0.61	305	132
086 Other disease symptoms and conditions	9.12	4.92	185	1,464
028 Malignant neoplasms of thyroid gland	0.87	0.49	175	110
.				
.				
.				
051 Ischemic heart disease	419.75	387.44	108	87,481
.				
.				
.				
081 Accidental poisoning, caustic corrosives necrosis	0.00	0.01	0	3

Index population–ICI, year(s) 1970-1977; standard population–England and Wales, year(s) 1972; category, all males.

in decreasing order of PMR so that the diagnoses of most concern can be picked out easily. The diagnostic groups have been chosen so as to scrutinize the cancer sites in some depth, while leaving the coronary and respiratory conditions in broad categories.

The usual criticisms of PMRs do not apply to this analysis. It is most unlikely that the proportion of one common diagnosis is so far from the national level as to distract attention from important but smaller divergencies. It is also unlikely that a high "all causes" SMR is being obscured, because the healthy-worker effect will have ensured that this SMR is well below 100. A more serious objection is that the data omits the important subset of past employees who left because of the conditions, or otherwise, and did not join the pension scheme. A similar objection is often applied to cohort studies that fail to follow up every member of the population. These objections appear to be based less on statistical theory than on one of Murphy's Laws, which states that "whatever can go wrong–will go wrong." In the case of vinyl chloride, it has been possible to compare the death statistics in the national study (Fox and Collier 1977) with those that could have been retrieved from the ICI pension records. Table 2 shows that the percentages of deaths in the various diagnostic groups are similar.

Table 2
Comparison of Traceable and Untraceable Death Records

Cause of death	Age -24	25-34	35-44	45-54	55-64	65-74	>74	total
			Traceable					
Cancer	0	1	2	6	9	16	1	35
Coronary	0	1	0	9	15	15	2	42
Cerebral	0	0	1	2	2	6	2	13
Respiratory	0	1	0	2	3	11	1	18
Accidental	1	0	0	1	0	0	0	2
Other	1	1	0	0	4	8	1	15
Total	2	4	3	20	33	56	7	125
			Untraceable					
Cancer	0	0	3	6	18	13	6	46
Coronary	0	0	3	9	13	17	2	44
Cerebral	0	0	1	1	3	6	1	12
Respiratory	0	1	0	4	2	5	3	15
Accidental	1	4	1	3	0	1	1	11
Other	2	0	3	6	5	9	8	33
Total	3	5	11	29	41	51	21	161

The course subdivision of the company into divisions has had the effect of generating many significant PMRs, but it is easy to argue that these are more likely to reflect geographic or social class effects than chemical exposures, because the effects of any chemical exposures will have been severely diluted. It is obvious that a necessary further step is to extend the analysis to works, or plants, or other smaller, self-contained locations. This, in the fashion of mapping or regression analysis, will generate as many hypotheses for further testing as any epidemiological team could possibly wish for. It would be advisable to subject these significant findings to a filtering process before embarking on a case-control study (Kupper et al. 1975) for each one. Two possibilities suggest themselves, but, as neither has been subjected to peer review, it would be unwise for too much reliance to be placed on them. The simpler approach is to plot approximately normally distributed figures on probability paper and accept as significant only those values that diverge appreciably from a straight line sketched through the points. The obvious statistic for such purpose is $(O - E)/\sqrt{E}$ based on Daniel's idea (Daniel 1959) of the half-normal plot, which was such a welcome addition to the analysis of factorial designs. This does not overcome the following problem, that is, because cancer is divided up into so many subsets it is probable that some cancer sites will top the lists of PMRs. A more adventurous approach would be to use a Bayesian analysis in which prior probabilities for relative risks (RR) have been ascribed by an expert panel before the data are analyzed. It is very strange that the same people who are very skeptical, or very convinced, after the event, are unwilling to place their bets before the event. Lacking such approaches, it becomes a question of playing hunches or choosing the largest numbers.

In Table 3, the results of the PMR analysis are shown for an abbreviated list of diagnostic categories for male ex-employees of ICI vs males in England and Wales. The first impression is that this table provides further evidence of a relationship between exposure to chemicals and the incidence of cancer. There are, however, several alternative interpretations of the figures in Table 3. As the excess is as marked for monthly staff as for weekly staff, it may simply reflect geographical variations. The table may be exhibiting a deficit of cases for diseases that preclude work, rather than an excess of cases of diseases attributable to work. At the other extreme, as the "other" category is mostly respiratory disease, which may also be occupational, the excess of cancer may really be even greater than that displayed. This table, like so many similar ones, exposes a problem without helping to resolve it.

Regardless of how the significance of excesses is assessed, the best method for the pursuit of those clusters selected for further study is a case-control approach. It is at this stage that the frailties of the supporting record systems are exposed. If the records can be found at all, they are likely to contain archaic and vague job descriptions, and there will be virtually no indication of exposure to chemicals. In a small study within one section of one works in ICI, 91

Table 3
Ranked PMRs for Selected causes (age-adjusted), All Age Groups

	ICI weekly staff			ICI monthly staff			
	observed deaths	expected deaths	PMR	observed deaths	expected deaths	PMR	England and Wales—observed deaths
006 Benign and unspecified neoplasm	2.44	1.69	143	1.55	0.92	168	596
001 Cancer	202.22	180.71	111	102.44	92.85	110	59,384
003 Cerebral	92.66	90.06	102	42.88	42.85	100	31,775
002 Coronary	314.11	310.94	101	173.66	157.30	110	105,422
004 Accident	21.77	24.07	90	11.22	13.57	82	10,769
005 Rest	194.00	219.67	88	82.00	106.21	77	77,733

Index population–ICI, year(s) 1970-1977; standard population–England and Wales, year(s) 1972; Category, all males.

locations within the company, other than the works in question, were found in the records of 235 decedents. In assessing the exposure of fertilizer workers to nitrates, Fraser et al. (1980) found references to 100 jobs for 676 employees. On a sample page of 50 deaths from our 1950-1969 deaths listing, it is rare to find any occupation mentioned more than once. These examples asre displayed not to demonstrate the difficulties inherent in case-control studies, but to lead into a discussion of the extreme problems that occur in the conduct of cohort studies in a large, complex chemical company.

In adopting objective (2)–is any *X* related to any *Y* among any group *Z*?–for strategic solution, the readily available information for many of the objectives in (1)–does *X* cause *Y* among employees *Z*?–already will have been sifted and the hypothesis already will have been rejected en passant. The information for the diagnoses most frequently associated with chemical exposure–liver cancer, bladder cancer, and leukemia, for example–will have been examined for clusters in some detail. The chemicals and groups of employees will also have been looked at, by implication, by looking at works, and perhaps calendar years, unless the chemical or occupational group is divided into several geographically and organizationally remote subsets. The strategy for objective (1) could be to list and reassess the relevant information from objective (2) and, if necessary, to carry out a modified case-control study more appropriate to the specific hypothesis. In many instances, the death certificates available do not show a single case of the diagnosis in question for employees exposed to the suspect compound. Unfortunately, such a discovery, with its obviously very imprecise estimate of maximum relative risk, is not given very much weight in comparison with the animal, bacterial, or clinical episode material that has led to the hypothesis being proposed. Industry is persuaded towards the cohort approach despite the weaknesses in the data that will be used to create the cohort and the comparatively vast expenditure of manpower that will be necessary.

THE IMPERFECTIONS OF COHORT STUDIES

Let us evaluate the cohort alternative in the context under discussion. In the first place, the conduct of cohort studies for all suspect chemicals cannot be simplified and formalized. In correspondence with the Office of Populations, Censuses and Surveys (OPCS), ICI has requested that all employees who leave the company without joining the pension fund should be tagged in the Department of Health and Social Security (DHSS) record system. OPCS have rightly refused to agree to this request pending an examination by committee of the logistic problems that would arise if other large companies made similar requests. The same information could be sought by constructing cohorts for a multiplicity of compounds, and including the unexposed employees in control groups, but this would be a poor use of everyone's time. Once it is made necessary to justify each cohort study, it is surprising how easy it becomes to identify the problems that beset them. First of all, most members of cohorts associated with compounds still in use, and identified from records at the plants, are still alive. They do no more than contribute to person-years at risk and hold out the prospect of providing one death at some future date.

The idea that such studies test hypotheses, rather than generate them, is also of dubious validity. All industrial cohort studies are afflicted by the healthy-worker effect. This effect is often used to dismiss low "all cause" standardized mortality ratios (SMRs) or to draw attention to specific SMRs of about 100. One of the few papers to explore the effect in depth is that of Fox and Collier (1977). It is clear that the effect can materialize in quite subtle ways and, that if Fox and Collier's suggestions for overcoming it are followed, then the cohorts that should be studied will be those most difficult to identify. The cohort study has benefitted from its successful application to the dyestuffs industry (Case et al. 1954), vinyl chloride, smoking, and asbestos. In each of these cases, the RRs of the exposed groups are so high that almost any analysis would have reached the same conclusions. These conclusions would have been less acceptable to the scientific community if they had not been reached in cohort studies. In less straightforward cases, the results of cohort studies have been challenged as vigorously as those of mortality studies and case-control studies. Does vinyl chloride cause any deaths apart from those due to liver cancer? Is acrylonitrile a proven human carcinogen? Of course, it is not the purpose of this paper to denigrate the cohort study, but it may not be so much superior to alternatives as is suggested.

CONCLUSIONS

If epidemiology is to make its full contribution to the debate about carcinogens in the environment, its techniques must be used strategically rather than piecemeal. Whilst the cohort study is regarded as the unique tool for the testing of hypotheses, industry will continue to be persuaded towards the technique to which its records are least suited. The most valuable records available in industry are the death records and the occupational histories, but the latter are so devoid of exposure data that they need to be interpreted on an individual basis. Techniques for the extraction of clusters of cases, supported by careful use of case-control studies, form the best strategy for industry until such time as computerized records become established.

REFERENCES

Case, R.A.M., M.E. Hosker, D.B. McDonald, and J.E. Pearson. 1954. Tumours of the urinary bladder in workmen engaged in the manufacture and the use of certain dyestuff intermediates in the British chemical industry. *Br. J. Ind. Med.* 2:75.

Daniel, C. 1959. Use of half-normal plots in interpreting factorial two-level experiments. *Technometrics* **1**:311.

Fox, A.J. and P.F. Collier. 1977. Mortality experience of workers exposed to vinyl chloride monomer in the manufacture of polyvinyl chloride in Great Britain. *Br. J. Ind. Med.* **34**:1.

Fraser, P., C. Chilvers, and J. Fox. 1980. Human relevance–Epidemiology and occupational exposure. *Oncology* **37**:278.

Kupper, L.L., A.J. McMichael, and R. Spirtas. 1975. A hybrid epidemiological study design useful in estimating relative risk. *J. Amer. Stat. Soc.* **70**:524.

Ott, M.G. 1977. Linking industrial hygiene and health records. *J. Occup. Med.* **19**:383.

Paddle, G.M. 1980. Epidemiological and animal data as a basis for risk assessment. *Arch. Toxicol.* (Suppl.) **3**:263.

Pell, S. 1968. Epidemiological studies in a large company based on health and personnel records. *Public Health Rep.* **5**:399.

COMMENTS

McMICHAEL: If Dr. Adelstein had been here, Dr. Paddle, I think he probably would have asked you a question about accounting for social class in the calculation of these ratios. I think you were using the total population of England and Wales in your calculations. Fox and Adelstein in 1978, demonstrated that, for most major causes of death, quite a substantial proportion of the apparent occupational associations could be explained by what he calls "social class confounding."

I would have thought that the British system of vital statistics, relatively luxuriant as it is, would have allowed industry in Britain, particularly, to make allowance for social class in the sort of calculation of expected events that you have presented here, and to thereby get more valid ratios.

I think it probably doesn't affect your office staff, because they come from the middle-of-the-road. You might see some different ratios for your production workers if you did that.

PADDLE: Yes, I appreciate that point. What I described was the first step in a filtration process. I am hoping to find, first of all, very large clusters that are independent of social class, that is they stick out, regardless of social class. You could say that we were very diligent, or perhaps we went on a wild goose chase, but the largest PMR of any size, in terms of expected-to-observe numbers in Table 3 were for stomach cancer (or "151" as I tend to refer to it because I'm not a medical man), and we have a very large excess of that compared with the population of England and Wales. There are some who say this is due to chemical dust and fumes, so we did a case control study based on dustiness and fuminess in various plants, and we found absolutely nothing.

Now, these people come from a social class who have a high level of stomach cancer, and so perhaps we were wasting our time. It's a bit of a toss-up because ICI in certain parts of the country is a very large employer and creates almost its own social class.

STEWART: What qualification do you need to be on your pension staff? For instance, does a worker have to work 10 years to qualify for a pension? Does he get a lump sum if he's ill?

PADDLE: That's another awkward question because it has changed over the years. In fact, now the qualification period is extremely short. The British system for pensions is not that you have to leave your pension in little bits around the country, but that you can actually transfer it. From an epidemiological point of view this causes problems. By British standards, or by any standards, it is really quite a comprehensive pension system.

STEWART: It could even affect your case control studies, couldn't it?

PADDLE: That's true.

ACHESON: Dr. Paddle, could you tell us roughly what proportion of the deaths in persons ever employed you lose? What is not clear to me is to what extent you are helped by your pension system.

PADDLE: The length of service of people in ICI is like that in most large companies, I think. It is called the "bathtub" distribution. Once you get into ICI and have worked there a couple of years you can't afford to leave. Once employees have passed the first 18 months, they tend to stay about 35 years. We do lose a lot of people, but they are the short service people. This gives us also a large chunk of people with 25-30 years of service. I did a little bit of work with the vinyl chloride cohort that Fox and Collier reported. In that cohort we had about 45% follow-up. It's not a good study to look at because for liver cancer—you've either got the one case or you haven't, so it doesn't tell whether or not the problem was found.

One could say that it's the good 50%—the long service people with interesting histories. Perhaps you could say it's the bad 50% because you lose the people who can't take the noxious fumes and leave their jobs earlier.

GAFFEY: It seems to me that you're reporting on the combination of a PMR as a screening device and then a case control study. The problem with case control studies is you have to place your bets in advance. While with your PMR, you're sort of fishing—when you find something then, in combination with the PMR you use the case control to follow up on the leads you might have.

PADDLE: That's right, yes. In fact, I do do the odd cohort study, but I have to have my arms sort of up here somewhere in a half Nelson (indicating).

R. PETO: You have asked why you're not given the facilities of the Office of Population Censuses and Surveys. These obviously would be of advantage to you because they could give you, not only deaths, but also incident cases of cancer. But the OPCS certainly were concerned that they would be giving information to a company, and they would have no check on whether the data were used honestly.

Now, they are prepared, on principle, to collaborate with independent bona fide medical researchers, but not with people who might want to suppress inconvenient data. You as an individual are probably as honest as the next man, but ICI has a very big financial interest in the outcome of these investigations.

Could you comment on what precautions you think OPCS should require? Perhaps there should be some kind of representation, at least of the sort of independent government statistics section, in your analyses and what you do with the data, I think. I think that's a fair viewpoint for them to take.

PADDLE: Well, one aspect of it is—I expect our American friends do know this, but if they don't—that the Southport system is not computerized. If ICI, followed by BP, followed by Shell, were to give people this amount of work, they would need to take on extra staff. Now, ICI would be willing to pay for extra staff, but I understand they would fall over one another, because they actually cannot get to the files to do the work. That's the view I have been given, that they just can't have more clerks in that place, therefore they can't do more work. We don't have the best record-keeping system. The difficulty we always have, even when doing joint research, is that the researcher must publish results immediately. We must first report to the workforce and management and then sort out what the results are. That process can take quite a long time.

R. PETO: ICI might be exceptional, compared with other companies. If they give it to one company they must give it to others. Perhaps ICI is better than others.

WAXWEILER: I assume you have been working on the excesses you found. Are there an excess of brain neoplasms?

PADDLE: No. I have not managed to get my medical officers interested in motley collections. There might be something there, but I need an awful lot of help because I'm a simple statistician, and it takes time.

REFERENCES

Fox, A.J. and A.M. Adelstein. 1978. Occupational mortality: Work or way of life? *J. Epidemiol. Community Health* **32**:73.

SESSION 3:
Industry-Wide Cancer Experience — Methodological Problems

Introduction — Developing Protective Strategies

MICHAEL A. SILVERSTEIN, Chairperson
International Union, United Auto Workers

I think that if one of the underlying aims of this meeting is to substitute one set of estimates with another, it would be an unfortunate mistake, however important the quantitative exercise may be. If, by the same token, a goal of this meeting is to seek specific consensus on a set or sets of numbers, I think that would be an inappropriate and ill-advised gesture.

Let me give you an example of what I mean. I found the numbers and the discussions surrounding the asbestos issue yesterday to be extremely challenging and interesting. But I–and I suspect that my feelings are shared by some others–would like the opportunity to be able to think carefully about what I have heard, to see material in writing, and to have a chance to give some careful thought, in particular, to the policy implications of what was raised.

As we enter a somewhat more speculative set of presentations, a sense of perspective of this sort becomes even more important. We must keep in mind, first, Irving Selikoff's opening comment that, because our current estimates inevitably rest on evidence that is at hand, it is hardly likely that we know all the occupational carcinogens or even, for that matter, all the important ones. We know even less about the populations at risk.

Second, we must consider the fact that this meeting, as broadly designed as it is, is forced to touch on a relatively narrow spectrum of chemical exposures and industrial processes.

Third, there have been enormous new fields of investigation opened for exploration in the recent past and there are many studies in progress now that are really still too rough, too unfinished for full discussion. For example, just surveying the corner of the industrial landscape with which I am most familiar, automotive manufacture and related metalworking industries, there have been recent findings generating hypotheses about work-related cancer. Some examples are in iron foundries and in machining plants where cutting-fluid mists and oil smokes are of concern, in certain plating and die-casting operations, in spray painting, in model and pattern making, and in automobile assembly plants themselves. In other words, these are huge areas of basic industry, largely unstudied in the past, yet involving hundreds of thousands of our UAW members alone, and beyond the UAW, hundreds and hundreds of thousands additionally.

Investigations are underway in all these areas, many of which are grappling with some very basic and difficult issues of study design and data availability. It is, therefore, appropriate that we move now into a series of papers, some of which involve the basic methodological considerations that may help to determine how we go about moving in the immediate future from these preliminary findings and these early hypotheses to more precise judgments and to protective strategies. From my perspective, the bottom line is that last note—the search for protective strategies.

Mortality Studies on Lung, Pancreas, Esophageal, and Other Cancers in Louisiana

MARISE S. GOTTLIEB AND JEAN K. CARR
Department of Medicine
Tulane University School of Medicine
New Orleans, Louisiana 70112

Louisiana has been shown to have a high mortality rate for cancers of all sites combined for 1950-1969, particularly among males, and more specifically for cancers of the lung, pancreas, and bladder (Mason and McKay 1974). These high cancer mortality rates are more marked in certain parishes and in local areas. These increased rates are noted primarily in parishes (counties) bordering the Mississippi River and the Atchafalaya Basin, which is the natural outlet for the Mississippi River, therefore several etiologic hypotheses have been proposed (Blot and Fraumeni 1976; Blot et al. 1977). Because there is heavy industrialization by petroleum refining, chemical, and petrochemical industries, particularly in the parishes located along the Mississippi River, we were interested in investigating the possible contribution of these industries to the observed cancer mortality rates.

To pursue this hypothesis, it was necessary to include the following variables: industry of occupation and occupation, particularly as the high mortality rate was being noted mainly among males; drinking water source, because many of the residents in the river parishes obtain their drinking water from the Mississippi River; and genetic susceptibility, as many of the residents of this region are Acadian in origin and have maintained their identification with this group, both by marriage and by cultural traditions.

Although the importance and contribution of cigarette smoking to the etiology of these cancers was recognized, we sought a rapid means to assess some of the other influences, because we believed that the increased rates of these cancers in Louisiana as compared with other states in the United States could not be accounted for solely by differences in cigarette smoking patterns.

METHODS

A death certificate survey was undertaken for these cancer sites for 1960-1975 in parishes selected as having high mortality rates for cancer of the lung and pancreas and whose residents had greater than 1% of their working population employed in the petroleum, chemical, and paper industries (Gottlieb et al. 1979; Pickle and Gottlieb 1980). To avoid uncontrollable effects of large urban areas, only parishes with small populations were included.

As a readily available comparison group to control for effects of drinking water source and Acadian ancestry, deaths from all other noncancer causes were selected from within the same parish of usual residence at death and matched to the cancer death by age at death (± 5 years), year of death (± 1 year), race, and sex. (In general, the drinking water sources for residents within a parish have similar origins and quality.) These were compared to the lung, pancreas, and bladder cancer deaths for frequency of employment in various industries as defined by the U.S. Census Classification of Industry and Occupation (Bureau of Census 1971). This procedure may have overcontrolled on industry of occupation, which would possibly decrease the observable risk for industry of occupation and cancers. To assess the possible bias of using deaths as a control group, the distribution of deaths from causes other than cancer in the selected population was compared to the statewide distribution of these deaths for the same time period. There were no significant differences in these distributions. This indicates, within reason, that the control deaths used for comparisons may not be subject to a bias operating to suggest or obscure associations with industry of occupation.

In a second study designed primarily to look at the possible contribution of drinking water source to their etiology, additional cancer sites were studied (Gottlieb 1981; M. S. Gottlieb et al., in prep.). Except for selecting the deaths for comparison from several parishes to ensure the availability of a distribution of water source types, the study design, variables included, and information obtained was similar to the first study. All of these parishes were from southern Louisiana. Some of the larger urban parishes were sampled to include them and to maintain a balance in availability of subjects by water source. Observations on several of these sites with regard to possible contributions of occupation to risk of disease are included.

Usual industry of occupation is reported routinely on Louisiana death certificates. However, it is not coded or kept on tape. Therefore, each death certificate was abstracted individually for usual industry and occupation, parish of birth, residence at death, as well as family surnames, to enable the development of a method to assess roughly the possible contribution of Acadian ancestry or culture to the susceptibility to cancer. Occupation and industry were reported on 81% of the certificates, with no differences in rate of reporting for the cancer death and noncancer death. However, persons employed in more than one industry during their lifetime will have only one detected, as only one is recorded on the death certificate.

The petrochemical industry first became a major employer in Louisiana in the mid-1960s. Therefore, it is now possible to use the period of deaths covered in these studies to begin to assess the impact of this industry on mortality in

Louisiana. Those employed in the petroleum industry are reported to follow the migration of the industry and maintain employment within the industry, despite perhaps changing companies.

The odds ratio is used to express the level of risk; and, the 95% confidence intervals (CI) and chi-square statistic, the likelihood of risk occurring by chance.

RESULTS

First Study

There were 3327 lung cancer deaths in the 19 parishes of the first study, 2805 of whom were male. Figure 1 indicates the parishes included in the study. The chemical and petroleum industry-related deaths are shown in Table 1,

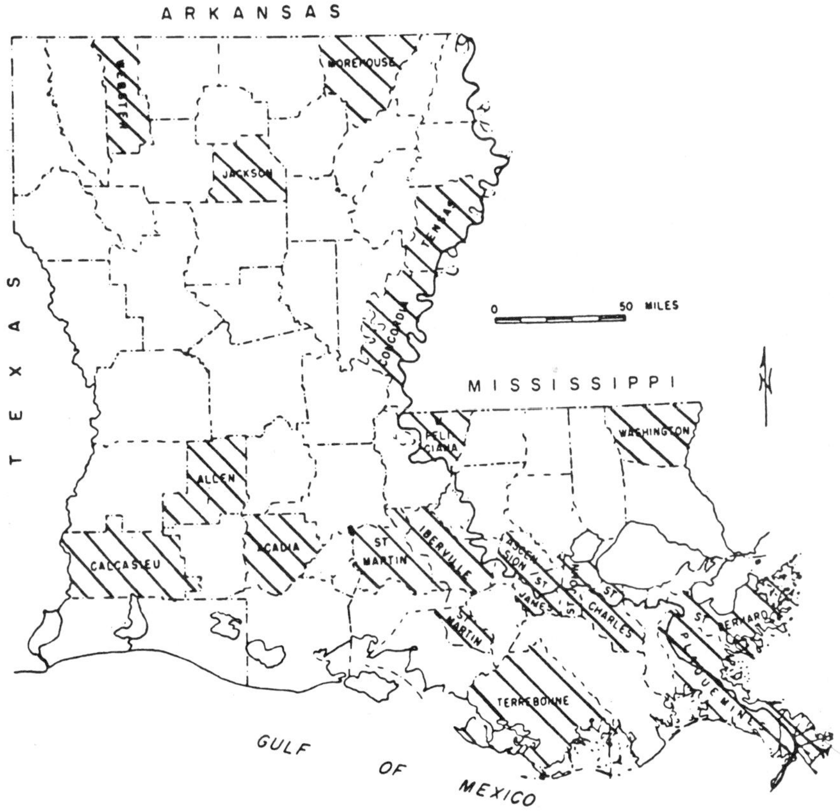

Figure 1
(▨) Louisiana parishes included in this study.

Table 1
Odds Ratios for Selected Industries for Lung Cancer and Controls among Males by Age

	Code	Cases	Controls	Odds ratio (95% CI)
Crude oil extraction	049	128	116	1.10 (0.95, 1.27)
< Age 63		75	87	0.85 (0.74, 0.97)
⩾ Age 63		53	29	1.83 (1.20, 2.79)
Chemical	347-369	38	34	1.11 (0.85, 1.44)
< Age 63		24	19	1.25 (0.85, 1.85)
⩾ Age 63		14	15	0.92 (0.66, 1.31)
Oil refining	377-378	76	58	1.31 (1.04, 1.65)
< Age 63		38	38	0.99 (0.79, 1.25)
⩾ Age 63		38	20	1.90 (1.13, 3.19)
Fishing	028	72	40	1.81 (1.27, 2.58)
< Age 63		28	17	1.64 (0.99, 2.71)
⩾ Age 63		44	23	1.91 (1.18, 3.12)

distributed above and below the mean age at death for cases of lung cancer included in the study.

Odds ratios of greater than 1.5 are found in the older oil mining extraction and refining workers, and the CI indicates an almost three-fold risk at the upper limits. Of all deaths from lung cancer, 7% list a usual occupation in either petroleum mining or refining. This is likely to be very much an underestimate of the true occupational exposures to these industries.

Except for a marginal increase in the odds ratio to 1.3 among younger chemical workers, this study does not demonstrate an occupational risk associated with lung cancer. The small numbers may reflect the recent entry and growth of the industry in this area, as well as the fact that it may be too early to measure its possible impact on disease by the use of death certificates. The observation of the slight increase among younger workers indicates a possible effect that would be worthwhile to continue to observe and perhaps to study by incidence studies.

The observation of the increase in the odds ratio to reflect an almost two-fold risk among fishermen, with 1.0 excluded in the 95% CI, is most intriguing, especially as it is a relatively frequently listed occupation. Moreover, it is a very common avocation in this area. It is reported that the vicinity of the oil rigs is a good fishing area, as the fish are attracted to the underwater conduits.

Of those workers employed in the petroleum mining and refining industries, the greatest increase in risk is found among the operator categories and oil field workers—the welders, operators, and boiler makers, (Table 2)—

Table 2
Risk of Lung Cancer Mortality by Specific Occupations in the Petroleum Industry by Age

Occupation	Cases	Controls	Odds ratio (95% CI)
Oilfield worker	26	15	1.7 (0.99, 3.01)
<60	6	5	
$\geqslant 60$	20	10	1.99 (0.93, 4.25)
Welder	8	2	4.0 (0.22, 72.98)
<60	5	1	
$\geqslant 60$	3	1	
Skilled, pumping, refining	54	36	1.5 (1.08, 2.07)
<60	29	26	1.1 (0.82, 1.50)
$\geqslant 60$	25	10	2.5 (1.01, 6.17)
Subtotal	88	53	1.67 (1.25, 2.24)
Other Petroleum	112	117	
Total	200	170	1.2 (1.04, 1.34)

where one can demonstrate an odds ratio in excess of 1.5 (1.67) and a CI not including 1.0 (1.25,2.24) (Gottlieb 1980).

The excess risk in this industry is clearly seen among older workers in the operator occupations, where there is a twofold risk. Because the accident rate is noted to be so high among younger workers in this industry, the observed rate among older workers is even more striking.

Although the deaths available for the study of cancer of the pancreas (399 white males) were much smaller than for lung cancer, as seen in Table 3, a similar excess risk was found among white males employed in oil refining (15 cases, 7 controls) 2.21 (0.83,6.48). A similar pattern is also noted for cancer of the bladder. Among 176 white males with bladder cancer, six cases, compared with one control, reported working in the oil refining industry (Gottlieb and Pickle 1981).

Table 3
Risk of Cancer of the Lung, Pancreas, and Bladder in Oil Refinery Workers

		Mean age at death (years)	Oil refinery cases (*n*)	Oil refinery controls (*n*)	Odds ratio (95% CI)	Total cases
Lung	males	63	76	58	1.31 (1.04, 1.65)	2805
Pancreas	white males	67	15	7	2.21 (0.83, 6.48)	399
Bladder	white males	71	6	1	6.12 (0.73-283.1)	176

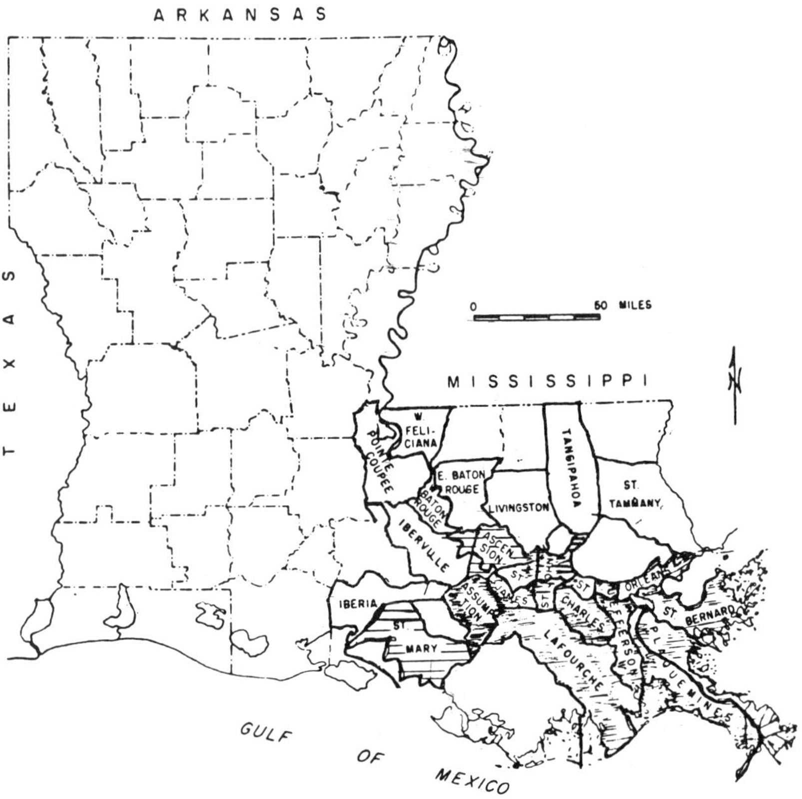

Figure 2
Location of parishes. (□) Ground water parishes; (▩) surface water parishes; (▨) mixed ground and surface water parishes.

Second Study

Figure 2 indicates the parishes included in the second study. Many cancer sites were screened to determine if there was a drinking water contribution to their etiology. The sites shown in Table 4 were found to be associated with the chemical industry.

Brain and kidney cancer showed an association with chemical industries with an odds ratio of 3.5 for brain (the CI does not include 1.0). One-half of the 14 brain cancer cases died at younger than 50 years of age, whereas none of the controls were so young at death.

Kidney, esophageal cancers and leukemia were noted to be associated with the petroleum refineries and petrochemical industries (Table 5). In Louisiana, many of these industries manufacture both pure chemical and petrochemical

Table 4
Risk of Cancer of the Brain and Kidney for Workers in the Chemical Industry

Site	Mean age (years)	Chemical cases (n)	Industry controls (n)	Odds ratio (95% CI)	χ^2 (p)	Total cases
Brain	46.0	14	4	3.52 (1.09, 14.8)	<.025	497
Kidney	58.6	6	1	6.06 (0.73, 279.6)	<.10	351
Total		20	5	4.03 (1.46, 13.8)	<.005	

Table 5
Risk of Cancer by Occupation in the Petroleum or Petrochemical Industry, for Kidney and Esophageal Cancer and Leukemia

		Petrochemical			
Cancer Site	Mean age (years)	cases (n)	controls (n)	Odds ratio (95% CI)	χ^2 (p)
Kidney	58.6	22	10	2.27 (1.01, 5.43)	<.05
Esophagus	63.2	23	8	3.19 (1.35, 8.37)	<.005
Leukemia	52.1	41	24	1.70 (0.99, 2.92)	<.05

products. Because it was impossible to distinguish the exposure of a given person, these industries were grouped for this analysis. Except for leukemia, where the odds ratio is only 1.7, the other odds ratios are in excess of 2.0—kidney at 2.3 (significant at $p < 0.05$) and esophagus at 3.2 (significant at $p < 0.005$).

The combined risk for kidney cancer by either the petroleum or chemical industries workers is reflected in an odds ratio of 2.66, which does not include 1.0 in the CI and is significant at $p < .01$. If one combines both brain and kidney cancers the risk is reflected in an odds ratio of 4.03 and significant at $p < 0.005$.

Among kidney cancer deaths, 7% were employed in the chemical, petroleum, and petrochemical industries, and similarly 7% of esophageal cancer deaths were employed in the petroleum and petrochemical industries.

The mean age at death among these cancers is 63 years for esophageal and lung cancer patients, 67 years for pancreas cancer, 71 years for bladder cancer, 59 years for cancer of the kidney, 52 years for leukemia, and 46 years for cancer of the brain.

DISCUSSION

When discussing cancer, the most important possible confounder for most mortality studies, such as the ones presented here, is cigarette smoking history. As there is no way of obtaining the smoking history of the decedents from death certificates, it is possible that heavier smoking habits might be associated with certain occupational groups, which could then predispose them to an increased chance of cancer. Using a death certificate data base, there is no way to refute this possibility conclusively, although internal evidence might be cited to make the possibility less likely. A majority of the control deaths, as is to be expected, died of circulatory system disease, diseases that are also associated with cigarette smoking. This might provide a control for cigarette smoking. The association of lung cancer with petroleum workers in the operations jobs closely related to the product, but not in operations jobs in other industries where workers are reported to have a similar cigarette smoking rate, suggests an occupational exposure rather than a smoking effect. The clear differential risk by industry appears to override a purely cigarette smoking effect, which would tend to obliterate these differences. The presence of the risk exclusively among those older than the mean age of 63 is somewhat more perplexing. It is possible that the somewhat lesser degree of cigarette smoking among older workers does not obscure the effect of industry as much as in younger workers, although this could also reflect a dose-response to length of exposure in the industry. While this pattern is present for both oil extraction and oil refining, it is not the case among fishermen, where the risk is present in both age groups. It is also interesting that an increased risk is seen with pancreatic cancer as well, although the numbers of cases and controls are too small to be conclusive.

The results from the second mortality study reinforce those from the first study, although the parishes studied were different and not selected because of high mortality rates for specific cancer sites. The study design introduced more variability in the residence at death, because the cases and controls were not matched on parish at death. The highly significant association of brain cancer with occupation in the chemical industry echoes associations reported elsewhere and in other studies, and, although the numbers are small, the effect is large enough to achieve significance. It was also observed that one-half the brain cancer cases were 50 years old or less when they died, while none of the controls was younger than 50 years old at death (by the design of the study, they had the same likelihood of being young). This might indicate an increasing risk with time. This association was marked for the purely chemical industries, and no risk at all was observed in the petroleum or petrochemical industries for brain cancer. For kidney cancer, on the other hand, a risk was seen for both industry types—a risk which was highly significant when the two industry types were combined. In addition to kidney cancer, a significant risk for esophageal cancer was observed in workers in the petroleum and petrochemical industries. The odds ratio for esophageal cancer is greater than 3 and is highly significant. By far, this was the largest occupational risk observed for any site in these studies. There is also a somewhat lower risk for leukemia, which is not quite as significant but demonstrates twice as many cases as controls in the petroleum industry.

The use of a mortality data base entails many obvious problems, which can only be partially overcome by careful study design. For an assessment of occupational risk, there is the clear inadequacy of the occupational history recorded on the death certificate, along with the biases possible in its recording. The use of noncancer deaths for controls to reflect the age-race-sex distribution of the population at risk is also not optimal because it is possible that some other very common disease, like heart disease, might make up enough of the noncancer deaths to give the distribution of the controls the characteristics of the risk factors for that disease.

The observations on these studies for 1960-1975 mortality data for Louisiana are consistent with observations based on aggregate analyses of the U.S. 1950-1969 mortality data by county. Also, the proportion of the cancer cases attributed to the various industries is very likely to be an underestimate because only one industry is recorded on the death certificate. These may be undetected by this methodology.

A small number of these cases and controls were followed up by contacting next-of-kin for more definitive information. For each cancer death, the death certificate diagnosis was confirmed. However, we found on follow-up a number of deaths, which did not report cancer on the death certificate and were employed in the chemical or petrochemical industries, to include cancer as a diagnosis. Also a number of the cancer deaths not recorded as employed in these industries on death certificates reported these exposures in response to a mail questionnaire. Inaccuracies in the opposite direction were not as common, resulting in a "corrected" risk estimate greater than the previous estimate. Therefore, it is likely that the estimate of 7% of people dying from these cancers and associated with these industries is very much an underestimate and the risk ratio is likely to be higher as well. Unfortunately, a better estimate of population risk is not able to be calculated from currently available data.

Although all of these are admitted and well-known problems, and although the estimates are probably lower than actual, the case-control mortality study still can and did contribute a great deal in examining a large field of variables, such as those found in South Louisiana, and narrowing down the investigation to those found to be the most likely contributors to the etiology of the disease.

ACKNOWLEDGMENT

This work was supported by NCI contract ICP 61058 and EPA grant number R805110 and the Louisiana Department of Health and Human Resources.

REFERENCES

Blot, W.T. and J.F. Fraumeni, Jr. 1976. Geographic patterns of lung cancer: Industrial correlations. *Am. J. Epidemiol.* **103**:539.

Blot, W.T., L.A. Brinton, J.F. Fraumeni, Jr. and B.J. Stone. 1977. Cancer mortality in U.S. counties with petroleum industries. *Science* **198**:51.

Gottlieb, M.S. 1980. Lung cancer and the petroleum industry in Louisiana. *J. Occup. Med.* **22**:384.

______. 1981. "Water source and risk of cancer mortality, Louisiana." EPA Grant No. R 805 11001-02.

Gottlieb, M.S. and L.W. Pickle. 1981. Bladder cancer mortality in Louisiana. *J. La. State Med. Soc.* **133**:6.

Gottlieb, M.S., L.W. Pickle, W.J. Blot, and J.F. Fraumeni, Jr. 1979. Lung cancer in Louisiana: Death certificate analysis. *J. Natl. Cancer Inst.* **63**:1131.

Mason, T.J. and F.W. Mc Kay. 1974. *U.S. cancer mortality by county: 1950-69.* DHEW Publ. No. (NIH) 74-615. U.S. Government Printing Office, Washington, D.C.

Pickle, L.W. and M.S. Gottlieb. 1980. Pancreatic cancer mortality in Louisiana. *Am. J. Public Health* **70**:256.

Bureau of Census. 1971. *1970 census of population. Alphabetical index of industries and occupations.* U.S. Government Printing Office, Washington, D.C.

An Estimate of the Percentage of Occupational Cancer Among a Group of Rubber Workers

RICHARD R. MONSON AND ELIZABETH DELZELL*
Department of Epidemiology
Harvard School of Public Health
Boston, Massachusetts 02115

We do not know whether it is possible to quantify the percent of cancer that is due to occupation, but we do know that any effort at quantification will be severely criticized. Our efforts at quantification follow the dictums of John Graunt who used three empiric methods to estimate the population of London in 1662 (Graunt 1939):

1. On the basis of the number of teeming women, the estimate was 384,000.
2. On the basis of the number of parishes within the walls, the estimate was 384,000.
3. On the basis of the amount of housing within the walls, the estimate was 380,160.

Graunt recognized that, although his methods were crude, his data gave no support to the belief that there were millions of people in London.

In 1978 investigators from the National Cancer Institute (NCI), the National Institute of Environmental Health Sciences (NIEHS), and the National Institute for Occupational Safety and Health (NIOSH) estimated that the percentage of future cancer attributable to past occupational exposure may be at least 20% (Bridbord et al. 1978). The methods used for this estimate were more complicated than those used by Graunt, however the quantitative estimate was not substantially more believable.

Bridbord et al. pointed out that of the previous "estimates only 1% to 5% of total cancers in the United States are attributable to occupational factors have not been scientifically documented." In this report we attempt to document our estimates of the percent of occupational cancer among a group of rubber workers.

*Present address: Duke University Comprehensive Cancer Center, Durham, NC 27710.

METHODS

Our data have been previously published (Monson and Nakano 1976; Monson and Fine 1978; E. Delzell and R. R. Monson 1981). The study population consists of 15,643 white male union members who worked in the Akron, Ohio, plant of the B.F. Goodrich Company. All were members of Local #5, United Rubber Workers. Each of these men had worked for at least 2 years in the plant between January 1, 1940, and July 1, 1971. Many had started employment in the early 1900s and were still active in 1940. Follow-up started on January 1, 1940, or the second anniversary of employment, whichever was later, and continued until death or July 1, 1978. Deaths were ascertained from company pension records and from the Social Security Administration (SSA).

Both external and internal comparisons were made. In the mortality analyses, expected numbers of cancer deaths were computed on the basis of age-time-cause-specific mortality rates for U.S. white males. In the morbidity analyses, rubber workers were stratified into persons who had worked in specific work areas and into residual workers. Directly standardized cancer morbidity rates were computed for the several groups using the age-time, person-years distribution of all white male union rubber workers. The results of these two modes of comparison were in general similar.

Our methods in this paper derive from a principle laid down by John Graunt: One should reduce data "into a few perspicuous Tables . . . without any multiloquious Deductions." We have taken the observed and expected numbers of cancer from our previous analyses and have examined them according to cause and several characteristics of exposure and follow-up: Age and year started working, number of years worked, latency (years between year of first employment and year of death), and age and year of death. We feel no need to justify our methods beyond the need to explore alternate means of quantifying the excess of occupational cancer among this group of rubber workers. For each method we suggest one criticism that the method leads to an estimate that is too high or too low.

RESULTS

In Table 1, we examine the overall observed and expected deaths among all workers for all cancers and all non-cancers. If one postulates that the standardized mortality ratios (SMRs) for these two categories of cause of death should be equal, the estimate of excess cancer is 13%.

In Table 2, we examine among all workers the specific cancers for which the SMR is greater than 100. Based on the excess cancers from these subtractions, the estimate of excess cancer is 3.5%. If an SMR of 90 is used as the "correct" comparison, the estimate of excess cancer is 3.9%. (Only one additional cancer would be added to Table 2: Brain cancer has an SMR of 91).

Table 1
Estimate of Excess Cancer among 15,643 Rubber Workers Based on Overall Observed and Expected Causes of Death

Data					
cause of death	observed deaths	expected deaths	O/E	Estimate of excess cancer	Criticism
Cancer	1352	1414.4	0.96	$0.96 \div 0.85 = 1.13$	estimate of excess too high because healthy-worker
Noncancer	5445	6400.8	0.85	excess = 13%	effect stronger for noncancer than for cancer

Table 2
Estimate of Excess Cancer among Rubber Workers Based on Cancers with an SMR Greater Than 100

Data					
cause of death	observed deaths	expected deaths	O – E	Estimate of excess cancer	Criticism
Esophagus cancer	36	34.3	1.7		estimate of excess too low because SMR of 100 is improper baseline
Stomach cancer	110	106.8	3.2		
Large intestine cancer	144	136.5	7.5		
Rectal cancer	58	56.4	1.6		
Biliary and liver cancer	40	35.8	4.2		
Prostate cancer	121	118.4	2.6		
Bladder cancer	60	51.5	8.5		
Lymphatic cancer	60	54.1	5.9		
Leukemia	68	56.3	11.7		
Total	697	650.1	46.9	$(46.9 \div 1352) \times 100 = 3.5\%$	

In Table 3 we examine among specific groups of workers the incident cancers that were judged previously as having some likelihood of being causal and for which some stable number of cases had been identified. The selection of these data was based on an extensive examination of the data available to us and not at all on prior knowledge. For each of these excesses, we assigned an arbitrary probability that the excess was causal: This probability was based primarily on knowledge of the rubber-making process and on knowledge available from other studies of rubber workers. We have no vested interest in the magnitude of any of these probabilities, but we firmly believe that some modification of the total number of excess cases of cancer is indicated. Based only on the crude numbers in Table 3, the estimate of excess cancer is 10.3%. Based on the modified numbers, the estimate of excess cancer is 5.8%.

In Tables 4-6, we examine excess cancer according to six methods of comparison of observed and expected numbers. The data were analyzed using 5-year strata and are grouped in Tables 5 and 6. Latency was the characteristic that most strongly discriminated between observed and expected numbers. As seen in Table 4, prior to 30 years of latency, expected numbers exceeded observed numbers. After 30 years of latency, there was a consistent excess of observed numbers. Based on the sum of these excesses, the estimate of excess cancers is 5.1%.

As seen in Tables 5 and 6, the other five characteristics of work and follow-up discriminated poorly or not at all between observed and expected numbers. The excess of cancer among men dying at age 75 and above is a reflection of these men having the longest latencies.

In Table 7, we summarize the estimates from Tables 1-6 and the criticisms of these estimates. We find it difficult to justify an estimate of excess cancer of greater than 10% from these data and believe that 5-6% is the best estimate. We judged that this group of rubber workers is not atypical of employed males in heavy industry with respect to exposure to chemicals that may be carcinogenic. We judge that workers in heavy industry are likely to have more exposure to chemical carcinogens than the average male. Therefore, based on the data available to us, we estimate that among American white males approximately 5% of cancer is due to occupational exposures.

DISCUSSION

We have conducted this exercise as one approach to the quantification of the percentage of cancer due to occupational exposures. We make no apologies for our estimate, but neither do we defend it to the teeth. Epidemiology is at best a semiquantitative science, and epidemiologic data must be interpreted with caution. Further, it is clear that any quantitative estimate is subject to a large dose of subjective judgment. However, we applaud the organizers of this conference and agree with the observation of John Graunt that ". . . a clear

Table 3
Estimate of Excess Cancer among Rubber Workers Based on Judgmental Evaluation of Excess Cancer Incidence According to Work Area

Data					Estimate of excess cancer (there were a total of 1359 incident cases)	Criticisms
cancer	work area	excess cases	probability[a]	likely excess[b]		
Stomach	rubber making	7.1	0.8	5.7		a. not all excesses are likely to be causal
	solid tires	1.1	0.5	0.5		
Large intestine	–	21.8	(0.69)[c]	15.1		b. not all causal excesses were identified
Pancreas	–	8.8	(0.16)	1.4		
Lung	tire curing	16.9	0.8	13.5		a. + b. probabilities are incorrectly judged
	tire molds	5.0	0.5	2.5		
	fuel cells/deicers	16.9	0.6	10.0		
Skin	tire assembly	10.2	0.9	9.2		
Brain	tire assembly	6.1	0.2	1.2		
Other	–	46.3	(0.43)	20.0	a. $(140.2/1359) \times 100 = 10.3\%$	
Total	–	140.2	(0.56)	79.1	b. $(79.1/1359) \times 100 = 5.8\%$	

[a]Arbitrary likelihood that excess is causal.
[b]Likely excess = excess cases × probability.
[c]Probabilities in parentheses are average probabilities based on more than one work area.

Table 4
Estimate of Excess Cancer among Rubber Workers Based on Latency (years between year of first employment and year of death)

Data						
years of latency	observed cancers	expected cancers	O/E	O − E	Estimate of excess cancer	Criticism
0	12	20.6	0.6			there are likely to be causal excesses among subgroups with less than 30 years of latency
5	26	37.8	0.7			
10	48	64.0	0.8			
15	82	105.8	0.8			
20	128	162.9	0.8			
25	190	224.0	0.9			
30	257	232.0	1.1	25.0		
35	184	183.1	1.0	0.9		
40	182	169.8	1.1	12.2		
45	128	121.1	1.1	6.9		
50	74	64.1	1.2	9.9		
55+	41	27.2	1.5	13.8		
Total	1352	1412.4[a]		68.7	(68.7/1352) × 100 = 5.1%	

[a]This differs from the total excess in Table 1 because of differences in the computer algorithm.

Table 5
Estimate of Excess Cancer among Rubber Workers Based on Age First Employed, Year First Employed, and Total Years of Employment

Data									
age first employed			year first employed			total years employed			
age	Observed cancers	O/E	year	Observed cancers	O/E	years	Observed cancers	O/E	Estimate of excess cancer
<30	625	0.9	<1925	383	0.9	<15	374	0.9	these three characteristics of employment did not discriminate between observed and expected numbers. The data were examined in 5-year strata and are grouped for presentation.
30-44	576	1.0	1925-39	545	1.0	15-29	486	1.0	
⩾45	151	1.0	⩾1940	424	1.0	⩾30	492	1.0	

Table 6
Estimate of Excess Cancer among Rubber Workers Based on Age At Death and Calendar Year of Death

Data						
age at death			year of death			
age	Observed cancer	O/E	year	Observed cancer	O/E	Estimate of excess cancer
<60	365	0.8	<1955	207	0.8	Year of death did not discriminate between observed and expected numbers. Age at death discriminated less than did latency, with which it is highly correlated.
60-74	682	1.0	1955-69	626	1.0	
⩾75	305[a]	1.2	⩾1970	519	1.0	

[a]Expected number = 264.5; excess number = 40.5; estimate of excess cancer = 3.0%.

Table 7
Summary Estimates of Excess Cancer among Rubber Workers and Generalization to Other Workers

Summary				
method	estimate of excess	criticism	Generalization	The bottom line
Overall SMR for all cancer	13%	too high	to other rubber workers–no reason to believe this group is atypical	
Overall SMRs for individual cancers	3.5%	too low	to other workers in heavy industry–the average rubber worker is judged to have at least as much exposure to chemicals as the average worker in other heavy industries	
Judgment on cancer incidence by work area				
Excess cases	10.3%	too high		
Likely excess	5.8%	about right	to all white males–the average worker in heavy industry is judged to have more exposure to chemicals than the average white male	based on these data from mortality between 1940 and 1978 among 15,643 white males who were employed for at least 2 years in one rubber plant, the percent of occupational cancer among U.S. white males is not likely to be greater than 5%
Latency	5.1%	about right		

knowledge of all these particulars . . . is necessary in order to good, certain, and easie Government."

ACKNOWLEDGMENTS

Supported by a contract with the B.F. Goodrich Company and the United Rubber, Cork, Linoleum and Plastics Workers of America. Dr. Delzell was also supported by a traineeship from the National Institute of Occupational Safety and Health (5 T15 OHO 7096)

REFERENCES

Bridbord, K., P. DeCoufle, J.F. Fraumeni, Jr., D.G. Hoel, R.N. Hoover, D.P. Rall, U. Saffiotti, M.A. Schneiderman, and A.C. Upton. 1978. "Estimates of the fraction of cancer in the United States related to occupational factors." NCI, NIEHS, NIOSH, September 15, 1978.

Delzell, E. and R. R. Monson. 1981. Mortality among rubber workers. III. Cost-specific mortality, 1940-1978. 5. *J. Occ. Med.* (in press)

Graunt, J. 1939. In *Natural and political observations made upon the bills of mortality* (ed. W.F. Willcox), Johns Hopkins Press, Baltimore.

Monson, R.R. and K.K. Nakano. 1976. Mortality among rubber workers. I. White male union employees in Akron, Ohio. *Am. J. Epidemiol.* **103**:284.

Monson, R.R. and L.J. Fine. 1978. Cancer mortality and morbidity among rubber workers. *J. Natl. Cancer Inst.* **61**:1047.

COMMENTS

GAFFEY: I had one reaction to your first three methods. In each of them, you look at a lot of SMRs, some of which are bigger than 100 and some of which are less; you throw away the ones that are less than 100, save the ones that are bigger, and use those to estimate. Thus, even if there is nothing wrong with the mortality experience of the cohort, you will always find an excess cancer, except for the unlikely event where all the SMRs are less than 100.

MONSON: Yes, I think some of the things that are negotiable are whether or not one would even want to do this method. I merely wanted to go through things that were possible and that were simple. As I said, in the second method, if one looks at specific cancers using 100 as an arbitrary cutoff, one could say, "Well, maybe you should use 110, maybe one should use 90, or whatever." I think that sort of points the finger at where you want to look further.

STEWART: I notice that we are constantly talking about the healthy-worker effect, which is expected to fade. I wonder if this is really correct. If you recruit exceptionally healthy people into any population, they should stay there. For instance, we don't expect the top social class will go and get worse off as it gets older. Everybody is going to die, but it will retain its advantage. I am wondering how much this assumption (that there is, in fact, a sort of initial advantage which disappears), isn't a reflection of extra work risks.

MONSON: I don't feel that way. Certainly, there is screening of employment when people with current illness are not entered into the work force.

STEWART: I don't think screening really does very much. I am not talking particularly about your industry. There are very few industries that systematically turn a man away because he has got high blood pressure. They can't afford to do this. There are lots and lots of industries that can't afford any initial examination. Yet you will always find that you have, to some extent, the healthy-worker effect. You might even argue that you have to be fit to apply for the job. I am just wondering whether we have gone wrong in assuming that this is a temporary phenomenon.

MONSON: Well, I think it is temporary, but the temporariness of it takes a fairly long time.

STEWART: Why?

MONSON: You know, if you look at specific causes of death in large numbers of occupational groups, it is always the same causes of death that are greatly underrepresented in early years—chronic respiratory disease, chronic digestive disease. It is really remarkable how you have extremely low SMRs for those illnesses in almost any industrial cohort, at least early on.

RADFORD: I would just like to enter a cautionary point about generalizing from the rubber workers to the whole occupational picture. What I think you may very well have demonstrated is that there are no prominent candidate carcinogens in the rubber industry that are likely to distort the cancer rates very greatly. But I don't think you can generalize that. Evidently you don't have much asbestos in the rubber industry, therefore, you don't see any asbestos cancers. Yet, as we saw yesterday, they could easily account for 1-2% of all cancers.

MONSON: Yes, I think the way one wants to approach it is to get estimates from various industries and then do some sort of weighing. I am not suggesting that rubber workers are typical or should be used as a model. But I am saying, if one assumes they are, this is what one would get. Again, that is a negotiable sort of thing.

ACHESON: Did all of these men work in one city?

MONSON: Yes, all in one plant in Akron.

ACHESON: And your standard was the United States rate?

MONSON: When I first did this I got Ohio rates as well. Ohio rates and U.S. rates were exactly the same on cancers for which there were data on both Ohio and the United States. Subsequently, the cancer maps for the United States came out; and Summit County, which is where Akron is located, is quite typical of the United States. In my opinion, there is no great error introduced by using U.S. rates.

ACHESON: I was particularly concerned about stomach cancer, which has very marked socioeconomic relationships. I wondered how you have taken care of that.

MONSON: Summit County doesn't have any atypical stomach cancer excesses. The excesses of stomach cancer that were seen in this group were limited to one work area, the rubber makers, which is a fairly small work area. That is where excess has been found in British rubber workers. Tony, isn't there some stomach cancer excess in some UNC study, too?

McMICHAEL: There is a case-control study showing an association that was done on the four companies that UNC was working with.

MONSON: Yes, so it is the same association in three different groups of rubber workers, not overall, but just related to work area. That is some persuasive evidence, I think.

KARRH: Regarding the healthy-worker question, prior to the Rehabilitation Act of 1973 in the United States, industrial workers were selected very carefully by a physical examination process and, in many cases, by a testing procedure. This was no longer possible after the Rehabilitation Act came into effect. So a cohort that existed prior to that time would have been more carefully selected from a physical examination standpoint.

McMICHAEL: I think, since we are talking about selection at a single point in time, either as a result of self-selection by the candidate to work or by the employer—that is, as a cross-sectional effect at that moment in time—we would expect, at least statistically, given the random nature of human health and departures therefrom, some regression to the main in the subsequent decades. The further we get past that initial point of selection, the more that is likely to operate.

STEWART: In the same group?

McMICHAEL: I think so. I think also there are, obviously, very likely to be cumulative effects of living and of working. But I think there is this statistical element in it, given some of the stochastic processes at work.

MONSON: Part of it gets into relative vs absolute differences, too. If you look at RRs or SMRs, they go from quite low toward 1. But if one looks at absolute differences, they really don't change that much, at least in the data I have. So part of it is simply a matter of the aging of the population, in that the advantage gets relatively smaller as the underlying death rate goes up.

STEWART: I suppose, really, what is worrying me is whether or not anybody has really thought out how much of this change is due to the occupation. It is too easily taken for granted that you are just expecting it to fade, because, as I say, if you think of it in terms of social class, it doesn't fade.

MONSON: If you look at any group, you see the same sort of thing. They have a very low SMR early on, and as they age, it goes up, to some extent.

SCHNEIDERMAN: Has anyone ever identified as a specific group, and done a follow-up on, the unhealthy nonworker group, so we can really see if we add up to an SMR of 1.

J. PETO: John Fox has done this in England. He has looked at mortality rates of people when they leave the industry.

MONSON: When you do studies of hospitalized groups, you do survival studies. When you do studies of healthy groups, you do mortality studies. Survival studies always have relative survivals, and you are trying to get it up to 1.

McDONALD: I am worried about the blanket treatment of the healthy-worker effect. There is one type of selection that we have come across in two or three cohorts–that is, high SMRs in workers–in heavy industry who have had short exposure. My interpretation is that there is a tendency for men of poor health to be allocated to light jobs in which they don't stay long.

WEN: Considering the increased length of observation or follow-up, if there is an early healthy-worker effect operating at the very early stage then there are two factors causing an increased SMR. First, the age structure is changing. Second, given a similar life expectancy amongst the cohort group, which is closed (i.e., everybody would die at the end), the SMR would increase to compensate for the early deficit, if the life expectancy is about the same between the study population and the general population.

SCHNEIDERMAN: But it is not. If these other people are dying off early, then the life expectancy of the two groups can't be the same.

WEN: The experience shows that they are about the same, or even a little better.

SCHNEIDERMAN: You mean the people with high SMRs have the same life expectancy as people with low SMRs?

GAFFEY: They can.

CAIRNS: Surely it is obvious that our ability to predict somebody is healthy must be greater for their health next year than for their health 20 years from now. Therefore, I am sure it is inevitable that the healthy-worker effect must gradually disappear in the later years of employment.

MONSON: I feel that way. You know, cancer is a disease that occurs at age 40 or 50 or older. You don't select that much for cancer, because there aren't any predictors at age 20, whereas people get a lot of chronic non-malignant illnesses early on. That is where I think most of the selection occurs.

STEWART: But it does demand the dead to rise from their graves.

RADFORD: This healthy-worker effect is going to be a theme running through all of the discussions. Take, for example, the alcohol-related diseases, which have extremely low SMRs in the working population, age 20-30, because it is easy to select against people who have alcohol problems at the outset. One would anticipate that the kind of random phenomenon that Dr. McMichael mentioned could play a role. In other words, the alcohol disease rate, say from cirrhosis, could climb with time, because workers get into trouble and they start to drink. There is a case where the rate might be tending toward the mean because the worker is changing himself and not just simply the workplace.

STEWART: The work may have driven him to drink.

SCHNEIDERMAN: I think that may happen to epidemiologists.

ENTERLINE: My experience is that industries, particularly in a large metropolitan area, tend to compete for workers. If we want to generalize from particular industries, we have to really understand where that industry stands in the competition for its work force in terms of desirability, strength of the union, wages, and so forth. In some areas, there are leftover workers who don't compete well in some of the bigger industries and who must work elsewhere. They have very curious mortality experience. As a result, industries competing with each other for workers have different worker mortality experiences, not because of anything in the industry, but because of the way they draw workers from the labor market.

Thus, to extrapolate from a particular industry, you have to understand how that industry stands in competition for workers in Akron.

WAXWEILER: I thought Fox's article on the healthy-worker effect was an excellent one, but I think there is more than one force going on that accounts for the healthy-worker effect. An example of one-time selection having an incredible healthy-worker effect is the studies Gil Beebe made of World War II veterans. They had incredibly low mortality, even in spite of lead flying for a few years, and actually for 10, 15, 20 years after World War II.

STEWART: That, surely, is survival of the fittest. This is another way of creating a healthy population; just kill off the susceptible.

SILVERSTEIN: I understand that the studies that you were referring to are really a portion of a much broader selection of studies in the rubber industry, which included not only epidemiology, but industrial hygiene evaluations. Can you make any comments about the ability to relate the epidemiology to the exposure information?

MONSON: IARC is having a meeting this summer on the rubber industry and we will try to do it then.

A Survey of Availability of Epidemiologic Data on Humans Exposed to Animal Carcinogens

MYRA KARSTADT, RENEE BOBAL, AND IRVING J. SELIKOFF
Environmental Sciences Laboratory
Mount Sinai School of Medicine
of The City University of New York
New York, New York 10029

Effective estimation of the risk of cancer due to exposure to environmental contaminants depends on the availability of good data on exposure and the effects of exposure. We have investigated the availability and likely availability of epidemiologic data concerning carcinogenic effects in humans of exposure to chemicals that had been determined by committees of experts organized by an authoritative scientific body to be carcinogenic in animals.

The International Agency for Research on Cancer (IARC), a constituent agency of the World Health Organization (WHO), conducts a monograph program sponsored by the National Cancer Institute (NCI). Expert committees are convened to review data on effects of human and animal exposures to potentially carcinogenic agents or processes. When the committees meet, they review available data and report a consensus determination as to whether or not these data support a finding of carcinogenicity in animals and (or) humans. The first IARC monograph volume was published in 1972. By early 1981, 25 volumes and 2 supplements had been published covering more than 500 chemicals, groups of chemicals, or industrial processes.

In this paper, we discuss our investigation of the availability of epidemiologic data for chemicals classified by IARC as carcinogenic in animals, but for which data were insufficient for IARC committees to draw a firm conclusion as to carcinogenicity in humans. We sought the epidemiologic data from U.S. manufacturers, processors, and importers of agents deemed by IARC to be animal carcinogens. The survey was carried out in late 1980.

METHODS

IARC Monographs Supplement 1 (IARC 1979) summarizes the first 20 monograph volumes. We used Supplement 1 to select chemicals determined by IARC committees to be carcinogenic in animals, but for which data were insufficient to draw a conclusion as to carcinogenicity in humans.

Volumes 1-20 of the IARC monographs reviewed 442 chemicals, groups of chemicals, and industrial processes. IARC reviewed data for individual chemicals where carcinogenic effects could be identified with specific chemicals. They reviewed data for groups of chemicals (as soots, tars, and mineral oils; chromium and certain chromium compounds) where it was not possible to identify the specific compound responsible for carcinogenicity. The committees also reviewed data for certain industrial processes such as underground hematite mining or manufacture of isopropyl alcohol by the strong acid process, in which, again, a specific compound could not be identified with the carcinogenic effects observed.

Of the 442 chemicals, groups of chemicals, and industrial processes, there were 142 chemicals or groups of chemicals with sufficient evidence of carcinogenicity in animals. Epidemiologic data were identified for 60 of the 442 chemicals, chemical groups, and industrial processes. Epidemiologic data were identified by IARC for 24 of the 142 animal carcinogens. IARC determined 10 chemicals or groups of chemicals to be carcinogenic in both animals and man.[1] Thus, 132 chemicals or groups of chemicals were determined by IARC to be carcinogenic in animals, but epidemiologic data were not sufficient for a firm judgment of carcinogenicity in humans.

One of us (IJS) reviewed the list of 132 chemicals or groups of chemicals and determined that for 21 of these chemicals,[2] current human data were sufficient to permit some judgment, either positive or negative, about carcinogenic effects in humans. No further consideration was given to these 21 chemicals in our study.

Table 1 lists the 111 IARC animal carcinogens reviewed in our study. We used several sources to determine which of the 111 chemicals or groups of chemicals were in commerce in the United States. We considered a chemical in commerce if it were manufactured or processed in the United States, or imported into the United States, moved in interstate commerce, or otherwise came under the jurisdiction of the federal government.

Our principal source of information on commercial availability of IARC animal carcinogens was the Toxic Substances Control Act (TSCA) Chemical Substance Inventory (Environmental Protection Agency 1979). The Toxic Substances Control Act (1976) provided for an inventory, with data submitted by companies that fell under the jurisdiction of the Act, of chemicals in commerce

[1] The following chemicals and groups of chemicals were determined by IARC to be carcinogenic in animals and humans: 4-aminobiphenyl; asbestos; benzidine; *bis*(chloromethyl)ether; chromium; diethylstilbestrol; melphalan; β-naphthylamine; soots, tars, and mineral oils; vinyl chloride (IARC 1979).

[2] The following chemicals were dropped from our study after review by IJS: acrylonitrile; aflatoxins; benz[*a*]anthracene; benzo[*a*]pyrene; beryllium; beryllium oxide; beryllium phosphate; beryllium sulfate; cadmium; cadmium chloride; cadmium oxide; cadmium sulfate; cadmium sulfide; calcium chromate; chlorambucil; cyclophosphamide; lead acetate; lead phosphate; lead subacetate; nickel; nickel subsulfide.

Table 1
IARC Animal Carcinogens Reviewed in This Study

IARC animal carcinogens[a]	In commerce in United States
Actinomycins	X
ortho-Aminoazotoluene	X
2-Amino-5-(5-nitro-2-furyl)-1,3,4-thiadiazole	
Amitrole (aminotriazole)	X
Aramite	X
Azaserine	X
Benzo[*b*] fluoranthene	
Benzyl violet 4B	X
β-Butyrolactone	
Carbon tetrachloride	X
Chlordecone (Kepone)	X
Chloroform	X
Citrus Red No. 2	
Cycasin	
Daunomycin	X
N,N'-Diacetylbenzidine	X
4,4'-Diaminodiphenyl ether	X
2,4-Diaminotoluene	X
Dibenz[*a,h*] acridine	
Dibenz[*a,j*] acridine	
Dibenz[*a,h*] anthracene	X
7H-Dibenzo[*c,g*] carbazole	
Dibenzo[*a,e*] pyrene	
Dibenzo[*a,h*] pyrene	
Dibenzo[*a,i*] pyrene	
1,2-Dibromo-3-chloropropane	X
3,3'-Dichlorobenzidine	
3,3'-Dichloro-4,4'-diaminodiphenyl ether	
1,2-Dichloroethane	X
Diepoxybutane	X
1,2-Diethylhydrazine	
Diethyl sulfate	X
Dihydrosafrole	X
3,3'-Dimethoxybenzidine	X
para-Dimethylaminoazobenzene	X
trans-2(Dimethylamino)methylimino)-5-(2-(5-nitro-2-furyl)vinyl)-1,3,4-oxadiazole	
3,3'-Dimethylbenzidine (o-tolidine)	X
Dimethylcarbamoyl chloride	X
1,1-Dimethylhydrazine	X

Table 1—*Continued*

IARC animal carcinogens[a]	In commerce in United States
1,2-Dimethylhydrazine	
Dimethyl sulfate	X
1,4-Dioxane	X
Estradiol-17β	X
Estrone	X
Ethinylestradiol	X
Ethylene dibromide	X
Ethylenethiourea	X
Ethyl methanesulfonate	X
2-(2-Formylhydrazino)-4-(5-nitro-2-furyl)thiazole	
Glycidaldehyde	
Hexachlorobenzene	X
Hexamethylphosphoramide	X
Hydrazine	X
Indeno(1,2,3-cd)pyrene	
Iron dextran	X
Isosafrole	X
Lasiocarpine	
Merphalan	
Mestranol	X
2-Methylaziridine	X
Methylazoxymethanol acetate	
4,4′-Methylene *bis*(2-chloroaniline)	X
4,4′-Methylene *bis*(2-methylaniline)	
Methyl iodide	X
Methyl methanesulfonate	X
N-Methyl-*N*′-nitro-*N*-nitrosoguanidine	
Methylthiouracil	X
Mirex	X
Mitomycin *c*	X
Monocrotaline	
5-(Morpholinomethyl)-3-((5-nitro-furfurylidene)-amino)-2-oxazolidinone	
Niridazole	X
5-Nitroacenaphthene	X
1-(5-Nitrofurfurylidene)amino)-2-imidazolidinone	
N-(4-(5-Nitro-2-furyl)-2-thiazolyl)acetamide	

Table 1—*Continued*

IARC animal carcinogens[a]	In commerce in United States
Nitrogen mustard and its hydrochloride	X
Nitrogen mustard *N*-oxide and its hydrochloride	
N-Nitrosodi-*n*-butylamine	X
N-Nitrosodiethanolamine	X
N-Nitrosodiethylamine	X
N-Nitrosodimethylamine	X
N-Nitrosodi-*n*-propylamine	X
N-Nitroso-*N*-ethylurea	X
N-Nitrosomethylethylamine	
N-Nitroso-*N*-methylurea	X
N-Nitroso-*N*-methylurethane	X
N-Nitrosomethylvinylamine	
N-Nitrosomorpholine	
N-Nitrosonornicotine	
N-Nitrosopiperidine	X
N-Nitrosopyrrolidine	X
N-Nitrososarcosine	
Oil Orange SS	X
Polychlorinated biphenyls	X
Ponceau MX	X
Ponceau 3R	
1,3-Propane sultone	X
β-propiolactone	X
Propylthiouracil	X
Safrole	X
Sterigmatocystin	
Streptozotocin	X
Testosterone	X
Thioacetamide	X
Thiourea	X
Toxaphene	X
Tris(aziridinyl)phosphine sulfide (thiotepa)	X
Tris (2,3-dibromopropyl)phosphate	X
Trypan Blue (commercial grade)	X
Uracil mustard	X
Urethane	X

[a]For definition, see text.

in the United States at approximately the time the Act went into effect (January 1, 1977). The inventory was published in spring 1979 and generally covered chemicals in commerce between January 1, 1975, and May 1, 1978. The published version of the inventory did not include data that would permit identification of manufacturers. However, with the cooperation of Region II, Environmental Protection Agency, New York City, we were able to obtain the data we needed.

The TSCA inventory covers industrial chemicals; pesticides, foods, drugs and cosmetics are not included. The 1978 Directory of Chemical Producers was our primary source for manufacturers of pesticides and other chemicals not covered under TSCA. Physicians' Desk Reference (1975, 1980, 1981) was used to locate drug manufacturers, and we wrote to the Bureau of Drugs, Food and Drug Administration (A. Guarino, pers. comm.) for assistance in locating manufacturers of several drugs.

In all, we found that 75 of the 111 IARC animal carcinogens were reported to be in commerce in the United States. Table 1 also lists the IARC animal carcinogens in commerce in the United States.

Once the companies manufacturing, processing, or importing the IARC animal carcinogens were identified, we located parent companies for each to reduce multiple inquiries to single corporations. Standard and Poor's Encyclopedia of Corporations, Directors and Executives (Standard and Poor's Corporation 1981) and the Directory of Chemical Producers (SRI International 1978) were used to locate parent companies.

We sent a letter to each parent company requesting information on their knowledge of epidemiologic studies of the chemicals in which we were interested. The letter asks: "Are you aware of any epidemiological studies either accomplished or under way, by your own or other companies or agencies, in relation to (name of chemical or chemicals)? It would be very helpful if you could let me know whether or not such investigations have or have not been made, at least according to information available to you. If they have not, it would be of additional assistance if you could provide your judgment as to whether or not such an investigation could be profitably made."

We defined "epidemiological study" broadly, to include any formally structured investigation of mortality or morbidity, designed in such a way that conclusions could be drawn about carcinogenicity in humans. By implication, some statistical analysis would be included in an epidemiological study. A review of medical records without some formal study design or without statistical analysis was not considered to be an epidemiological study. Similarly, monitoring of biological indicators or environmental monitoring was excluded unless the data obtained were related to possible studies of carcinogenicity. We did not analyze the epidemiologic studies or other studies submitted as regards design, validity of conclusions, etc.

In all, 142 letters were mailed to parent companies[3] between August and October 1980; if no response was received, a follow-up letter was sent approximately 4 weeks after the first mailing.

By late March 1981, we had received a total of 99 responses. Four letters were returned as "undeliverable." More than 40 respondents reported that they no longer dealt in at least one of the chemicals about which we inquired; 11 companies reported that they had never dealt in the chemicals at all. These latter statements were in conflict with our sources, particularly the TSCA initial inventory.

RESULTS

We studied availability of epidemiologic data for chemicals designated by IARC as animal carcinogens, but for which published human data were insufficient to permit a firm conclusion as to carcinogenicity, by conducting a survey of U.S. manufacturers, importers, and processors of the chemicals.

We found that manufacturers-importers-processors had performed or contracted for completed epidemiologic studies of 8 of the 75 chemicals about which we inquired (Table 2); 6 of the studies have been published and studies of 6 more chemicals were in progress at the time of our inquiry (fall 1980) (Table 3). A study of tris and ethylene dibromide was reported as going through peer review in fall 1980, and was therefore close to completion at that time. There were medical surveillance programs or reviews of worker health records for 13 chemicals (Table 4). Allowing for duplication of chemicals in the three categories, 23 different chemicals were reported as being under some sort of formal or informal review. Thus, fewer than one-third of the 75 chemicals about which we inquired have been or are being subjected to study that was, is, or could become an epidemiologic study. These results are summarized in Table 5.

We received anecdotal reports of health effects of exposure to several chemicals (Table 6). The anecdotal reports included reports on acute effects of exposure, statements that cancer incidence had not been increased in industrial use of the chemicals over a long period of time, or, in the case, of safrole, that elevated cancer incidence was not apparent in sassafras oil workers in Brazil. These statements were listed as anecdotal because supporting data and references were not supplied.

We received approximately two dozen responses to our question as to whether epidemiologic studies could be carried out in a scientifically profitable manner. Most of these replies stated that studies could not be carried out in a scientifically profitable manner, or studies in progress would not yield

[3] Of the 142 companies, 141 were U.S. companies. One company, Fisons Limited, is a United Kingdom corporation that supplies iron dextran to U.S. distributors.

Table 2
Epidemiologic Studies of IARC Animal Carcinogens—Studies Completed As of Fall 1980

		Dissemination of report and references	
Company number	Chemical name (CAS number)	published	transmitted to U.S. government agency
16	dimethylcarbamoyl chloride (79-44-7)	Hey et al. 1974; Frentzel-Beyme et al. 1976	
	1,2-dichloroethane (107-06-2)	Frentzel-Beyme et al. 1978	
31	1,4-dioxane (123-91-1)	Buffler et al. 1978	
	ethylene dibromide (106-93-4)	Ott et al. 1980	
32	dimethyl sulfate (77-78-1)		Pell 1976
	4,4′-methylene *bis*(2-chloroaniline) (101-14-4)	Linch et al. 1971	
69	Mirex (2385-85-5)		
93	hydrazine (302-01-2)	Roe 1978	

Table 3
Epidemiologic Studies of IARC Animal Carcinogens—Studies in Progress As of Fall 1980

Company number	Chemical name (CAS number)	Comments
5	chlordecone (Kepone) (143-50-0)	long-term follow-up by NIOSH
32	hexamethyl phosphoramide (680-31-9)	
50	toxaphene (8001-35-2)	
95	3,3′-dimethylbenzidine(*o*-tolidine) (119-93-7)	
96	Brominated compounds including tris (2,3-dibromopropyl) phosphate (126-72-7) and ethylene dibromide (106-93-4)	study complete; peer review in progress fall 1980

Table 4
IARC Animal Carcinogens—Medical Surveillance Programs, Review of Health Records from Surveillance

Company number	Chemical name (CAS number)	Record review	Medical surveillance program	Comments
5	carbon tetrachloride (56-23-5)	X		includes death certificates
	chloroform (67-66-3)	X		includes death certificates
	2,4-diaminotoluene (95-80-7)		X	
8	2,4-diaminotoluene (95-80-7)		X	
	4,4′-methylene *bis*(2-chloroaniline) (101-14-4)		X	
	thiourea (62-56-6)		X	
	tris (aziridinyl) phosphine sulfide (52-24-4)		X	
31	hexachlorobenzene (118-74-1)	X		
42	1,2-dichloroethane (107-06-2)	X		system being set up for review of records all pharmaceutical workers
58	propylthiouracil (51-52-5)		X	
62	actinomycin D (50-76-0)		X	
	nitrogen mustard (hydrochloride) (51-75-2)		X	
81	mestranol (72-33-3)		X	

Table 5
IARC Animal Carcinogens—Summary of Epidemiologic Studies

Status	Number of chemicals
Completed	8
In progress	6
Medical surveillance program or review of health records	13
Total	27[a]

[a]Due to duplications within the group of chemicals studied, 23 different chemicals are represented in this total.

Table 6
Anecdotal Reports of User or Worker Experience with IARC Animal Carcinogens

Company number	Chemical name (CAS number)
4	ethylenethiourea (96-45-7)
59	*N*-nitroso-*N*-methylurea (684-93-5)
73	safrole (94-59-7)
97	1,2-dichloroethane (107-06-2) carbon tetrachloride (56-23-5) chloroform (67-66-3)

meaningful data. The reasons given, which are set out in detail in Table 7, include: (1) insufficient time elapsed since beginning of exposure (new plant, new process); (2) small work force; (3) difficulties in tracing workers (change of ownership, workers left company); (4) low volume of production, formulation or use; (5) little or no exposure (closed system, sales only with no handling); (6) short exposure periods during manufacture or use; and (7) miscellaneous.

The miscellaneous reasons were, most typically, judgments that the chemicals about which we inquired did not pose health hazards. In one case, we were informed that a former user of 1,3-propane sultone had completed a study of the user plant and found no excess of deaths from any cause (the study was not designed to evaluate propane sultone). However, the Manager of Toxicology Services for this company stated that: ". . . we consider the existing data [presumably, animal data (MK)] sufficient to regard the compound as a potential human carcinogen so further supporting data would not change our attitude in the matter. Negative data, on the other hand, would probably not convince us to resume its use in our process."

Table 7
IARC Animal Carcinogens—Reasons Given Why Epidemiologic Studies Would Not Be Profitable and Limitations on Studies Planned or in Progress

Company number	Chemical name (CAS number)
Insufficient time elapsed since beginning of exposures (new plant, new process)	
3	2,4-diaminotoluene (95-80-7)
5	1,2-dichloroethane (107-06-2)
32[a]	hexamethyl phosphoramide (680-31-9)
93	1,1-dimethylhydrazine (57-14-7)
Small work force	
5	carbon tetrachloride (56-23-5)
	chloroform (67-66-3)
	2,4-diaminotoluene (95-80-7)
26	carbon tetrachloride (56-23-5)
32	several chemicals
38	iron dextran (9004-66-4)
63	1,3-propane sultone (1120-71-4)
82	1,2-dibromo-3-chloropropane (96-12-8)
	1,2-dichloroethane (107-06-2)
89	tris(2,3-dibromopropyl) phosphate (126-72-7)
93	1,1-dimethylhydrazine (57-14-7)
95	uracil mustard (66-75-1)
Difficulties in tracing workers (change of ownership, workers left company)	
29	toxaphene (8001-35-2)
95[a]	3,3′-dimethylbenzidine(*o*-tolidine) (119-93-7)
Mixed exposures (including batch process manufacturing)	
25	Benzyl Violet 4B (1694-09-3)
	Trypan Blue (72-57-1)
26	carbon tetrachloride (56-23-5)
32	several chemicals
78	hexachlorobenzene (118-74-1)
82	1,2-dibromo-3-chloropropane (96-12-8)
93	Aramite ® (140-57-8), 1,1-dimethylhydrazine (57-14-7)
95	3,3′-dimethylbenzidine(*o*-tolidine) (119-93-7)
Low volume of production, formulation, or use	
27	1,2-dibromo-3-chloropropane (96-12-8)
84	1,2-dichloroethane (107-06-2)
88	hexamethyl phosphoramide (680-31-9), propylthiouracil (51-52-5)
93	Aramite ® (140-57-8)
Little or no exposure (closed system, sales only with no handling)	
5	carbon tetrachloride (56-23-5)
	chloroform (67-66-3)
26	carbon tetrachloride (56-23-5)
38	iron dextran (9004-66-4)
44	thiourea (62-56-6)
66	1,2-dichloroethane (107-06-2)

Table 7—*Continued.*

Company number	Chemical name (CAS number)
	ethylene dibromide (106-93-4)
93	1,1-dimethylhydrazine (57-14-7)
	Short exposure periods
88	propylthiouracil (51-52-5), hexamethylphosphoramide (680-31-9)
93	1,1-dimethylhydrazine (57-14-7)
95	uracil mustard (66-75-1)
	Miscellaneous
13	1,2-dibromo-3-chloropropane (96-12-8) data on health effects based on chemical of unknown purity; DBCP previously studied contaminated with epichlorhydrin; technical DBCP has unknown contaminants
38	iron dextran (9004-66-4) clinical observations show no causal relationship between iron dextran injections and sarcomas (low incidence)
58	propylthiouracil (51-52-5) "to date . . . no evidence of adverse medical conditions or evidence of toxicity in . . . employees . . ."
63	1,3-propane sultone (1120-71-4) study of 3700 employees in plant where compound was used for 5 years showed no excess of deaths; chemical is potential human carcinogen
69	Mirex (2385-85-5) do not produce chemical anymore; study of worker health several years ago showed no adverse effects
89	tris(2,3-dibromopropyl)phosphate (126-72-7) has not handled chemical for some time
95	streptozocin (18883-66-4) human data indicate chemical is not a human carcinogen or only a weak human carcinogen
	1,4-dioxane (123-91-1) ". . . 1,4-dioxane is not a serious chronic toxicity risk, and it might be noted that the ACGIH[b] states that it should be excluded from consideration as a carcinogen . . . 1,4-dioxane has been shown to be an experimental carcinogen, but at very high doses."
97	carbon tetrachloride (56-23-5)
	chloroform (67-66-3)
	1,2-dichloroethane (107-06-2) "Based on the extended usage in industry of these chemicals without evidence of carcinogenic response, we believe that they are not human carcinogens."

[a]Epidemiologic studies in progress; limitations on data as noted.
[b]American Conference of Governmental Industrial Hygienists.

Table 8
Economic and Other Reasons Given for Not Undertaking Epidemiologic Studies of IARC Animal Carcinogens

Company number	Chemical name (CAS number)
Economic considerations (costs of study too great given return on trade in chemical; reduction in production volume)	
36	safrole (94-59-7)
66	ethylene dibromide (106-93-4)
	1,2-dichloroethane (107-06-2)
Importers: depend on supplier for health data	
37	diethyl sulfate (64-67-5)
94	hydrazine (302-01-2)

We were also informed of reasons why individual companies would not undertake epidemiologic studies of chemicals, reasons which had more to do with economics and the structure of the chemical industry than with scientific considerations. Table 8 sets out these economic and other reasons why studies would not be carried out. The reasons included low or declining production, with costs of study great relative to return on sales, and importers' reliance on manufacturers for toxicity data.

DISCUSSION

Results of our survey of manufacturers, processors, and importers of IARC animal carcinogens indicate that relatively few–less than one-third–of the 75 carcinogens in commerce in this country have been or are now under some sort of review of health effects. Only 8 of the 75 chemicals are covered by completed epidemiological studies.

The companies with which we corresponded offered good reasons why it would not be profitable to carry out epidemiologic studies of the IARC animal carcinogens, or why epidemiologic studies now in progress would be limited in their usefulness. In certain of the situations, it should be possible to overcome the obstacles to performance of epidemiologic studies, while in other cases the obstacles would range from difficult to impossible to overcome. Whether problems can be solved in the short- or long-term is also important, as data needed for regulation are required in a much shorter time frame than are data to be used for research unrelated to regulation. Table 9 sets out the obstacles to performance of epidemiologic studies, some possible solutions to these problems, and the feasibility of achieving a solution within the short or long term.

Table 9
Obstacles to Performance of Epidemiologic Studies of Worker Groups Exposed to IARC Animal Carcinogens—Problems and Possible Solutions

		Feasibility	
Problem	Possible solution	research	regulation
Small work force in individual company	pool cohorts, industry-wide studies	yes	yes
Insufficient time elapsed since beginning exposures (latent period)	prospective studies	yes	no
Exposures infrequent or level characterized as "low"	uncertain—may be possible to pool cohorts	uncertain	uncertain
Mixed exposures	rare tumor (as, angiosarcoma), preferably coupled with animal data	yes, in special circumstances	yes, in special circumstances
Records unobtainable: facility closed or sold, workers transferred, etc.	better tracing of workers—obtain from sources like union records or "shoe leather epidemiology"	yes	yes

Some of the limitations noted by our correspondents can be overcome. Pooled industry cohorts can be used to overcome the problem of small worker cohorts in individual companies (Selikoff 1977). Such pooled studies must be designed very carefully to avoid sampling bias, and the use of pooling may be limited by variations in exposures among different company cohorts.

Better tracing of workers who were employed at facilities that had been closed or sold, or workers who have left the employ of a company that has not maintained records on its workers, is possible. The Internal Revenue Service (IRS) and Social Security Administration (SSA) data bases include the best American data on work histories of individuals, but access to these federal data bases to trace workers for epidemiologic studies is restricted in scope. Limitations on access to the IRS and SSA data bases, varying data retention policies among companies, the special data retention problems of small businesses, and difficulties in tracing groups such as migrant farm workers could represent a major problem. The Environmental Sciences Laboratory has had success over the years in locating workers. Often, using a combination of union records and "shoe leather epidemiology," worker cohorts have been traced very satisfactorily.

As regards time needed to trace workers, IRS and SSA files would provide the speediest access to individuals. However, those files are not generally available. Use of the other methods listed above for tracing workers would be feasible for research purposes, and, possibly, for regulation as well.

Certain limitations are more difficult to overcome, both in theoretical and practical terms, and may, in fact, present insurmountable obstacles to performance of epidemiologic studies. For example, long latent periods (Selikoff et al. 1980) before appearance of cancer present an important and difficult problem. Several correspondents stated that studies would not be profitable at this time because exposures had begun too recently—often within the previous 5 years—for effects to be noted. Since latent periods may be 20 years or longer, prospective studies of workers with recent first exposures to chemicals may be suitable for research purposes, but are not useful for regulatory purposes. Difficulties, both practical and ethical, associated with delaying regulation while conducting prospective epidemiologic studies, are discussed elsewhere (Karstadt 1975).

Mixed exposures constitute a major problem in studies of worker groups for association between cancer and exposure to a given chemical. In a workplace atmosphere in which there are many chemicals, unless monitoring data are available to establish with certainty exposure of workers to the chemical in question, epidemiologic data might be at best suggestive. However, the occurrence of unusual cancers, such as asbestos-associated mesothelioma or vinyl chloride-associated angiosarcoma of the liver, can help resolve complex environmental exposures. Such unusual cancers are infrequently discovered, and the elucidation in a complex environment of carcinogenic exposures that result in more common cancers (as, broncogenic carcinoma) would be more difficult. Overall, it is probably not very likely that the problem of resolution of mixed exposures will be overcome.

One of the most important problems in cancer biology is development of information on effects of exposure to low levels of carcinogens; low exposure levels, along with infrequent exposures or closed systems, were reported as reasons why epidemiologic studies would not be profitable.

Documenting exposure levels is an important part of any epidemiologic survey, but exposure data, particularly data relating to past exposures, are frequently unavailable. It is especially difficult to obtain data on "low" levels of exposure, yet asbestos levels sufficient to give a 1-in-1000 lifetime risk of cancer, by no means a trivial risk given the number of people exposed, are so low they could not be measured with the current OSHA-approved sampling method (W. J. Nicholson, pers. comm.).

Other exposures not monitored include infrequent exposures, accidental exposure in maintenance of closed systems, and dusting or other accidental loss of material in such places as importers' warehouses, where relabeling may be the only process carried on and no exposure is anticipated.

For situations in which exposures are classified as "low" or are poorly documented but assumed to be low, a solution might be the establishment of very large study cohorts. However, worker populations large enough to achieve statistical significance for at least some of the chemicals with low-level exposures are unlikely to be available.

Finally, nonscientific considerations were reported as reasons for not carrying out epidemiologic studies. These reasons were economic in nature or dealt with the special position of importers in the U.S. chemical industry. Importers told us they rely on manufacturers to perform necessary tests and studies and supply toxicology data. Consideration of importers' responsibilities for performing, participating in, or obtaining data on epidemiologic studies is a matter for the regulatory agencies. On the other hand, chemical companies have been developing means to pool financial resources to carry out toxicological and epidemiologic studies. Large chemical companies have formed the Chemical Industry Institute of Toxicology (CIIT), while the much smaller companies which comprise the fragrance industry have formed the Research Institute for Fragrance Materials. Economic problems may be among the easier obstacles to overcome. In another paper (M. Karstadt et al., in prep.), we discuss the availability of epidemiologic data relative to production volume of individual chemicals and company size and type.

CONCLUSIONS

Few epidemiologic studies of human populations exposed to chemicals deemed by IARC expert committees to be animal carcinogens have been performed by

U.S. manufacturers, processors, or importers of the chemicals. Given the obstacles to performance of such studies, it is unlikely that many of the remaining chemicals could be studied using epidemiologic techniques, and alternative sources of information must be used for regulatory decisions. In these circumstances, animal data represent the best available information on carcinogenic effects of chemicals. Use of these data, on a qualitative rather than quantitative basis, for regulatory purposes, has been discussed and supported elsewhere (McGinty 1977; Rall 1979).

ACKNOWLEDGMENTS

We wish to thank the following companies for their participation in our study: A. & S. Corporation; Aceto Chemical Co., Inc.; Air Products and Chemicals, Inc.; Akron Chemical Company; Allied Chemical; Alpine Laboratories, Inc.; AmeriBrom, Inc.; American Cyanamid Company; American Hoechst Corporation; American International Chemical, Inc.; American Research Products Company; The Ames Laboratories, Inc.; Amvac Chemical Corporation; Anderson Development Company; Ashland Oil, Inc.; BASF Wyandotte Corporation; Bemis Company, Inc.; Borden Inc.; Bristol-Myers Company; Browning Chemical Corporation; Buckman Laboratories, Inc.; Byk-Gulden, Inc.; Carey Industries, Inc.; Celanese Corporation; CIBA-GEIGY Corporation; C-I-L Chemicals, Inc.; Columbia Organic Chemicals Company, Inc.; Conoco Inc.; Cook Industries, Inc.; Diamond Shamrock Corporation; The Dow Chemical Company; E. I. du Pont de Nemours & Company Incorporated; Eastman Kodak Company; Ethyl Corporation; FMC Corporation; Fairmount Chemical Co., Inc.; Fallek Chemical Company; Fisons Limited; Fritzsche Dodge & Olcott Inc.; GAF Corporation; Givaudan Corporation; The B.F. Goodrich Company; Great Lakes Chemical Corporation; Gulf Oil Corporation; Haarmann & Reimer Corp.; J. E. Halma Company, Inc.; Henkel Corporation; Henley & Co. Incorporated; Hercofina; Hercules Incorporated; Holtrachem, Inc.; I C C Industries, Inc.; I. C. D. Group, Inc.; C. Itoh & Co. (America) Inc.; Kalama Chemical Inc.; Kyowa Hakko U. S. A., Inc.; International Dyestuffs Corporation; Eli Lilly and Company; Mackenzie Chemical Works, Inc.; V. Mane Fils, Inc.; M C B Manufacturing Chemists, Inc.; Merck Sharp & Dohme; 3M; Mitsui and Co. (USA) Inc.; Mobay Chemical Corporation; Mobil Oil Corporation; Napp Chemicals, Inc. (Organon, Inc.); Naval Sea Systems Command; Occidental Petroleum Corporation; Olin Corporation; Orbis Products Corporation; Pennwalt Corporation; Polarome Manufacturing Company, Inc.; Polychemical Laboratories, Incorporated; Polyesther Corporation; P P G Industries, Inc.; Realco Chemical Company; Rhone-Poulenc Inc.; Richardson-Merrell Inc.; R. S. A. Corporation; G. D. Searle & Co.; Shell Oil Company; S. S. T. Corporation; Stauffer Chemical Company; Steuber Company Incorporated; Sumitomo Shoji America, Inc.; Synarome Corporation of America; Syntex

(U. S. A.) Inc.; Tenneco Chemicals; Tridom Chemical, Inc.; Ungerer & Company; Union Carbide Corporation; Uniroyal, Inc.; United Mineral & Chemical Corporation; The Upjohn Company; Velsicol Chemical Corporation (Northwest Industries, Inc.); Vulcan Materials Company; Warner-Lambert Company; Whittaker Corporation.

We are especially grateful to Dr. Robert Anthony, Vice-President, R. S. A. Corporation, and Dr. Bruce W. Karrh, Corporate Medical Director, E. I. du Pont de Nemours & Company, for their interest in our study and their gracious responses to our requests for information.

We also wish to thank our colleagues who reviewed drafts of our manuscript and made suggestions for revisions. Drs. David P. Rall, Marvin Schneiderman, Kenneth Bridbord, and William J. Nicholson, were most generous with their time, and we are very grateful to them.

REFERENCES

Buffler, P.A., J.M. Wood, L. Suarez, and D.J. Kilian. 1978. Mortality followup of workers exposed to 1,4-dioxane. *J. Occup. Med.* **20**:255.

Environmental Protection Agency (EPA). 1979. *Toxic Substances Control Act (TSCA) chemical substance inventory.* Environmental Protection Agency, Office of Toxic Substances, Washington, D.C.

Frentzel-Beyme, R. and A.M. Thiess. 1976. Mortality of workers exposed to dimethylcarbamoyl chloride (DMCC) and diethylcarbamoyl chloride (DECC). Report #14 from the Medical Department of BASF AG, Ludwigshafen, Germany.

Frentzel-Beyme, R., T. Schmitz, and A.M. Thiess. 1978. Mortalitätsstudie bei VC/PVC-Arbeitern der BASF Aktiengesellschaft, Ludwigshafen am Rhein. *Arbeitsmedizin, Sozialmedizin, Präventivmedizin* **10**:218.

Hey, W., A.M. Thiess, and H. Zeller. 1974. Zur frage etwaiger Gesundheitsschadigungen bei der Herstellung und Verarbeiterung von Dimethylcarbaminsäure-chlorid. *Zentralblatt für Arbeitsmedizin und Arbeitsschutz* **24**:71.

International Agency for Research on Cancer (IARC). 1979. IARC monographs on the evaluation of the carcinogenic risk of chemicals to humans: Chemicals and industrial processes associated with cancer in humans. *IARC Monographs* **1-20** and suppl. 1.

Karstadt, M. 1975. Protecting public health from hazardous substances: Federal regulation of environmental contaminants. *Environmental Law Reporter* **5**:50165.

Linch, A.L., G.B. O'Connor, J.R. Barnes, and A.S. Killian, Jr. 1971. Methylene-bis-Ortho-Chloroanile (MOCA): Evaluation of Hazards and Exposure Control. *Am. Ind. Hyg. J.* **32**:802.

McGinty, L. 1977. Controlling cancer in the workplace. *New Sci.* **76**.

Ott, M.G., H.C. Scharnweber, and R.R. Langner. 1980. Mortality experience of 161 employees exposed to ethylene dibromide in two production units. *Br. J. Ind. Med.* **37**:163.

Pell, S. 1976. "Mortality of worker exposed to dimethyl sulfate, 1932-1974." Report submitted by E.I. du Pont de Nemours and Company to the National Institute for Occupational Safety and Health.

Physicians' Desk Reference. 1975, 1980, 1981. Medical Economics Company, Oradell, New Jersey.

Rall, D.P. 1979. The role of laboratory animal studies in estimating carcinogenic risks for man. *IARC Sci. Publ.* **25**:179.

Roe, F.J.C. 1978. Letter to the editor: Hydrazine. *Ann. Occup. Hyg.* **21**:323.

Selikoff, I.J. 1977. Perspectives in the investigation of health hazards in the chemical industry. *Ecotoxicology and Environmental Safety* **1**:387.

Selikoff, I.J., E.C. Hammond, and H. Seidman. 1980. Latency of asbestos disease among insulation workers in the United States and Canada. *Cancer* **46**:2736.

SRI International. 1978. *Directory of Chemical Producers.* SRI International, Menlo Park, California.

Standard and Poor's Corporation. 1981. *Standard and Poor's encyclopedia of corporations, directors and executives. Corporations,* vol. 1. Standard and Poor's Corporation, New York.

Toxic Substances Control Act. 1976. P.L. 94-469, 90 Stat. 2003.

COMMENTS

ACHESON: In Southampton, (U.K.) we did an exercise in which we started with the 142 chemicals in which there was "sufficient evidence" of carcinogenicity in mammals and tried to assign priorities in terms of the need for industrial cohort studies. We took into account, first, whether studies were already reported from IARC as being underway elsewhere; second, whether a group of experts advised us that we were likely to find a population that had been exposed to the particular chemical and not to other confounding chemicals; and, third, an estimate of the scale of exposure of the population as a whole to the substance in question.

To give an example, we found that, in respect to safrole, there was thought to be only two men exposed in manufacture. It seems that there is a need for a formal attempt to try to determine priorities in a field where resources are limited, both in terms of money and trained research workers. I wonder whether it would be possible for estimates of scale of production in the United States of substances carcinogenic in animals to be provided.

I would like to ask Rodolfo Saracci also whether IARC might in future send information.

KARSTADT: I didn't present the production and use data, but we did trace production data wherever they were available for the chemical. We also tried to define uses of the chemicals to get an estimate of exactly what we were looking at, which was potential exposure.

Some of the chemicals turned out to be very interesting, because there are changing patterns of use and production in the chemical industry. For instance, chloroform and carbon tetrachloride are feedstocks for some of the chlorofluorocarbons, and their production is somewhat irregular because of proposed regulations, which I guess are sort of on and off these days. There is an estimate for overall decline over the next few years in production of those two chemicals. There are other chemicals whose use, of course, is on the way up. Vinyl chloride, which is not on our list, has shown production increases, despite regulatory activity earlier in the mid-1970s.

I mentioned that a number of the chemicals are produced on a scale of a few kilograms per year. For example, you have experimental carcinogens that are essentially used as positive controls in bioassays. They are produced in very small quantities by one or two companies in this country, and the human exposure is very limited.

We tried to look at other cohorts, for example, at some of the drugs, to see whether there were sufficient treated populations. We have some data on the drugs, on the potential use of the drugs, and I would expect that we will publish those data. I would be very interested, if your data are available, Dr. Acheson, in seeing how to set the priorities.

I think what we have established here are potentials—opportunities for working around some of these problems, whether by combining cohorts on a multicompany basis or taking other steps to isolate exposures, as well as ways to consider the effect of other exposures. I am not an epidemiologist, but I am intrigued by this on an information-collection basis. I would be very interested in ideas you or others would have on how to extend these results to improve data collections.

ACHESON: In the end, we are finding that the limiting factor is the ability to negotiate with the firm and the work force a study relating to the things in which we are interested.

KARSTADT: We have tried to define a terminology for this field of exposure assessment, and then to get some parameters together for determining the best ways to assess and estimate exposures, given the very limited information in this country and abroad.

My studies of data bases, like the National Occupational Hazards Survey, tend to demonstrate difficulties in even determining qualitative exposure. The quantitative nature of exposure is one level beyond where I have been able to get. I am trying to find out what people are exposed to in a given workplace and trying to estimate realistically the extent of their exposure. That is a real difficulty and is more or less inherent in some of the monitoring schemes and in the regulatory schemes in this country and abroad.

KARRH: I noticed that acrylonitrile was on the list of chemicals for which you thought there was sufficient evidence to label them carcinogenic in humans. We did a study on acrylonitrile, and the only way we saw an excess was after we used a 20-year latency period. We interpret that study in combination with the animal data as raising a serious suspicion that acrylonitrile may be a human carcinogen. But we really are waiting for other studies to confirm or refute that.

Our perspective is that it is premature to classify acrylonitrile as a human carcinogen.

Regarding Dr. Acheson's point, I think that the exposure part of the information contained in the IARC monographs is certainly the one with which we feel the least satisfied; it is very difficult information to acquire, so we would certainly like to expand that area and make it much more factual. However, there is no explicit program in that direction.

We can also use this scale of priorities to look at different types of studies, as you were mentioning. There are studies that can have a high priority from a research viewpoint, but not from a public health sense. You have studies that may qualify as high priority for one enterprise, and others that you mentioned for putting together resources. From our viewpoint, there are some studies that may lend themselves particularly well to international levels, because, in our experience, for some situations you can get the people to collaborate more easily within a framework of an international study.

PADDLE: I can understand the reply of "mixed exposure" as being a reasonable response to your letter, Myra, but industry should not rely on the mixed-exposure argument for not doing epidemiology. The answer arises from the toxicologist's view of life, that is, to do one compound at a time. I don't think that is the way to try to sort out hazards in the chemical industry as we know it. We have got to try to develop and use the techniques that Richard Waxweiler has made available to us.

SIEMIATYCKI: How do your findings compare as between small and large companies?

KARSTADT: That question is interesting, and I have started looking at it because I want to try to correlate the response rate with the size of the firms. The types of responses were different, depending on the size of the firm. Smaller companies were more likely to respond either saying they didn't know, they didn't have the information, or they would refer us to other people. Larger companies were more likely to send us substantive responses. The epidemiology we received was generally from the largest companies, although there were smaller chemical companies who did send us epidemiologic studies. The epidemiologic studies from those companies generally did not meet the criteria we had here, in that they did not go to the long-term effect, specifically cancer, that we were looking for.

A Prospective Study of Morbidity and Mortality in Petroleum Industry Employees in the United States — A Preliminary Report

DAVID SCHOTTENFELD, M. ELLEN WARSHAUER, ANN G. ZAUBER, JANE G. MEIKLE, AND BONNY R. HART
Epidemiology and Preventive Medicine Service
Memorial Sloan-Kettering Cancer Center
New York, New York 10021

The American Petroleum Institute (API)-Memorial Sloan-Kettering Cancer Center (MSKCC) Prospective Morbidity and Mortality Study has been concerned with petroleum industry employees from 19 U.S. companies who are involved in four activities: Petroleum refining, petrochemical manufacturing, research and development, and quality control. It is a concurrent rather than historical prospective investigation and, therefore, its concern is with illnesses and deaths as they occur rather than with an attempt to reconstruct past events through linkage of employment and vital records.

The specific aims of the study may be summarized as follows:

1. Concurrent morbidity and mortality in a defined population of active workers in the petroleum industry will be identified. For previously employed annuitants, only patterns of mortality will be studied.
2. Suitable "control" populations will be selected for comparison. These will be derived from appropriate subgroups in the U.S. general population, other industrial population studies, and the pooled experiences of the study employees of the petroleum industry.
3. If aberrant patterns of morbidity and (or) mortality are demonstrated, epidemiologic studies will be conducted to determine whether groups of employees are at special risk. With the cooperation of industry, cohorts of workers of particular interest will be delineated and studied (e.g., benzene, coking, asphalt).
4. A system of data collection and management with suitable quality controls that will enable compliance with the previously described specific aims will be developed.

The study population is defined by the population census. This consists of basic demographic and employment information on every individual who is attached to a division or plant that has been entered into the study. All full-time, active employees at these units are listed in the initial population census and constitute the "active study population." Individuals who are annuitants of these plants and divisions constitute the "annuitant population." Basic demographic data and employment information also are collected as part of the initial census on annuitants. Deaths that occur among the annuitants are reported to MSKCC. However, as they are no longer actively employed, reports of illness or cancer incidence are not being collected routinely.

Because the design of our study is prospective, we are interested in monitoring changes in the status of the study population. We have, therefore, developed a system of updating information on the population census that records the addition of new employees, and the number of retirees, transfers, and job changes. This allows us to maintain a record of the dynamics of the study population and will be useful in addressing questions of population turnover that have troubled other studies of occupational groups.

Let us now turn to the nature of the information that is collected about sickness and death in this population. There are three components to the reporting system: Morbidity, mortality, and cancer incidence.

All illnesses that cause employees to lose 5 scheduled days from work are being reported. When an employee returns to work after such an episode, a Morbidity Reporting Form is completed and submitted to MSKCC. Information on the cause of absence is recorded, including the final diagnosis, whether the individual was hospitalized, and whether surgery was performed. The source for reporting this information is to be recorded. This serves as a means of assessing the reliability of the diagnostic information. Diagnostic information is coded according to the 8th revision of the International Classification of Diseases.

The second component of the study is registration of incident cancers. Every newly diagnosed case of cancer occurring in the active employee study population is reported using the Cancer Registry Reporting Form. This form includes, in addition to company and individual identifying codes and birth date, the primary anatomic and histopathologic diagnosis. The date of diagnosis and histopathologic description determine whether this is indeed an incident case, as opposed to recurrence of a previously diagnosed malignancy or one prevalent at the inception of the study. We regard verification of selected cancer diagnoses as an important function of the cancer surveillance registry. For selected cases, records are requested from the employee's physician and hospital, including slides of biopsy material, excerpts of the hospital record, and surgery and pathology reports. Release of this material to MSKCC of course requires specific permission from the employee. These materials are to be reviewed and evaluated at MSKCC with the assistance of a consulting pathologist.

The final component of the reporting system is concerned with mortality. Deaths are recorded in active employees and annuitants. The death certificate is coded at MSKCC as to underlying cause according to nationally standardized practices.

Table 1
Population Census Profile

	N	Percent
Sex		
Male	86,820	90.7
Female	8,881	9.3
Total	95,701	
Race		
White	79,825	83.4
Spanish	3,756	3.9
Black	10,622	11.1
Other	1,498	1.6
Total	95,701	

Population defined as initial population and all new hires added through December 12, 1979 (ever in study).

Table 1 shows the sex and race distribution of the entire study population who were actively employed at any time during the study. The study population is predominantly male (90.7%) and white or Hispanic (87.3%). The tabulations represent the initial analysis of all cases of mortality and cancer incidence among the 76,336 white and Hispanic male employees from 114 plants who were employed any time during January 1, 1977, to December 31, 1979.

Other demographic characteristics of the study population are summarized in Tables 2-5. About 72% of the population are engaged in petroleum refining, while 19% are involved in petrochemical manufacturing (Table 2). The petrochemical workers generally have come into the study later than refinery employees and, therefore, have been followed for a shorter period of time (Table

Table 2
Population Census Profile—White and Spanish Surname, Males

	All workers	
Division at entrance into study	N	percent
Research and development	5,188	6.8
Refinery	55,007	72.1
Petrochemical	14,729	19.3
Quality control	1,410	1.9
Missing	2	
Totals	76,336	

3). Overall, 41% of all workers (30% of petrochemical and 44% of refinery workers) have been employed for approximately 20 years or more (Table 4). The age distribution at entrance into the study for the active workers analyzed in this report is summarized in Table 5. The refinery has a greater proportion of older employees than the petrochemical plants. In particular the refinery has a lower proportion of workers in the 30-39 age group and a higher proportion of those in the 50-59 and 60-69 age group than those in the petrochemical plants.

METHODOLOGY

Standardized mortality ratios (SMRs) for all deaths and standardized incidence ratios (SIRs) for cancer were used to compare the observed deaths and incident cancers with the numbers expected in the general population. The current sample size enabled only a comparison of employees in petroleum refining with those in petrochemical manufacturing. In the current presentation, API mortality was compared with that of the U.S. white, male, age-specific mortality for 1977, which is the most recent year available. API cancer incidence was compared with U.S. age-specific cancer incidence rates. The U.S. standard was based upon the population-based cancer registration of the Surveillance, Epidemiology, and End Results (SEER) program of the National Cancer Institute for 1977 (J. Young, pers. comm.).

Exact person-years at risk were calculated for each person. The person-years began when the individual entered the study either on the initial population census or subsequently if he was newly hired or transferred into a reporting site. In the mortality analysis, the person-years were counted until the individual died, left the company, or transferred into a nonparticipating unit. If none of the above occurred, person-years were counted to the end of the study period. Active members who subsequently retired were assumed to be alive on December 31, 1979, unless a mortality form was received.

In the cancer incidence analysis, person-years of observation were terminated when an individual died, left the company, transferred to a non-participating unit, or retired. If none of these events occurred, person-years were counted to the end of the study period. Incidence data were collected on employees only while active. Consequently, cancers diagnosed subsequent to retirement were not included in the incidence analysis, but were analyzed, when applicable, in the mortality analysis.

Expected number of cases was calculated for those causes of death or cancer sites for which there were five or more observed cases. An exception was made for selected cancer sites of particular interest based upon reports in the literature or their relative rarity (e.g., ocular melanoma).

Altogether, over 200 individual tests of significance were performed. The observed number of cases was considered to be distributed in accordance with the Poisson distribution with the mean equal to the expected number. Whether

Table 3
Population Census Profile—White and Spanish Surname, Males

Year of entrance into study	All workers N	All workers percent	Refinery N	Refinery percent	Petrochemical N	Petrochemical percent
1977	30,983	40.6	24,369	44.3	3,420	23.2
1978	33,017	43.3	22,348	40.6	8,076	54.8
1979	12,123	15.9	8,148	14.8	3,191	21.7
1980	213	0.3	142	0.3	42	0.3
Totals	76,336		55,007		14,729	

Table 4
Population Census Profile—White and Spanish Surname, Males

Year first employed	All workers N	All workers percent	Refinery N	Refinery percent	Petrochemical N	Petrochemical percent
Before 1960	31,094	40.7	24,239	44.1	4,380	29.7
1960 or after	45,233	59.3	30,762	55.9	10,346	70.2
Missing	9		6		3	
Totals	76,336		55,007		14,729	

Table 5
Population Census Profile—White and Spanish Surname, Males

Age at entrance into MSKCC-API study	All workers N	All workers percent	Refinery N	Refinery percent	Petrochemical N	Petrochemical percent
20	703	0.9	445	0.8	207	1.4
20-29	20,198	26.5	14,316	26.0	4,163	28.3
30-39	17,527	23.0	11,765	21.4	4,239	28.8
40-49	12,703	16.6	9,017	16.4	2,425	16.5
50-59	20,488	26.8	15,801	28.7	3,060	20.8
60-69	4,709	6.2	3,661	6.7	630	4.3
Missing	8		0		5	
Totals	76,336		55,007		14,729	

the observed is significantly different from the expected can be determined from the Poisson distribution. When many tests are performed, some could yield significant results purely by chance. Tukey (1977) suggested that in multiple testing within the same study, a *p* level of 0.05 divided by the number of tests be used as a more conservative criterion for significance testing. Caution is indicated when interpreting significant results out of many tests on the same data. Conversely, not all nonsignificant results reflect a true absence of a significant difference between the observed and expected. When the observed number of events is small, there is generally insufficient power to detect a small or even moderate excess or deficit.

MORTALITY

The current mortality analysis was based upon 502 deaths and 122,607 person-years of observation. The crude average annual mortality ratio was 4.1/1000. This rate was considerably lower than that reported in mortality studies of other industrial populations. For example, the crude annual mortality rate among white male steelworkers was 9.1/1000 (Lloyd and Ciocco 1969); the death rate among petroleum workers in the United States (Tabershaw and Cooper 1974) was 8.5/1000 and in the United Kingdom 7.7/1000 (Rushton and Alderson 1980).

Overall, the age-sex-race-standardized mortality of the study population was significantly lower than that of the U.S. standard (SMR=55) (Table 6). Mortality for each of the nonmalignant causes of deaths was significantly lower than expected in all instances; heart diseases (SMR=55), strokes (SMR=41), and accidents (SMR=57) were decreased significantly. The all causes SMR in the study of steelworkers was 86 (Lloyd and Ciocco 1969), whereas in the mortality studies of petroleum refinery workers cited previously, the SMRs ranged from 69 to 84 (Tabershaw and Cooper 1974; Rushton and Alderson 1980).

The API-MSKCC crude mortality figures should be considered preliminary and may be lower than expected because of the following factors:

1. There was a relatively short period of observation to date, with each worker having been followed on an average of 1.6 person-years.
2. Only annuitants who retired since each company joined the study were included in the mortality analysis. Had the population of former employees who are identified as annuitants in the initial population census been included, it is expected that the crude mortality rate would not be as low when compared with the U.S. population and other cohorts of industrial workers. As an example, only 0.7% of the 122,607 person-years of observation are for workers 65 years of age and older, and only 9.3% of the person-years are for workers 60 years of age and older.
3. There was underreporting of deaths. As the average lag time between the date of death and the receipt of a death certificate has been 4-5 months, the

Table 6
Mortality—White and Spanish Surname, Males

	All workers				Refinery				Petrochemical			
Site	O	E	SMR	*P*	O	E	SMR	*P*	O	E	SMR	*P*
All deaths	502	912.78	55.00	< .01↓[b]	393	701.21	56.05	< .01↓	74	130.38	56.76	< .01↓
All cancer	156	217.60	71.69	< .01↓	127	168.77	75.25	< .01↓	17	29.48	57.66	.02↓
Digestive	39	52.88	73.75	.06	31	41.12	75.39	.12	6	7.06	85.02	.88
Stomach	6	7.67	78.23	.71	6	5.95	100.85	.99	—	1.04	—	—
Colon	14	18.03	77.65	.41	10	14.02	71.34	.35	3	2.41	124.50	.87
Rectum	6	4.64	129.26	.64	4	3.61	110.75	.97	2	.62	323.36	.26
Pancreas	11	11.38	96.69	.99	10	8.85	112.96	.79	—	1.51	—	—
Lung	57	83.57	68.21	< .01↓	48	65.07	73.77	.03↓	6	11.07	54.19	.15
Melanoma	5	4.44	112.66	.91	3	3.35	89.63	.99	—	.69	—	—
Prostate	5	6.73	74.28	.67	5	5.30	94.32	.99	—	.84	—	—
Bladder	3	4.21	71.19	.79	3	3.30	91.01	.99	—	.54	—	—
Brain	8	6.41	124.77	.63	8	4.90	163.18	.25	—	.94	—	—
Lymphoma[a]	3	7.01	42.80	.16	2	5.39	37.11	.19	—	1.00	—	—
Hodgkin's disease	2	2.18	91.81	.99	2	1.62	123.53	.96	—	.37	—	—
Leukemia	4	7.83	51.09	.22	4	5.98	66.91	.58	—	1.15	—	—
Heart	187	338.45	55.25	< .01↓	152	262.72	57.86	< .01↓	25	45.53	54.91	< .01↓
Stroke	14	34.39	40.71	< .01↓	10	26.66	37.51	< .01↓	4	4.66	85.82	.99
Accident	46	80.32	57.27	< .01↓	29	58.76	49.35	.01↓	17	14.58	116.63	.59
Suicide	15	32.32	46.41	< .01↓	12	23.82	50.38	< .01↓	1	5.65	17.70	.05↓
Homicide	5	14.54	34.38	< .01↓	4	10.50	38.10	.04↓	1	2.76	36.18	.47

U.S. mortality rates.
[a]Non-Hodgkin's.
[b]↓, Significantly less than expected.

magnitude of underreporting can be determined more accurately through methods that enable independent ascertainment of vital status, such as the social security system.

4. The healthy-worker effect is reflected in overall age-standardized mortality that is 10-40% lower than that expected in the general population. This effect of selection into a working population is less striking for malignant neoplasms, presumably because the risk of cancer increases as a function of age and becomes expressed clinically after a long induction-latency period.

CANCER MORTALITY

The mortality due to all categories of cancer was significantly lower than expected (SMR=72) (shown in Table 6). For the subgroups, the SMR for refinery workers was 75 and for petrochemical workers 58. As a comparison, in other published cohort studies of petroleum workers, the SMRs for total cancers ranged from 81 to 92.

The SMR for lung cancer was significantly less than expected among all workers (SMR=68) and among the petroleum refinery employees (SMR=74). This observation is in agreement with the Tabershaw and Cooper (1974), Rushton and Alderson (1980), and Theriault and Goulet (1979) studies of petroleum workers, but not with the historical cohort study of Hanis et al. (1979), nor the U.S. county mortality studies of Blot et al. (1977) and Gottlieb et al. (1979), which suggested that lung cancer mortality was increased significantly.

SMRs for other causes of cancer mortality were not significantly increased or decreased. The subsequent discussion of mortality patterns is intended to summarize relationships of potential interest. For example, brain cancer mortality (8 observed deaths compared with 6.4 expected) exhibited an increase of 25% over the expected for all workers combined, and an increase of 63% for the refinery workers. Rushton and Alderson (1980) and Blot et al. (1977) reported lower than expected brain cancer mortality. B. Karrh (pers. comm.) and C. P. Wen (pers. comm.) concluded in their cohort studies that brain cancer frequency was essentially the same as in the general population. Theriault and Goulet (1979), Thomas et al. (1980) and Alexander et al. (1980) have raised the possibility of an excessive risk of brain cancer among oil refinery and petrochemical plant workers, although no specific causative agent has yet been identified. The surveillance of the API-MSKCC work force will continue to monitor for aberrant patterns of brain cancer incidence and mortality.

Digestive tract mortality was diminished in all workers (74) and within the subgroups working in refining (75) and petrochemical manufacturing (85). For cancer of the rectum, the SMR was increased in all workers (129) and within both subgroups, refining (111) and petrochemical manufacturing (323) (Table 6). For colon cancer, the SMR was diminished for all workers (78) and for workers in refining (71), but was increased for those in petrochemical manufacturing (125). Pancreatic cancer was not increased for all workers (97), but was elevated for the subgroup in refining (113). None of these ratios were statistically significant. Hanis et al. (1979) observed that refinery workers had twice the risk of nonrefinery workers for cancer of the large intestine (rectum and colon combined). Blot et al. (1977) observed significantly higher mortality from stomach and rectal cancer in petroleum counties. The SMR for cancer of the pancreas was raised, but not significantly. Rushton and Alderson (1980) showed slightly raised SMRs for each site of the digestive tract, except for the pancreas, which was slightly lower than expected.

SUMMARY OF MORTALITY STUDY

The results of the mortality study to date indicate decreased age-standardized mortality ratios for the major classifications of diseases within the International Classification of Diseases. Lung cancer mortality was decreased significantly in all workers and in the subgroup of refinery workers. As we have discussed, there is a number of factors that may have contributed to an underestimation of mortality.

CANCER INCIDENCE

Of the cancer cases considered in the analysis, 52% were confirmed either by reviewing their hospital records and (or) by reviewing slides of biopsies at MSKCC. This follow-up is dependent upon receipt of a signed release form from each employee-patient that allows MSKCC to request slides and records from the employee's physician. In addition to confirming the primary site and histopathology for the cancer, the follow-up also provided a precise date of diagnosis, which was essential for determining an accurate number of observed incident cases per year.

The current analysis of cancer incidence was based upon 307 events and 118,566 person-years of observation. The crude average annual cancer incidence rate was 2.6/1000. As a comparison, in the study by Pell et al. (1978), among male DuPont employees during the period 1956-1974 there were 2905 incident cancer cases (excluding nonmelanoma skin cancers) and 1,616,457 person-years of observation for a crude annual cancer incidence rate of 1.8/1000.

In the total group of white and Spanish-surnamed employees and for the subgroups, refinery workers, and petrochemical workers, all of whom were actively employed at any time during the study period, the age-sex-race-standardized cancer incidence ratio was less than the U.S. standard (SIR=85, 86, 86, respectively). As a comparison, in the study by Pell among DuPont employees, the SIR for all sites combined was 79, using the U.S. Third National Cancer Survey (TNCS) as the standard.

Table 7
Cancer Incidence—White and Spanish Surname, Males Dx 1977-1979

	All workers				Refinery				Petrochemical			
Sites	O	E	SIR	*P*	O	E	SIR	*P*	O	E	SIR	*P*
All cancers	307	362.18	84.76	< .01↓[a]	240	278.72	86.11	.02↓	44	50.88	86.47	.37
Digestive organs	64	83.51	76.63	.03↓	50	64.66	77.33	.07	9	11.33	79.41	.61
Colorectal	49	49.31	99.37	.99	35	38.15	91.74	.68	9	6.71	134.13	.47
Colon	37	31.24	118.45	.34	28	24.14	115.98	.48	6	4.28	140.11	.52
Rectum	12	18.08	66.39	.18	7	14.01	49.95	.06	3	2.43	123.29	.88
Stomach	5	11.14	44.87	.07	5	8.62	57.97	.28	–	1.51	–	–
Respiratory system	87	101.67	85.57	.15	68	78.80	86.30	.24	14	13.71	102.11	.99
Larynx	16	12.08	132.41	.32	12	9.36	128.17	.47	3	1.64	183.41	.45
Lung and bronchus	70	87.15	80.32	.07	55	67.57	81.39	.13	11	11.72	93.87	.99

Hematopoietic tissues												
Leukemia	14	9.93	140.98	.26	11	7.56	145.47	.29	–	1.48	–	–
Monocytic	–	0.45	–	–	–	0.45	–	–	–	0.07	–	–
Lymphocytic	7	3.31	211.39	.10	7	2.56	273.52	.03↑[b]	–	0.46	–	–
Other	7	6.17	113.45	.84	4	4.55	87.91	.99	–	0.96	–	–
Genitourinary organs												
Kidney	11	11.05	99.54	.99	8	8.48	94.33	.99	2	1.56	127.83	.93
Prostate	27	31.47	85.81	.49	21	24.77	84.79	.52	5	3.90	128.10	.70
Testis	5	8.15	61.33	.36	4	5.79	69.06	.63	–	1.64	–	–
Bladder	14	22.86	61.24	.07	10	17.69	56.54	.07	3	3.12	96.19	.99
Lymphatic tissues												
Multiple myeloma	6	4.02	149.35	.44	2	3.11	64.23	.80	3	0.54	552.03	.04↑
Hodgkin's disease	6	5.01	119.77	.77	4	3.63	110.07	.98	1	0.94	106.43	.99
Non-Hodgkin's lymphoma	7	12.63	55.44	.13	7	9.61	72.87	.52	–	1.88	–	–
Other sites												
Eye (includes melanoma)	2	1.23	163.26	.69	1	0.94	106.59	.99	–	0.18	–	–
Melanoma of the skin	16	13.26	120.66	.52	13	9.86	131.90	.39	2	2.19	91.29	.99
Brain	9	9.25	97.31	.99	9	6.97	129.08	.53	–	1.44	–	–
Lip	4	4.17	95.93	.99	4	3.20	124.89	.80	–	0.59	–	–

U.S. incidence rates, 1977.
[a]↓, Significantly less than expected.
[b]↑, Significantly greater than expected.

In our study, statistically significant increases in cancer incidence were observed for (Table 7):

1. Acute and chronic lymphocytic leukemias in refinery workers (SIR=274);
2. Multiple myeloma among petrochemical workers (SIR=552); and
3. Cutaneous melanoma among workers in the Middle Atlantic region (SIR=278).

Although these results may suggest problems associated with the industry, they must be interpreted cautiously. For example, acute and chronic lymphocytic leukemias were significantly elevated in the refinery workers (7 observed cases compared with 2.6 expected, SIR=274) but no cases were recorded in the petrochemical workers. Nonlymphocytic leukemias, in particular the granulocytic or myelogenous leukemias, were increased in all workers (SIR=113), but not significantly. This is of interest because ionizing radiation, alkylating agents, and benzene have been implicated previously in the etiology of acute nonlymphocytic and chronic myelogenous leukemias, but not in the pathogenesis of chronic lymphocytic leukemia. Multiple myeloma, also attributed in part to ionizing radiation exposure, was elevated significantly in the petrochemical workers but not in the refinery workers.

Melanoma of the skin (16 observed cases compared with 13.3 expected) was increased in all workers (121) and in the subgroup of refinery workers (132), but was decreased in the petrochemical workers (91). None of these deviations were statistically significant. In the Middle Atlantic region, which contains 15% of the population at risk (white male employee population: 11,382), 8 of the 16 total cases of melanoma were reported, and the SIR was increased significantly (278). Of the remaining 8 incident cases of cutaneous melanoma, 4 were reported in the West South Central region (white male employee population: 39,383) and 4 in the Pacific region (white male employee population: 14,504). During 1977-1979, 2 cases of ocular melanoma were observed outside of the Middle Atlantic region (SIR=163). Whereas cutaneous melanoma was increased significantly in the Middle Atlantic region, the SIR in this region for all cancers (110) was not increased significantly, although it did exceed the corresponding SIR for all workers in all regions (85).

In the study by Pell et al. (1978), the highest SIR was reported for melanoma of the skin (SIR=123). The higher incidence was observed for both wage and salaried employees. In the studies of the petroleum industry by Blot et al. (1977), Thomas (1980), and Bahn et al. (1976), excesses in melanoma mortality were reported. Albert and Puliafito (1977) reported 3 ocular melanomas in an Ohio Valley chemical plant and these were interpreted as excessive. The workers were exposed to hydrazine, dimethylsulfate, and 4, 4′-methylene dianiline. Various experimental animal systems have shown that polycyclic hydrocarbons can give rise to melanomas when administered by various routes to different rodent species.

The digestive organs included 64 cases in all workers (SIR=76) which was decreased significantly (Table 7). The SIRs for large intestine (99), colon (118), and rectum (66) were not statistically significant. For the refinery workers, the SIRs were large intestine (92), colon (116), and rectum (50). For the petrochemical workers, the SIRs were large intestine (134), colon (140), and rectum (123). Whereas large bowel (colon and rectum) tended to be elevated for the petrochemical workers, there was a contrasting pattern of elevated colon cancer incidence and diminished rectal cancer incidence for the refinery workers. These deviations were not statistically significant, but they do suggest a trend within the petrochemical workers that requires further monitoring.

SUMMARY OF CANCER INCIDENCE

Cancer incidence analyses indicate decreased age-standardized incidence ratios overall and within the major cancer categories of the International Classification of Diseases. Statistically significant increases in cancer incidence were observed for lymphocytic leukemia in the refinery workers, multiple myeloma in the petrochemical workers, and cutaneous melanoma in plants reporting from the Middle Atlantic region.

We believe that all of these results, including certain trends that fall short of statistical significance, should be viewed as preliminary because the period of observation to date has been quite short, the number of older workers included in this analysis has been limited, and the degree of underreporting, particularly of mortality, is unknown. Future reports will review the patterns of illness giving rise to 5 or more days of absence from work among the total population of workers who were ever actively employed (current population census of 95,702) and the patterns of mortality in the annuitants (current population census of 16,679) who retired prior to their company joining the study. In addition, we plan to make internal comparisons of the API population, with stratification for occupational classification and years of employment.

REFERENCES

Albert, D.M. and C.A. Puliafito. 1977. Choroidal melanoma: Possible exposure to industrial toxins. *N. Engl. J. Med.* **296**:634.

Alexander, V., S.S. Leffingwell, J.W. Lloyd, R.J. Waxweiler, and R.L. Miller. 1980. Brain cancer in petrochemical workers: A case series report. *Am. J. Industrial Med.* **1**:115.

Bahn, A.K., I. Rosenwaike, N. Herrmann, P. Grover, J. Stellman, and K. O'Leary. 1976. Melanoma after exposure to PCBs. *N. Engl. J. Med.* **295**: 450.

Blot, W.J., L.A. Brinton, J.F. Fraumeni, Jr., and B. J. Stone. 1977. Cancer mortality in US counties with petroleum industries. *Science* **198**:51.

Gottlieb, M.S., L. Pickle, W.J. Blot, and J.F. Fraumeni, Jr. 1979. Lung cancer in Louisiana: Death certificate analysis. *J. Natl. Cancer Inst.* **63**:1131.

Hanis, N.M., K.M. Stavraky, and J.L. Fowler. 1979. Cancer mortality in oil refinery workers. *J. Occup. Med.* **21**:167.

Lloyd, J.W. and A. Ciocco. 1969. Long term mortality study of steelworkers. I. Methodology. *J. Occup. Med.* **11**:299.

Pell, S., M.T. O'Berg, and B.W. Karrh. 1978. Cancer epidemiologic surveillance in the DuPont Company. *J. Occup. Med.* **20**:725.

Rushton, L. and M.R. Alderson. 1980. *An epidemiological survey of eight oil refineries in the UK: Final report.* Institute of Cancer Research, Division of Epidemiology, Sutton, Surrey, England.

Tabershaw, I. and W.C. Cooper. 1974. *A mortality study of petroleum refinery workers.* Tabershaw/Cooper Associates. Bethesda, Maryland.

Theriault, G. and L. Goulet. 1979. A mortality study of oil refinery workers. *J. Occup. Med.* **21**:367.

Thomas, T.L., P. Decoufle, and R. Moure-Eraso. 1980. Mortality among workers employed in petroleum refining and petrochemical plants. *J. Occup. Med.* **22**:97.

Tukey, J.W. 1977. Some thoughts on clinical trials, especially problems of multiplicity. *Science* **198**:679.

COMMENTS

SILVERSTEIN: Let me ask one quick question: How is that you become notified of deaths among workers who have left employment?

WARSHAUER: When an employee is entitled to any kind of benefit the company is notified and we get the death certificate from the benefit department.

SILVERSTEIN: Are the definitions of eligibility uniform across the different companies?

WARSHAUER: I think so.

MILHAM: What is the most recent year of hire that enters into the mortality cohort?

WARSHAUER: In this analysis it would have to have been prior to 1980. The study is still going on, so we are adding workers as they are newly hired.

MILHAM: Well, I think that accounts for your really low standardized mortality ratios (SMRs), in that the recent hires will inflate your person-years to accumulate any deaths. I think you should keep your analysis to those men hired, at the latest, before 1965.

WARSHAUER: Well, we hope to move to this. We are going to stratify by year joined the company and by other factors. This was just a first look at the data to try to determine what the problems were and to familiarize ourselves with what we had.

GAFFEY: Do you have any idea how good your ascertainment is on your cancer morbidity? Do you have any method of checking on that to see how well you are doing in getting it?

WARSHAUER: Overall, we feel we are getting a good accounting of cancer incidence. We have a separate form for cancer incidence, but we are picking up some additional cases through our normal morbidity forms. The ones we would be missing are primarily those that do not result in an absence of work for 5 days or more. We know we would be low, for example, on nonmelanoma skin cancers, which we have excluded. But I think we feel we are picking up any absence that causes 5 or more days lost from work.

AUSTIN: Are you tracing workers who have short periods of employment.

WARSHAUER: We are not tracing any workers at the present time. We are trying to institute some procedures for tracing all workers through Social Security and through the National Death Index. At this point we are not doing that. We have no individual names or Social Security numbers, so we cannot do that ourselves at this time.

AUSTIN: Are your SMRs just taken out of follow-up when they terminate?

WARSHAUER: In computing the SMRs for mortality, no, because we assume that the company will be notified of their death. For the cancer incidence, yes. As soon as they leave the company, person-years are terminated.

STEWART: Do you hear of a death just because benefits have been awarded to them?

WARSHAUER: Correct.

STEWART: Then presumably the man has subscribed to this benefit while working. Can workers opt for a lump sum benefit payment when they leave?

RADFORD: Yes.

STEWART: This is a great catch, because sick people are most likely to do this. They won't wait. They want their money in their pockets.

WARSHAUER: This would be interesting to follow up. I don't know how large that population is, but I think we will try to get some estimate from the various companies.

SILVERSTEIN: As Ellen knows, we have been trying to grapple with the same issue in the automotive industry, where the benefits are structured such that, using this type of strategy for a study design, you can lose a fairly substantial portion of deaths among those who may have worked for as much as 12, 14, 15 years, left employment, have a vested pension, but who are not eligible for life insurance benefits, and therefore would not come to the routine attention of the company. It sounds like it may be a bit different in the petrochemical industry.

McMICHAEL: One quick point of information and then a comment. Dr.

Monson and myself both found, when looking at various rubber industry populations, that it was the lymphocytic, rather than the myelogenous, leukemias that were the most raised.

WARSHAUER: Both acute and chronic, or just acute?

McMICHAEL: I think it was the chronic lymphocytic, particularly, but I have to check that. In a case-control study drawing on a number of those companies subsequently, we reported a dose-response element across three estimated levels of exposure to organic solvents, particularly benzene.

You are looking at lots of SMRs and they do stray around a lot. When looking at the colon and rectum you should have questions relating to those things that are considered the major determinants–diet and perhaps alcohol consumption, life-style factors.

WARSHAUER: It also could be just differences in classification of the sites within the large bowel.

McMICHAEL: That, too.

GOTTLIEB: Are you using the Surveillance, Epidemiology, and End Results (SEER) program for your comparison base for the incidence data?

WARSHAUER: Yes.

GOTTLIEB: Do you have any estimate as to the proportion of people in those SEER areas that are employed in the petrochemical industries? Is that a good base to use?

WARSHAUER: Well, it is the only base to use. We have 114 plants spread throughout the United States, and the SEER program is the only program that really includes data for all areas. The Middle Atlantic region only includes the Connecticut rates for a basis of comparison. We did not use the entire SEER population. We hope, as we move to looking at rates in various regions, we will use the SEER registries for that region as a comparison, rather than the total United States, for the ten areas.

GOTTLIEB: How many of your plants fall within the SEER areas?

WARSHAUER: Offhand, I cannot answer that.

BEAUMONT: I had a question about person-years calculations for the mortality part for people who left employment. Were there just certain workers that were eligible, once they left employment, for a benefit for their survivors?

WARSHAUER: Only those workers who were benefit eligible and retired were kept in the person-year calculations for the mortality analysis since the companies would only be aware of deaths among those receiving benefits. Person-years were terminated for workers leaving for any other reason besides retirement. I believe that the definition for eligibility for pension benefits is fairly uniform across the different companies.

PADDLE: What do you hope to learn from the sickness-absence data that you are collecting?

WARSHAUER: We would like to see if there are different patterns of illnesses, and not only cancer, in different activities or in different regions. The petroleum industry itself is quite interested in looking at this. We are not only going to talk about it generally; we have been coding it and we will look at cause specific absences to see if there are any patterns in illnesses in the industry. I think loss from work is a concern. We also may explore some of the factors contributing to this.

PADDLE: If you do find something, it will be very interesting, because I think general opinion in the United Kingdom is that it is merely a data collection exercise.

WEN: The death certificates were collected only on those deceased in active service or those on a retirement pension.

WARSHAUER: Yes. Those terminated were not included.

WEN: The table that you presented did not include any so-called long-term retirees. The retirees were not included. All those were active service deceased people.

WARSHAUER: Correct. I mentioned that previously. It is only those who retired sometime between 1977 and 1979. We have not yet looked at the previous annuitant population that retired prior to the beginning of the study.

WEN: So I am not sure there is an overestimation of person-years as long as you follow up the individual at the time of separation, which you can control.

WARSHAUER: If he left the company—that is right—we did end the person-years at that time. It is only if he retired that we kept them on. However, if workers did opt for a lump-sum retirement benefit instead of normal retirement, they would be contributing person-years and the companies would not be aware of their deaths. Therefore, there may be a slight overestimate of person-years. As I said before, we will look into this.

SESSION 4: Cancer in the U.S.: Recent Trends and Proportion Due to Occupation

Trends in U.S. Cancer Onset Rates

RICHARD PETO
Nuffield Department of Clinical Medicine
Radcliffe Infirmary
Oxford University
Oxford OX2 6HE, England

BACKGROUND: METHODOLOGY

It has been claimed, especially by people who wish to emphasize the importance of the control of occupational and environmental pollutants, that there is at present a generalized increase in U.S. cancer onset rates over and above that which could plausibly be attributed to cigarette smoking. The assessment of trends, however, is a difficult business, requiring comparison of either incidence or mortality rates recorded in 1 year with the corresponding rates recorded at some later year, and both the available incidence data and the available mortality data are subject to various quite substantial errors which themselves may change with time. Before presenting and interpreting the apparent trends, I shall therefore outline the separate pitfalls inherent in these two separate types of data, incidence, and mortality.

We have recently completed (Doll and Peto 1981) a review of the sources of such data, of the trends that they suggest, and of the implications of these apparent trends. Rather than reproduce in full the extensive discussions therein, I shall merely draw on the main conclusions. Readers requiring more detailed substantiation of any points in the text of this paper are referred in particular to Appendices C, D, and E of it (Doll and Peto 1981).

AGE STANDARDIZATION

First, and most obviously, the available rates have to be examined on an age-specific basis, or standardized for age (for details, see Doll and Peto 1981, Appendix A) to allow for the effects of the changing proportions of old people in the population.

This raises the question of population estimation. The U.S. population in general is not recorded accurately by the decennial census, and the errors (a small percentage in whites and 10-20% in blacks) are not constant from census to census. These changes, unless allowed for, themselves generate artefactual trends in cancer rates. Population estimates that have been corrected for census undercount are available from the U.S. Bureau of the Census (Doll and Peto 1981, Appendix B) and should be used routinely for the calculation of trends in U.S. national mortality rates.

I have no information on the accuracy of the (uncorrected) population estimates that are used for calculating incidence rates for the particular parts of the United States that collaborated in the Second National Cancer Survey (SNCS), the Third National Cancer Survey (TNCS), or the Surveillance, Epidemiology and End Results (SEER) program, but presumably errors at least as great as in the national population estimates affect them, too.

METHODOLOGY

Incidence Data

By definition, cancer *incidence* comprises all cases of cancer, fatal or nonfatal. There are two chief pitfalls in assessing trends in cancer onset rates by trends in cancer incidence registration rates in the particular areas served by cancer registries. First, not all cancers that are diagnosed among people who normally live in the catchment area of a cancer registry get notified to that registry, but the proportion that was notified rose, perhaps by 10 or 20% (see Table 1), during the 1950s and 1960s, although probably not during the 1970s, which has caused an artefactual increase in recorded incidence rates since 1950.

Second, by old age, many people's bodies contain one or more lumps that will not be diagnosed as cancer during the remainder of their natural life-span but that would be described as "cancer" by a histologist if they were specially looked for, excised, and examined microscopically. Fox (1979) has described such lumps in the breast as "histologically cancer but biologically benign". The prevalence of such lumps is high—perhaps of the same order of magnitude as the cumulative incidence of clinically apparent cancer—and any increase in the care with which people are scrutinized by their doctors, therefore, may artificially increase the number of "cancers" that are counted. This certainly happens as a result of breast cancer screening programs (Gastrin 1980); it is, however, too soon to know whether the excision of tens of thousands of quiescent lumps that are histologically "breast cancer" will have any material effect on future breast cancer rates, but it certainly has a large effect on current "incidence" rates.

Another type of tumor whose incidence rate is likely to be affected by the increasing search for lumps is cancer of the prostate. Whereas the cumulative incidence of clinically diagnosed prostate cancer by the age of 70 is 2-3%, this is merely one-tenth of the prevalence of what a histologist would call "prostate

Table 1
Percentages of Patients Whose Cancers Were Ascertained by Death Certificate Only and for Whom No Medical Details Subsequently Could Be Found

	Cancer							
	lung		breast	prostate	colon		pancreas	
Years	male	female	female	male	male	female	male	female
1935-39	32	38	24	39	33	35	46	54
1940-44	28	36	15	23	24	32	30	45
1945-49	24	19	10	15	17	19	32	29
1950-54	17	21	7	12	13	14	24	25
1955-59	15	13	6	9	11	11	21	24
1960-64	8	6	3	5	4	6	9	9
1965-69	2	3	1	2	1	2	4	5
1970-74	2	2	1	1	1	1	2	5

The percentages that would not have been registered but for the death certificate are higher than the percentages cited in this table. (This is because in some instances finding the death certificate may have directed attention to a medical record that would otherwise have been overlooked.) The cited percentages, moreover, are percentages of *all* tumors, fatal or nonfatal, that were ascertained by death certificate only, and so are not as high as the percentage of *fatal* tumors that would not have been registered but for the death certificate. The percentages of nonfatal tumors that were not registered is, of course, not known directly but may also have been large in the earlier years.

Reprinted from Doll and Peto (1981).

Data from Connecticut Cancer Registry, 1935-74.

cancer" in the prostates of 70-year-old men who have died of unrelated causes (Breslow et al. 1977). Consequently, the invention and wide introduction of some practical means of detecting such lesions in vivo would cause an artefactual increase in prostatic cancer incidence rates of about 1000%! Phenomena related to this may underly the marked divergence in recent years between the trends recorded for the incidence and mortality from prostatic cancer (Fig. 1), for there have been no substantial improvements in its availability over this period.

Indeed, although in recent decades there have been spectacular improvements in the therapy for various uncommon types of tumor such as Hodgkin's disease and childhood or embryomal tumors, there has been disappointingly little progress in curative (as opposed to merely palliative) treatment for the common types of cancer. Consequently, if incidence and mortality data were both reliable one would expect the trends suggested by each to be roughly parallel, but they are not.

The recorded incidence rates are rising quite rapidly compared with the recorded mortality rates (as in Fig. 1, though the divergence is less extreme for most other types of cancer) and the most plausible explanation is that most of this divergence is because of artefactual increases in the recorded

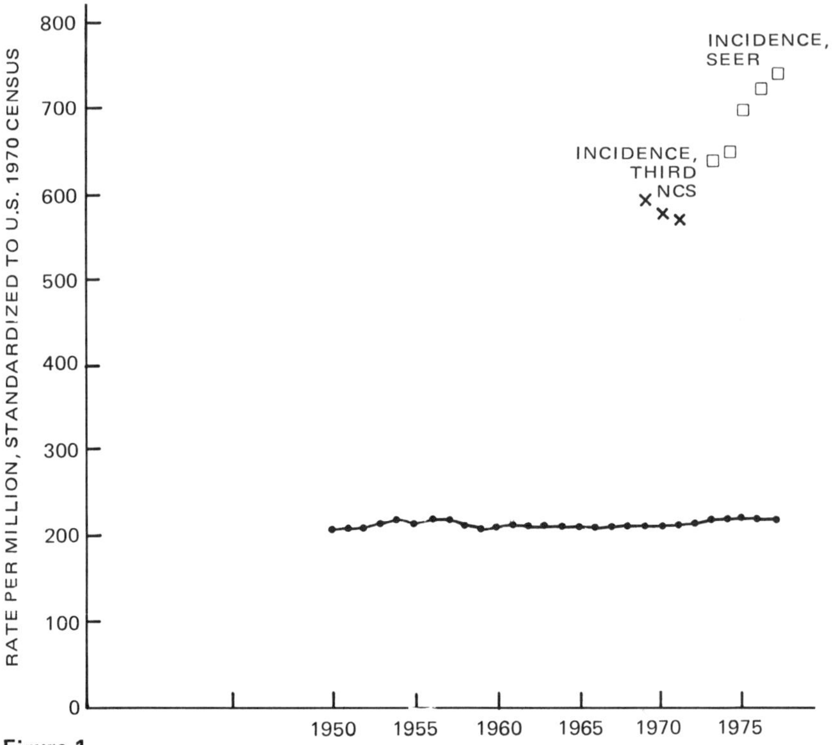

Figure 1
Trends in age-standardized (to U.S. 1970) recorded rates for prostatic cancer, indicating discrepancy between marked upward trends in recorded U.S. incidence rates and roughly flat trends in U.S. death certification rates. Since curative therapy has not changed greatly, the trends in mortality are probably roughly correct, so the large upward trends in incidence are probably wrong. Note that even now only about 10% of histologically malignant prostatic cancers arising by age 70 get diagnosed, so there is plenty of room for artefactual increases in "incidence" to be caused by progressively more thorough medical investigation of old people.

The incidence data are based on approximately one-tenth of the whole U.S. population, so purely random errors are relatively unimportant–indeed, the standard errors for each annual estimate of incidence would be smaller than the sizes of the symbols that have been used.

incidence rates. Consequently, I am reluctant to accept as informative any of Marvin Schneiderman's interpretations (Davis et al., this volume) of trends in recorded *incidence* rates, for the errors inherent in the methodology appear to be greater in many cases than the true effect that is to be studied.

Mortality Data

Mortality data depend on the death certificate being correctly filled in, which in turn depends on the degree of medical attention a dying person is likely to receive. Even as far back as the 1950s, a person dying in youth or middle age from cancer would probably be investigated in a hospital, and (with the chief exception of the diffuse neoplasms) the methods of diagnosis avilable then were not much worse than today. The chief change probably has not been in the diagnosis of the young, but rather in that of the old, who, in recent years, partly as a result of the "war on cancer," have received increasingly careful medical attention. This must artefactually affect the trends in cancer death *certification* rates among the old, so that if trends in cancer mortality are to be used to estimate the true trends in cancer onset rates it is prudent to restrict attention to the trends among people under the age of 65, as these are less subject to error.

This is not to say that deaths after the age of 65 do not matter, nor that nonfatal cancers do not matter, nor that industrial chemicals will not cause deaths among old people (although the *relative* effect of new environmental pollutants and of most new industrial processes is likely at first to be greater among people under 65 than among older people, just as was the case when cigarettes first began to affect strongly national rates of lung cancer). It is merely that, except for the gross effects of smoking on cancers of the mouth, throat, and lung, most of the trends in cancer incidence are likely to be moderate rather than extreme. So, it is difficult to estimate them reliably unless attention is directed chiefly to the most reliable parts of the available data, i.e., the trends in age-standardized *mortality* at ages *under* 65. (For further methodological details, see Doll and Peto 1981, Appendix C.)

Smoking

The final point of methodology that must be introduced concerns the effects of smoking. There are at present large increases in lung cancer, as a delayed effect of widespread adoption of cigarette smoking by Americans earlier this century. Whether the changes in lung cancer over the last few decades are, as I believe, almost wholly due to changes in the amount and method of tobacco usage is a matter for debate, as is the question of whether the mixture of much smaller increases and decreases that are seen among the remaining few dozen types of tumors constitute any evidence for a generalized increase. What is not open to debate, however, is whether it is advisable to mix up these two questions by looking at the aggregate of lung and all other cancers. Of course, if one does that, one sees increases, but this is helpful in answering neither question. Thus, none of the analyses of trends in *total* cancer presented by Marvin Schneiderman (see Davis et al., this volume) bear directly on the question of whether there is any generalized increase in progress over and above the effects of smoking.

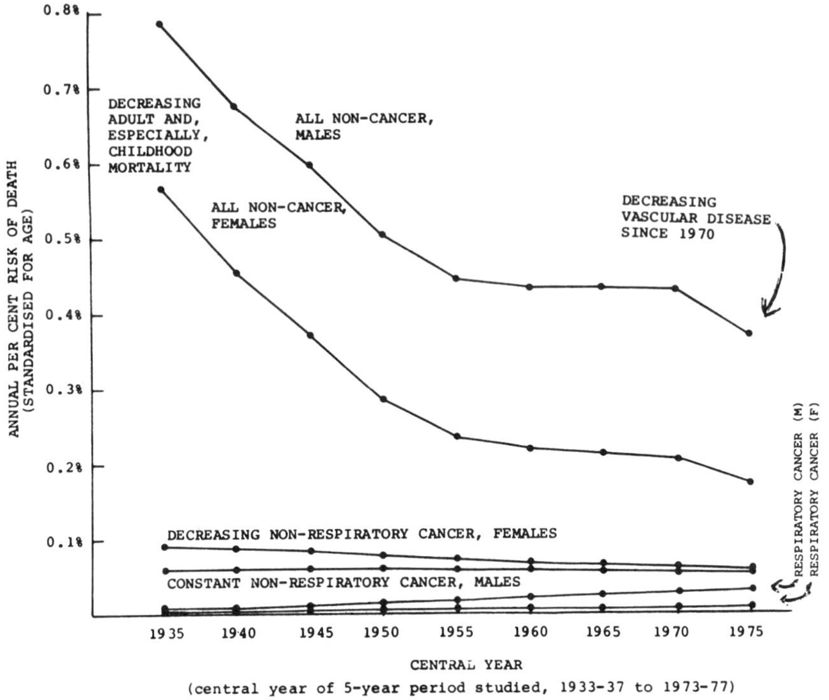

Figure 2
Annual age-standardized death rates, 1933-1977, among Americans under 65 years of age.

ACTUAL DATA

I shall now review some of the relevant data, chiefly emphasizing the trends in age-standardized mortality among people aged under 65 years. First, non-neoplastic deaths have been decreasing for half a century and are still doing so (Fig. 2). If the effects of tobacco on respiratory and vascular diseases could be allowed for, the decrease since 1950 in nonneoplastic mortality would be even greater. Close examination of Figure 2 shows that for the past half century the aggregate of all nonrespiratory cancer has been decreasing among females (chiefly because of the steady decrease in mortality from uterine cancer) but fairly constant among males, although, even in males, over the last 10 to 15 years there has been a slight decrease in total nonrespiratory cancer rates that is not visible on the large scale of Figure 2.

Respiratory cancer mortality, however, is increasing rapidly in both sexes. Much of the increase before 1950 is artefactual, produced by the improving ability of doctors to diagnose lung cancer in people dying of it (many of whom previously might have been certified as dying of some cause other than lung cancer, such as tuberculosis or pneumonia). The increase in respiratory cancer death rates since 1950 is, however, largely real, and largely due to tobacco (Doll and Peto 1981, Appendix E).

In considering nonrespiratory cancers, however, it makes little sense to bracket together diseases as different as cancer of the brain, bone, bladder, etc. Their causes are likely to be substantially different, so the trends in each type need to be considered separately (Figs. 3 and 4).

A clear picture emerges from these figures and from the detailed numerical tabulations of the data that underly them (available in Doll and Peto 1981, Appendix D):

1. Large increases at those sites (mouth, throat, and lung) that are strongly affected by tobacco.
2. Large decreases in cancer of the stomach and of the uterus.
3. Decreases due to improving treatment of Hodgkin's disease and (to a lesser extent) leukemia.
4. Otherwise, various minor ups and downs with no generalized pattern clearly evident in either sex.

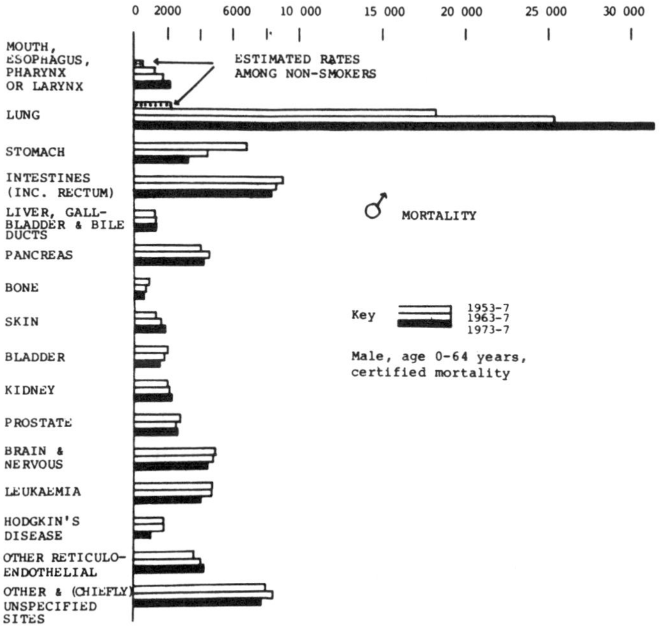

Figure 3
Certified mortality per 100 million males, ages 0-64 years (standardized for age to U.S. 1970 population).

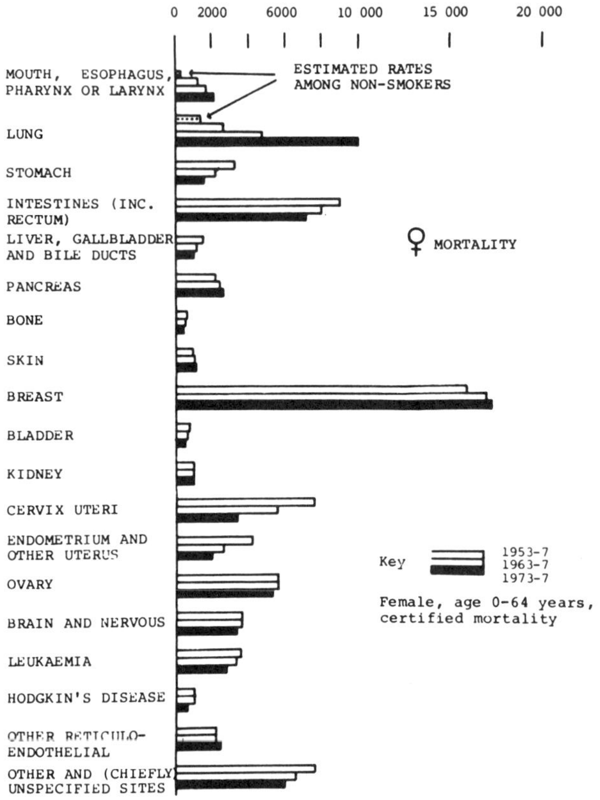

Figure 4
Certified mortality per 100 million females, ages 0-64 years (standardized for age to U.S. 1970 population).

For discussion of the separate reasons for these various trends, see Doll and Peto 1981. Note particularly the lack of increase recorded in cancers of the liver (although this may be artefactual) and bladder, two sites where large effects of occupational factors might be expected. Moreover, were it not for smoking the decrease in bladder cancer mortality would presumably be even more marked, as might the recent decrease in male pancreatic cancer (but, as seen below, the decrease in pancreatic cancer may partly be caused by recent changes in tobacco usage).

It should be noted particularly that mortality from cancer of the brain, a disease commonly supposed to be increasing, appears to be decreasing. This illustrates the importance of directing attention chiefly to people below 65 years of age, for among old people brain tumors commonly were misdiagnosed as other types of brain change. Correction of an increasing proportion of such errors may be the chief reason for the contrast between decreasing rates under 65 and increasing rates over 65 in both sexes.

Another factor that affects both brain and bone tumors, especially in old age, and which accounts for some or all of the apparent decrease in bone cancer mortality is a decreasing tendency to misdiagnose secondary deposits at those sites as primary tumors of those sites.

Another apparent change of somewhat dubious significance is the increase in death certification rates for the aggregate of all the non-Hodgkin's lymphomas, a category that includes myeloma. At least part of this increase must be an artefact of improving diagnostic technology, but whether most of the apparent increase can be attributed to this remains uncertain.

The decreases in male pancreatic cancer death certification rates since 1965 are intriguing, and again are not widely recognized. Because this trend is not apparent among females, it is unlikely to be merely a diagnostic artefact. Since the disease remains almost entirely incurable, its decrease cannot be due to improved therapy. If it is due to the changes since the 1950s in tar yields of cigarettes, then, because the increase appeared in all middle-aged groups of males simultaneously, this suggests that tobacco acts primarily on rather a late stage of the process of pancreatic carcinogenesis.

LUNG CANCER

Each change is interesting. Each deserves separate discussion. But by no stretch of the imagination can one claim in these data any evidence of a generalized increase in cancer, unless *either* lung cancer is combined with nonrespiratory cancer *or* attention is directed chiefly to the over-65's, *or* incidence registration rates are used instead of death certification rates. These are the chief respects in which my analysis differs from that of Marvin Schneiderman (see Davis et al., this volume). The final respect in which we differ is in our interpretation of the lung cancer trends.

The epidemiological studies of smoking and lung cancer have shown three things:

1. Cigarettes are far worse than other forms of tobacco.
2. If you stop smoking there is rapid benefit (at least in terms of avoidance of any further increase in incidence), so that one would expect substantial benefits to be enjoyed already as a result of people stopping smoking or switching to low-tar brands over the past quarter-century.
3. If you really want to give yourself lung cancer, it pays to start smoking when you're really young (Fig. 5).

This third point implies that what happens to you in your teens and twenties imprints on you a susceptibility to the effects of smoking in later life.

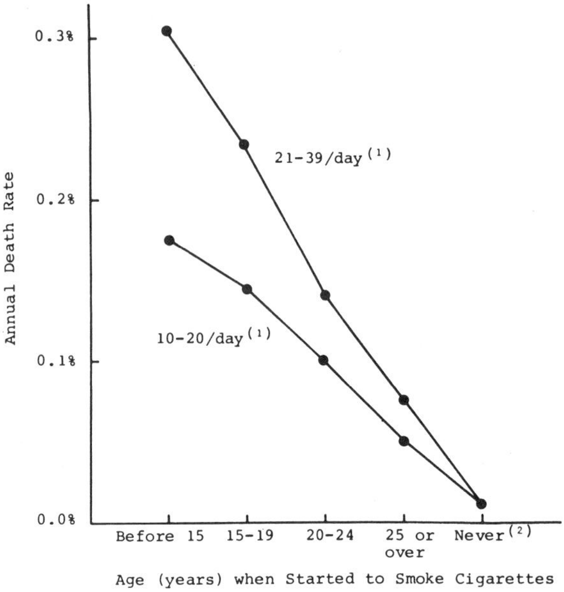

Figure 5
Data on U.S. veterans (Kahn 1966). Lung cancer mortality at ages 55-64 among current smokers of cigarettes only, in relation to the age when cigarette smoking first began (though this was perhaps not when regular consumption of substantial numbers of cigarettes first began).

[1] The figures 10-20 and 21-39/day refer to the maximum rate at which the subject ever normally smoked cigarettes; the lifelong average may, of course, be much less than this.
[2] Subject may previously have smoked "once in a while but not every day."

This, in turn, implies that the sudden, permanent increase in U.S. cigarette consumption that coincided with World War II (Fig. 6) will not have its full effect on U.S. lung cancer among people in their 30s until about 1960, on people in their 40s until about 1970, on people in their 50s until about 1980, and so on. Thus, the increases in lung cancer currently seen among American men aged over 50 are, qualitatively at least, what one would expect as a delayed consequence of the rapid increase in U.S. cigarette consumption during the World War II. If this is so, increases in lung cancer among Americans aged over 75 probably will continue until at least the turn of the century.

Schneiderman's analysis tries to interpret lung cancer trends without taking explicit account of the delayed effects of the increase in cigarette consumption by the young 30 to 50 years ago. This is impossible. Superposed on the pattern of increases in lung cancer (at least among men aged over 50) due to the delayed effects of the wartime increase in cigarette consumption is the pattern of decreases due to decreasing tar yields. The net effects of these two opposing tendencies are: (1) net increases in U.S. male lung cancer mortality above age 50 and (2) net decreases below age 50 (Fig. 7).

It is noteworthy that the rates in the older age groups have not yet caught up with British male rates, for British males started to smoke substantial numbers of cigarettes somewhat earlier than did U.S. males even though we now smoke less.

Before comparing this analysis of lung cancer rates with that proposed by Schneiderman (Davis et al., this volume), it should be noted that if the lung cancer rate due to smoking is increasing then the proportion of all lung cancer that is due to smoking must also be increasing, and *not* (as Schneiderman, considering only the late stage, i.e., quick-acting, effects of tobacco, predicted from recent changes in tobacco consumption and tar yields) staying constant or decreasing. Once this is accepted, no evidence remains for any increase over and above that which could plausibly be attributed to cigarettes.

The trouble with this argument, of course, is that we don't know *exactly* what the effects of tobacco would have been if nothing else had changed. Maybe, if all factors but tobacco had been constant, the decreases at ages under 50 would have been somewhat different in magnitude, or maybe the increases at ages over 50 would have been different. One cannot say for sure. We know on other grounds that some important increases (e.g., the change from a few hundred asbestos-induced lung cancers per year in the 1950s to a few thousand nowadays) due to agents other than tobacco do lie concealed in the lung cancer trends, however.

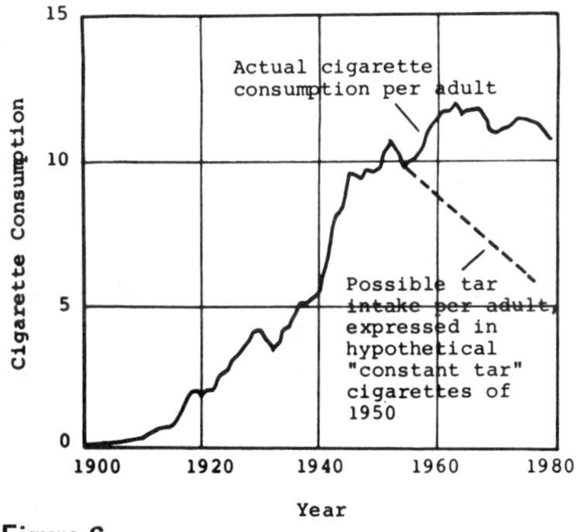

Figure 6
Mean daily sales of manufactured cigarettes per U.S. adult over 18 years of age (Public Health Service 1980), together with a crude estimate of tar yield per adult, based on Owen (1976). The estimate of tar yield allows approximately for decreases since 1954 in tar yield per cigarette smoked in a standard manner (but not for any hypothetical compensatory increases in number of puffs per low-nicotine cigarette).

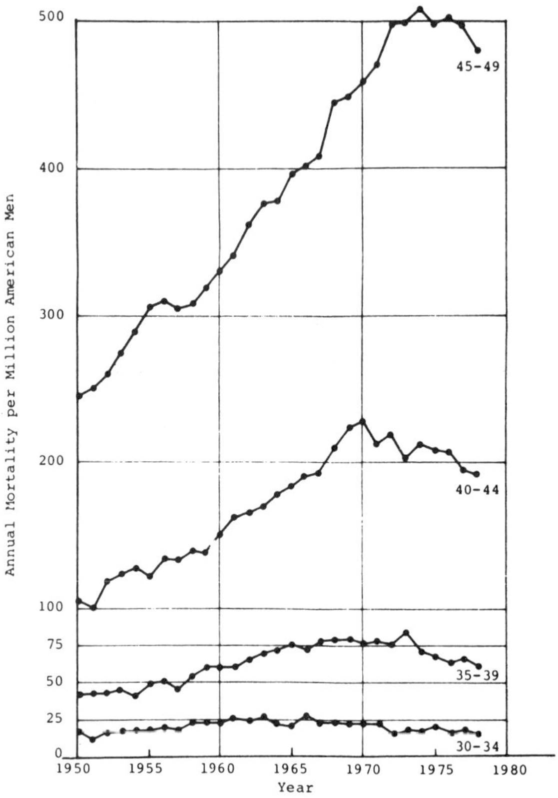

Figure 7
Trends since 1950 in lung cancer mortality in U.S. males at young ages; recent decreases are shown for the age groups 30-34, 35-39, 40-44, and 45-49 years.

Thus, I am not arguing that I have proved that all is well. Still less am I arguing that all will be well in the future. I have argued merely that the lung cancer data *of themselves* do not offer any evidence for an increase in exposure to any important lung carcinogen other than tobacco smoke, and that the suggestion by Davis et al. (this volume) that they do is not well-founded.

INTERNATIONAL COMPARISONS

At the moment, America is not at the top of the international lung cancer league. Britain is, in most age groups. However, this is because the full effect of the post-World War II increase in U.S. tobacco usage has not made itself felt yet. When it does, after the turn of the century, American lung cancer rates probably will be the worst in the world. An indication that this will be so is in the relationship between manufactured cigarette consumption in 1950 in various countries and recent lung cancer rates among people who were *young adults* in 1950 (Fig. 8), i.e., among those whose susceptibility to future damage if they continued to smoke was imprinted on them by their exposure to cigarette smoke in about 1950. This American excess in early middle age will presumably eventually spread to older age groups indicating that for America, the worst is yet to come.

CONCLUSION

There is no good evidence for any generalized increase in U.S. cancer rates over and above that due to smoking. This is not, however, a guarantee that all is well. Although it makes the attribution of *large* percentages of U.S. cancer to relatively new occupational or environmental pollutants implausible, even plausibly small percentages represent large absolute numbers of affected people. Still less is the lack of evidence for any recent generalized increase in U.S. cancer rates beyond that due to smoking a guarantee that all in the future will be well. However, the most direct evidence of what the trends in total cancer rates among people aged 55-64 will be during the 1990s are the trends in total cancer rates among people aged 35-44 during the 1970s, and these were remarkably favorable (Doll and Peto 1981, Table D6). Indeed, these decreases at younger ages have even led Schneiderman (this volume) to speculate that some aspect of the modern U.S. diet or life-style is conferring a generalized protection against cancer. So, it is difficult to believe that evidence for any generalized adverse effect of new pollutants is likely to be contained in these data.

One question of interest that remains is why so many people have come to opposite conclusions. The use of data on people aged over 65, or of incidence data, or of data on the aggregates of lung and other tumors, has been mentioned, as has the failure to expect a long delay between the increase in cigarette usage and the full resultant increase in lung cancer. In addition, some commentators, particularly Epstein and Swartz (1981), in a paper that they circulated to all participants at this meeting, have attempted to base inferences about cancer onset rates on trends in such misleading statistics as the crude cancer rate, the percentage of all deaths due to cancer, or the lifelong probability of getting cancer. All of these are grossly biased by the decrease in causes of death other than cancer, and the increase in the proportion of older people.

A more fundamental reason, however, may be that people positively *wish* to believe ill of the modern world, for the same sort of reasons that Prometheus was chained to a rock, and are surprised to learn that longevity is still increasing. This increase would have been even more pronounced, of course, were it not for the few hundred thousand U.S. deaths (well over 10% of the U.S. total) that nowadays are caused each year by tobacco. Furthermore, cancer

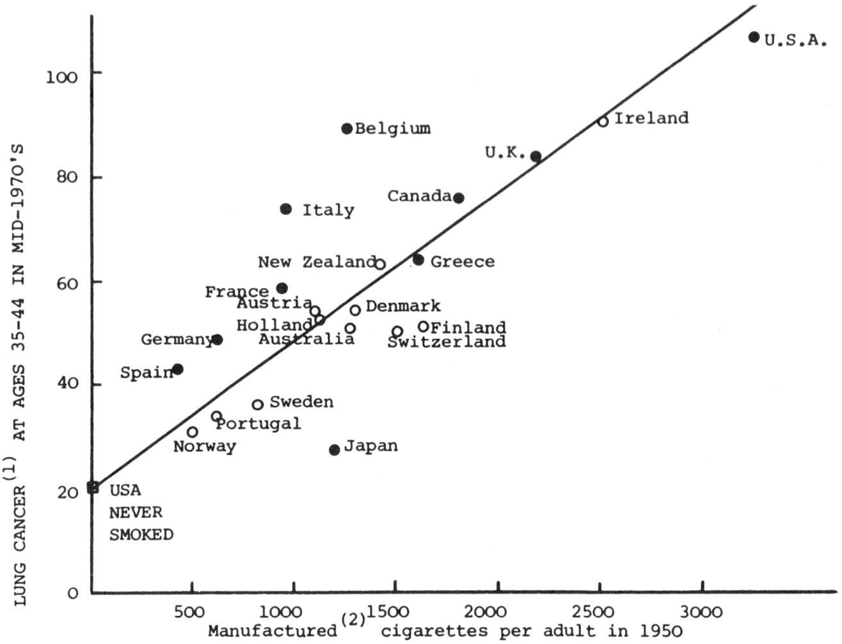

Figure 8

International correlation between manufactured cigarette consumption per adult in 1950 while one particular generation was entering adult life (in 1950) and lung cancer rates in that generation as it enters middle age (in the mid-1970s). (•) Rates based on over 100 deaths; (○) rates based on 25-100 deaths; (□) U.S. nonsmokers 1959-1972.[3] Comparison has been restricted to developed countries (i.e., excluding Africa, all of Asia except Japan, and all except North America) with populations > 1 million, to improve the accuracy of the observed death certification rates as indicators of the underlying risks of lung cancer among people aged 35-44.

[1] Lung cancer death certification rates per million adults aged 35-44 are from WHO (1977, 1980). These rates are the means of the male and female rates for all years (1973, 1974, or 1975) reported in WHO (1977), except for Greece (which was not reported in WHO [1977] and thus was taken from WHO [1980] and Norway), for which the rates in WHO (1977) and WHO (1980) were based on only 11 and 14 cases, respectively; for statistical stability, these were averaged.

[2] Manufactured cigarettes per adult are from Lee (1975) for the year 1950 (except for Italy, where consumption data are available in 5-yr groups only; to avoid the temporary postwar shortages, data for 1951-1955 have been used). This excludes handrolled cigarettes, which in most countries accounted for only a small fraction of all cigarette tobacco in 1950.

[3] U.S. nonsmoker rates were estimated by fitting straight lines (on a double logarithmic scale) to the relationships between lung cancer mortality and age reported for male and for female lifelong nonsmokers by Garfinkel (1980) and averaging the predicted values at age 40. (Although the average of the male and female rates actually observed at these ages is similar to this estimated value, these observed rates are each based on fewer than 5 cases [Garfinkel 1980] and so might have been inaccurate.)

is talked about now far more than in the past. Friends or public figures with cancer no longer make the disease a private, secret fact. Also, any odd details of cancer research are newsworthy now. Traces of nitrosamines in whisky, undetectable 20 years ago, now make headline news (in complete disregard of the fact that the alcohol in whisky is probably far more carcinogenic than the nitrosamines).

In discussing mistaken arguments based on the available data, it is tempting to be over-definite as to what the data do and do not say. Although there is in these data no good evidence for any generalized increase in cancer, there is no guarantee against some more moderate effect. National trends are crude tools, and their examination should have little place in the quantification of things like occupational factors that probably account for only a small percentage of all cancers.

SUMMARY

The estimation of trends in cancer onset rates is fraught with difficulties. Unless these are all allowed for in one analysis, errors will arise that are of the same order of magnitude—or even greater—than the true trends. At present, the U.S. data demonstrate large and continuing increases in respiratory cancer that are due chiefly to the delayed rapid effects of people starting to smoke cigarettes still outweighing the lesser (though important) effects of recent decreases in tar yields and cigarette usage. The U.S. data also indicate large decreases in cancer of the stomach and uterus, large relative increases in melanoma, and a mixture of minor increases and decreases in the various other nonrespiratory cancers, with liver cancer mortality constant and bladder cancer mortality decreasing much faster than can be accounted for plausibly by improvements in cancer therapy. Future trends may differ substantially from recent trends, of course, but at present the U.S. data contain no clear evidence for any generalized increase in cancer over and above that due to the delayed effects of tobacco. Opposite conclusions by other commentators appear to derive chiefly from methodological oversights. Such an examination of national trends does provide suggestive evidence against the view that a large percentage of today's cancers are due to occupational and environmental factors that were introduced during this century, but does not provide evidence against the more reasonable view that a *small* percentage are. But, even a small percentage of all cancers may represent several thousand U.S. cancer deaths a year. This is a large enough absolute number to justify efforts to seek out and reduce or eliminate any likely causes of substantial future numbers of cases of occupational cancer.

REFERENCES

Breslow, N., C.W. Chan, G. Dhom, R.A.B. Drury, L.M. Franks, B. Gelei, Y.S.

Lee, S. Lundberg, B. Sparke, N.H. Sternby, and H. Tulinius. 1977. Latent carcinomas of prostate at autopsy in seven areas. *Int. J. Cancer* **20**:680.

Doll, R. and R. Peto. 1981. The causes of cancer: Quantitative estimates of avoidable risks of cancer in the United States today. *J. Natl. Cancer Inst.* **66**:1191.

Epstein, S. and J.B. Swartz. 1981. Fallacies of lifestyle cancer theories. *Nature* **289**:127.

Fox, M. 1979. On the diagnosis and treatment of breast cancer. *J. Am. Med. Assoc.* **241**:489.

Garfinkel, L. 1980. Cancer mortality in nonsmokers: Prospective study by the American Cancer Society. *J. Natl. Cancer Inst.* **65**:1169.

Gastrin, G. 1980. Programme to encourage self-examination of breast cancer. *Br. Med. J.* **1**:193.

Kahn, H.A. 1966. The Dorn study of smoking and mortality among U.S. veterans. Report on eight and one-half years of observation. *Natl. Cancer Inst. Monogr.* **19**:1.

Lee, P.N. 1975. *Tobacco consumption in various countries.* Research paper Number 6 (4th ed.) Tobacco Research Council, London.

Owen, T.B. 1976. Tar and nicotine from U.S. cigarettes: Trends over the past twenty years. In *Proceedings of the Third World Conference on Smoking and Health. Modifying the risk for the smoker.* Vol. 1. (ed. E.L. Wynder et al.) p. 73. DHEW (NIH) 76-1221. Government Printing Office, Washington, D.C.

Public Health Service. 1979. *Smoking and Health. A report of the Surgeon General.* DHEW publication number (PHS) 79-50066. Government Printing Office, Washington, D.C.

———. 1980. *Smoking and Health. The health consequences of smoking for women. A report of the Surgeon General.* GPO publication number 0-326-003. Government Printing Office, Washington, D.C.

———. 1981. *The health consequences of smoking. The changing cigarette.* DHEW publication number DHHS (PHS) 81-50156. Government Printing Office, Washington, D.C.

World Health Organization (WHO). 1977. *World health statistics annual: Vital statistics and causes of death.* WHO, Geneva.

———. 1980. *World health statistics annual: Vital statistics and causes of death.* WHO, Geneva.

Estimating Cancer Causes: Problems in Methodology, Production, and Trends

DEVRA LEE DAVIS
Environmental Law Institute
Washington, D.C. 20036

KENNETH BRIDBORD
National Institute for Occupational Safety and Health
Washington, D.C.

MARVIN SCHNEIDERMAN
Clement Associates, Inc.
Washington, D.C. 20007

What public health strategies might effectively reduce future cancers and other diseases (Davis and Ng 1981)? Considerable debate surrounds the relative importance of life-style (Higginson and Muir 1979; Whelan 1979, 1981; Cimino and Demopoulos 1980; Wynder 1980) and industrial chemical factors (Epstein 1974; Epstein and Swartz 1981; Hueper 1979) for human cancer rates. Obviously both factors are consequential.

This three-part paper reviews difficulties in allocating the proportion of cancers attributable to specific causes: The first part briefly notes problems associated with allocating causes of cancer, including a discussion of previous efforts to make such estimates based on epidemiological studies. The second part discusses recent trends in production, consumption, and use of materials known or suspected to be carcinogens. The third part examines trends in the 1970s of cancer incidence and mortality within the United States and speculates about explanations for the decline in cancer in people under age 45 and the increases in those over 45. The possible contributions of cigarette smoking and industrial exposures also are examined.

Those claiming that most cancers are caused by life-style factors, such as smoking and nutrition, point to the lack of drastic increases in cancer rates as evidence that high-volume industrial production has not had an important impact on cancer rates (Higginson 1980). Following this viewpoint, reducing future cancer rates requires changes in life-style factors, rather than regulation of chemical production, use, and disposal. Of the numerous documented causes of cancer, ranging from sunlight to cigarette smoking to early and frequent sexual intercourse with many partners, (Clayson 1967, 1977; Doll 1977; Epstein 1972, 1974; Fraumeni 1977; Lancet 1977; Wynder and Gori 1977; Higginson and Muir 1979; Habs and Schmahl 1980; Jacobson 1980), toxic chemicals in the workplace are among the very few controllable by law. As Doll and Peto (1981) note, if two particular agents account for a similar percentage of all cancer deaths, that which is the more easily controlled is obviously of greater public health significance.

The effort to estimate the causes of human cancer gained prominence when attempts to regulate carcinogens began in earnest. Some had suggested that between 1% and 5%, or no more than 15% of cancer (in males), could be related to the workplace (Higginson 1969; Higginson and Muir 1976; Cole 1977). It would appear that many of these estimates relied on the delphi method, whereby a group of experts polls itself.

ESTIMATING CANCER CAUSES

The Estimates Paper

In 1978, the Occupational Safety and Health Administration (OSHA) held hearings on its proposal to identify and regulate carcinogens generically, and in 1980 a standard was promulgated (Federal Register 1980). In an effort to assess systematically the possible contribution of workplace exposures to cancer, scientists from the National Cancer Institute (NCI), the National Institute of Environmental Health Sciences (NIEHS), and the National Institute for Occupational Safety and Health (NIOSH) prepared and submitted a paper for the OSHA hearings (Bridbord et al. 1978). The paper applied a population attributable risk percent (PARP) model to estimating the fraction of cancer in the United States related to occupational factors (Cole and Merletti 1980). As is well known to participants at this meeting, the cancer estimates paper generated considerable controversy and discussion (Stallones and Downs 1978; Higginson and Muir 1979; Maugh 1979; Morgan 1979; Abelson 1980; Cole and Merletti 1980; Higginson 1980; Peto 1980; Epstein and Swartz 1981).

Out of the then 26 chemicals or substances identified as human carcinogens, the estimates paper developed a "worst-case" scenario for six high-volume workplace carcinogens. Based on risk factors and estimated previous occupational exposures to these carcinogens, the paper projected possible future occupational contributions to cancer. The analysis considered best available estimates of occupational exposure to asbestos, arsenic, benzene, chromium, nickel, and petroleum fractions (including aromatics). It estimated that subsequent occupationally related cancers may be 20% or more of future total cancer mortality. Table 1 indicates available estimates of full- or part-time workers exposed to five of these substances in 1974 (DHEW 1974), along with

Table 1
Risk Factors Associated with Workplace Exposures to Five High-volume Confirmed Human Carcinogens

Chemical	Target organs in humans	Other chronic health effects	Occupations at risk	Latency period for cancer (yr)	Risk ratios for cancer	Estimated number of workers exposed annually
Arsenic	skin, lung, liver, lymphatic system	gastrointestinal disturbances, hyperpigmentation, peripheral neuropathy, hemolytic anemia, dermatitis, bronchitis, nasal system ulceration	miners, smelters, insecticide makers and sprayers, chemical workers, oil refiners, vintners	10+	3-8	1,500,000
Asbestos	lung, pleural and peritoneal mesothelioma, gastrointestinal tract	asbestosis (pulmonary fibrosis, pleural plaques, and pleural calcification), anorexia, weight loss	miners, millers, textile, insulation, and shipyard workers	4-40	1.5-12	1,600,000 2,522,000
Benzene	bone marrow (leukemia)	central nervous system and gastrointestinal effects, blood abnormalities (anemia, leukopenia, and thrombocytopenia)	explosives, benzene and rubber cement workers, distillers, dye users, printers, shoemakers	6-14	2-3	2,000,000 1,900,000
Chromium	nasal cavity and sinuses, lung, larynx	dermatitis, skin ulceration, nasal system ulceration, bronchitis, bronchopneumonia, inflammation of the larynx and liver	producers, processors, and users of Cr–acetylene and aniline workers; bleachers; glass, pottery, and linoleum workers; battery makers	5-15	3-4	1,500,000 (chromium oxides) 175,000 (chromium VI)
Nickel	nasal cavity and sinuses, lung	dermatitis	nickel smelters, mixers, and roasters, electrolysis workers	3-30	5-10 (lung), 100+ (nasal sinuses)	1,400,000 (oxides) 25,000 (inorganic nickel)

[a]Data from Davis and Rall (1981).

risk ratios of past industrial exposures (Davis and Rall 1981). Asbestos comprised by far the largest contributor to these estimated cancers, considering exposures in shipyards during World War II and later exposures in the construction and auto industries, etc.

Before commenting on the estimates paper, it is necessary to consider exactly what is involved in talking about causes of cancer. Cancer is many diseases with multiple, interdependent causes. To go about the business of doing epidemiology, analysts assume perfect isolation among complex interacting systems. In an absolute sense, causation remains a guiding idealization: "Strict and pure causation works nowhere and never. . . . Causal hypotheses are no more (and no less) than rough, approximate, one-sided reconstructions of determination. . . ." (Bunge 1959).

Several related methodological problems pointed out by Cole and Merletti (1980) are noteworthy in any effort to estimate cancer causes. In fact, contributing causes of cancers are interdependent, so that a reduction of smoking-caused cancer could increase the proportion of occupationally related cancers, although the amount of the latter remained the same. Further, although every cause is partially distinct, every sufficient cause is in fact a constellation of component causes (Cole and Merletti 1980). Thus, if the overall cancer rate declined 25% following the elimination of cigarette smoking, this does not mean that smoking alone caused 25% of cancer. Rather, it means that smoking contributed to the causation of 25% of all cancer.

As the estimates paper noted in 1978, in a PARP model the sum of component causes exceeds 100% because multiple factors can contribute to the same case of cancer. Theoretically, a given case of cancer could be prevented by intervening in any number of ways, reflecting these multiple contributing factors. In this regard, there is no theoretical upper limit to the sum of attributable causes. This aspect has made many uncomfortable with such an approach, preferring instead to focus preventive efforts on predominant causal factors, that is factors in the absence of which the greatest number of cancers might be prevented (Higginson 1980). However, focusing exclusively upon predominant causes may miss many important opportunities to prevent disease by reducing other contributing risk factors.

Complicating and Confounding Issues

In developing estimations of cancer causes, the estimates paper noted some major complicating issues, many of which continue to be relevant:

- Many previous estimates of the causes of cancer relied on the delphi method and generally gave limited consideration to workplace factors and underestimated the number of occupationally exposed individuals. The latter is especially the case regarding asbestos exposure in shipyards during World War II.

- Previous estimates of cancer etiology sometimes neglected complex interactions and arrived at the occupational contribution largely by subtraction, assuming for example that because 80-90% of lung cancer was related to smoking, and therefore only 10-20% could possibly be "due to" all other causes.
- The problem of cancer estimates is further complicated by the fact that most physicians and other health professionals have not been trained to take adequate occupational histories; consequently, such professionals rarely inquire as to the existence of possible occupational factors contributing to the etiology of disease. This is understandable because treatment is rarely dependent upon etiology. However, lack of adequate occupational histories slows recognition of suspected workplace correlates of cancer.
- Perhaps the two most important limitations of the 1978 paper were that it considered a limited number of known hazards and a small number of cancer sites known to be related to occupational exposures.
- The paper did not consider such known occupational carcinogens as radiation or pesticides; rather the analysis only considered one-fifth of those substances or processes considered by the International Agency for Research on Cancer (IARC) at the time to cause cancer in humans. In addition, the paper did not include workers who might develop cancer from exposure to high-volume industrial substances or processes that are carcinogenic to animals. A large number of industrial materials have been identified as carcinogens in laboratory studies, but have not been investigated in human populations. On this point, Karstadt (this volume) makes the important observation that most animal carcinogens now in commerce have not been and are not likely to be subject to epidemiological study. For these substances, waiting for epidemiological confirmation becomes waiting for Godot.
- As to the limited number of cancer sites studied, the paper did not consider skin or bladder cancers known to be occupationally related. Further, the paper could not have considered the most recent epidemiologic studies in which excess cancer incidence has been reported, sometimes without identification of a specific etiologic agent (Tables 2 and 3). Further, the estimates paper only considered cancer risk, even though carcinogens may also affect other target organs, as shown in Figure 1.
- A methodological catch-22 also confounded the estimates paper. The study generally applied the excess risks observed in published epidemiologic studies of past highly exposed groups to all current full- and part-time exposed workers. In this regard, epidemiology studies are not generally available for groups exposed to low levels of carcinogens. This failure to consider exposure reductions inflated the estimates of risk. As R. Peto has pointed out at this meeting (R. Peto, this volume), in the case of nickel workers such an approach was clearly inappropriate. The estimates paper did not consider

Table 2
Recent Epidemiologic Studies Suggestive of a Relationship Between Occupation and Cancer

Type of cancer	Occupation, industry, exposure	Reference
Prostate	rubber and tire workers	Goldsmith et al. (1980)
Bowel and rectum	paint and coatings manufacturing	Morgan et al. (1981)
Stomach, brain, leukemia, and multiple myeloma	petroleum refining and petrochemical plants	Thomas et al. (1980)
Respiratory system	welders, shipfitters, and metal-trades workers	Beaumont and Weiss (1980)
Soft-tissue sarcomas	phenoxyacetic acids and chlorophenols	Hardell and Sandstrom (1979) Honchar and Halperin (1981)
Stomach cancer and leukemia	ethylene oxide, ethylene dichloride	Hogstedt et al. (1979a, b)
Malignant lymphoma, lung cancer, and pancreas	aluminum reduction plant workers	Milham (1979)
Lymphatic leukemia	rubber workers	Wolf et al. (1981)
Lung-bronchus, esophagus, and lymphatic-hematopoietic	plumbers and pipefitters	Kaminski et al. (1980)
Brain cancer	petrochemical workers	Alexander et al. (1981)
Choroidal malignant melanoma	chemical workers	Albert et al. (1980)
Kidney and genitals	female laundry and dry cleaning workers	Katz and Jowett (1981)
Lung and uterine-cervical cancers	laundry and dry cleaning workers	Blair et al. (1979)
Bladder cancer	leather and leather products manufacturing	Decoufle (1979)
Lung cancer	spray painters, zinc chromate primer-paints	Dalager (1980)
Digestive organs and lungs	smelter and battery plant workers, lead	Kang et al. (1980)
Respiratory cancer	arsenic-exposed workers	Pinto et al. (1978)
Lung cancer	beryllium	Cole and Merletti (1980)
Prostate, kidney, and lung	cadmium	Cole and Merletti (1980)
Lung cancer	automobile manufacture (casting and plating)	Silverstein et al. (1981)

Table 3
Occupational Groups in Which Excess Cancer Incidence Has Been Reported Without Identification of a Specific Etiologic Agent

Occupational groups	Cancer site	Percent excess reported	Reference
Coal miners	stomach	40	Rockette (1977)
Chemists	pancreas,	64	Li et al. (1969)
	lymphomas	79	
Foundry workers	lung	50-150	Koskela et al. (1976); Gibson et al. (1977)
Textile workers	mouth and pharynx	77	Moss and Lee (1974)
Printing pressmen (newspaper)	mouth and pharynx	125	Lloyd et al. (1977)
Metal miners	lung	200	Wagoner et al. (1963)
Coke by-product workers	large intestine,	181	Redmond et al. (1976)
	pancreas	312	
Cadmium production workers	lung,	135	Lemen et al. (1976)
	prostate	248	
Rubber industry			
Processing	stomach,	80	Monson and Nakano (1976)
	leukemia	140	
Tire building	bladder,	88	Monson and Nakano (1976)
	brain	90	
Tire curing	lung	61	Monson and Nakano (1976)
Furniture workers	nasal cavity and sinuses	300-400	Acheson (1976)
Shoe workers	nasal cavity and sinuses,	700	Acheson (1976); Brinton (1977)
	leukemia	100	Aksoy et al. (1974)
Leather workers	bladder	150	Cole and Goldman (1975)

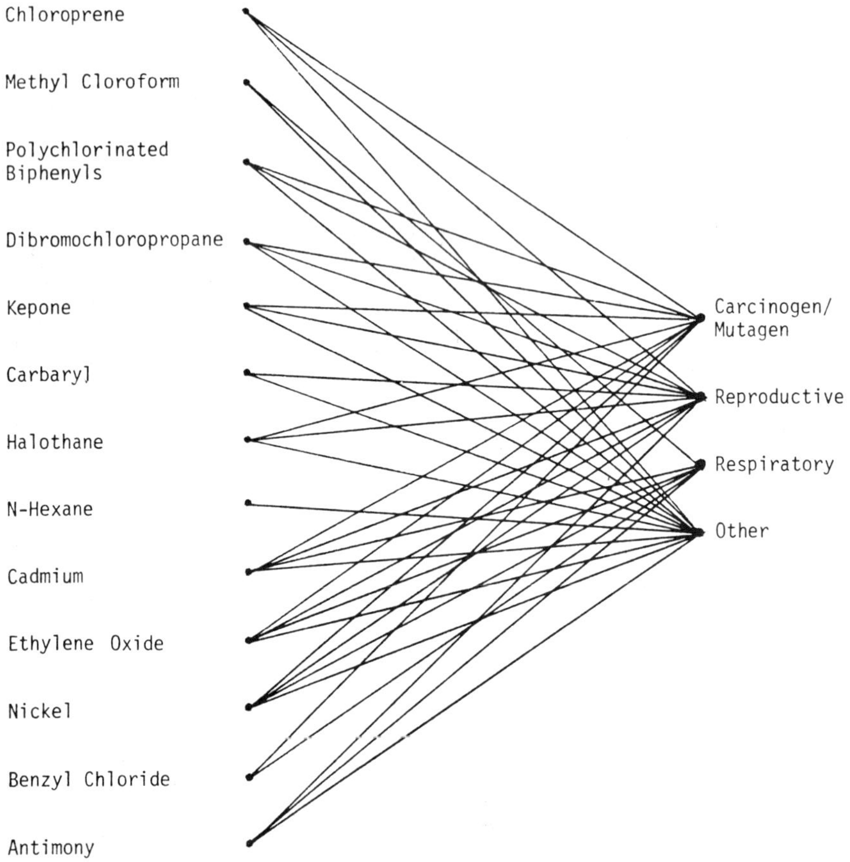

Figure 1
Multiple chronic effects of environment chemicals

consider that some of the exposures that led to excess risks might have since been reduced or controlled–and thus risks to currently exposed populations should be less than previously seen. For any given previously identified carcinogen, Hoerger (this volume) suggested that in larger industries there is less exposure to workers per unit production.

- The estimates paper relied largely on epidemiologic studies that may only detect those cancers that develop early, as cohorts generally have not been followed for a lifetime.
- Further, as the above suggests, exposure assessment problems are pivotal. The estimates of exposed workers were not based on measurements of actual levels of exposure, durations, or doses of exposure. These data are not available generally. The estimations may have double-counted workers exposed to more than one of the agents considered. Conversely, the

employment estimates did not fully consider turnovers in the work force, which would have added to the potential population at risk.

- The estimations did not isolate smoking or other potentially confounding variables. The general population control groups used in virtually all cohort mortality studies include many individuals exposed to carcinogens on the job, thus understating the risk compared to "nonexposed" persons. This is analagous to comparing the risk of lung cancer in smokers to that in the general populations, which includes a large percentage of smokers.

In summary, recent research indicates that the estimates paper probably overestimates the contributions of these six substances to the overall cancer rate. Some of the original assumptions about exposure have since been shown to be incorrect. However, we believe that the basic PARP approach remains a valid technique for estimating the contribution of occupational exposures to the overall cancer rate. Other papers presented at this meeting suggest specific instances of inflation in the original estimates. Ultimately, these will be fully aired and subject to further discussion. In the meantime, we wish to draw attention to recent changes in chemical production that suggest important increases in potential exposure to known carcinogens.

CHEMICAL PRODUCTION PATTERNS

Estimating future cancer risks is complicated by the fact that since World War II, and particularly since 1960, there has been a dramatic change increase in the use of chemicals in the workplace and in the general environment (Fig. 2). IARC has estimated that about 350 chemicals are suspect human carcinogens based upon studies in experimental animals and limited human observations (Tomatis et al. 1978). Fewer than 60 chemicals have been evaluated as cancer hazards in humans through epidemiologic studies (IARC 1980). This is largely due to the fact that most occupational exposures have not been adequately evaluated epidemiologically, if at all. Chemicals introduced into the workplace since 1960, or chemicals whose use has greatly increased since 1960, for example, could not possibly be ruled out as human carcinogens based upon epidemiologic studies conducted in 1980 due to latency considerations and unavailability of suitable study populations. (Epstein 1974; Ember 1976; Cairns 1977; Harris et al. 1977; Eisenbud 1978; Davis and Magee 1979; Environmental Defense Fund 1979; Rall 1979; Doll and Peto 1981).

To some, the lack of an explosive increase in cancer mortality now exonerates individual chemicals as causes of cancer (Whelan 1979). This view ignores the fact that production and normal use of many carcinogenic, bioavailable, and otherwise hazardous substances has reached very high levels only since the early 1960s (Fig. 2). Fewer than 10% of all chemicals in commerce have been even minimally tested.

In light of the average 20-year or more latency period for most cancers to become clinically evident, the bulk of industry-associated cancers in the 1980s stems from initiating exposures that occurred typically before 1960

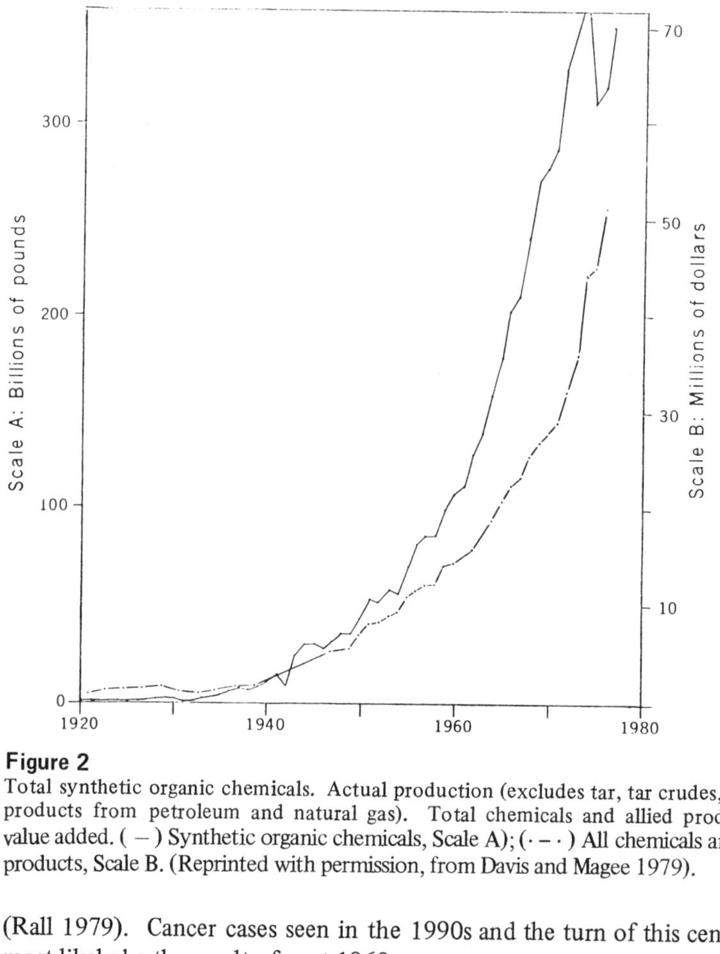

Figure 2
Total synthetic organic chemicals. Actual production (excludes tar, tar crudes, and primary products from petroleum and natural gas). Total chemicals and allied products, annual value added. (—) Synthetic organic chemicals, Scale A); (· — ·) All chemicals and allied products, Scale B. (Reprinted with permission, from Davis and Magee 1979).

(Rall 1979). Cancer cases seen in the 1990s and the turn of this century would most likely be the result of post-1960 exposures.

Under our direction, Brian Magee, Mary Supler, and Jennifer Douville have gathered and compiled statistical production data on a variety of high-volume inorganic and organic chemicals. For most of these chemicals, no direct estimates on human exposures are available. Indeed, human exposure to a chemical is not simply related to production or use. But the recent, large increases in chemical use (and disposal) certainly have been associated with greater human exposures to a complex of substances, stricter environmental and occupational controls notwithstanding (Davis and Magee 1979).

Aggregate trends of production for the chemical industry are potentially misleading because individual chemicals do not have identical public health impacts. Annual production statistics are not available for many of the chemicals listed in the Environmental Protection Agency's (EPA) inventory of substances in commercial use.

There is a consistent and remarkable production pattern for many hazardous chemicals, with exponential growth in the 1960s and later. Figure 3 shows the production histories of benzene and vinyl chloride, both class-I IARC human carcinogens, as well as acrylonitrile, an IARC class-II probable carcinogen based upon animal and limited human data (IARC 1980), along with perchloroethylene, a suspected carcinogen and a confirmed neurotoxin. Approximately 374,000 full- and part-time workers are exposed potentially to varying levels of acrylonitrile (NIOSH 1981). Vinyl chloride is carcinogenic in mice, rats, and hamsters, producing tumors at several sites, including angiosarcoma of the liver (IARC 1979). In humans, vinyl chloride has been identified as the causative agent of angiosarcoma of the liver and tumors of the brain, lung, and hemolymphopoietic system (IARC 1979). The annual production rate of vinyl chloride is expected to rise more than 10% per year through the 1980s; approximately 30,000 full-time workers have been exposed to varying levels of this carcinogen (NIOSH 1981). Exposure to vinyl chloride both per unit produced and in total has been reduced dramatically following regulatory efforts

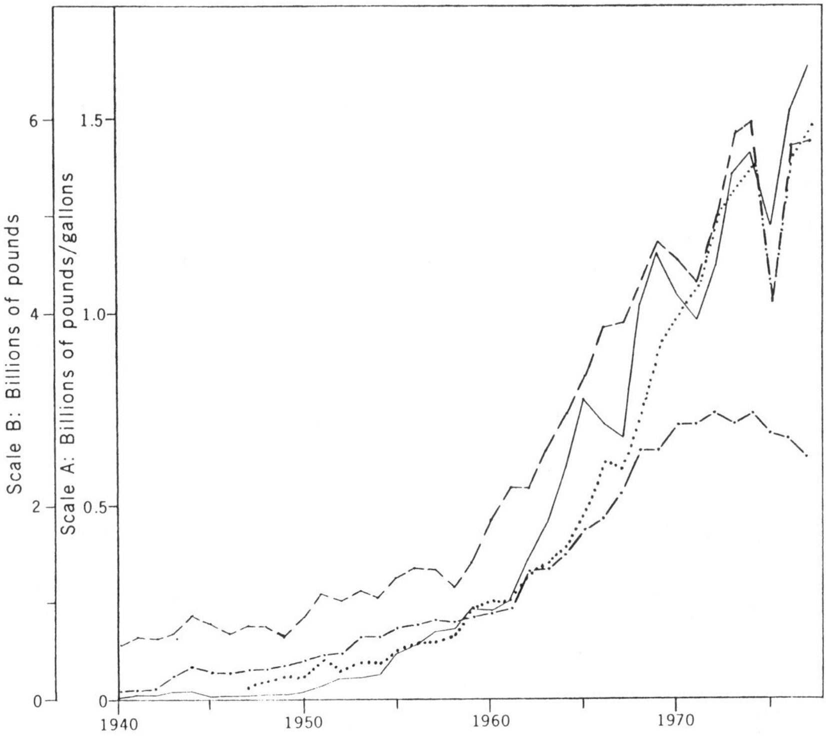

Figure 3
Annual production of selected carcinogenic substances. (–) Acrylonitrile, Scale A in pounds; (– – –) Benzene, Scale A in gallons; (· – ·) Perchloroethylene, Scale A in gallons; (· · ·) Vinyl chloride, Scale B in pounds. (Reprinted, with permission, from Davis and Magee 1979).

in the mid-1970s. Benzene causes chromosomal damage. Epidemiological studies have identified it as a leukemogen (Infante et al. 1977). Approximately 1.5 million people in the United States are exposed to benzene in the workplace, including workers in gasoline stations and numerous small businesses (NIOSH 1981). Similar production data are available for chloroform, carbon tetrachloride, ethylene oxide, dibromochloropropane, ethylene dibromide, and trichloroethylene, all of which also are suspect carcinogens.

Although potential widespread human exposure has occurred only since the 1960s, some occupational cancers have already been linked to these chemicals. Even if these chemicals have had only a small effect on the current overall cancer rate, they may still have a very large effect on the rates of future cancer and other diseases (Davis and Magee 1979). Furthermore, it is incorrect to associate these chemicals only with occupational exposures, as many of these toxicants are incorporated into high-volume consumer products, pharmaceuticals, and foods.

The relatively recent history of rapid production growth of the chemicals shown in the figures here is not unusual. Figure 4 shows that the production of several classes of bioavailable substances was also significantly greater after 1960 than before. These four categories of chemicals: plastics, and resin materials, plasticizers, flavors and perfumes (benzenoid and napthalenoid), and food, drug, and cosmetic dyes all have the common characteristic of being present in products designed for uses in, on, or very near to humans. Any toxic or potentially toxic chemical substances contained therein are likely to be consumed by or absorbed into the body of the product user (Davis and Magee 1979). Because the population-at-large is exposed to these bioavailable compounds, it will be hard to find unexposed control populations, thus making it difficult for epidemiological surveys to detect relationships between exposure and effects. As an illustration of this problem, one study recently reported that 85% of people sampled in the United States showed pentachlorophenol in their urine (IARC 1979).

There is no simple way to estimate the amount of carcinogenic chemicals to which humans are exposed occupationally or environmentally. Routinely collected statistics indicate domestic production and (or) consumption. These production measures do not quantify how much of an agent comes into contact with the population, rather they reflect only the amount of a chemical potentially available for exposure. It is reasonable to assume, however, that increased production and use means that more people come into contact with the agent at more different points (Davis and Rall 1981). Hoerger reported that Dow Chemical Company provides a cleaner, more protective, and more efficient workplace today.

To the extent that any reported decrease in workplace exposures stems from increased use of protective clothing, however, the problems of noncompliance and ineffective protective clothing must be stressed. A recent

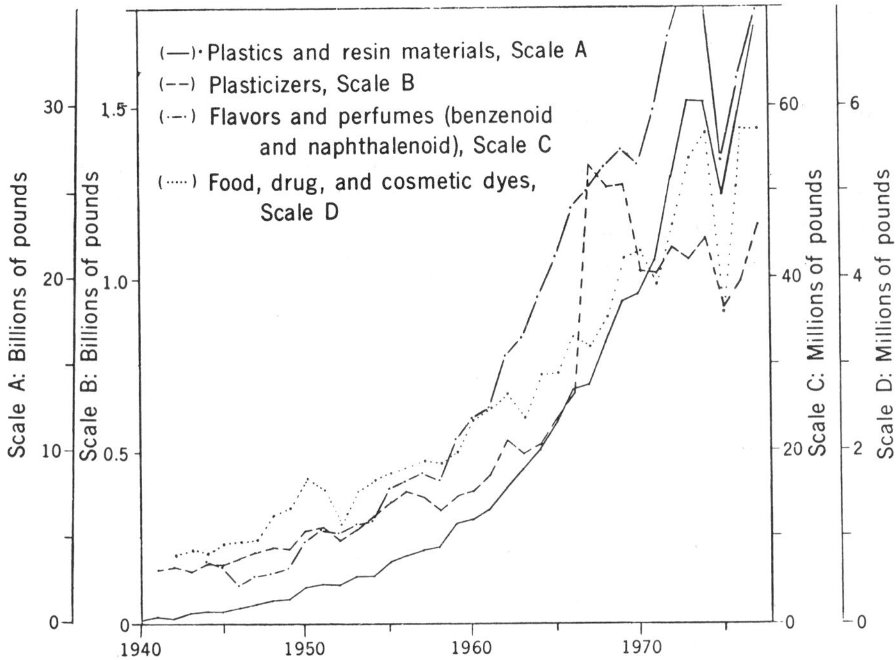

Figure 4
Annual production of selected bioavailable classes of chemicals. (–) Plastics and resin materials, Scale A; (- -) Plasticizers, Scale B; (• - •) Flavors and perfumes (benzenoid and haphthalenoid), Scale C; (• • • •) Food, drugs, and cosmetic dyes, Scale D. (Reprinted, with permission, from Davis and Magee 1979.)

NIOSH study indicates that materials currently used in the manufacture of protective garments may be inadequate to protect workers handling halogenated ethanes and a polychlorinated biphenyl (PCB) mixture (NIOSH 1981). The preliminary report assessed a number of materials commonly used for protective clothing. The three liquid halogenated ethanes studied are high-volume, widely used industrial solvents, with reported evidence of carcinogenicity in animal studies. Breakthrough times for a PCB mixture and the halogenated ethanes ranged from periods of less than 10 minutes to 24 hours (NIOSH 1981). For those chemicals that are carcinogens, it is also reasonable to assume that increased handling combined with ineffective protective clothing may be reflected, years later, by increased incidences of cancer.

In light of the relatively recent increase in the production of some carcinogenic and other bioavailable hazardous substances, it is not now possible to determine the extent to which chemical exposures will influence future cancer and other disease rates. However, if the incidence pattern is similar to that between lung cancer and cigarette smoking, it may be expected that the 1980s, 1990s, and the turn of the century will show the effects of increases in exposures that occurred during the 1960s.

RECENT TRENDS IN CANCER INCIDENCE AND MORTALITY

It is clear that the effects, if any, of the increases in production and use of carcinogens since the 1960s are unlikely to be reflected in current overall cancer incidence and mortality rates. Nonetheless, it is worthwhile to examine recent trends in cancer for possible early indications of an increase.

This section considers recent trends of several sets of data—data relating to the sum of all cancers, data related to individual sites, and data related to specific age groups. We look first at overall patterns, and then attempt to break these down into appropriate categories. Changes in site-specific incidence and mortality can help clarify contributing causes, such as postmenopausal estrogens, cigarette smoking, sociological factors (such as important public figures having a diagnosis of breast cancer), industrial exposure, etc. We examine both mortality and incidence data, although we prefer incidence data where and when they are available. Incidence data are important for several reasons. First of all, incidence reflect failed prevention—our major concern. Second, incidence data are important for assessing the chronic aspects of cancer. People fear not only death, but also long and painful illness. Costs to society are measured not only by death, but also by disability and hospitalization, as for example in illnesses like arthritis and mental disease, which cause few deaths but much pain and much cost in medical care. Finally, incidence data from the Third National Cancer Survey (TNCS) and for the Surveillance and End Results (SEER) program of the National Cancer Institute, can only lead to more accurate reporting (both in total, and especially for specific sites) than the mortality reporting derived from death certificate data (Percy et al. 1981).

Total cancer mortality data over all ages, races, and both sexes are also important because such totals are more likely to be correct than subdivisions, or breakdowns. That is not to say that details should be disregarded. On the contrary, age, sex, race, and site differences tell us a great deal, and to neglect these data is as unwise as it is to neglect the total data. Although scientific resolution of cancer causes is more likely to stem from considering details, disease prevention strategies may derive from larger patterns. To concentrate on either one alone, however, is sure to mislead. For long-term trends, however, we rely on mortality data, because incidence data in the United States do not exist earlier than 1935. Further, increased mortality reflects failed diagnosis and treatments, as well as increased incidence.

With these ideas in mind, we have considered the following: Cancer mortality, both in total and in some detail for this whole century (in the United States); available data on cancer incidence with emphasis on changes in the

1970s for the portion of cancers attributable to cigarette smoking; and finally, by inference, the changes in incidence and mortality for the remainder of cancers that cannot be attributed to cigarette smoking.

Mortality Trends

For all races, ages, and both sexes standardized to the U.S. population of 1940, cancer mortality has been increasing at a decreasing rate throughout this century (Fig. 5). There was a period from about 1950 to 1965 when the slope was quite small and the increase was slight, but since 1965 the slope has grown, and the increase is currently at about 1% a year. Mortality changes have not been uniform by race and sex. Table 4 shows the substantially greater increases in nonwhites.

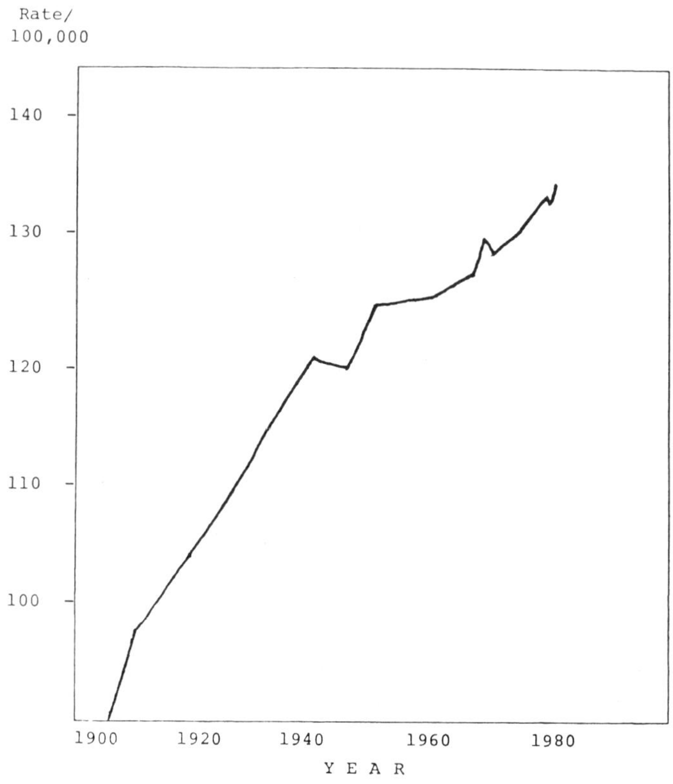

Figure 5
Age-adjusted cancer mortality, United States (1900-1980) (adjusted to 1940 U.S. population). 1979, Provisional; 1980, estimated from 10% sampling, January-December 1980.

Table 4
Trends in Cancer Mortality, 1968-1977

				Percent increase	
Race	Sex	1968	1977	annual	10 yr
White	male	196.6	210.4	0.8	8.3
	female	133.1	134.5	0.2	2.0
Black	male	237.8	282.9	2.0	21.9
	female	149.6	158.6	0.6	6.6
Total		163.2	168.6	0.5	5.1

Age = adjusted U.S. population, 1970.
[a]From fitted curves.

In looking at detailed data by age, the most striking finding is the decline in mortality among persons under 45 since the 1950s (Fig. 6). This reflects both declines in incidence and improvements in treatment, especially for leukemias and lymphomas. For older persons, substantial increases in mortality and incidence have occurred in the age groups 45-64, 65-74, and much smaller increases in persons over 75.

Interestingly, there are differences in trends in the age-specific cancer incidence and mortality rates, with rates declining most in the youngest persons, and increasing most in the 65-74 year age group (for both incidence and mortality). Mortality increases in the 65-74 age group have been relatively steady since 1950. The age group with the next largest increases was the 45-64 year group. The over-75 group showed increases beginning later than the two next younger age groups.

These differences in trend by age are of considerable consequence. We offer two possible explanations for the differential mortality of younger persons compared with older persons: (1) Reduction in mortality through improved diagnosis and treatment and (2) reductions in incidence for reasons outlined below. Treatment improvements have been greater in cancers of young persons. This is particularly true of acute lymphocytic leukemia (as a childhood disease) and Hodgkin's disease (as a disease of young adults), and cancer of the uterine cervix (a disease of relatively younger women; 30-45% of all new cases occur in women under age 45). Treatment outcomes for cancers more common to older persons have not changed as much as have those for younger persons.

As to factors that may account for reductions in incidence among younger persons, three immediately come to mind. First, the substantial declines in infectious diseases of all types and extensive immunization programs mean that younger persons have less exposures to viral infections than older persons. To the extent that viral sources initiate cancers, then younger persons have had less exposure to these initiators. Second, the diets of younger persons may contain

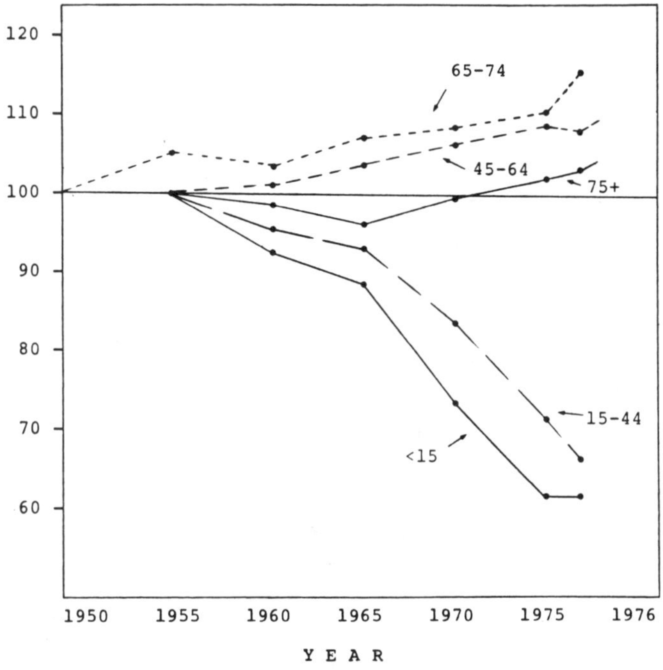

Figure 6
Cancer mortality, United States, all rates, both sexes, 1950-1976 (1950 = 100)

more anticarcinogens in fresh and frozen fruits and vegetables. Finally, the reduction in the proportion of adults who smoke cigarettes and reductions in tars and nicotine in those cigarettes should be noted. Because of increased smoking by young persons, most of these effects however should have been seen in somewhat older persons. In any case, the change in smoking and cigarette type should affect only the cigarette-related cancers and should not explain declines in so many of the noncigarette-related cancers.

Incidence Trends

There is some internal evidence of possible underreporting of incidence by the TNCS program in 1970-1971. The arguments are detailed in Appendix I. This has two consequences. Incidence comparisons from the Second National Cancer Survey (SNCS) to the TNCS tend to understate increases (and overstate decreases), whereas comparisons of TNCS with SEER tend to overstate increases (and understate decreases). To avoid these problems, our incidence comparisons are made wherever possible only with the SEER data set (1973 onward).

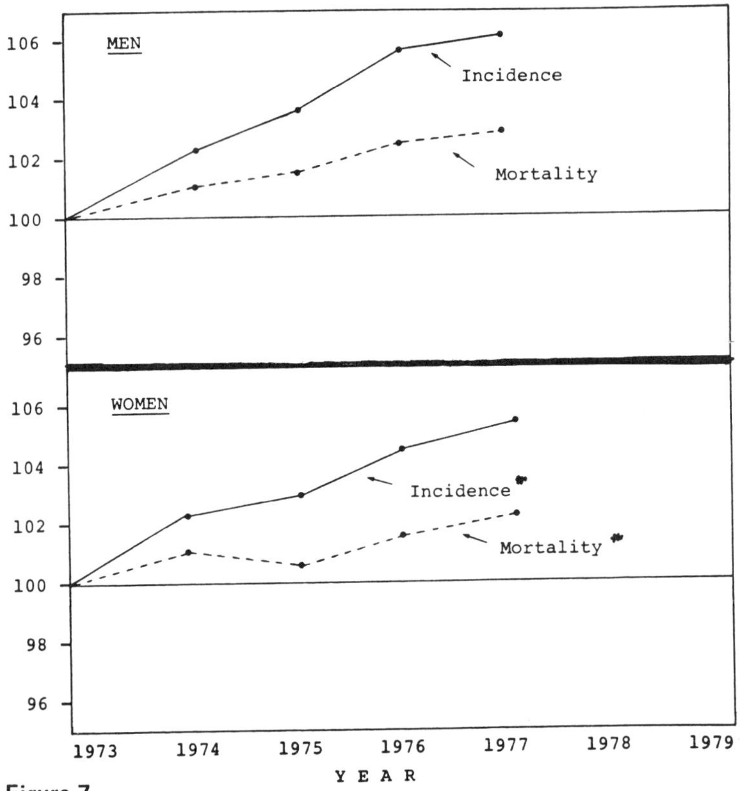

Figure 7
Cancer trends, whites, 1973-1977, 1978 (1973 = 100). Data age-adjusted to 1970. (*) Excluding breast and uterine corpus. (Data from NCI-SEER Program.)

For white men and women in the 1970s, reported incidence has increased somewhat more rapidly than mortality. Figure 7 shows these data for men and women. During this period, there are sharp increases in reported breast cancer and endometrial cancer. The incidence increase for breast cancer came mostly in 1974 and 1975 following the diagnosis of breast cancer in the wives of both the President and the Vice-President of the United States. The increased incidence of cancer of the endometrium, without a concomitant increase in mortality, has been ascribed (Walker and Jick 1979) to a sharp increase in the use of postmenopausal estrogens—probably cancer-promoting agents. The incidence of both these diseases has now been reduced. Figure 7 excludes these two diseases.

In looking at incidence trends, we confine ourselves to the 1970s and to white men and women for two reasons. First, we are most concerned with recent trends in incidence that are likely to reflect recent increases in exposures.

Second, we confine ourselves to whites because the data for blacks are subject to more reporting problems and this might be misleading. We do this despite the fact that mortality changes for blacks have been much greater than for whites. It is thus possible that the incidence changes we report for whites understate the changes for the country as a whole.

Cancer Rate Changes Associated with Smoking

Because some allege that cigarette smoking (by itself) accounts for most of the reported increase in cancer, it is important to explore systematically the role of smoking in recent changes in cancer mortality. If we now look at the incidence data for recent years, 1973-1977, we can ask the question of how much of the changes seen in this period are likely to have been related to cigarette smoking (Fig. 7). In view of the mortality and incidence ratio data presented in Appendix I, it might be reasonable to use the incidence data for 1969 to compare with 1973-1977. However, because some epidemiologists have expressed concern that the 1973-1977 data, having been collected differently from the 1969 data and therefore might be noncomparable, we will confine our attention to the 1973-1977 period. So short a time span does not give much information about trends, however.

To accomplish this examination we did the following:

1. We identified the following sites as probably having some portion of the incidence attributable to cigarette smoking (Hammond et al. 1976; Seidman and Hammond 1980): Lung, bladder, pancreas, buccal cavity and pharynx, esophagus, larynx, and kidney.
2. The attributable risks (ARs) assigned to each of these were derived from and are given in Table 5. The Seidman data are for whites. For blacks, we compared blacks and whites for average ages started smoking, proportion of smokers before 1970, and amount smoked per day. Blacks, especially black males, started smoking at later ages than whites and smoked fewer cigarettes per day. The differences between black and white women were small.

The Seidman and Hammond (1980) ARs for women seemed to us to be particularly low. For lung cancers, we estimated that one-third of the white females smoked, and that the relative risk (RR) for (women) smokers compared with nonsmokers was 8 (compared with 10 or 11 for men). This gives an excess AR of:

$$\text{AR} = \frac{p(R-1)}{1+p(R-1)} \qquad (1)$$

$$= .70$$

where $p = .33$, the proportion exposed, and $R = 8$, RR of exposed persons. We

Table 5
Smoking-related Sites—ARs

Site	Males			Females		
	white (Seidman and Hammond)	black (Davis et al.)		white (Seidman and Hammond)	black (Davis et al.)	
Lung	.828	.83	.75	.43	.70	.67
Bladder	.49	.45	.41	.10	.25	.24
Pancreas	.48	.55	.50	.11	.30	.29
Buccal cavity and pharynx	.81	.75	.68	.44	.70	.67
Esophagus	.67	.55	.50	.50	.30	.29
Larynx	–	.80	.72	–	.70	.67
Kidney	–	.30	.27	–	.15	.14

used this AR rather than the .43 reported by Seidman and Hammond (1980), and adjusted (upward) the ARs for all other sites. The effect of this change is to increase the estimate of the proportion of (new) cancers attributable to smoking and to increase the estimate of the proportion of the changes that can be attributed to cigarette smoking.

The data on white males are, in some sense, the best and most important data to examine. This is because males are more likely than females to have been exposed industrially; the data on females include the incidence increases for breast and endometrial cancers (although by 1977 much of that effect was dissipated); the data on blacks are less stable than the data on whites.

Nonetheless, we report in Tables 6 (men) and Table 7 (women) the changes in cancer incidence for all four sex-race groups. In addition, Tables 6 and 7 give the proportion of all cancers that can be attributed to cigarette smoking. Assuming that ARs for white men remained constant for the period 1973-1977, 18% of the increased incidence of cancer can be attributed to cigarette-related cancers. For white women, who have experienced a very sharp increase in lung cancer, the equivalent percentage is 45%. For blacks, where the data are more problematic, the corresponding percentages were 72 for males and 76 for females.

We have also done these computations for mortality changes for the same years—the cigarette-related cancers often being ones of high mortality. The proportions of the increases in mortality attributable to these cancers were higher than the attributable increases in incidence.

We find that slightly under 30% of the new cancers in men and about 10% of the new cancers in women are attributable to cigarette smoking. Overall (both sexes), this indicates that about one in five cancers (20%) are associated

Table 6
Cancer Incidence Changes, 1973-1977, for Men

	White			Black		
	1973	1977	Δ	1973	1977	Δ
Total	355.5	379.6	24.1	449.5	464.9	15.4
AR, smoking-related	103.3	107.7	4.3	122.2	133.4	11.2
Percent of total	29.1	28.4		27.2	28.7	
Proportion of increase in smoking-related sites	4.3/24.1 = .18			11.2/15.4 = .72		

Rates/100,000, age-adjusted 1970.

Table 7
Incidence Changes, 1973-1977, Women

	White			Black		
	1973	1977	Δ	1973	1977	Δ
Total	287.3	298.2	10.2	282.3	289.1	6.8
AR, smoking-related	22.3	27.2	4.9	26.4	31.6	5.2
Percent of total	7.8	9.1		9.4	10.9	
Proportion of increase in smoking-related sites	4.9/10.2 = 45			5.2/6.8 = .76		

Rates/100,000, age-adjusted to 1970.

with cigarette smoking. Our estimate for women may be high because of our use of substantially higher ARs than Seidman and Hammond would indicate.

These attributions to cigarette smoking are the maximum possible. The RRs for whites used in the computations were based on two papers derived from the Hammond and Garfinkel findings for cigarettes smoked in the 1950s and 1960s. The RRs for blacks were derived from sample data gathered by the Current Population Survey (CPS), with appropriate adjustments for quantity smoked and age started smoking. In this regard, this analysis did not account for the reduced smoking in the 1970s (mostly by adult males), the lower-tar and tobacco content of cigarettes smoked in the 1960s and 1970s, or for the differential mortality (excess) from other causes among smokers in the age range 55-65, which in time would remove the heaviest smokers from the population at risk at older ages. No allowance was made for the differential smoking by occupation which is discussed below. (The proportion of smokers is highest in those occupations that are most likely to involve occupational exposures to other environmental hazards). Allowance was not made for declining mortality from stomach cancer and cancer of the uterine cervix, nor for possible interactions of cigarette smoking and other possible carcinogenic hazards. Even where these other hazards exist, all the cancers that could possibly be attributed to cigarette smoking were so attributed.

Occupational Factors and Smoking

In addition, some of the cancers we have attributed to smoking are occupation-confounded, because smoking is confounded by occupation. The CPS reported 1970 smoking habits and history by occupation (cited by Sterling and Weinkham 1976, 1978). A crude possible hazard score to the occupations reported in the 75,827-person CPS data can be devised, with 1 being least hazardous and 5 being most hazardous: Professionals, 1; managers, farmers and farm laborers, 2; clerical, household, sales, not in labor force, 3; craftsmen, service workers, laborers, 4; operatives, 5. This scoring approach conforms to methods for ranking professions adapted by Hollingshead and Redlich (1958), Blau and Duncan (1978) and Kitagawa and Hauser (1973).

These crude occupational "hazard" rankings can be summed across current smoking classes by sex and race. Taking the CPS data for persons who ever smoked cigarettes, the indices of possibly hazardous employment that result are shown in Table 8. This is done by computing separately for each sex-race group

$$\frac{\sum_{j=0}^{1} \sum_{i=} w_i n_i (\% S_j)}{\sum_{i=} \sum_{j=0}^{1} n_i (\% S_j)} \qquad (1)$$

where w_i = hazard weight for each occupational group (e.g., w for professionals = 1); n_i = number of persons in the ith occupational group (for the specific sex-race category); $j = (0,1)$: 0 for nonsmokers, 1 for smokers so that

Table 8
Indices of Possibly Hazardous Employment

	White		Black	
	smoker	nonsmoker	smoker	nonsmoker
Male	3.26	2.89	3.71	3.37
Female	3.03	3.02	3.22	3.11

$$\sum_{0}^{1} (\%S_j) = 1 \qquad (2)$$

$\%S_j$ = percent of persons in the jth class. As can be seen, men have higher hazardous job scores than women. Blacks have higher hazardous job scores than whites. Smokers have higher hazardous job scores than nonsmokers.

Black-white differences in cigarette smoking are in the opposite direction from black-white differences in cancer incidence and mortality rates. Blacks (both smokers and nonsmokers) appear to be engaged, on the average, in more hazardous jobs. Hazardous jobs are positively correlated with cigarette smoking. In part, this may account for why black men who smoke less, who started smoking at a later age, and among whom there are a lower proportion who have ever smoked, nonetheless, have higher lung cancer rates than whites.

Problems in Trend Analyses

Some further caveats are in order. Some changes in reported mortality and incidence in the 1970s doubtlessly are due to increased diagnostic acumen and access to medical care. There is no question that some of these reported reductions in mortality are real, as in the treatments of childhood and adult leukemias, the treatment of Hodgkin's disease and probably many other of the lymphomas including multiple myeloma, the treatment of breast cancer in pre-menopausal women, the treatment of colon cancer, and possibly several others. There is also evidence of earlier diagnosis, which should lead to better survival statistics. The preliminary evidence is that the jump in diagnosis of breast cancer in the mid-1970s has been followed by decreases in mortality for breast cancer in 1980.

The 1980 census has uncovered some difficulties in the reporting of undocumented aliens, which also bear mention. The population reported in 1980 appears to be larger than previous demographic computations would have suggested (e.g., 1970 population, plus births, plus immigration, minus deaths, minus emigration). If the U.S. population base is in error as a result of this, there will be overstatements of death rates (and incidence rates), particularly among younger age groups. Existing information suggests that undocumented aliens are to be found mostly among the under 45 group, and more among whites than blacks. This means that the real decreases in mortality for those under 45 may be even greater than estimated, but that increases in older persons cannot be explained by undercounts in the census.

Despite these diverse influences on cancer rates in considering rate changes, the age group 45-75 is the key. In this regard, Doll and Peto's (1981) analysis for people under 65 of cancer mortality changes up to 1977 needs to be viewed with some reservations. Given the recent production surge of human carcinogens and the continuing growth in chemical production as reported here, people who were age 45 and under in 1977 have only been a part of the more heavily exposed industrial workforce for at most 17 years. For this group, it is unlikely to find much occupationally related cancer, given the average 20-year or more latency period for cancer to be manifest clinically. Further, by excluding people over 65 from their analyses, Doll and Peto (1981) remove from consideration a large group in whom occupationally related cancers may be more likely to occur, because they have had longer histories of exposure and longer latencies. Reported changes in cancer mortality in the early days of Medicare for those over 65 may well have reflected some of the artefacts identified by observers, such as improved diagnosis and access to medical care for this age group. However, changes within the past decade certainly cannot be attributed to such artefacts. Given the marked reduction in cancer mortality for people under 45, excluding people over 65 from an analysis of overall cancer trends, produces a final analysis that primarily reflects improvements in this younger age group. About half of all cancers in the United States occur in persons over 65. Until mortality and incidence rates are obtained for a broad representation of cohorts with greater exposures to industrial carcinogens and until those with 20 years or more exposure to new synthetic organic chemicals are studied, it is not possible to assess the full impact of chemicals on the cancer rate. Prudent public policy continues to dictate caution, in light of the volumes of substances in commerce for which no data are available and the lack of opportunity to study many of these exposures epidemiologically.

CONCLUSION

This review of problems, methods, and data for estimating the causes of cancer shows the profound and continuing difficulties of generating such estimates. Most investigators agree that it is difficult to estimate with accuracy what proportion of new cancers may be associated with industrial production, smoking, and life-style factors. The estimates paper of Bridbord et al. (1978) used the PARP model and relied on some assumptions about data that have been shown subsequently to be incorrect. Despite the data deficiencies of that paper, we believe its methodology remains appropriate. Beyond question, industrial exposure to known or suspect carcinogens remains a serious public health problem that requires preventive policies. If as few as 5% of all new cancers in the United States are related to industrial exposure, this still would represent a major public health problem resulting in 20,000 excess cancer deaths each year. As Legator (this volume) and others continue to note, epidemiology like any discipline, has its limitations. Despite these limitations, recent epidemiological studies have identified new substances or processes as carcinogenic to humans. Further, toxicological data implicate still others. Moreover, as Karstadt, Siemiatycki, Hoar, and others (all this volume) have indicated here, waiting for complete epidemiological studies may be an infinite regress.

The production data displayed at this meeting document the marked increase since the 1960s in chemical production of class-I and -II IARC carcinogens and other substances suspected of causing cancer and other chronic health effects.

The analysis of recent trends presented here indicates increases in total age-adjusted cancer incidence and mortality. These increases are only partially accounted for by the changes in rates for cancer attributed to cigarette smoking. For those under 45, cancer rates have declined markedly, while for those over 45, rates have increased at about 1% a year, in the past half decade. This reduction in mortality for the younger half of the population should be researched carefully and appropriate policies should be developed. The recent increases in cancer rates for the older group also merit careful study and the development of appropriate preventive policies. Given the greater exposures of the older half of the population, more detailed trend analyses of this age group needs to be undertaken, with special reference to those over age 65.

Methodological controversies will continue to characterize the study of occupational and environmental carcinogenesis, as befits an evolving science. The health effects of such recent increases in production are not likely to be fully expressed before the end of this century. In the meantime, these data, together with recent epidemiological and toxicological studies, suggest the need for both caution and vigilance. Where toxicological data on high-production volume chemicals warrant regulatory intervention, the economic and social costs of waiting for human studies (which often are not likely to be forthcoming) are inestimable. To wait renders industrial workers fodder for research, and subjects future generations to potentially irreversible risks. If this view is wrong, regulatory policies can be changed. If it is correct, lives will be saved (Davis 1979). Clearly, in our view, effective cancer prevention requires control of occupational and environmental hazards, as well as smoking and other life-style factors.

APPENDIX I: PROBLEMS IN INCIDENCE DATA

There is some internal evidence that incidence may have been underreported by the TNCS in the last 2 years of the survey, 1970 and 1971. Table 9 shows the mortality-to-incidence (M/I) ratios (U.S. total mortality, TNCS incidence, both age-adjusted to 1970) for the 3 years of the TNCS and for 5 years of the SEER programs (1973-1977).

If we exclude breast cancer and cancer of the endometrium because of their unusual changes during the 1970s, we find that the ratio of M/I increased from .56 in 1969 to .60 in 1971 for both men and women (white). This implies that either incidence was underreported in 1970 and 1971, mortality was over-reported, or treatment worsened. There is good reason to believe that treatments improved, and no reason to believe that there was a sudden excessive

Table 9
Cancer M/I, 1969-1977

	Whites	
	men	women[a]
TNCS		
1969	.56	.56
1970	.58	.59
1971	.60	.60
SEER		
1973	.57	.56
1974	.57	.56
1975	.56	.55
1976	.56	.55
1977	.55	.55

[a]Ratios exclude breast and uterine corpus.

increase in mortality. In view of the fact that the TNCS was planned as a temporary program, it is possible that reporting efficiency fell off with time.

Another possibility, of course, is that there was overreporting of incidence in 1969. As an indirect measure of this, we looked at the M/I ratio for the SEER program, 1973-1977. Those data are shown in the bottom half of Table 9. There the M/I ratios are closest to the 1969 M/I ratio and decline slightly with time, as one would expect if treatments were improving, and this has been reported (DeVita et al. 1981).

APPENDIX II: AN ATTRIBUTABLE RISK

The attributable excess risks were computed using the formula by Cole and MacMahon (1971):

$$\text{AR} = \frac{p\,(R-1)}{1+p\,(R-1)} \tag{2}$$

where p = proportion of persons in the population exposed and R = relative risk of exposed persons. RR for whites were derived from the data of Hammond and Seidman (1980) and the earlier report by Hammond (1976). Where RR were not computed separately, they were estimated for lung cancer in blacks from the approximate relationship for current smokers (Gart and Schneiderman 1980).

$$R = 1 + \frac{d}{2}\left[\frac{75 - A_B}{75 - A_w}\right]^5 \tag{3}$$

where d = average number of cigarettes smoked per day; A_W = average age of onset of smoking among whites; and A_B = average age of onset of smoking for blacks. For example, in the 1970 Household Interview Survey (National Center for Health Statistics) for white men $d = 21.73$, $A_W = 17.93$, $p_W = .4263$. For black men, $d = 15.00$, $A_B = 19.11$, $P_B = .5058$. Thus, a RR for white men (for lung cancer) approximates $1 + 21.73/2 = 11.87$, which is close to Hammond and Seidman's published RR. The AR computed from this would be

$$\text{AR} = \frac{.4263\,(10.87)}{1 + .4263\,(10.87)} = .823, \qquad (4)$$

which compares to the Hammond and Seidman (1980) figure of .828. For black men:

$$R = 1 + \frac{(15.00)}{(2)} \left[\frac{55.89}{57.07}\right]^{5} \qquad (5)$$

$$= 7.74$$

$$\text{AR} = \frac{.5058\,(6.74)}{1 + .5058\,(6.74)} = .77 \qquad (6)$$

The ARs for blacks' and whites' sites other than lung were assumed to be proportional to the lung cancer ARs.

ACKNOWLEDGMENTS

An effectiveness grant from the Hewlett Foundation and a development grant from the Andrew W. Mellon Foundation to the Environmental Law Institute partially supported this research. Harvey Babich provided immeasureable collegial assistance throughout this project. Brian Magee, Mary Supler, Jennifer Douville, and Margaret Cech painstakingly compiled and reviewed production data figures, and tables. John Horm, Paul Milvy, John Ficke, Ralph Tartaglioni, Peter Preuss, Paul White, Reid Adler, Jonathan Cain, and Jeremy Glaser provided thoughtful assistance in data generation and analyses. John Cairns, Harry Rosenberg, Alan Moshell, and Richard Peto made generally helpful comments. Without the dedicated assistance of Helen Burdette, preparation of this manuscript would not have been possible.

REFERENCES

Abelson, P.H. 1980. New directions in toxicology. *Food Cosmet. Toxicol.* 8:303.

Acheson, E.D. 1976. Nasal cancer in the furniture and boot and shoe manufacturing industries. *Prev. Med.* 5:295.

Aksoy, M., S. Erdem, and G. Dineol. 1974. Leukemia in shoe workers chronically exposed to benzene. *Blood* **44**:837.

Albert, D.M., C.A. Puliafito, A.B. Fulton, N.L. Robinson, Z.N. Zakov, T.T. Dryja, A. Blair-Smith, E. Ega, and S.S. Leffingwell. 1980. Increased incidence of choiroidal malignant melanoma occurring in a single population of chemical workers. *Am. J. Ophthal.* **89**:323.

Alexander, V., S.S. Leffingwell, J.W. Lloyd, R.J. Waxweiler, and A.L. Miller. 1981. Brain cancer in petrochemical workers: A case series report. *Am. J. Ind. Med.* **1**:115.

Beaumont, J.J. and N.E. Weiss. 1980. Mortality of welders, shipfitters and other metal trades workers in Boilermaker's Local No. 104, AFL-CIO. *Am. J. Epidemiol.* **112**:775.

Blair, A., P. Decoufle, and D. Grauman. 1979. Causes of death among laundry and dry cleaning workers. *Am. J. Public Health* **69**:508.

Blau, P. and O.D. Duncan. 1978. *The American occupational structure*, LC-50657. Free Press, N.Y.

Bridbord, K., P. Decoufle, J.F. Fraumeni, Jr., D.G. Hoel, R.N. Hoover, D.P. Rall, U. Saffiotti, M.A. Schneiderman, and A.C. Upton. 1978. "Estimates of the fraction of cancer in the United States related to occupational factors." National Cancer Institute, National Institute of Environmental Health Sciences, and National Institute for Occupational Safety and Health, September 15.

Brinton, L.A. 1977. A death certificate analysis of nasal cancer among furniture workers in North Carolina. *Cancer Res.* **37**:3473.

Bunge, M. 1959. *Causality*. The World Publishing Company, Cleveland, Ohio.

Cairns, J. 1977. Some thoughts about cancer in lieu of a summary. *Cold Spring Harbor Conf. Cell Proliferation* **4**:1813.

Cimino, J.A. and H.B. Demopoulos. 1980. Introduction: Determinants of cancer relevant to prevention, in the war on cancer. *J. Environ. Pathol. Toxicol.* **3**(4):1.

Clayson, D.B. 1967. Chemicals and environmental carcinogenesis in man. *Eur. J. Cancer* **3**:405.

———. 1977. Relationships between laboratory and human studies. *J. Environ. Pathol. Toxicol.* **1**:31.

Cole, P. 1977. Cancer and occupations: Status and needs of epidemiologic research. *Cancer* **39**:1788.

Cole, P. and M.B. Goldman. 1975. Occupation. In *Persons at high risk of cancer* (ed. J.F. Fraumeni, Jr.), p. 167. Academic Press, New York.

Cole, P. and B. MacMahon. 1971. Attributable risk percent in case-control studies. *Br. J. Prev. Soc. Med.* **25**:242.

Cole, P. and F. Merletti. 1980. Chemical agents and occupational exposures. *J. Environ. Pathol. Toxicol.* **3**:399.

Dalager, N.A., T.J. Mason, J.R. Fraumeni, R. Hoover, and W.W. Payne. 1980. Cancer mortality among workers exposed to zinc chromate paints. *J. Occup. Med.* **22**:25.

Davis, D.L. 1979. Science and regulatory policy. *Science* **203**:7.

Davis, D.L. and B.H. Magee. 1979. Cancer and industrial chemical production. *Science* **206**:1356.

Davis, D.L. and L.K.Y. Ng. 1981. Introduction. In *Strategies for public health. Promoting health and preventing disease.* Van Nostrand Reinhold, New York.

Davis, D.L. and D.P. Rall. 1981. Estimating risks as the basis for preventive policies. In *Strategies for public health: Promoting health and preventing disease* (ed. L. Ng and D.L. Davis). Van Nostrand Reinhold, New York.

Decoufle, P. 1979. Cancer risks associated with employment in the leather and leather products industry. *Arch. Environ. Health* **34**:33.

Department of Health, Education, and Welfare. 1974. *Current estimates from the health interview survey.* DHEW publication number (HRA) 74-1054, Series 10. Number 72. Government Printing Office, Washington, D.C.

DeVita, V.T., J.E. Henney, and S.M. Hubbard. 1981. Estimation of the numerical and economic impact of chemotherapy in the treatment of cancer. Proceedings of 1980 International Symposium on Cancer. In *Cancer achievements and prospects for the 1980s* (ed. J.H. Buchenal and I. Stratton), p. 859.

Doll, R. 1977. Strategy for detection of cancer hazards to man. *Nature* **265**: 589.

Doll, R. and R. Peto. The causes of cancer: Quantitative estimates of avoidable risks of cancer in America today. *J. Nat. Cancer Inst.* (in press).

Eisenbud, M. 1978. *Environment, technology, and health.* New York University Press, New York.

Ember, L. 1976. Environmental cancers: Humans as the experimental model? *Environ. Sci. Technol.* **10**:1190.

Environmental Defense Fund (EDF). 1979. *Malignant neglect.* Knopf Publishers, New York.

Epstein, S.S. 1972. Environmental pathology: A review. *Am. J. Pathol.* **66**: 352.

______. 1974. Environmental determinants of human cancer. *Cancer Res.* **34**:2425.

Epstein, S.S. and J.B. Swartz. 1981. Fallacies of lifestyle cancer theories. *Nature* **289**:127.

Federal Register. 1980. 45 *Fed. Reg.* 5002, (January 22, 1980).

Fraumeni, J.F., Jr. 1977. Environmental and genetic determinants of cancer. *J. Environ. Pathol. Toxicol.* **1**:19.

Gart, J.J. and M.A. Schneiderman. 1980. Low risk cigarettes: The debate continues. *Science* **204**:689.

Gibson, E.S., R.H. Martin, and J.N. Lockington. 1977. Lung cancer mortality in a steel foundry. *J. Occup. Med.* **19**:807.

Goldsmith, D.F., A.H. Smith, and A.J. McMichael. 1980. A case-control study of prostate cancer within a cohort of rubber and tire workers. *J. Occup. Med.* **22**:533.

Habs, M. and D. Schmahl. 1980. Diet and cancer. *J. Cancer Res. Clin. Oncol.* **96**:1.

Hammond, E.C. and H. Seidman. 1980. Smoking and cancer in the United States. *Prev. Med.* **9**:169.

Hammond, E.C., L. Garfinkel, H. Seidman and A. Lew. 1977. Some recent findings concerning cigarette smoking. *Cold Spring Harbor Conf. Cell Proliferation* **4**:101.

Hardell, L. and A. Sandstrom. 1979. Case-control study: Soft-tissue sarcomas and exposure to phenoxyacetic acids or chlorophenols. *Br. J. Cancer* **39**:711.

Harris, R.H., T. Page, and N.A. Reiches. 1977. Carcinogenic hazards of organic chemicals in drinking water. *Cold Spring Harbor Conf. Cell Proliferation* **4**:309.

Higginson, J. 1969. Present trends in cancer epidemiology. *Proc. Can. Cancer Congr.* 8:40.

______. 1980. Multiplicity of factors involved in cancer patterns and trends. *J. Environ. Pathol. Toxicol.* **3**(4):113.

Higginson, J. and C.S. Muir. 1976. The role of epidemiology in elucidating the importance of environmental factors in human cancer. *Cancer Detect. Prev.* **1**:79.

______. 1979. Environmental carcinogenesis: Misconceptions and limitations to cancer control. *J. Natl. Cancer Inst.* **63**:1291.

Hogstedt, C., O. Rohlen, B.S. Berndtsson, O. Axelson, and L. Ehrenberg. 1979a. A cohort study of mortality and cancer incidence in ethylene oxide production workers. *Br. J. Ind. Med.* **36**:276.

Hogstedt, C., N. Malmquist, and B. Wadman. 1979b. Leukemia in workers exposed to ethylene oxide. *J. Am. Med. Assoc.* **241**:1132.

Hollingshead, A.B. and F.C. Redlich. 1958. *Social class and mental illness: A community study.* John Wiley & Sons, New York.

Honchar, P.A. and W.E. Halperin. 1981. 2,4,5-T, trichlorophenol and soft tissue sarcoma. *Lancet* i:268.

Hueper, W.C. 1979. Some comments on the history and experimental explorations of mental carcinogens and cancers. *J. Natl. Cancer Inst.* **62**:723.

Infante, P.F., J.K. Wagoner, R.A. Rinsky, and R.J. Young. 1977. Leukemia in benzene workers. *Lancet* ii:76.

International Agency for Research on Cancer (IARC). 1979. Some halogenated hydrocarbons. *IARC Mongr. Ser.* **20**:308.

______. 1980. An evaluation of chemicals and industrial processes associated with cancer in humans based on human and animal data: IARC Monographs, volumes 1 to 20. *Cancer Res.* **40**:1.

Jacobson, M.F. 1980. Diet and cancer. *Science* **207**:258.

Kaminski, R., K.S. Geissert, and E. Dacey. 1980. Mortality analysis of plumbers and pipefitters. *J. Occup. Med.* **22**:183.

Kang, H.K., P.F. Infante, and J.S. Carra. 1980. Occupational lead exposure and cancer. *Science* **207**:935.

Katz, R.M. and D. Jowett. 1981. Female laundry and dry cleaning workers in Wisconsin: A mortality analysis. *Am. J. Publ. Health* **71**:305.

Kitagawa, E.M. and P.M. Hauser. 1973. *Differential mortality in the United States: A study in socio-economic epidemiology.* Harvard University Press, Cambridge.

Koskela, R.S., S. Hernberg, R. Karava, E. Jarvinen, and M. Nurinen. 1976. A mortality study of foundry workers. *Scand. J. Work Environ. Health* 2(suppl.)**1**:73.

Lancet. 1977. Are 90% of cancers preventable? *Lancet* i:685.

Lemen, R.A., J.S. Lee, J.K. Wagoner, and H.P. Blejer. 1976. Cancer mortality among cadmium production workers. *Ann. N.Y. Acad. Sci.* **271**:274.

Li, F.P., J.F. Fraumeni, Jr., N. Mantel, and R.W. Miller. 1969. Cancer mortality among chemists. *J. Natl. Cancer Inst.* **43**:1159.

Lloyd, J.W., P. Decoufle, and L.G. Salvin. 1977. Unusual mortality experience of printing pressmen. *J. Occup. Med.* **19**:543.

Maugh, T.H. 1979. Cancer and environment: Higginson speaks out. *Science* **205**:1363.

Milham, S. 1979. Mortality in aluminum reduction plant worker. *J. Occup. Med.* **21**:275.

Monson, R.R. and K.K. Nakano. 1976. Mortality among rubber workers; I. White male union employees in Akron, Ohio. *Am. J. Epidemiol.* **103**:284.

Moss, E. and W.R. Lee. 1974. Occurrence of oral and pharyngeal cancers in textile workers. *Br. J. Ind. Med.* **31**:224.

Morgan, W.K.C. 1979. Industrial carcinogens the extent of the risk. *Thorax* **34**:431.

Morgan, R.W., S.D. Kaplan, and W.R. Gaffey. 1981. A general mortality study of production workers in the paint and coatings manufacturing industry: A preliminary report. *J. Occup. Med.* **23**:13.

National Institute for Occupational Safety and Health (NIOSH). 1981. Permeation of protective garment material by liquid halogenated ethanes and a polyphlorinated biphenyl. DHHS (NIOSH) 81-110, Cincinnati, Ohio.

______. 1981. National Occupational Hazard Survey (NOHS). National Institute for Occupational Safety and Health, Cincinnati, Ohio. Provisional estimates.

Percy, C., E. Stanek III, and L. Gloeckler. 1981. Accuracy of cancer death certificates and its effect on cancer mortality statistics. *Am. J. Public Health* **71**:242.

Peto, R. 1980. Distorting the epidemiology of cancer: The need for a more balanced overview. *Nature* **284**:297.

Pinto, S., V. Henderson, and P. Enterline. 1978. Mortality experience of arsenic-exposed workers. *Arch. Environ. Health* **20**:325.

Rall, D.P. 1979. Occupational cancer risk. *Science* **203**:224.

Redmond, C.K., B.R. Strobino, and R.H. Cypess. 1976. Cancer experience among coke by-product workers. *Ann. N.Y. Acad. Sci.* **271**:102.

Rockette, H.E. 1977. Cause specific mortality of coal miners. *J. Occup. Med.* **19**:795.

Silverstein, M., F. Mirer, D. Kotelchuch, B. Silverstein, and M. Bennett. 1981. Mortality among workers in a die casting and electroplating plant. *Scand. J. Work Environ. Health* (in press).

Stallones, R.A. and T. Downs. 1978. *A critical review of "estimates" of the fraction of cancer in the United States related to occupational factors.* University of Texas School of Public Health, Houston.

Sterling, T.D. and J.J. Weinkham. 1976. Smoking characteristics by type of employment. *J. Occup. Med.* **18**:743.

———. 1976. Smoking patterns by occupation, industry, sex, and race. *Arch. Environ. Health* **18**:313.

Thomas, T.L., P. Decoufle, and R. Moure-Eraso. 1980. Mortality among workers employed in petroleum refining and petrochemical plants. *J. Occup. Med.* **2**:97.

Tomatis, L., C. Agthe, M. Bartsh, J. Huff, R. Montesano, R. Saracci, F. Walker, and J. Wilbourne. 1978. Evaluation of the carcinogenicity of chemicals: A review of the monograph program of the International Agency for Research on Cancer. *Cancer Res.* **38**:877.

Walker, A.M. and H. Jick. 1979. Cancer of the corpus uteri: Increasing incidence in the United States. 1970-75. *Am. J. Epidemiol.* **110**:47.

Wagoner, J.K., R.W. Miller, F.E. Lundin, Jr., J.F. Fraumeni, Jr., and M.E. Haji. 1963. Unusual cancer mortality among a group of underground metal miners. *N. Engl. J. Med.* **269**:284.

Whelan, E.M. 1979. Cancer and the politics of fear. *Toxic Subst. J.* **1**:78.

Wolf, P.H., D. Andjelkovich, A. Smith, and H. Tyroler. 1981. A case-control study of leukemia in the U.S. rubber industry. *J. Occup. Med.* **23**:103.

Wynder, E.L. and G.B. Gori. 1977. Contribution of the environment to cancer incidence: An epidemiologic exercise. *J. Natl. Cancer Inst.* **58**:825.

NCHS Data Resources for Studying Occupational Cancer Mortality

HARRY M. ROSENBERG
Mortality Statistics Branch
Division of Vital Statistics
Hyattsville, Maryland 20782

In this presentation, I would like to describe some of the existing and emerging data resources available from the National Center for Health Statistics (NCHS) that can be used to shed statistical evidence on some of the important issues with which this meeting is concerned. I will consider the availability of NCHS mortality data for the study of factors associated with deaths from malignant neoplasms in respect to: (1) existing resources, (2) imminent resources, and (3) potential resources.

NATURE AND SOURCE OF U.S. MORTALITY DATA

The principal source of mortality in the United States and in other nations is the death certificate, a legal and a statistical document. The relevant information regarding conditions present at the time of death and their reported causal sequence culminating in death are from the medical certification portion of the certificate as recorded by the attending physician, medical examiner, or coroner. Subsequently, this information is coded according to the conventional classification system of causes of death in use at the time the death occurred. Thus, for deaths occurring beginning with 1979, it is the practice in the United States to use the classification system promulgated by the World Health Organization (WHO), namely, the 9th revision of the International Classification of Diseases (ICD). Earlier during 1968-1978, we used the eighth revision adapted for use in the United States which was based on the classification system developed by WHO. Revisions in ICD are made once every decade since 1900 to reflect developments in medical and diagnostic knowledge.

From among the conditions reported on the death certificate it is the usual practice for statistical tabulation and analysis to select, according to a set of internationally agreed-upon rules, the single underlying cause of death believed to have set in motion the sequence of conditions reported on the certificate that culminated in the death. The United States and other nations publish most of their mortality statistics in terms of what is called the underlying cause of death.

Mortality statistics produced by NCHS are based on information obtained directly from copies of the original certificates received from the vital statistics registration offices in the states where records are filed. Each state provides the data to NCHS through the Cooperative Health Statistics System in which 44 states currently participate. For these states, part or all of the mortality is coded from the original certificates and provided to NCHS on computer tape. Moreover, seven states submit all mortality data, including cause of death, precoded on computer tape. The other states in the Cooperative System submit computer tapes with only preceded demographic data. They also provide NCHS with copies of the original certificates from which NCHS codes cause of death. For remaining states not in the Cooperative System, NCHS codes both the demographic and medical (cause of death) data directly from copies of the original death certificates.

EXISTING STATISTICAL RESOURCES

The major existing statistical resources for describing and analyzing national mortality patterns are monthly and annual cause-of-death statistics published by NCHS. Monthly data are published in the Monthly Vital Statistics Report approximately 3 months after the month of occurrence of the death. The cause-of-death information is based on a 10% sample of deaths classified for tabulation purposes into the 72 selected causes of death whose total accounts for all causes of death. The component conditions of cancer published in this monthly report and their corresponding classification numbers from ICD, 9th revision, are shown in Table 1.

Table 1
Component Conditions of Cancer Published in Monthly Vital Statistics Report

Cause of death	ICD number (9th rev.)
Malignant neoplasms, including neoplasms of lymphatic and hematopoietic tissues	140-208
Malignant neoplasms of lip, oral cavity, and pharynx	140-149
Malignant neoplasms of digestive organs and peritoneum	150-159
Malignant neoplasms of respiratory and intrathoracic organs	160-165
Malignant neoplasm of breast	174-175
Malignant neoplasms of genital organs	179-187
Malignant neoplasms of urinary organs	188-189
Malignant neoplasms of all other and unspecified sites	170-173,190-199
Leukemia	204-208
Other malignant neoplasms of lymphatic and hematopoietic tissues	200-203

The monthly figures are considered provisional. In contrast, final figures are based on the complete (nonsample) count of approximately 2 million deaths annually in the United States. The data are published in *Vital Statistics of the United States, Vol II, Mortality.* These final data from the complete file usually are available to the public about 1.5-2 years after the close of the data year in the form of an advance release, which signifies that all of the data are available to researchers. This is prior to publication of the buckram-bound volumes, which may not be distributed by the Government Printing Office until 1-2 years later. The two volumes that constitute the national published mortality data include over 100 tables of frequencies and rates for the nation, for geographic areas including counties and states, and for demographic subgroups (age, race, and sex).

NCHS uses several varied tabulation lists varying in detail for tabulating and analyzing underlying cause of death, but all are consistent with both the WHO classification system as well as with the WHO recommendations for tabulating cause of death. For cancer, the level of detail ranges from the nine broad groups shown in Table 1 to the over 370 categories of malignant neoplasms shown at the four-digit (most detailed) level. For tabulation and analysis purposes, an intermediate classification of malignant neoplasms, containing 50 mutually exclusive categories is shown in Table 2.

One of the most important and most flexible sources of mortality data from our total file is the public-use tapes for each data year from 1968-1978. The most detailed public-use tapes include a statistical record without identifiers for each death in the United States in a particular data year. Two other summary tapes, one focusing on geographic areas, the other on causes of death, also are produced by NCHS and are made available through the National Technical Information Service (NCHS 1980b). The content of these three sets of public-use tapes is shown in Table 3.

IMMINENT STATISTICAL RESOURCES

Two new NCHS initiatives will make available statistical tools that are of considerable potential for studying the correlates of cancer—the National Death Index (NDI) (Patterson 1980), and the multiple cause-of-death file annual mortality data for each death in the United States for which data would be available on each condition reported for the decedent rather than just the underlying cause of death.

For those of you who are unfamiliar with the NDI, it is a computerized listing of each death in the United States annually, effective with the 1979 data year, and the location of the actual death certificate. This file, to be used only for research and statistical purposes, can be matched against a study cohort to determine the likelihood that individuals in the study cohort are deceased and, if so, to learn the particulars of their deaths as reported on the original legal document filed with the states. The NDI is expected to go on

Table 2
NCHS Intermediate (282) Tabulation List for Malignant Neoplasms as Underlying Cause of Death, International Classification of Diseases, ICD, 9th Revision, Effective 1979

Cause of death	ICD number
Malignant neoplasms, including neoplasms of lymphatic and hematopoietic tissues	140-208
Malignant neoplasms of lip, oral cavity, and pharynx	140-149
Of lip	140
Of tongue	141
Of pharynx	146-149.0
Of other and ill-defined sites within the lip, oral cavity, and pharynx	142-145,149.1-149.9
Malignant neoplasms of digestive organs and peritoneum	150-159
Of esophagus	150
Of stomach	151
Of small intestine, including duodenum	152
Of colon	153
Hepatic and splenic flexures and transverse colon	153.0-153.1,153.7
Descending colon	153.2
Sigmoid colon	153.3
Cecum, appendix, and ascending colon	153.4-153.6
Other and colon, unspecified	153.8-153.9
Of rectum, rectosigmoid junction, and anus	154
Of liver and intrahepatic bile ducts	155

Liver, primary	155.0
Intrahepatic bile ducts	155.1
Liver, not specified as primary or secondary	155.2
Of gallbladder and extrahepatic bile ducts	156
Of pancreas	157
Of retroperitoneum, peritoneum, and other and ill-defined sites within the digestive organs and peritoneum	158-159
Malignant neoplasms of respiratory and intrathoracic organs	160-165
Of larynx	161
Of trachea, bronchus, and lung	162
Of all other and ill-defined sites within the respiratory system and intrathoracic organs	160,162-165
Malignant neoplasms of bone, connective tissue, skin, and breast	170-175
Of bone and articular cartilage	170
Of connective and other soft tissue	171
Melanoma of skin	172
Other malignant neoplasms of skin	173
Of female breast	174
Of male breast	175
Malignant neoplasms of genital organs	179-187
Of cervix uteri	180
Of other parts of uterus	179,181-182
Of ovary and other uterine adnexa	183
Of other and unspecified female genital organs	184
Of prostate	185

Table 2 *(Continued)*

Cause of death	ICD number
Of testis	186
Of penis and other male genital organs	187
Malignant neoplasms of urinary organs	188-189
Of bladder	188
Of kidney and other and unspecified urinary organs	189
Malignant neoplasms of other and unspecified sites	190-199
Of eye	190
Of brain	191
Of other and unspecified parts of nervous system	192
Of thyroid gland and other endocrine glands and related structures	193-194
Of all other and unspecified sites	195-199
Malignant neoplasms of lymphatic and hematopoietic tissues	200-208
Lymphosarcoma and reticulosarcoma	200
Hodgkin's disease	201
Other malignant neoplasms of lymphoid and histiocytic tissue	202
Multiple myeloma and immunoproliferative neoplasms	203
Leukemia	204-208
Lymphoid leukemia	204
Myeloid leukemia	205
Monocytic leukemia	206
Other and unspecified leukemia	207-208

Table 3
Summary of 1968-1977 Mortality Data Tapes, by Type of File

Detail	Local area summary	Cause-of-death summary
Data year	stub variables[a]	Stub variables[a]
Residence of decedent[a]	residence of decedent[b]	State of residence[b]
State	State	Sex
County	County	Race
City (250,000 persons or more)	City (10,000 persons or more)	1968 (7 categories)
Population size	Population size	1969-1975 (9 categories)
SMSA[c]	SMSA	Underlying cause of death:
Metropolitan-nonmetropolitan	Metropolitan-nonmetropolitan	each cause
Age at death (single years)	underlying cause of death	recoded to 281 cause-of-death groups
Month of death	Recoded to 69 cause-of-death groups	recoded to 69 cause-of-death groups
Day of death (1972-1977)	Recoded to 34 cause-of-death groups	Spread variables
Place of death (State, county)	spread variable	age at death
Race:	total number of deaths	5-year age groups
1968 (7 categories)		single years under 5 years of age
1969-1975 (9 categories)		Under 1 year:
Six		less than 1 day
Underlying cause of death		1-6 days
Each cause		7-27 days
Whether autopsy performed (1972-1977)		1-11 months
Whether findings used (1972-1977)		month of death

Table 3 *(Continued)*

Detail		Local area summary		Cause-of-death summary	
Record length	160	record length	28	record length	194
Block size	3,200	block size	1,400	block size	1,940
Approximate number of records	2,000,000	approximate number of records	180,000	approximate number of records	180,000
Number of reels		number of reels:		number of reels:	
1968	10	1968	1	1968	2
1969	10	1969	1	1969	2
1970	10	1970	1	1970	2
1971	10	1971	1	1971	2
1972	5	1972	1	1972	1
1973	10	1973	1	1973	2
1974	10	1974	1	1974	2
1975	10	1975	1	1975	2
1976	10	1976	1	1976	2
1977	10	1977	1	1977	2

Data from NCHS (1980b).

[a]All data items in the detail file are in EBCDIC code. The stub portion of all summary records consists of EBCDIC codes and the spread portion consists of a series of full-word binary fields containing numbers of deaths.

[b]Beginning in 1970, the place of residence for decedents who were nonresidents of the United States has been coded to the country of residence (8 categories). Formerly these deaths were considered resident deaths of the place of occurrence. The local area and cause-of-death summaries exclude data for nonresidents of the United States.

[c]Standard metropolitan statistical area.

line during 1981, and no doubt, when implemented, will be a major facilitator of epidemiological research in the United States.

Our multiple cause-of-death statistics program will make available on tape and in publications the multiple conditions reported on death certificates for the data years beginning with 1968, the first year of the eighth revision period (Rosenberg 1978). The first data year to be available will be 1976 followed by 1977-1979, 1969-1971, and 1968 and 1975. This information will be available during 1981 from the National Technical Information Service. The sequence will permit us to approach producing these data concurrently with our underlying cause-of-death statistics, and will make available data for the 1969-1971 period, when 1970 census data can be used to develop detailed death rates for special studies.

POTENTIAL STATISTICAL RESOURCES

Although the existing vital statistics system produces useful mortality data for biomedical and epidemiological research and while its utility will be enhanced considerably by the availability of the NDI and multiple cause-of-death statistics, there is considerable potential for additional augmentation to this data base. From an epidemiological point of view, a major limitation of currently available mortality data from the vital statistics system is the limited information on the characteristics of the decedent. Available characteristics are the basic demographic descriptors, namely, age, race, and sex, and the place of death (county or city). For research on the correlates of cancer, missing are needed data on those attributes of decedents that could reflect environmental exposures or other individual factors that may be associated with elevated risks. These could be, for example, occupational factors, socioeconomic factors, or life-style factors.

NCHS is actively considering two approaches to enriching existing vital statistics information to fill this need. One of these is to exploit more fully existing information reported on the death certificate. For example, two items of interest on the certificate are not routinely coded, namely, the occupation and industry of the decedent. Yet, similar information has been used decennially in Great Britain for studies of occupational mortality (Office of Population Censuses and Surveys 1978), and less frequently in the United States for special studies of occupational mortality. The last national U.S. study was in 1950 (Guralnick 1962). NCHS recently completed a study to determine the feasibility of coding the information reported on the death certificate with regard to the decedent's occupation and industry. It was found that existing coding procedures used by the Bureau of the Census were compatible with information reported on the death certificate (Rosenberg et al. 1979). With support from the National Institute for Occupational Safety and Health (NIOSH), NCHS is working with the Bureau of the Census to develop coding procedures that could be used by the states to produce these data on a uniform and routine basis. If these procedures are evaluated as compatible with state vital statistics processing, then this information may become an integral element within the annual mortality files released by NCHS.

Another approach to developing statistical information on the correlates of cancer mortality that has been implemented in the past by NCHS and has recently been reconsidered is called the follow-back approach. This is a survey that augments existing information on vital records. Currently NCHS has such a survey in the field for births and fetal deaths; similar surveys could be put into the field for deaths—surveys that could solicit from informants additional information about the circumstances of death and about decedents' characteristics such as work history and socioeconomic status. Surveys of this type were carried out during the early 1960s (NCHS 1962-1963). From an epidemiological point of view follow-back surveys are an efficient data collection mechanism because they permit one to collect information about events that are relatively low in terms of prevalence among the total population. Mortality is such a "rare" event, in that it occurs annually to less than 1% of the population. Cancer deaths occur to about 0.2% of the population annually.

Yet another potential source of data for examining the relation between cancer and occupational factors is through linking records, in particular mortality records with those in other files. For example, files containing information on occupational work histories and exposures could be linked to the fact and nature of death. Beebe (this volume) has alluded to a variety of possible files with which the death record can be linked to enrich its usefulness for epidemiological research. We are aware of the great value of such studies from the classic matching study that resulted in the American Public Health Association Monograph *Differential Mortality in the United States* (Kitagawa and Hauser 1973). In that study, a sample of death records were matched with corresponding Census records for 1960, the latter providing a wealth of social and economic information with which to augment the medical data and the limited demographic information on the death certificate. As Beebe has pointed out, record linkage for both small-scale epidemiological studies as well as larger-scale national studies such as the Kitagawa-Hauser study can be greatly facilitated by the NDI.

CONCLUSION

A principal source of statistical information for studying the relation between cancer and associated factors, such as occupation, is mortality data from the national vital statistics system. Imminent and potential enrichments to this long-standing, durable, and essential data source have been described. As these developments materialize, it is hoped that they will be used effectively to identify further correlates and causal factors related to cancer morbidity and mortality.

APPENDIX I: SPECIFIC COMMENTS ON DR. RICHARD PETO'S PRESENTATION

Dr. Peto has made an effective presentation of mortality trends due to cancer in the United States. I am particularly pleased with his procedure for segmenting the analysis by broad age groups in describing trends. This is a useful and valid departure from other presentations of trends in cancer mortality. In the case of cancer trends in the United States, it is particularly important not to use aggregate indices such as the crude death rate or the age-adjusted death rate for all age groups combined, as this obscures in a detrimental way important divergent trends among different age groups, broadly-speaking, between the younger and the older population, approximately distinguished as being below and above 45 years of age at the present time. Overall, cancer mortality trends are downward for the younger group, as shown in Table A, and upward for the older population.

The use of a single mortality index to describe mortality time series, where age-specific trends diverge, is undesirable as has been discussed in another paper (Curtin et al. 1979). Commendably, Dr. Peto has made an age differentiation in his analysis, between those below 65 years and those 65 years old and over. His analysis would be strengthened, I believe, by further differentiating the group under 65 years of age.

APPENDIX II: MORE RECENT CANCER MORTALITY TRENDS

It is of interest to have the most recent available national data on cancer mortality trends. These data for the years 1979 and 1980, available from the NCHS 10% Current Mortality Sample, have been published as provisional estimates (NCHS 1981). The NCHS provisional sample data are only for the broader component categories of cancer rather than for specific sites. This limits the analysis that can be made from these data. Three other limitations also characterize the generalizations that can be made from the data, namely, sample size, the absence of age-specific data, and changes in disease classification. The sample-size limitation means that each point estimate of the death rate is associated with sampling errors. The size of these sampling errors is described in the published report. The absence of age-specific data means that changes in death rates over time may reflect shifts in population composition rather than actual changes in health risk. Such a limitation is more important in comparisons of long-term trends than in the analysis of year-to-year changes; but nevertheless it warrants consideration, even in the short term.

The third consideration is related to the change in the classification of diseases and causes of death approximately every 10 years to reflect changes in medical knowledge and diagnoses. These changes are reflected in the successive revisions of the ICD. The new classification, the 9th revision, was implemented in the United States effective with the 1979 data year. This

Table A
Death Rates for Selected Causes of Death by Age: United States, 1968, 1977, and 1978

Cause of death (ICD, 8th revision, 1965)		Year	Total	Under 1 year	1-4 years	5-14 years	15-24 years	25-34 years	35-44 years	45-54 years	55-64 years	65-74 years	75-84 years	85 years and over
All causes		1978	883.4	1,434.4	69.2	33.9	117.5	135.5	238.9	609.7	1,416.3	3,027.2	7,187.8	14,700.7
		1977	878.1	1,485.6	68.8	34.6	117.1	136.2	247.5	620.7	1,434.9	3,055.6	7,181.9	14,725.9
		1968	967.9	2,265.7	89.6	43.0	123.7	157.2	319.8	751.3	1,704.4	3,724.0	8,293.5	19,582.7
Malignant neoplasms including neoplasms of lymphatic and hematopoietic tissues	(140-209)	1978	181.9	4.1	4.9	4.2	6.3	14.2	49.6	184.4	441.8	800.7	1,293.8	1,450.5
		1977	178.7	3.8	5.2	4.8	6.5	14.5	50.9	182.5	440.5	792.6	1,267.5	1,445.6
		1968	159.8	4.2	8.0	6.4	8.2	17.3	61.0	183.0	413.5	749.2	1,133.8	1,475.3
Malignant neoplasms of buccal cavity and pharynx	(140-149)	1978	3.8	0.0	0.0	0.0	0.1	0.2	1.0	5.5	11.8	16.4	13.7	22.1
		1977	3.9	0.0	0.0	0.0	0.1	0.2	1.0	5.4	12.7	16.6	19.6	24.1
		1968	3.7	0.1	0.0	0.0	0.1	0.1	1.1	5.7	12.0	14.9	20.6	13.9
Malignant neoplasms of digestive organs and peritoneum	(150-159)	1978	48.3	0.2	0.2	0.1	0.3	1.6	8.3	36.8	103.7	219.7	412.5	513.3
		1977	47.6	0.4	0.2	0.1	0.4	1.8	8.9	36.1	105.6	218.0	405.5	508.4
		1968	46.9	0.5	0.1	0.1	0.4	2.1	10.3	40.3	112.0	223.8	416.8	573.5
Malignant neoplasms of respiratory system	(160-163)	1978	45.8	0.1	0.0	0.0	0.1	0.9	10.1	56.6	142.3	227.3	246.6	158.6
		1977	44.0	0.1	0.0	0.0	0.1	1.0	10.6	55.1	137.3	219.2	237.3	156.3
		1968	31.8	0.2	0.0	0.1	0.2	1.1	11.0	43.3	107.8	166.3	159.5	116.8
Malignant neoplasm of breast	(174)	1978	15.9	0.1	–	–	0.1	1.7	8.7	26.4	44.0	56.5	83.9	109.5
		1977	16.1	–	–	0.0	0.0	1.8	8.9	27.0	44.1	58.3	85.1	117.0
		1968	14.6	0.1	0.0	0.0	0.0	2.0	10.8	27.7	40.8	53.4	74.6	117.1
Malignant neoplasms of genital organs	(180-187)	1978	20.7		0.0	0.0	0.6	1.7	5.0	15.2	38.3	88.7	187.7	242.4
		1977	20.5	0.0	0.0	0.1	0.7	1.9	5.0	15.0	39.9	88.4	185.5	237.6
		1968	20.5	0.1	0.1	0.1	0.8	2.8	8.5	20.6	43.2	94.7	179.8	259.2
Malignant neoplasms of urinary organs	(188,189)	1978	8.1	0.3	0.2	0.1	0.1	0.2	1.1	5.5	16.2	36.4	71.6	94.4
		1977	8.0	0.1	0.3	0.1	0.1	0.2	1.3	5.9	16.2	37.1	71.8	91.7
		1968	7.4	0.3	0.5	0.3	0.1	0.3	1.4	5.8	16.9	38.3	56.8	92.6
Malignant neoplasms of all other and unspecified sites	(170-173,190-199)	1978	22.4	1.9	2.4	1.5	2.2	3.9	9.1	24.7	52.8	88.0	144.2	171.8
		1977	21.9	1.9	2.6	1.8	2.3	3.7	9.2	24.0	51.3	87.6	138.0	174.9
		1968	18.7	1.8	3.0	2.2	2.6	3.9	9.2	23.3	47.2	76.0	112.0	162.6
Leukemia	(204-207)	1978	7.1	1.2	1.8	2.0	1.7	1.8	2.8	5.2	10.9	24.7	53.8	69.5
		1977	7.1	1.0	1.8	2.2	1.7	1.8	2.7	5.2	11.5	25.2	53.3	69.7
		1968	7.2	1.6	3.8	2.9	2.1	2.0	3.3	5.6	12.2	27.4	49.2	71.6
Other neoplasms of lymphatic and hematopoietic tissues	(200-203,208,209)	1978	9.9	0.3	0.2	0.4	1.1	2.1	3.4	8.6	21.6	42.9	74.0	68.9
		1977	9.7	0.2	0.2	0.5	1.1	2.1	3.3	8.8	22.0	42.1	71.2	65.9
		1968	8.9	0.3	0.4	0.7	1.9	3.1	4.9	10.6	21.5	39.5	54.4	48.0

Refers only to resident deaths occurring within the United States. Excludes fetal deaths. Rates per 100,000 population in specified group.
Data from NCHS (1980a).

Table B

Provisional Counts of Deaths in The 10% Current Mortality Survey and Provisional Death Rates for All Causes of Death and for Malignant Neoplasms, January-December 1979 and 1980: United States

		January-December			
		1980		1979	
Cause of death (ICD, 9th rev., 1975)		number[a]	rate	number	rate
All causes		197,745	892.6	189,538	866.2
Malignant neoplasms, including neoplasms of lymphatic and hematopoietic tissues	(140-208)	41,277	186.3	40,145	189.5
Malignant neoplasms of lip, oral cavity, and pharynx	(140-149)	846	3.8	783	3.6
Malignant neoplasms of digestive organs and peritoneum	(150-159)	10,900	49.2	10,799	49.3
Malignant neoplasms of respiratory and intrathoracic organs	(160-165)	10,734	48.5	10,188	46.6
Malignant neoplasm of breast	(174-175)	3,469	15.7	3,499	16.0
Malignant neoplasms of genital organs	(179-187)	4,597	20.8	4,482	20.5
Malignant neoplasms of urinary organs	(183-189)	1,746	7.9	1,754	8.0
Malignant neoplasms of all other and unspecified sites	(170-173,190-199)	5,177	23.4	4,982	22.8
Leukemia	(204-208)	1,696	7.7	1,619	7.4
Other malignant neoplasms of lymphatic and hematopoietic tissues	(200-203)	2,112	9.5	2,039	9.3

Rates are per 100,000 population.
Data from NCHS (1981).
[a]Figures for Connecticut are not included in the December sample for 1980.

necessarily introduces into time-series analysis of mortality certain discontinuities for certain causes of death where the classification had a major impact. The discontinuities would be between data for 1978 and 1979, the former being the end of the period when the 8th Revision was used in the United States (1968-1978). NCHS currently is measuring the size and the nature of these discontinuities through a double-coding "comparability study." From our published preliminary results from this study, we know that the discontinuity for all cancer sites combined is very small (NCHS 1980). For specific sites, it is greater.

Table B shows provisional cancer mortality data for the latest two data years 1979 and 1980 from our Current Mortality Sample. Taking into account the trend discontinuities associated with the introduction of the ninth revision of the ICD and the limitations of sample size, one can make some generalizations about cancer mortality trends, as follows.

The provisional death rate for all causes of death combined was slightly higher (1%) in 1980 than in 1979, resulting in large measure from the influenza epidemic in early 1980 and in December 1980, and from the lack of a major influenza epidemic in the previous year. Cancer mortality for all sites combined was also up over 2% between the 2 years, continuing the long-term upward trend in this cause of death. Some of the upward thrust may reflect the impact of the influenza epidemic with which mortality from other conditions, notably chronic conditions, is often correlated.

The largest site-specific increase between the 2 years was for respiratory cancer (malignant neoplasms of respiratory and intrathoracic organs), an increase of over 5% and thus continuing the long-term trend observed with this condition. There was also an increase in death rates due to leukemia; however, this is not consistent with the longer-term stable trend observed during the past decade and should be viewed with considerable caution until final (nonsample) data are available to reexamine the trend for this cause of death.

REFERENCES

Curtin, L., J. Maurer, and H. Rosenberg. 1979. "A comparison of alternative standards in computing age-adjusted death rates." Paper presented at the 1979 meeting of the American Statistical Association.

Guralnick, L. 1962. Mortality by occupation and industry, among men 20-64 years of age: United States, 1950. *Vital statistics–special reports,* vol. 53, no. 2.

Kitagawa, E. and P.M. Hauser. 1973. *Differential mortality in the United States.* Harvard University Press, Cambridge.

NCHS. 1962-1963. Socioeconomic characteristics of deceased persons, United States, 1962-63 deaths. *Vital and health statistics,* series 22, no. 9.

———. 1980a. Estimates of selected comparability ratios based on dual coding of 1976 death certificates by the eighth and ninth revisions of the International Classification of Diseases. *Monthly vital statistics report* vol. 28, no. 11.

______. 1980b. *Catalog of public use data tapes from the National Center for Health Statistics.* DHHS Publication No. (PHS) 81-1213, November.

______. 1981. Births, marriages, divorces, and deaths for January 1981. *Monthly vital statistics report* vol. 30, no. 1.

Office of Population Censuses and Surveys. 1978. *Occupational mortality, the Registrar General's decennial supplement for England and Wales, 1970-72.* Her Majesty's Stationery Office, London.

Patterson, J. 1980. The establishment of a National Death Index in the United States. *Banbury Rep.* **4**:443.

Rosenberg, H., D. Burnham, R. Spirtas, and V. Valdisera. 1979. Occupation and industry information from the death certificate: Assessment of the completeness of reporting. In *Statistical uses of administrative records with emphasis on mortality and disability research* (ed. L. Delbene and B. Scheuren), p. 83, Social Security Administration, Washington, D.C.

Rosenberg, H. 1978. "National multiple cause of death statistics." Paper presented at the 17th Biennial Meeting of the Public Health Conference on Records and Statistics, Washington, D.C., June.

SESSION 5:
Special Problems of Methodology

A Holistic Approach to Monitoring High-Risk Populations by Short-term Procedures

MARVIN S. LEGATOR
Division of Genetic Toxicology
Department of Preventive Medicine and Community Health
University of Texas Medical Branch
Galveston, Texas 77550

One of the major conclusions to be drawn from this meeting is that classical epidemiological studies are of limited value in identifying the carcinogenic effects of industrial chemicals. Several obvious shortcomings may affect epidemiologic studies of occupational or environmental cancer. First, it is difficult to assemble a sufficiently large group of workers (cohort), all suffering the same exposure, to draw a definitive conclusion concerning the risk of cancer at a particular site. Second, although cancer is a "major killer" in the United States and other developed nations, from a statistical or population point of view, death from a particular type of cancer is actually a "rare" event.

Thus, the incidence (rate of new cases) of lung cancer, for example, in the United States in 1970 was 40 cases/100,000; statistically speaking, the probability that an individual would contract lung cancer in the year 1970 in the United States was 1/2500 (DHEW 1970). Consequently, because of this low risk and unavoidable statistical variation, detection of a slight excess in incidence of lung cancer clearly would require access to records of tens of thousands of specifically exposed individuals.

A recent, well-designed epidemiologic study by O'Berg (1977) at Dupont compared the rates of cancer of the lung and of other sites in workers matched for age and smoking, who were exposed to acrylonitrile, and showed a significant increase in lung cancer mortality in the exposed workers. Yet, the number of exposed workers was quite small. Even more recently, this apparent excess in mortality from lung cancer in acrylonitrile-exposed workers was questioned because of the possibility of different smoking histories (degree and length of smoking) between exposed and unexposed workers, even though the study had been matched for smokers and nonsmokers (EPA 1979). Thus, when the risk is low and confounding effects by another important causative agent are present (such as smoking), epidemiologic studies require very large populations and extremely cautious design.

When a malignant tumor is rare in the absence of exposure to occupational agents such as vinyl chloride or asbestos (related to angiosarcoma of the liver and mesothelioma, respectively) and when the association of the agent to the disease is strong, it is easier to show an excess risk due to exposure. Otherwise, the amount of data that must be generated to designate a specific agent as a human carcinogen is formidable, and in many instances, such an assemblage is an insurmountable task. In addition to the large populations required, the long latency period for cancer induction (10-40 years) add a further problem to the epidemiologic method: Multiple exposure to other agents during this latency period confounds the study.

The main drawback of an epidemiologic study as a primary tool for safeguarding high-risk populations is that the results come too late or after the fact. Consider that in the few cases that an agent has been identified as a human carcinogen, it is only because a sufficiently large number of individuals has already developed the disease. It may be anticipated that many more will develop the disease after the symptomless latency period. Thus, classical epidemiologic studies cannot be considered as a primary tool for identifying carcinogens. Although such studies can provide proof and can corroborate animal and short-term tests, ideal studies are difficult to perform, and the information—when it does surface—comes too late to entertain remedial action.

In the ideal situation, animal studies would act as the surrogate for human experiments. Animal carcinogens should never reach the workplace; they should be eliminated if they are in commerce or in the case of necessary chemicals, measures should be taken to minimize human exposure.

A significant number of industrial chemicals have either not been tested in animals or have been tested inadequately for carcinogenic-mutagenic activity. In fact, there are numerous examples where known animal carcinogens are nevertheless being produced and significant human exposure is occurring even after adequate testing.

Given the present situation where the overwhelming majority of chemicals have not been evaluated for carcinogenic-mutagenic response in definite epidemiological studies or in many cases in animal studies, where even some chemicals that are known animal carcinogens are still being manufactured and used commercially, we must devise a new strategy for identifying and eliminating industrial carcinogens.

It is also highly likely, however, that several chemicals identified as being carcinogenic-mutagenic in nonhuman studies are not mutagenic or carcinogenic in man and therefore information that attests to the safety of a valuable chemical in relevant human studies is highly desirable.

THE IDEAL PROCEDURES FOR IDENTIFYING CARCINOGENS-MUTAGENS IN HIGH-RISK POPULATIONS

Given the large number of chemicals that have not been evaluated for carcinogenicity or mutagenicity and the severe limitations of classical epidemiologic studies, procedures are needed that would allow carcinogens in the workplace to be identified without recourse to the usual epidemiologic studies. Ideally, workers should be monitored continuously by relevant short-term procedures that could identify potentially harmful products and combinations of products long before clinical symptoms appear. The Utopian approach to this problem would be to have a number of accurate, economical tests that could be conducted in man that would not pose any danger to the human subject being tested, and that would yield results in a short period of time. Further, the results should serve as an advance warning system so that immediate action could be taken before any clinical symptoms occur.

In very general terms, the goal is to detect, quickly and accurately, those chemicals in the workplace that are potential carcinogens or mutagens long before any neoplasms or adverse birth effects are seen. The fact is that at this very moment such procedures are available. It is entirely conceivable that by using a number of available procedures and without any additional laboratory work, those chemicals in the workplace that are carcinogenic or mutagenic could be identified.

TECHNOLOGICAL BASIS FOR PROCEDURES USED TO DETECT CARCINOGENS IN THE WORKPLACE

What are these procedures? They are a series of short-term, noninvasive tests that can be conducted in high-risk populations, using blood, urine, or semen to determine whether recent exposure to carcinogens-mutagens has occurred. These procedures utilize the assumption that mutations are part of the carcinogenic process and that a high correlation exists between carcinogenic and mutagenic activities of chemicals. The theoretical basis for this association was recently reviewed (Stich and Acton 1979) and the most likely mutation model of carcinogenesis was presented. The mutation model indicated that a series of discrete actions must occur for a chemical to induce cancer:

1. Adduct formation with DNA, or other DNA damage.
2. Induction of gene mutations.
3. Induction of chromosome aberrations.
4. Shift of DNA repair from error-free excision-repair to error-prone systems to facilitate mutagenesis.
5. Reduced DNA repair to elevate the frequency of chromosome aberrations.
6. Suppression of DNA replication and mitosis in normal cells to facilitate clone formation of cells with a mutated regulator gene.

This series of events occurs in somatic cells for the induction of cancer. A similar series of events, including point mutation and chromosomal mutation, occurs in germinal cells, but the expression of the final outcome of the event is different. If a germinal mutation is not lethal, a live birth will occur, but the

Table 1
Carcinogens and Mutagens in High-risk Populations

Event	Procedures	Status
	Somatic cells	
1. Adduct formation with DNA (macromolecules)	alkylation of macromolecules	advanced developmental stage
2. Induction of gene mutations	body fluid analysis	available procedure
	HGPRT[a] variants	advanced developmental stage
3. Induction of chromosome aberrations	metaphase analysis	available procedure
	SCE	available procedure
4. Repair induction	alkaline elution	developmental stage
	unscheduled DNA synthesis	developmental stage
	Germinal cells	
1. Early or late fetal loss	increase in spontaneous abortion obtained by questionnaire	available procedure but difficult to derive significant differences
2. Unequal chromosome segregation	YFF sperm study	available procedure
3. Abnormal sperm	test for morphologic variants	available procedure
4. Aspermia or oligospermia	sperm count	available procedure

[a]Hypoxanthine-guanine phosphoribosyl transferase.

infant will have a genetic defect. If these events are lethal, however, this lethality may show up as early fetal loss, late fetal loss, abnormal sperm, or sperm lethality. All of the short-term procedures that are used to identify potential carcinogens and mutagens in the workplace capitalize on the spectrum of events that are induced either in somatic or germinal cells. The event that is measured can be classified as a component of the mutagenic process. These responses simply identify a phase in the overall process that might result in an abnormal outcome, such as cancer or a genetic defect. Table 1 lists the events and the procedures that can be used in human monitoring, as well as the practicality of using the procedure at present to monitor high-risk populations. From Table 1, it can be deduced that the procedures available for monitoring workers include determination of three events: Cytogenetic abnormalities, point mutations, and the spectrum of events in spermatogenesis, including the induction of the extra YF body.

DESCRIPTION OF AVAILABLE PROCEDURES

The premier procedure for evaluating adverse effects of chemicals in a human population is cytogenetic analysis. This technique, used with a sufficient number of cells and sufficient number of subjects in exposed and control groups, is probably the most powerful tool available for evaluating high-risk groups. In a recent presentation, the summary of the assessment of cancer risks by the International Agency for Research on Cancer (IARC 1980) was correlated with cytogenetic studies (R.W. Kapp, pers. comm.). Of the 442 chemicals evaluated by IARC since it began providing information on chemical carcinogens in 1968, sufficient evidence of carcinogenicity in animals had been accumulated in 112, but, only 53 chemicals had been tested in human studies. These 53 chemicals are categorized as: (1) Chemicals carcinogenic for humans (17, total), (2) chemicals probably carcinogenic for humans (18, total), and (3) chemicals for which data are insufficient (18, total).

Of the 17 chemicals or chemical processes classified as carcinogenic for humans, 4 have been tested for cytogenetic aberrations in humans and were found to be positive: Arsenic compounds (Nordenson et al. 1978; Beckman et al. 1979), benzene (Tough et al. 1970; Picciano 1979b), *bis*(chloromethyl)ether and technical-grade (chloromethyl) methyl ether (Zudova and Landa 1977), and vinyl chloride (Ducatman et al. 1975; Funes-Gravioto et al. 1975). Of the 18 chemicals and chemical processes classified as probably carcinogenic for humans, 3 have been tested for production of cytogenetic aberrations in humans and results were positive: Cyclophosphamide (Etteldorf 1976), epichlorohydrin (Kucerova et al. 1977; Picciano 1979a), and tris(1-azirdinyl)phosphine sulfide (thio-TEPA) (Silezneva and Korman 1973).

Of the 18 chemicals and chemical processes that could not be classified as to their carcinogenicity for humans, although data from animal studies would indicate their potential carcinogenic activity, 4 were found to be positive for cytogenetic aberrations: Chloroprene (Katosova 1973; Sanotskii 1976), ethylene oxide (Garry 1979), lead and lead compounds (Forni and Secci 1972; Garza-Chapa et al. 1977), and styrene (Meretoja 1977). Each of these agents is a cancer suspect, and in every case where human cytogenetics studies have been reported, the results indicate significant chromosomal damage.

The evaluation of an exposed and nonexposed group for chromosomal abnormalities is a comparatively simple procedure; it requires a trained cytogeneticist, a light microscope, and several milliliters of blood. Presently, two types of analysis can be performed. The traditional method is to determine chromosome aberrations in metaphase cells. In this study, the identification and classification of chromatid and chromosome abnormalities are carried out and both numerical and structural changes are identified.

The second procedure is a new method that is referred to as sister chromatid exchange (SCE). SCE involves a crossing over of sister chromatids either at the time of (or after) DNA replication. With certain chemicals, this procedure has been found to be more sensitive than the standard metaphase analysis. There are classes of active chemicals, however, that do not increase SCE, and the genetic basis for this procedure is not fully understood. Although metaphase analysis is the preferred method, analysis for SCE can be a valuable adjunct.

Another procedure that can be carried out concurrently with cytogenetic analysis is the analysis of body fluids for the presence of genetically active compounds. In this procedure, samples of blood or urine or both are either tested directly or are concentrated and then evaluated for the presence of mutagenic agents. *Salmonella typhimurium* is used often as the indicator organism to detect the presence of chemicals that can induce gene mutations; this analysis is a valuable addition to the cytogenetic tests, because it can identify compounds that cause gene mutations. Agents that have been identified with the indicator organism *S. typhimurium* in the urine assay include cyclophosphamide (Sievert and Simon 1973), epichlorohydrin (Legator et al. 1979a), ethyleneimine imine (T.H. Connor, unpubl.), metronidazole (Dobias 1980), and niridazole (Legator et al. 1979b).

Recently a unique procedure has been developed that allows detection of the increase in the frequency of Y chromosomes in sperm, indicating a disjunctional error of the Y chromosome. If mature spermatozoa are stained with quinacrine dihydrochloride, the Y chromosome is visible under conventional fluorescent microscopy, with the Y body appearing as a single, bright spot within the sperm. When the Y chromosome has failed to separate normally at anaphase, there are two Y chromosomes and, therefore, two fluorescent bodies. The presence of two fluorescent bodies in a normal-size spermatozoa indicates the existence of two Y chromosomes due to a disjunctional error in spermatogenesis at anaphase. This technique has already detected an increase in the frequency of sperm bearing two Y bodies in persons exposed to chemotherapeutic agents, radiation, and dibromochloropropane. This procedure not only detects a compound that could induce cancer but it also shows a specific effect in germinal cells (Kapp et al. 1980).

Sperm analysis for abnormal morphology is an additional procedure that can be used. Several known mutagens-carcinogens have been identified in both animals and man with this procedure. The genetic validity of this test, however, has yet to be established and the background rate in man is quite high.

The above-described procedures form a comprehensive battery of tests that, used properly, should identify the majority of hazardous substances that could induce cancer and genetic abnormalities. There can be little doubt that the success record of these procedures to date has been rather remarkable, and to the best of my knowledge, false positive results have not been found. These procedures almost can be considered diagnostic for hazardous materials in the workplace, and can serve as advance warning signs with chemicals, much as a radiation badge tells us that we are being exposed to harmful radiation. It should be emphasized that these effects occur well in advance of clinical symptoms. These tests are noninvasive and comparatively economical, and the answers are forthcoming shortly after the tests are performed. These studies can be conducted with comparatively small numbers of individuals, and there is no compelling reason why these procedures should not be incorporated as an integral part of a medical surveillance program in industry.

JUSTIFICATION OF SHORT-TERM PROCEDURES IN A MEDICAL SCREENING PROGRAM

In medical screening procedures, a list of criteria have been developed that should be met to justify a screening program:

1. The disease must have a major and significant effect on the quality or length of life.
2. The disease must have an asymptomatic period in which detection and treatment significantly reduce morbidity and mortality.
3. Treatment in the asymptomatic phase must result in a better prognosis than after symptoms appear.
4. Tests must be available to detect the disease.
5. Incidence of the disease must be great enough to justify screening for it.

In addition to the above five criteria, other considerations include the progression of the disease, sensitivity and reliability of tests, cost of detection, benefit from treatment, and risk factors.

If we look upon the described battery of tests that can be instituted to detect carcinogens in the workplace, it quickly can be seen that they meet the established criteria to justify a screening program.

1. Cancer and genetic abnormalities affect both the quality and length of life.
2. Induction of cancer includes a latency period ranging from 5 to 40 years; induction of genetic effects spans several generations. Indeed, a long asymptomatic period must pass between the chemical insult and the resultant syndrome.
3. If we can remove the individual or curtail his exposure to environmental carcinogens, there is little doubt this can reduce greatly the probability of having cancer or genetic abnormalities.
4. We have a series of tests that presently are available that can detect these hazardous chemicals.
5. Certainly, the incidence of cancer and mutagenic abnormalities will justify any screening.

As to other criteria for consideration—the progression of the disease, the sensitivity and the reliability of the tests, the cost of detection and benefit from early treatment—all would further argue for using these procedures. In fact, it is hard to describe any commonly used screening test carried out in human subjects that is as ideally suited for detecting future adverse effects as are the procedures described above.

INTERPRETATION OF THE DATA

There is a key difference between the procedures described above and other methods that are used to detect malignancies in high-risk groups. The short-term procedures, for the most part, cannot be interpreted on an individual basis. The individual who is exposed to a hazardous substance and is showing an increase in any one of the short-term end points is not necessarily going to exhibit a malignant tumor or experience an adverse outcome in giving birth; therefore, these procedures must be interpreted from a population standpoint. If we find, for instance, that the cytogenetic test reveals a increase in either stable or unstable configurations among an exposed group, as compared with a control group, we can deduce from that study that the exposed group has been in the presence of a chemical that has the potential to cause genetic damage, including cancer.

As with every other biological method, the information that can be derived from these techniques depends upon utilization of a proper experimental design, including statistical analysis. In cytogenetic studies, a number of variables have to do with inter- and intralaboratory variation. Exposure of individuals to drugs, viruses, radiation, selection of a proper nonexposed control group, seasonal variation, the number of cells that are counted, and a variety of other factors can influence the experimental outcome. It should be emphasized, however, that for almost any technique conducted either in animals or in man, a series of variables can be listed that are similar in many instances to those listed for the cytogenetic procedure. If the variables are understood and adjusted appropriately and if the work is carried out by competent investigators, interpretation of the data as to the exposure of a group of individuals to a deleterious agent is valid. The major problem, as in most testing procedures, is the possibility that because of faulty design, a toxic chemical will not be detected.

Our limited experience with cytogenetic analysis in high-risk populations would attest to the power of this procedure. When combined with the other procedures previously discussed, it is my opinion that we have the tools to prevent substantially the induction of cancer and genetic abnormalities in the occupational setting and probably in the population as a whole. It is entirely possible that we now have tools at our disposal for human monitoring that do not suffer from the severe limitations of the classical epidemiological approach and where relevancy is hard to challenge because these tests are carried out directly in man. One of the major advantages of such studies is the fact that they can be conducted prior to the onset of any clinical symptoms. The outlined battery of tests probably offers the best approach to meeting the challenge of establishing a safe work environment in the specific area of chronic toxicity having to do with carcinogenicity and mutagenicity.

REFERENCES

Beckman, G., L. Beckman, I. Nordenson, and S. Nordstrom. 1979. Chromosomal aberrations in workers exposed to arsenic. In *Genetic damage in man caused by environmental agents* (ed. Kare Berg), p. 205. Academic Press, New York.

Department of Health, Education, and Welfare (DHEW). 1970. *Vital statistics of the United States, vol. 2, Mortality*. Public Health Service, Washington, D.C.

Dobias, L. 1980. Human blood mutagenicity for *Salmonella typhimurium* tester strains after oral application of entizol. *Mutat. Res.* **77**:357.

Ducatman, A., K. Hirschhorn, and I.J. Selikoff. 1975. Vinyl chloride exposure and human chromosome aberrations. *Mutat. Res.* **31**:163.

Environmental Protection Agency (EPA). 1979. Carcinogen assessment group: Assessment of acrylonitrile. PB80-146301, December.

Etteldorf, J.N., C.D. West, J.A. Pitcock, and D.L. Williams. 1976. Gonadal function, testicular history and meiosis following cyclophoychamide therapy in patients with nephrotic syndrome. *J. Pediatr.* **88**:206.

Forni, A. and G.C. Secci. 1972. Chromosome changes in preclinical and clinical lead poisoning and correlation with biochemical findings. In *Proceedings of the International Symposium Environmental Health Aspects of Lead,* p. 473, Elsevier, Amsterdam.

Funes-Cravioto, F., B. Lambert, J. Lindsten, L. Ehrenberg, A.T. Natarajan, and S. Osterman-Golkar. 1975. Chromosome aberrations in workers exposed to vinyl chloride. *Lancet* **i**:459.

Garry, V.F., J. Hozier, D. Jacobs, R.L. Wade, and D.G. Gray. 1979. Ethylene ozide: Evidence of human chromosomal effects. *Environmental Mutagens* **1**:375.

Garza-Chapa, R., C.H. Leal-Garza, and G. Molina-Ballesteros. 1977. Analysis eromosomico en personas professionalmente expuestas a contaminacion con plomo. *Arch. Invest. Med.* **8**:11.

International Agency for Research on Cancer (IARC). 1980. Long-term and short-term screening assays for carcinogens: A critical appraisal. *IARC Monogr. Eval. Carcinog. Risk Chem. Hum.* **Suppl. 2**:227.

Kapp, W.R., Jr., N.S. Benge, D. Picciano, D.J. Killian, M.S. Legator, and C.B. Jacobson. 1980. Monitoring Y chromosomal nondisjunction in human with the YFF sperm test. In *Proceedings of workplace and methodology for assessing reproductive hazards in the workplace* (ed. P.F. Infante and M.S. Legator), p. 307. PHHS (NIOSH) Publication No. 81-100, Government Printing Office, Washington, D.C.

Katosova, L.D. 1973. Cytogenetic analysis of peripheral blood of workers engaged in the production of chloroprene. *Gig. Tr. Prof. Zabol* **10**:30.

Kucerova, M., V.S. Zhurkor, Z. Polivkova, and J.E. Ivanove. 1977. Mutagenic effect of epichlorohydrin, II. Analysis of chromosomal aberrations in lymphocytes of persons occupationally exposed to epichlorohydrin. *Mutat. Res.* **48**:355.

Legator, M.S., L. Truang, and T.H. Connor. 1979a. Analysis of body fluids including alkylation of macromolecules for detection of mutagenic agents. *Chem. Mutagens* **5**:1.

Legator, M.S., T.G. Pullin and T.H. Connor. 1979b. The isolation and detection of mutagenic substances in body fluids and tissues of animals and body fluids of human subjects. In *Handbook of mutagenicity testing procedures* (ed. B. Kilbey et al.), p. 149. Elsevier, Amsterdam.

Meretoja, T., H. Vainio, M. Sorse, and H. Harkonen. 1977. Occupational styrene exposure and chromosomal aberrations. *Mutat. Res.* **56**:193.

Nordenson, I., G. Beckman, L. Beckman, and S. Nordstrom. 1978. Occupational and environmental risks in and around smelter in northern Sweden, II. Chromosomal aberrations in workers exposed to arsenic. *Hereditas* **88**:47.

O'Berg, M.T. 1977. Epidemiological study of workers exposed to acrylonitrile. Preliminary results submitted to NIOSH, OSHA, EPA, DDA, NCI, and IARC.

Picciano, D. 1979a. Cytogenetic investigation of occupational exposure to epichlorohydrin. *Mutat. Res.* **66**:169.

———. 1979b. Cytogenetic study of workers exposed to benzene. *Environ. Res.* **19**:33.

Sanotskii, I.V. 1976. Aspects of the toxicology of chloroprene: Immediate and long-term effects. *Environ. Health Perspect.* **17**:85.

Sievert, D. and U. Simon. 1973. Cyclophosphamide pilot study of genetically active metabolites in the urine of a treated human patient: Induction of mitotic gene conversion in yeast. *Mutat. Res.* **19**:65.

Silezneva, T.G. and N.P. Korman. Analysis of chromosomes of somatic cells in patients treated with antitumor drugs. *Sov. Genet.* **9**:1575.

Stich, H.F. and A.B. Acton. 1979. Can mutation theories of carcinogenesis set priorities for carcinogen testing programs? *Can. J. Genet. Cytol.* **21**: 155.

Tough, I.M., P.G. Smith, W.M. Court Brown, and D.G. Harden. 1970. Chromosome studies in workers exposed to atmospheric benzene, the possible influence of age. *Eur. J. Cancer* **19**:49.

Zudova, Z. and K. Landa. 1977. Genetic risk of occupational exposures to haloethers. *Mutat. Res.* **46**:242.

An Industry-sponsored Mortality Surveillance Program

SUSAN G. AUSTIN
Union Carbide Corporation
270 Park Avenue
New York, New York 10017

Increasing concerns regarding the relationship of occupational factors to health status have stimulated many large corporations to implement company-sponsored morbidity or mortality surveillance programs. Although there is increasing interest in surveillance programs that will monitor the health status of active employees to detect hazards in the immediate work environment, such programs have not been forthcoming due to the absence of valid biological indicators or "precursors" of disease in man. When a company employs a sufficiently large number of workers, surveillance programs that monitor the mortality experience of certain segments of the population become a feasible and practical alternative. This report describes a mortality surveillance program being developed at Union Carbide Corporation (UCC).

PURPOSE

The purpose of UCC's Mortality Surveillance Program is to provide management with an internal warning system for identification of potential health hazards, past or present, in the work environment. It is termed a "surveillance program," rather than a "mortality study," to signify its emphasis on hypothesis generation rather than on hypothesis testing. Comparison of the mortality profile of one plant with some predetermined reference population may provide an indication of where a more in-depth investigation, such as a cohort or case-control study, is needed.

SCOPE

Because this program is relatively new (started in 1977), mortality surveillance is at present limited to numerator data (that is, deaths only) occurring among active and former employees. This includes those categories of deaths known to the employer on a systematic basis. Although there has been speculation that the study of these deaths may lead to an underrepresentation of certain types of

Table 1
Terminations and Deaths Known to Union Carbide per Year

Employee status	Number of terminations	Number of deaths
Active (at death)	375	375
Retired	2,500	700
Disabled	300	150
Other	9,000	75
Vested	1,350	75
Nonvested	7,650	0
Total	12,175	1,375

deaths, i.e. malignant neoplasms (Redmond and Breslin 1975), there is at present no basis for such speculation. Although some bias may indeed be introduced from the exclusion of employees who terminate from a company without any disability or pension benefits, little research has been directed at this question.

In Table 1 are shown the segments of the employee population that can be followed readily for mortality surveillance. This table indicates the total number of employees who terminate each year by reason for termination and the total number of deaths per year that occur in each population group. The total active UCC population is about 80,000 persons. There is a turnover of about 13-15% per year, or 12,000 persons in 1980. Of these, approximately 375, or 3%, are due to death. All of these deaths are known to the company. Another 2500 (20%) retire each year. There are currently about 20,000 retirees among whom there are approximately 700 deaths each year, all of which are known to the corporation. There are approximately 300 total and permanent disabilities per year and from this population (about 5000) there are approximately 150 deaths, all of which are also known to the company. There are approximately 9000 terminations per year for reasons other than death, retirement, or disability. Approximately 15% of these are "vested," meaning generally that they have 10 or more years of company service and are entitled to a pension at retirement age. (Vesting requirements changed in 1973 from 15 years to 10 years company service). These deaths are also known to the company. Either the employees' survivor will notify the company in the event of death or the company will attempt to contact the employee at age 65 to determine why the pension has not been matured.

METHODS

The methods employed in the Carbide Surveillance Program fall under four categories: (1) notification; (2) data collection; (3) data storage; and (4) data analysis.

Notification

Notification of deaths among active and inactive employees is obtained from two sources–the payroll department and the benefits department. The payroll department is the only source of notification of deaths among active employees not covered under the group life insurance program. This represents a small but important number of deaths among active employees. The remainder of death notifications are received through the benefits department.

Data Collection

Data collection (Fig. 1) for the mortality surveillance program is derived from two documents–the death certificate and the Mortality Survey Questionnaire. In most instances, a death certificate is supplied by the Group Insurance Department. Where it is not, it can usually be obtained by writing to the appropriate state health department (provided that does not happen to be New York City). Underlying and contributory causes of death are coded by the Statistics Department of the Metropolitan Life Insurance Company and the underlying cause is selected through the Automated Classification of Medical Entities computer program (ACME). Deaths prior to January 1, 1980 are coded to the International Classification of Diseases (ICD), 8th revision, and deaths after January 1, 1980 are coded to the 9th revision.

Upon receipt of a death notification, a questionnaire is initiated by the Epidemiology Data Group and sent to the plant where the employee last worked. The complete work history is obtained from the plant employee relations department, and a limited health history is obtained from the plant

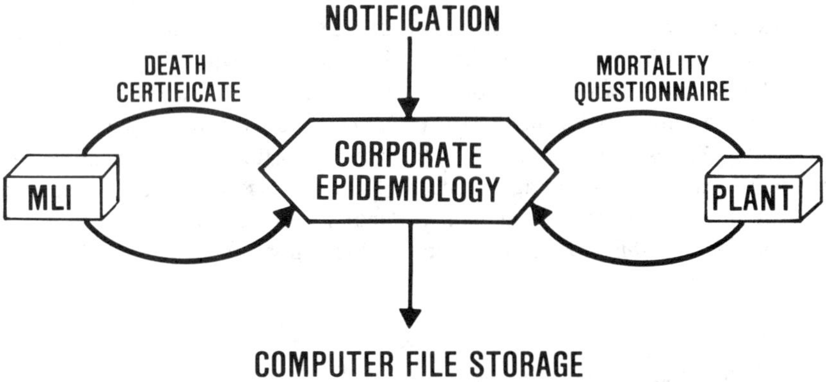

Figure 1
Data collection

Table 2
Contents of MMR

Personal identifiers	Work history	Medical information
Name	date of hire	smoking history
Social Security number	date of termination	causes of death
Date of birth	payroll status	autopsy
Date of death	plant locations	location of death
Sex	termination reason	
Race		

medical department. Upon completion, the questionnaire is returned to the corporate headquarters.

Data Storage

Data for the surveillance program is stored alphabetically in hard copy files and an abstract of the information received pertaining to the employee death is completed for input into the computerized Master Mortality Register (MMR). Updates and edits of the file are performed weekly. The data content of this file is listed in Table 2.

Analyses

On a periodic basis, proportionate mortality ratios (PMRs) and proportionate cancer mortality ratios (PCMRs) can be generated from the MMR file by division or plant. Because collection of death certificates by the Corporate Medical Department only began in 1977, the early 1970s are not as well represented in the MMR as are the later years in the decade. For analysis purposes, each individual is classified to the last plant at which he or she worked.

All deaths for white males on the file between 1970 and 1979 are used in the computation of PMRs and PCMRs using the 1975 white male death rates for the United States as the source of reference proportions. These analyses are indirectly standardized for age at death by 5-year age intervals. A separate analysis is done for each plant with a minimum of 50 cancer deaths, as the principal focus of this program has been on cancer mortality.

RESULTS

Table 3 shows an example of the results of this program for one plant. Both PMRs and PCMRs are calculated for the sake of comparison. It is clear from all of our analyses that the cause-specific PMRs overestimate the underlying cancer

Table 3
Analysis of Plant-specific PMRs and PCMRs for White Male Deaths January 1, 1970-June 30, 1979

Cause of death	Number observed	PMR	PCMR
All causes	207		
Malignant neoplasms	50	111.8	
Buccal cavity	1	72.5	67.9
Digestive organs	18	153.0	137.5
Respiratory system	17	102.2	93.3
Genital-urinary system	6	92.5	85.8
Lymphatic tissues	5	125.3	111.4
Other	3	59.4	52.1

risk and are influenced by the distribution of deaths in other categories, such as respiratory diseases, cardiovascular diseases, and accidents. The PCMR is much lower than the PMR for each cause-specific cancer category and provides a better indication of a possible cancer excess.

Table 4 illustrates the comparison of PMRs for all malignant neoplasms across six divisions. This suggests a slight excess of cancer deaths as a proportion of all deaths compared with expectation based on the U.S. population—again, a result likely attributable to the deficit of deaths in other disease categories (i.e., circulatory and respiratory) that have been associated with the healthy-worker effect in most studies of employed populations.

Table 5 compares lung cancer PCMRs across divisions. Some variation can be seen here, although one must remember that these ratios are not directly comparable because of the indirect method of age standardization used. Some of the variation may be attributable to differing age distributions. As with the PMR, the PCMR is also influenced by the relative excesses or deficits of deaths

Table 4
Comparison of PMRs for All Malignant Neoplasms among Six Divisions: January 1, 1970-June 30, 1979

Division	Observed	Expected	PMR
A	124	117.2	105.7
B	50	44.7	111.8
C	75	64.2	116.7
D	266	223.1	119.2
E	437	392.6	111.3
F	186	175.0	106.2

Table 5
Comparison of Site-specific PCMRs by Division—Lung Cancer Deaths: January 1, 1970-June 30, 1979

Division	Observed	Expected	PCMR
A	46	43.2	106.4
B	16	17.4	92.0
C	16	24.9	64.0
D	120	99.2	120.9
E	126	157.9	79.7
F	73	65.0	112.2

in other cancer categories, and it is not possible to identify whether a proportion is elevated because the underlying rate is elevated or because some other underlying rate may be depressed. Although this system has its limitations, it can and is being used to determine directions for further research.

Discussion

In discussing the utility of the PMR statistic in a surveillance system, the fundamental difficulty with such a proportion is that it is numerator data and as such cannot be used to indicate an underlying rate or the underlying risk of dying from a particular disease. It is virtually impossible to distinguish between a PMR that is elevated because the underlying population death rate is elevated or one that is elevated because some other underlying (disease-specific) death rate is too low. This is of particular concern in occupational studies in our industry where we know that the underlying death rates for cardiovascular and respiratory diseases are significantly lower than those of the general population (due in part to preemployment screening and self-selection), yet the death rate from malignant neoplasms is generally comparable. For a typical employee group, therefore, one can expect the PMRs for malignant neoplasms to be overstated due to the proportionate overrepresentation of these deaths relative to other causes. The use of the PMR statistic in a cancer surveillance program is therefore somewhat misleading because it will almost always produce a high rate of false positive results that could be avoided in part by calculation of the PCMR.

The existence of this program serves to provide some assurance to employers and employees that health hazards in the workplace will be identified. The success of the attainment of this goal is yet to be proved. Some disease excesses may escape identification because not all of the deaths of former employees are covered. In addition, because of the methodology used (i.e., proportions) some excesses may be hidden by even larger excesses. There is always the problem of the inaccuracy of death certificate diagnoses and the inability to identify some important diseases (e.g., skin cancer) that do not lead routinely to death or appear on the death certificate.

There are other problems peculiar to the internal system. The classification of an employee to the last location at which he or she worked ignores the fact that he may have had multiple plant assignments in his company history. This is a problem only for salaried employees who tend to transfer frequently from plant to plant. (We are now coding up to 5 plant assignments on the analysis file to alleviate this particular problem.)

There are other problems that have been identified and for which we are seeking solutions. We have created a data base that should be useful not only for surveillance but for special case-control studies as well as cohort mortality studies.

Future plans include the expansion of this program to a population-based surveillance system that will enable calculation of standardized mortality ratios (SMRs) for all employees with a minimum of 1 year of company service.

Special Study

I would like to mention briefly a pilot study underway that is rather unique and interesting for several reasons.

This study population was defined as all hourly or salaried workers employed in one division on January 1, 1974, who had at least 10 years of company service, meaning that they were all vested. We restricted the cohort to 2220 white males and have followed this group using Social Security searches through the end of 1977. In Figure 2 is indicated the current status determined from follow-up. In all, 65% are still active; there have been 781 terminations during the 6-year period January 1, 1974, through December 31, 1979. Of these, all but 34, or 4%, terminated in one of the categories that would be readily traced through the company (death, retirement, disability). Social Security found only one death that was not known through company sources and this was an example of a vested employee who died at the age of 55. The company would not normally know about his death until he would have been 65. Another three deaths among retirees and apparently not known to the company were reported by Social Security. When these were investigated (benefits department sent an investigator to the alleged decedents' homes, it was discovered that the three retirees in question were alive and well and that their next of kin were not fraudulently collecting pension checks on their behalf.

The overall PMRs and SMRs for this cohort are shown in Table 6. It is immediately apparent that there are either some deaths that have been missed or there is an extreme healthy-worker effect in operation. It is not likely that any deaths have been missed in this group and, therefore, the low SMRs are probably a valid statement regarding the health status of a group of employees who are

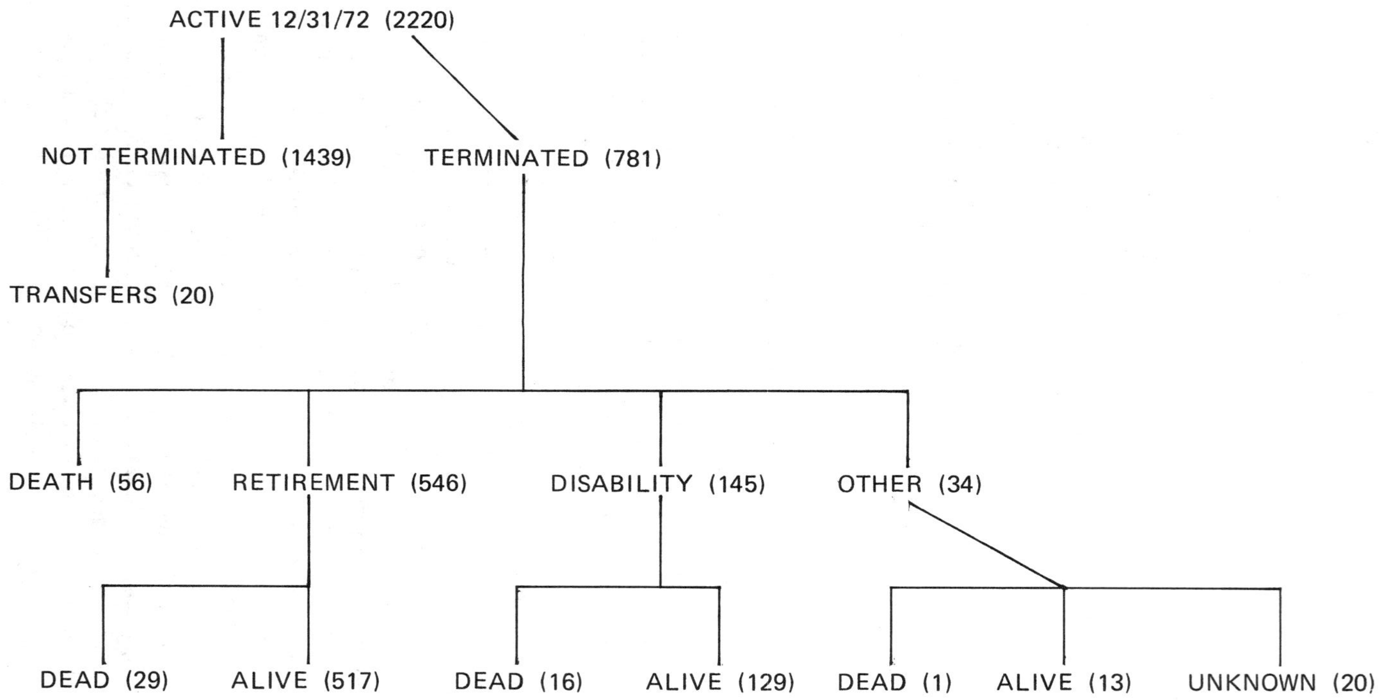

Figure 2
Status of special study cohort.

Table 6
PMRs and SMRs in a Cohort of 2220 White Males

All causes	PMR	SMR
All causes		58
All malignant neoplasms	128	71
Digestive system	159	87
Respiratory system	113	64
Genital-urinary system	164	77
Lymphopoeitic system	183	107
Circulatory diseases	116	64
Respiratory diseases	21	10
Digestive diseases	59	39
Genital-urinary diseases	139	72
External causes	58	42

unusual in that they have remained with the same company for 10 or more years. The stability of the group may have a relationship to a less stressful or more healthy life-style that is readily exhibited in the overall mortality experience.

REFERENCES

Redmond, C.K. and Breslin, P. 1975. Comparison of methods for assessing occupational hazards. *J. Occup. Med.* **17**:313.

COMMENTS

SILVERSTEIN: I am wondering, with respect to this last investigation that you described, whether or not there is an equivalent group of workers who had 10 years of service with the company and were alive in 1973 but were not active employees at that time. If so, do you have any idea how large that group might be?

AUSTIN: This group was selected as sort of a pilot test. We were thinking of developing a surveillance program that would be based only on people who had 10 years of employment. There was a computer tape available on this division–the end of the year payroll tape in 1973. We don't have the kind of data that you are talking about now, so I can't answer that question. But that is why we originally looked at this group.

McMICHAEL: We all seem to use different terminology when referring to proportionate mortality ratio. Many use PMR when they should use SPMR. They are both age standardized but we refer to it differently. Perhaps we should all decide on similar terminology.

AUSTIN: Yes. You are right. To clarify, the figures I have presented are age standardized.

ACHESON: Am I correct to assume that the National Death Index will be able to report on all the employees who left and that studies like yours will be available as well? What percentage of the employees in your study left before they were vested?

AUSTIN: 63% left.

ACHESON: Right. Now, when the National Death Index is available you will be able to report on what happened to these people? Is that true of all industrial cohort studies?

AUSTIN: I would think that would be true. You have to start with the vested employees. What makes it attractive to follow them is that the company usually keeps a file with their Social Security numbers, because they are entitled to payment. The vested employees that left maybe 8 years ago may still be able to be traced if the company still has the Social Security numbers on those employees.

PADDLE: I wonder if I can offer a comment that I hope will be helpful. I think any chemical company that is brave enough to give itself a

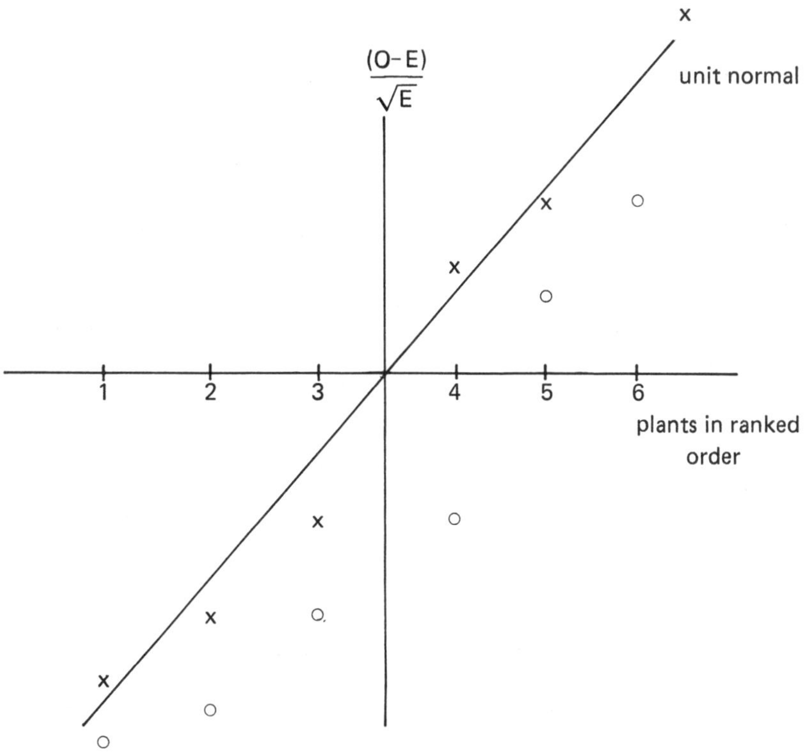

Figure A
PMR analysis of company data. (○) SMRs; (x) PMRs.

hypothesis-generating system ought also to have a hypothesis-destructive system.

What you can, in fact, do with data such as Susan has presented is to take an ordinary piece of probability graph paper and calculate $O - E/\sqrt{E}$ as being something that is approximately normal (Fig. A). One can then draw the normal distribution mean zero S. D. 1. Then one can find the expected value for the lowest, next lowest, next lowest, up to the highest value of any number of SMRs (○) or PMRs (x) that are calculated. It is better with PMRs, because they will go through the origin. The SMRs will be lower down. So let's take PMRs, because the standard normal line is a reasonable one to use.

For the six plants that Susan had with six lung cancer rates, she might say "I am a bit worried about that one, but, fortunately, that one is low, so ought we to look at them any further." If she takes from tables the expected value for the lowest of six, next lowest of six, next lowest of six, etc., this will give her six points to plot. In this case three of them were negative and three were positive. They might very well come quite close to a straight line.

So, she could say, instead, "We ought to look at that one, but it is, after all, only the sixth highest of six normally distributed values. Perhaps it is not too worrying after all. But, we have got a defense mechanism that says, if you look often enough, you will find something that big quite often."

You can do it equally well for one plant and all the diseases. You can take the lowest disease, the next lowest disease, etc. You can do it for 55 diseases, 10 diseases, any number of diseases–a couple of points, for clarification. You don't need all the points that come in near zero because you can't see them and they are unimportant. But you can take the highest few of the 55. These numbers are tabulated, and you can take them out of any decent book of tables. And if the figures are near a straight line, then you can say this looks like normally distributed data.

We ought to be worried about these high values, particularly if we have got prior information that makes us worried about them. But at least it is some sort of defense mechanism that will keep the legislators and unions and other people off your backs while you are looking at the data.

I am not saying to generate hypotheses and then just chuck them in the bin, I am saying have a defense mechanism because it makes statistical sense that most of them will be false positives.

An Epidemiologic Study of Workers Potentially Exposed to Brominated Chemicals: With a Discussion of Multifactor Adjustment

OTTO WONG
Biometric Research Institute
1010 Wisconsin Avenue, N.W.
Washington, D.C. 20007

Recently, attention has been focused on the human toxic effects of exposure to a number of brominated compounds, including 1,2-dibromo-3-chloropropane (DBCP), Tris (2,3-dibromopropyl)phosphate, and polybrominated biphenyls (PBB). These chemicals are suspected of producing a number of toxic effects, including cancers in animals and sterility in humans.

Because of these concerns, an epidemiologic study of chemical workers potentially exposed to these brominated chemicals was conducted. (In addition, these workers were also potentially exposed to trimethylene chlorobromide [TMCB], various organic and inorganic bromides, and DDT.) The primary goals of this study were to determine the cause-specific mortality experience of these workers and to establish an epidemiologic data base on the current employees so that their health can be monitored prospectively on a periodic basis. This report will focus on the mortality experience of the workers.

METHODS AND MATERIALS

The cohort consisted of chemical workers from locations where potential exposure to brominated compounds existed. Included in this study were persons who had been employed between 1935 and 1976 at three manufacturing plants (two in Michigan and one in Arkansas) and a research facility in Michigan.

The personnel records maintained generally included the following information: Name, social security number, sex, date of birth, date of hire, date of separation, and summary work history. Race was also recorded on some records. Dates of death and some death certificates were available for a few persons who died while employed or after retiring. The employment records maintained at the research facility did not have summary work histories, but separate personnel action forms giving the employees' names, dates of birth, dates of hire, present status, and proposed status changes. These were used in reconstructing work histories. All personnel records were microfilmed or photocopied.

By using the microfilmed or photocopied personnel records, the following items for each employee were abstracted onto a coding form for entry into a computer:

1. name,
2. social security number,
3. date of birth,
4. sex,
5. state of residence,
6. race (when available),
7. date of hire,
8. date of separation,
9. date of death (if applicable),
10. employment status (e.g., active, separated, retired, etc.),
11. vital status,
12. vital status source,
13. summary work history (department and date of transfer),
14. film reference.

At the onset of the study, there were 508 individuals who were known to be living as of the study cutoff date (December 31, 1976). Of the 508, 507 were actively employed as of December 31, 1976. The remaining individual was known to be living as of that date, because he died subsequently.

In addition, 11 persons were identified as deceased (with death certificates) by the employment records. However, it was necessary to conduct vital status follow-up on 3695 former employees who had terminated their employment prior to the study cutoff date. The follow-up consisted of a local inquiry and a search through the files of both the Social Security Administration (SSA) and the motor vehicle bureaus (MVBs) of several states.

The local follow-up process involved contacting the former employees or their families, their former coworkers, known friends, or other reliable sources and asking whether the person was living or deceased. By this process, 2004 persons were determined to be living and 364 were identified as deceased. Whenever possible, information on place and date of death was obtained for the deceased. Of the 2004 persons identified as living, 11% (220) were contacted directly, while family members were contacted for 78% (1564), and coworkers, friends, or neighbors were contacted for 11% (220). For each of these 2004 individuals, the specifics of the follow-up, including the names of persons contacted, telephone numbers, and dates, were documented. Thus, the vital status can be verified independently.

Follow-up using the SSA files was conducted for the remaining 1327 persons of unknown vital status. The 364 persons identified as deceased were also submitted to the SSA to obtain additional information on date and place of death. A total of 1640 punch cards was submitted to the SSA; 51 persons were excluded because of unknown social security numbers.

From the 1640 social security numbers submitted, 560 employees were identified as deceased, as death claims had been filed, and 736 persons were identified as living as of December 31, 1976. For 344 persons, SSA was unable to provide any information. Among these 344, 33 persons were previously identified by local follow-up as deceased. Upon the completion of the SSA vital status follow-up, there were 362 (344 - 33 + 51) persons of unknown vital status.

Vital status follow-up through various state MVBs was pursued after the SSA follow-up was completed. Driving records were requested from the state MVBs, and persons were considered living if they had renewed their driver's licenses after December 31, 1976. Additional follow-up by telephone was conducted for those persons who had renewed their licenses prior to the study cutoff date by obtaining their telephone numbers at the addresses listed on their driving records. Requests were made for a total of 349 individuals. Thirteen unknowns were excluded from this follow-up because their dates of birth, a necessary identifier for MVB follow-up, were unknown. It was necessary to conduct MVB follow-up in seven states. As a result, 83 persons were identified as living.

Upon the completion of all vital status follow-up, 279 persons were still of unknown vital status. These 279 persons comprised 6.62% of the study population; 72 of the 279 were females and 207 were males. Thirteen unknowns (1 female and 12 males) were excluded from final analysis because their dates of birth were unknown. A total of 3331 persons (2827 males and 504 females) or 79.05% of the study population was determined to be living as of December 31, 1976, and 604 persons (14.33%) were identified as deceased. Of the deceased, 26 were females and 578 were males. Figure 1 summarizes the results of the various follow-up procedures.

Death certificates were requested for all persons identified as deceased from the appropriate state vital statistics departments. In all, 561 death certificates (93.05%) were obtained; 21 (80.77%) death certificates were obtained for the 26 deceased females and 541 (93.60%) death certificates were obtained for the 578 deceased males.

STATISTICAL ANALYSIS

Cohort Description

There was a total of 2214 individuals included in the follow-up. Among this group, there were 602 females. Because males and females have considerably different mortality experiences, and because the number of females is too small for a separate statistical analysis (only 26 known deaths among the females), the females are not included in the following analysis.

Also excluded from the following analysis are 33 males whose dates of birth were not available from employment records. As such, there was insufficient information to include these 33 in the mortality analysis.

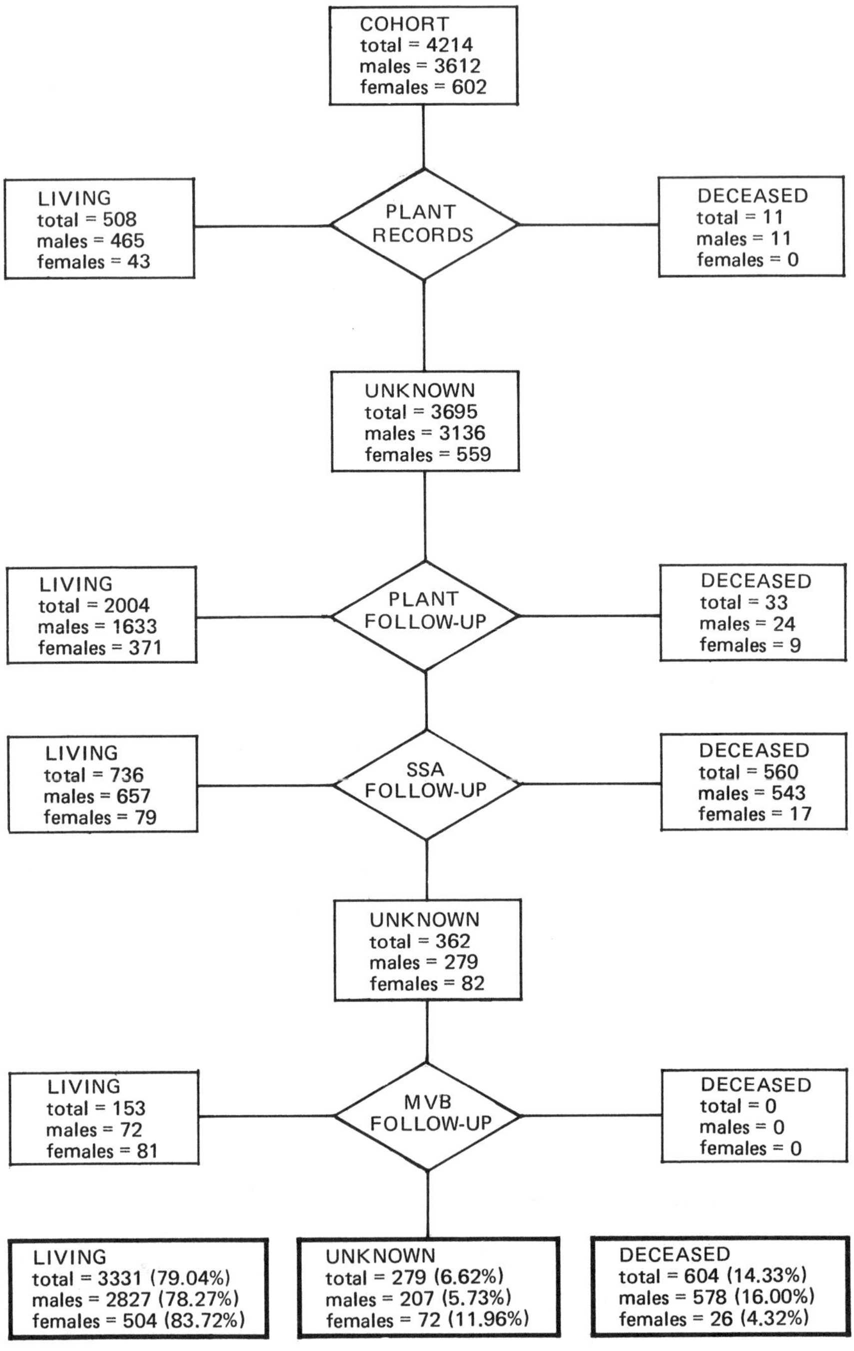

Figure 1

Summary of vital status follow-up

Race identification was not recorded on all employment records. However, a company officer indicated that "there has never been a higher figure than about 4% (of minorities). No blacks were ever employed at the plant. The predominant minority hire(d) was Spanish American and that did reach a figure in the area of 4% at times." Because Spanish Americans are classified in the broad category "white" in the national mortality statistics, the entire cohort will be assumed to consist of white males only.

Table 1 shows the distribution of the 3579 male workers by employment status as of December 31, 1976. In the entire cohort, only 461 (12.88%) males were employed actively as of December 31, 1976. On the other hand, there were 2949 (82.40%) male workers who had terminated their employment between 1935 and 1976. In addition, there were a few individuals who left for various other reasons, such as retirement, disability, leave of absence, transfer, and death. The distribution of the cohort by length of employment is presented in Table 2. The distribution demonstrates a high turnover rate. Almost half (44.87%) of the cohort worked for less than 6 months, and the majority (53.56%) worked for less than a year. Only 11.40% of the cohort worked for more than 10 years. The average length of employment was 3 years and 9 months.

Mortality Analysis for Entire Cohort

In the previous chapter, the procedure for vital status determination was described. As shown in Table 3, of the 3579 males included in the cohort for analysis, the vital status of 195 (5.45%) individuals remained unknown at the end of the study. A total of 2806 male workers (78.40%) was identified as living. Of the 578 (16.15%) identified deaths, death certificates were obtained for all but 37 cases (6.40%).

Table 1
Distribution by Employment Status of 3579 Male Workers Potentially Exposed to Brominated Chemicals

Employment status	Frequency	Percent
Active	461	12.88
Separated	2949	82.40
Retired	85	2.37
Disabled	28	0.78
Leave of absence	3	0.08
Transferred	3	0.08
Died while employed	50[a]	1.40
Total	3579	99.99

[a]11 with death certificates.

Table 2
Distribution by Length of Employment of 3579 Male Workers Potentially Exposed to Brominated Chemcials

Length of employment	Frequency	Percent
1 month	586	16.37
1-5 months	1020	28.50
6-11 months	311	8.69
1-4 years	954	26.66
5-9 years	297	8.30
10-14 years	132	3.69
15-19 years	81	2.26
20-24 years	86	2.40
25-29 years	56	1.56
30-34 years	42	1.17
35-39 years	8	0.22
40 years	3	0.08
Unknown	3	0.08
Total	3579	99.98

Causes of death were coded by a trained nosologist according to the 8th revision of the International Classification of Diseases (ICD). Among the males, a total of 541 deaths was coded.

The most common summary index for assessing the risk of death in a population studied prospectively is the standardized mortality ratio (SMR). Basically, the number of deaths occurring in the study population is compared with the number of deaths that would have been expected if the study population had, adjusting for age and time period, the same mortality experience as a comparable nonexposed population. During the observation period of the study, the cohort members entered the study at different points in time; some

Table 3
Distribution by Vital Status (as of 12/31/76) of 3579 Male Workers Potentially Exposed to Brominated Chemicals

Vital status	Frequency		Percent	
Living	2806		78.40	
Deceased	578		16.15	
With Death Certificates		(541)		(93.60)
Without Death Certificates		(37)		(6.40)
Unknown	195		5.45	
Total	3579		100.00	

died, and some were lost to follow-up. For all these reasons, cohort members are observed for various lengths of time and, therefore, do not contribute equally to the "population at risk." To utilize fully the period of observation for each member and to weigh properly the SMR, the concept of person-years is used in the analysis. The basic unit of computation is the number of years each employee was followed, from the date of first employment to the end of the study period, or to the date of death. Each year contributed by an individual worker is classified by age and calendar year, and these person-years are then summed up by age and calendar year. The U.S. national age-sex-race-year-cause-specific mortality rates for 5-year time periods from 1925 to 1975 are applied to those person-years to obtain the number of deaths from a particular cause to be expected from an equal number of person-years similar in age, sex, race, and calendar year. SMRs can be computed by expressing the actually observed deaths as percentages of the expected. An SMR higher (lower) than 100 indicates an excess (a deficit) in mortality. The deviation from 100 is tested to determine whether it is statistically significant. The statistical analysis was performed using a standard computer program (Monson 1974; an updated version of this program was used in the present study). This program computes an SMR for every cause of death included, even if only one death is attributed to that cause. Some epidemiologists and biostatisticians prefer not to calculate SMR when the number of deaths is two or less (or even five or less), because of the large amount of variability associated with such a small number of deaths. The approach in this report is to provide all SMRs and their confidence intervals (CI). If the number of deaths is small, the corresponding variance, and hence, the CI, will be large. In this case, unless the SMR is extremely high, the result will not be statistically significant. As such, the significance test takes into account the small number involved. However, one concern is that for rare diseases, one or two cases will be adequate for statistical significance. Whereas for rare diseases expected deaths can be calculated down to a small fraction, in reality deaths occur in whole numbers. As such, statistically significant SMRs with only one or two observed deaths should be interpreted with caution.

Because, according to plant personnel, no blacks had ever been employed at the large Michigan plant, which contributed approximately 95% of the cohort, the mortality rates for U.S. white males were used in the analysis. Individuals with unknown vital status and those presumed dead but without a death certificate or a date of death were treated as lost to follow-up on the last day of contact (termination). Deaths with a known date of death but without a death certificate were included in the overall mortality analysis but not in the cause-specific analysis.

The observed deaths, expected deaths, and SMRs by cause for the entire cohort are listed in Table 4 (pages 366-367). The limits of the 95% CI for the SMRs also are presented. If the lower limit is higher than 100, there is a significant mortality excess at the 0.05 level. If the upper limit is lower than 100,

Table 4
Observed and Expected Deaths by Cause, SMRs, and Their 95% Confidence Limits for the Entire Cohort of 3579 Male Workers Potentially Exposed to Brominated Chemicals

Cause of death (8th ICDA)	Observed deaths	Expected deaths	SMR	Lower limit	Upper limit
All causes	543	614.34	88[b]	81	96
Infective and parasitic diseases (000-139)	6	11.37	53	19	115
All cancers (140-209)	112	110.29	102	84	122
Cancer of buccal cavity and pharynx (140-149)	3	3.73	81	16	235
Cancer of digestive system (150-159)	18	32.58	55[b]	33	87
Cancer of stomach (151)	2	7.07	28	3	102
Cancer of large intestine (153)	6	9.78	61	22	134
Cancer of rectum (154)	2	3.93	51	6	184
Cancer of liver (155)	3	2.41	124	25	363
Cancer of pancreas (157)	5	6.00	83	27	195
Cancer of respiratory system (160-163)	46	34.07	135	99	180
Cancer of larnyx (161)	1	1.69	59	1	330
Cancer of lung (162-163)	42	31.95	131	95	178
Cancer of prostate (185)	11	6.71	164	82	293
Cancer of testis (186)	2	1.04	193	22	697
Cancer of bladder (188)	3	3.25	92	19	270
Cancer of kidney (189)	4	2.76	145	39	370
Cancer of brain (191)	5	3.78	132	43	309

Lymphatic and hematopoietic cancer (200-209)	13	11.73	111	59	190
Hodgkin's disease (201)	1	1.95	51	1	286
Leukemia and aleukemia (204-207)	9	4.83	187	85	354
Diabetes mellitus (250)	19	8.65	220[b]	132	343
Diseases of blood and blood-forming organs (280-289)	1	1.61	62	1	346
Diseases of nervous system and sense organs (320-389)	6	5.59	107	39	234
Diseases of circulatory system (390-458)	258	309.03	83[b]	74	94
Chronic rheumatic heart disease (393-398)	4	7.54	53	14	136
Arteriosclerotic heart disease (including coronary heart disease (410-413)	184	209.87	88	75	101
Cerebrovascular disease (430-438)	37	42.03	88	62	121
Nonmalignant respiratory disease (460-519)	26	32.32	80	53	118
Pneumonia (480-486)	6	13.15	46[a]	17	99
Emphysema (492)	9	7.76	116	53	220
Asthma (493)	1	1.52	66	1	366
Diseases of digestive system (520-577)	15	31.44	48[b]	27	79
Cirrhosis of liver (571)	4	15.83	25[b]	7	65
Diseases of genito-urinary system (580-629)	8	10.47	76	33	151
Symptoms, senility, and ill-defined conditions (780-796)	4	6.52	61	17	157
Accidents, poisonings, and violence (E800-E999)	79	77.27	102	81	127
Accidents (800-949)	55	54.67	101	76	131
Motor vehicle accidents (810-827)	35	26.59	132	92	183
Suicide (950-959)	20	16.66	120	73	185

Person-years = 68,821.7; persons = 3579.
[a]Statistically significant at 0.05 level.
[b]Statistically significant at 0.01 level.

there is a significant deficit. Similarly, the 99% CI also have been calculated for selected SMRs, but not presented in the table. A total of 543 deaths was included in the analysis (two with date of death but no death certificate). As 614.34 deaths were expected, the overall SMR is 88, indicating that these male workers enjoyed a mortality deficit of 12%, compared to U.S. white males. This deficit is statistically significant at the 0.01 level because the upper limit of the 99% CI is less than 100.

A total of 112 deaths was attributed to malignant neoplasms, practically identical to the expectation of 110.29 based on the U.S. white male cancer mortality rates. However, the site-specific cancer mortality observed in this cohort of male workers deviated from the expected, although only in one case is the deviation statistically significant at the 0.05 level. For cancer of the digestive system, 18 deaths were observed, compared to an expected 32.58. The corresponding SMR is 55 ($p < 0.01$). That is, the digestive cancer mortality of this cohort is only 55% of the expectation based on a comparable group of U.S. white males similar in age during the same period of time. The deficit appears to have come from cancer of the stomach.

None of the other site-specific cancer SMRs examined is statistically significant. However, it should be noted that 46 deaths from cancer of the respiratory system occurred, while only 34.07 were expected. The corresponding SMR of 135 is very close to statistical significance ($p \approx 0.05$). In addition, there were 11 observed deaths from prostate cancer, compared to 6.71 expected (SMR = 164, nonsignificant), and 9 observed leukemia deaths, compared to 4.83 expected (SMR = 187, nonsignificant).

For diabetes mellitus, 19 deaths were observed, with only 8.65 expected based on the U.S. experience, adjusting for age, race, sex, and calendar time. The corresponding SMR is 220, statistically significant at the 0.01 level. Additional analysis and discussion on diabetes mellitus will be given below.

As shown in Table 4, there are three other causes of death that show a significant deficit when compared to the U.S. population. For diseases of the circulatory system, the cohort as a whole experienced only 83% of the expected (SMR = 83, $p < 0.01$). The SMR for pneumonia is 46 (6 observed vs 13.15 expected, $p < 0.05$) and for diseases of the digestive system is 48 (15 observed vs 31.44 expected, $p < 0.01$).

When mortality was analyzed by plant, it was found that among the 134 Arkansas employees, only 1 death (motor vehicle accident) occurred. The remaining cohort came primarily from the large Michigan plant, with a very small contribution from the small Michigan plant and the Michigan laboratory. Therefore, the results for the entire cohort are in essence those of these three Michigan facilities. Because of the record-keeping practices, there is no easy way of separating the Michigan facilities. In the remaining analysis, only the Michigan facilities will be included.

Table 5 provides mortality analysis by length of employment for the Michigan facilities. Such an analysis will eliminate the dilution effect of including short-term employees and will also indicate whether a longer employment at the plants could, in fact, be associated with a more adverse mortality experience. It should be pointed out that the basic unit of calculation in these tables is person-years. For example, if an employee left after 9 years of service and subsequently died, the first 5 years would be included in the first 5-year interval and the remaining years till death in the second interval. In this example, the death would be counted in the second interval.

For the group with less than 5 years of employment, 36 deaths from cancer of the respiratory system were observed, whereas 25.15 were expected. The corresponding SMR is 143, and statistical significance is right at the 0.05 level (lower limit = 100). However, when persons with longer employments were examined, such statistical significance was not found. Nor is there any indication of a trend in respiratory cancer mortality.

A statistically significant mortality excess from cancer of the prostate was also detected in the group with less than 5 years of employment. Ten prostatic cancer deaths were observed, compared to an expected of 4.73 (SMR = 211, $p < 0.05$). However, a similar significant excess was not found in groups with longer length of employment. In fact, only one case of prostatic cancer was found among the other groups. It should be pointed out here that the prostatic cancer decedents all died at a fairly old age and worked for a very short period of time. (A discussion on these deaths will be given in the Discussion and Conclusions section.)

When other causes of deaths were examined, no significant excess mortality was found. For the group with less than 5 years of employment, significant deficits were observed in the following causes of death: All causes, cancer of the digestive system, diseases of the circulatory system, and diseases of the digestive system.

Table 6 shows the cause-specific SMRs for the Michigan facilities by year of hire—before 1945, 1945-1954, and after 1954. One notable finding is that significant mortality excess in diabetes mellitus was observed among those hired prior to 1945 (SMR = 364, $p < 0.01$). (A detailed discussion on diabetes mellitus will be found in the Discussion and Conclusions section.) Among those hired between 1945 and 1954, 7 deaths were attributed to leukemia, compared to 2.41 expected. The corresponding SMR was 290, significant at the 0.05 level. No other significant cause-specific mortality excess was observed.

For many chronic diseases, there is usually a long latent period between first exposure and death. Therefore, it would be logical to examine mortality experience after a certain lag period has elapsed. Cause-specific SMRs by latency for the Michigan facilities are presented in Table 7. The only consistent excess comes from diabetes mellitus. The other significant excess was found in diseases of the nervous system and sense organs (SMR = 427, $p < 0.05$) among those with a lag time of at least 25 years. (An examination of the 5 decedents with diseases of the nervous system and sense organs will be presented in the Discussion and Conclusions section.)

Table 5
Observed Deaths and SMRs by Cause and Length of Employment for Male Workers Potentially Exposed to Brominated Chemicals at Three Michigan Facilities

	Length of employment in years									
	< 5		5-9		10-14		15-19		20+	
Cause of death (8th ICDA)	O	SMR	O	SMR	O	SMR	O	SMR	O	SMR
All causes	397	87[a]	52	91	35	83	34	132	24	86
All cancers (140-209)	86	105	8	80	9	124	5	103	4	65
Cancer of digestive system (150-159)	13	54[b]	2	63	1	43	2	137	0	–
Cancer of respiratory system (160-163)	36	143[c]	2	69	5	252	1	64	2	86
Cancer of lung (162-163)	33	140	2	74	5	270	1	69	1	45
Cancer of prostate (185)	10	211[b]	1	153	0	–	0	–	0	–
Cancer of brain (191)	4	137	1	306	0	–	0	–	0	–
Lymphatic and hematopoietic cancer (200-209)	10	112	1	97	1	143	0	–	1	181
Leukemia and aleukemia (204-207)	6	164	1	230	1	327	0	–	1	479
Diabetes mellitus (250)	11	171	3	370	2	335	2	540	1	251
Diseases of nervous system and sense organs (320-389)	3	69	0	–	2	673	1	528	0	–
Diseases of circulatory system (390-458)	176	78[a]	31	105	18	74	20	141	13	88
Arteriosclerotic heart disease (410-413)	132	86	18	93	13	83	13	132	8	72
Nonmalignant respiratory disease (460-519)	20	84	3	104	1	41	1	67	1	61
Diseases of digestive system (520-577)	10	42[a]	3	104	1	53	1	80	0	–
Accidents, poisonings, and violence (E800-E999)	67	107	3	46	1	31	4	199	3	147

[a] $p < 0.01$.
[b] $p < 0.05$.
[c] $p = 0.05$.

Table 6
Observed Deaths and SMRs by Cause and Date of Hire for Male Workers Potentially Exposed to Brominated Chemicals at Three Michigan Facilities

	Year of Hire					
	before 1945		1945-1954		after 1954	
Cause of death (8th ICDA)	O	SMR	O	SMR	O	SMR
All causes	229	81[a]	272	94	41	107
All cancers (140-209)	40	80	64	119	8	130
Cancer of digestive system (150-159)	9	55	7	47[b]	2	145
Cancer of respiratory system (160-163)	16	114	27	151	3	156
Cancer of lung (162-163)	15	114	25	148	2	110
Cancer of prostate (185)	6	142	5	212	0	–
Cancer of brain (191)	1	81	4	184	0	–
Lymphatic and hematopoietic cancer (200-209)	2	44	11	179	0	–
Leukemia and aleukemia (204-207)	2	99	7	290[b]	0	–
Diabetes mellitus (250)	15	364[a]	4	100	0	–
Diseases of nervous system and sense organs (320-389)	3	135	2	70	1	208
Disease of circulatory system (390-458)	125	80[b]	121	87	12	94
Arteriosclerotic heart disease (410-413)	84	84	91	92	9	96
Nonmalignant respiratory disease (460-519)	10	62	15	103	1	68
Disease of digestive system (520-577)	7	55	7	43[b]	1	47
Accidents, poisonings, and violence (E800-E999)	16	73	47	112	15	120

[a] $p < 0.01$.
[b] $p < 0.05$.

Table 7
Observed Deaths and SMRs by Cause and Latency for Male Workers Potentially Exposed to Brominated Chemicals at Three Michigan Facilities

	Latency in years					
	15		20		25	
Cause of death (8th ICDA)	O	SMR	O	SMR	O	SMR
All causes	374	93	274	95	152	92
All cancers (140-209)	74	95	53	92	33	97
Cancer of digestive system (150-159)	11	50[a]	5	31[b]	4	43
Cancer of respiratory system (160-163)	35	133	29	143	17	140
Cancer of lung (162-163)	32	129	27	141	16	139
Cancer of prostate (185)	7	134	5	123	2	77
Cancer of brain (191)	2	88	1	63	1	118
Lymphatic and hematopoietic cancer (200-209)	8	107	5	93	4	131
Leukemia and aleukemia (204-207)	5	166	3	139	3	245
Diabetes mellitus (250)	16	280[b]	14	336[b]	7	290[a]
Diseases of nervous system and sense organs (320-389)	6	201	5	238	5	427[a]
Disease of circulatory system (390-458)	192	88	145	91	80	87
Arteriosclerotic heart disease (410-413)	136	88	99	87	54	81
Nonmalignant respiratory disease (460-519)	23	97	17	94	11	101
Disease of digestive system (520-577)	12	60	8	56	3	39
Accidents, poisonings, and violence (E800-E999)	33	103	18	89	8	82

[a] $p < 0.05$.
[b] $p < 0.01$.

In an attempt to correlate mortality with exposure, a job or department title dictionary consisting of all job or department titles encountered during the coding process was created. A copy of the dictionary was given to the company industrial hygienists and plant personnel, who were asked to classify each department or job title into several major exposure categories. Because little industrial hygiene data existed in the past, it was felt that it would not be possible to assign any exposure levels. However, with this broad exposure classification, it was possible to identify the potential exposures of the cohort members through their work histories.

Cause-specific mortality analysis was carried out for departments with common exposures. These exposures included DBCP, TMCB, Tris, PBB, organic and inorganic bromides, and DDT. However, because of space limitation, the results will not be presented here, but will be the subject of a separate publication.

DISCUSSION AND CONCLUSIONS

The overall mortality of this cohort of male chemical workers at the bromination facilities was 12% less than what one would have expected from a group of U.S. white males similar in age during the same time period. This mortality deficit is statistically significant at the 0.05 level. This observation of a deficit in overall mortality is quite common in occupational epidemiologic studies. This healthy-worker effect may be the result of several factors: Preemployment selection through physical examinations, self-selection by those who are physically fit to work, and economic stability enjoyed by regularly employed individuals.

To determine whether any of the potential occupational hazards has an adverse health effect, one needs to examine the cause-specific SMRs. For the entire cohort, the observed mortality from cancer of all sites was very similar to the expected. When site-specific cancer mortality was examined, a significant deficit was found in cancer of the digestive system. A total of 46 respiratory cancer deaths was observed, compared to an expected 34.07; this excess is of borderline statistical significance ($p \approx 0.05$). All other site-specific cancer SMRs are within the expected range.

Diabetes mellitus was the only cause of death with a statistically significant excess for the cohort as a whole. There were 19 deaths due to this condition, when only 8.65 were expected (SMR = 220, $p < 0.01$), using the U.S. white males as the standard. Diabetes mortality rates vary considerably by state. For males, the average annual age-adjusted Michigan diabetes mortality rate for 1969-1971 ranked third and was 47% higher than the national average (DHEW 1976). For whites, the Michigan rate ranked second and was again 47% higher than the national rate. In view of this considerable regional difference, it would be more appropriate to compute an SMR based on Michigan rates. Using the 1970 Michigan white male rates as the standard, a total of 13.81 diabetes deaths would have been expected for the entire cohort as a whole, and the corresponding SMR is 138 (not significant). Therefore, the significant diabetes mortality excess observed in the cohort as a whole can be attributed to the regional variation between Michigan and the U.S. However, it should be pointed out that, even after adjusting for regional variation, there was still a nonsignificant excess for the entire cohort.

The overall mortality deficit in the entire cohort discussed above comes primarily from diseases of the circulatory system (SMR = 83, $p < 0.01$). However, this deficit in the entire cohort would not rule out that some of the subgroups would experience adverse mortality from diseases of the circulatory system. For the entire cohort, mortality from pneumonia and diseases of the digestive system was also significantly less than that of the overall U.S. white male population.

An analysis by length of employment for the three Michigan facilities did not reveal any increasing trend in any of the causes of death examined. In fact, the cause-specific mortality excess appeared to have come only from the group with less than 5 years of employment. The excess in cancer of the respiratory system is of borderline significance. However, the excess in cancer of the prostate is significant at the 0.05 level (10 observed vs 4.73 expected, SMR = 211). According to the National Cancer Institute, the average annual age-adjusted mortality rate for U.S. white males during 1950-1969 was 17.84 per 100,000, and for Michigan 18.62 (Mason and McKay 1974). It is unlikely that this small difference would account for the excess. An examination of the work histories or exposures of the 10 cases does not indicate any unusual work experience. One notable point is that 4 of this group were employed for less than 2 months, and 8 for less than 2 years. The fact that the excess comes from those employees who worked only for an extremely short time does not support the interpretation that these prostatic cancers were related to employment at the bromination facilities.

When mortality experience was examined by date of hire, it was found that diabetes mellitus was significantly high among those hired prior to 1945 (SMR = 364, $p < 0.01$). Using the 1970 age-specific diabetes mellitus mortality rates among Michigan white males as the standard, the SMR was reduced to 216, a figure which is still statistically significant at the 0.05 level.

There was a total of 19 cases of diabetes mellitus deaths in the entire cohort. In addition to the 15 employees hired prior to 1945, two were hired in 1945, one in 1946, and the remaining one in 1949. No death due to diabetes mellitus was found among those employees hired after 1950.

Among the 15 diabetes mellitus decedents hired before 1945, 9 worked in the maintenance departments. In fact, the cause-specific mortality analysis for the maintenance departments shows that there was a significant excess (10 observed vs 2.54 expected, SMR = 394) in diabetes mellitus in these departments. With the exception of two cases, these maintenance workers were long-term employees. Again, if the Michigan rates were used, the SMR would become 244 ($p < 0.05$). Thus, the excess among the maintenance workers can be partly, but not entirely, explained by regional variation in diabetes mortality.

Based on the above discussion, the excess in diabetes mellitus appears to have come from the maintenance group hired in the early 1940s. However, the work histories do not permit any further detailed investigation, and no specific etiologic agents associated with occupation can be identified, if any indeed exist. An examination of the list of chemicals present at the plants did not reveal any known pancreatic toxin. We are not aware of any occupational hazards that would induce diabetes mellitus. However, chromium is mentioned as one of the risk factors in a recent National Institutes of Health publication (Public Health Service 1979). Welders potentially are exposed to chromium, but none of the diabetes decedents were specifically engaged in welding. Based on our current knowledge of diabetes, the major etiologic factors are genetic and obesity. An investigation in this direction would be beyond the scope of the current study.

Among those hired between 1945 and 1954, leukemia mortality was significantly elevated (SMR = 290, $p < 0.05$). An examination of the work histories of the 7 decedents did not reveal any exposure in common.

Long latent periods usually are required for chronic diseases to develop. In many situations, it would be more appropriate to examine the mortality experience only after a certain lag period has elapsed. Significant mortality excess in diseases of the nervous system and sense organs was detected when mortality was examined 25 years after the date of hire, regardless of length of employment (5 observed vs 1.17 expected, SMR = 427). In fact, 3 of the 5 worked for less than 2 years (1, 5, and 19 months). The remaining 2 died at very old ages (81 and 88). A review of the work histories does not show any common exposure. No occupational factor, if one exists, can be identified as responsible for the statistical association.

Before closing, let us focus on one methodological issue of quantification of chronic diseases in occupational epidemiology. In this paper, we have examined separately mortality by length of employment and latency because the cohort would not be large enough for a two-factor analysis. In addition to these two factors, other investigators have analyzed mortality rates by age at first exposure, duration of exposure, number of years since first exposure, level of exposure (either ranking or numeric grouping), and cumulative exposure defined as the summed products of concentration and duration of exposure. Most of the time, these factors are examined one at a time, even though these study variables are interrelated or confounded.

For example, when occupational exposure is measured in terms of cumulative exposure, there is a confounding effect between the latter parameter and the latency required to induce chronic diseases. On the average, those workers in the higher cumulative exposure groups are also those with a longer latency or a longer time lapse since first exposure. The reason is that a longer time is required to accumulate enough exposure for entry into higher cumulative exposure categories, presumably before the workers have had the time to respond to earlier exposures. The presence of such a confounding effect on respiratory cancer mortality among uranium miners has been suggested by the observation that the risk of excess respiratory cancer mortality increases with time after first exposure and that a positive association exists between the latter and cumulative exposure (Lundin et al. 1971). One solution is to adjust the mortality rates for the effect due to latency by either the direct or the indirect method. However, there are limitations in using the direct and indirect procedures for multifactor adjustment. For example, the factors of interest may be age at first exposure and cumulative exposure. The data (numbers of deaths and person-years at risk) can be presented in a two-way table. The rates specific to age at first exposure and directly adjusted for cumulative exposure can be computed, with the standard cumulative exposure distribution being that of the total cohort. The direct method has a nice property in that both sets of adjusted rates yield the same overall adjusted rate. However, this overall adjusted rate does not necessarily equal the overall crude rate. In the indirect adjustment, the set of crude rates specific to age at first exposure can be used as standard rates. However, the two sets of adjusted rates do not yield the same overall adjusted rates, and the indirectly adjusted rates can be totally out of range of the corresponding specific rates. As a means of correcting these anomalies, Mantel and Stark (1968) have proposed a modified indirect procedure in which the set of standard rates is derived internally from the observed data. This procedure has been successfully applied to mongolism rates with adjustment for maternal age and birth order (Mantel and Stark 1968; Fleiss 1973). This technique had also been used in calculating adjusted cause-specific rates between 1951 and 1966 among coke-oven workers, who were employed in 1951-1955 in seven steel plants in Allegheny County, in relation to age at entry to study, cumulative exposure to coke-oven emission, and length of exposure (Wong 1975).

Table 8 shows lung cancer mortality rates among nonwhite coke-oven workers. The crude rates for all three factors show an upward trend. After adjustment, however, the trend in length of exposure disappears, but the trends in cumulative exposure and in age persist. The dose-response relationship is with cumulative exposure and not with length of exposure.

Table 9 shows similar rates for cardiovascular renal diseases and clearly demonstrates that there is no dose-response relationship with either cumulative exposure or length of exposure. This brief discussion is intended to call the attention of other epidemiologists to the problem of simultaneous multifactor adjustment. Details of the method can be found in the above cited references.

In closing, it should be pointed out that there are several limitations in this study, most of which are typical of an historical mortality study of industrial populations. Although both the percent lost to follow-up and the proportion of outstanding death certificates are reasonably low, it is possible, but unlikely, that deaths from certain rare causes might have been missed. A termination date was missing for a considerable number of workers for whom the length of employment might have been over-or under-estimated. In several cases, work histories in the employment records did not provide enough details to pinpoint specific exposures. Historical exposure levels were inadequate for the chemicals

Table 8
Crude and Adjusted Death Rates per 1000 from Lung Cancer among Nonwhite Coke Oven Workers (1951-1966).

	Crude rates	Adjusted rates
Cumulative exposure (mg/m^3-months)		
< 200	2.3	2.0[a]
200-499	12.9	7.5[a]
500-699	31.0	26.7[a]
700+	68.4	89.6[a]
Age at entry to study (years)		
< 35	7.1	10.9[b]
35-44	13.9	15.5[b]
45-54	36.4	30.5[b]
55+	86.0	68.7[b]
Length of exposure (years)		
< 10	3.2	20.3[c]
10-19	23.6	31.0[c]
20-30	24.5	6.7[c]
30+	62.2	6.4[c]

Data from Wong (1975).
[a]Adjusted for age at entry to study and length of exposure.
[b]Adjusted for cumulative exposure and length of exposure.
[c]Adjusted for age at entry to study and cumulative exposure.

Table 9
Crude and Adjusted Death Rates per 1000 from Cardiovascular Renal Diseases among Nonwhite Coke Oven Workers (1951-1966)

	Crude rates	Adjusted rates
Cumulative exposure (mg/m^3-months)		
< 200	42.7	67.6[a]
200-499	69.4	65.9[a]
500-699	73.8	62.3[a]
700+	79.8	42.2[a]
Age at entry to study (years)		
< 35	14.9	13.1[b]
35-44	61.2	59.9[b]
45-54	128.5	134.9[b]
55+	231.2	232.5[b]
Length of exposure (years)		
< 10	40.7	64.5[c]
10-19	76.3	73.0[c]
20-30	53.9	44.6[c]
30+	129.2	64.2[c]

Data from Wong (1975).
[a]Adjusted for age at entry to study and length of exposure.
[b]Adjusted for cumulative exposure and length of exposure.
[c]Adjusted for age at entry to study and cumulative exposure.

under investigation. Thus, no quantification of exposure is possible. Many of the workers were exposed potentially to a multitude of chemicals, and it is impossible to examine mortality by "pure" exposure. For a couple of conditions, the number of study subjects in some of the subgroups was smaller than desirable, and its difficult to draw any definitive conclusion. Nor was the study large enough for simultaneous multifactor adjustment. Being a mortality study, the investigation not only inherits all the problems associated with death certificates, but also suffers from the lack of in-depth clinical information. Employment other than that with this specific company has not been considered. Nor was it feasible to include smoking history in the analysis.

In spite of limitations, the study has identified several potential health problems in this cohort. It is recommended that this study be updated in the future. A larger observation period will not only increase the statistical power of the study, but also establish any trend in mortality, if one exists, in the cohort.

REFERENCES

Department of Health, Education and Welfare (DHEW). 1976. *Report on the National Commission on Diabetes,* vol. III, Part 1. DHEW Publication No. (NIH) 76-1021, Government Printing Office, Washington, D.C.

Fleiss, J.L. 1973. *Statistical methods for rates and proportions.* John Wiley & Sons, New York.

Lundin, F.E., J.K. Wagoner, and V.E. Archer. 1971. *Radon daughter exposure and respiratory cancer, quantitative and temporal aspects.* DHEW, Public Health Service Publication, Government Printing Office, Washington, D.C.

Mantel, N. and C.R. Stark. 1968. Computation of indirect-adjusted rates in the presence of confounding. *Biometrics* 24:997.

Mason, T.J. and F.W. McKay. 1974. *U.S. cancer mortality by county, 1950-1969.* DHEW Publication No. (NIH) 74-615, Government Printing Office, Washington, D.C.

Monson, R.R. 1974. Analysis of relative survival and proportional mortality. *Computers and Biomedical Research* 7:325.

Public Health Service, National Institutes of Health. 1979. *Diabetes data, compiled 1977.* NIH Publication No. 79-1468, Government Printing Office, Washington, D.C.

Wong, O. 1975. *Adjustment of mortality rates in the presence of confounding factors and competing risks in occupational health studies.* Doctoral Dissertation, University of Pittsburgh. University Microfilm, Ann Arbor, Michigan.

Quantification of Differences Between Proportionate Mortality Ratios and Standardized Mortality Ratios

RICHARD J. WAXWEILER, MARIE K. HARING,
SANFORD S. LEFFINGWELL AND WILLIAM H. HALPERIN
Industrywide Studies Branch
Division of Surveillance, Hazard Evaluations and Field Studies
National Institute for Occupational Safety and Health
R.A. Taft Laboratories
Cincinnati, Ohio 45226

Two epidemiologic methods are particularly suitable for studying cancer mortality among industrial populations. Standardized mortality ratios (SMRs), computed from retrospective cohort mortality studies, are advantageous because they permit calculation of cause-specific mortality rates; however such studies require expensive cohort follow-up. Standardized proportionate mortality ratios (PMRs), computed from analysis of available death certificates without any follow-up, can be determined quickly and inexpensively, but are not always predictive of the SMRs.

If we can understand why a PMR differs from an SMR and identify conditions under which a PMR is likely to be a good risk estimator, we may be able to allocate scarce epidemiological resources much more effectively. Following this reasoning, there are three specific objectives in this presentation:

1. To describe the reasons a cause-specific PMR differs from an SMR;
2. To quantify the magnitude of these PMR/SMR differences in a specific example; and to some extent, in general,
3. To propose conditions under which a PMR is likely to be a good indicator of an excess risk.

Additionally, we would like to emphasize four key variables that we will use in this presentation:

1. SMR, or standardized mortality ratio. It equals 100 times the observed number of deaths divided by the expected number of deaths in a cohort study. It is based on complete follow-up of a cohort.
2. RSMR, or relative standardized mortality ratio as defined by Kupper et al. (1978). A cause-specific RSMR equals the SMR for the same cause of death divided by the all-causes SMR, both of which are based on complete follow-up of a cohort.

3. PMR_{ALL}, or standardized proportionate mortality ratio. It is based on the observed divided by the expected relative frequencies of cause-specific deaths. It is computed from *all* deaths ascertained by complete follow-up of a cohort.
4. PMR_{EBP}, or standardized proportionate mortality ratio computed only from deaths ascertained through routine administration of a typical company employee benefits program. No other follow-up is used to ascertain deaths.

Because the PMR studies usually are carried out on readily available death certificates, such as those ascertained through an employee benefit program, our ultimate goal is to compare the PMR_{EBP} with the SMR.

The difference between the PMR and SMR can be divided into three components (Table 1). When added together, these three components completely account for the total difference. The first component is the total force of mortality. It can be measured by the difference between a cause-specific SMR and the corresponding cause-specific RSMR. If the all-causes SMR equals 100, there is no difference between the cause-specific SMRs and RSMRs. However, in an industrial population, the total force of mortality usually is low because of the healthy worker effect, i.e. selection of healthy people into industry and selection of unhealthy people out of industry. Thus the all-causes SMR is below 100, which forces the cause-specific RSMRs to be greater than their corresponding cause-specific SMRs.

The second component of the difference between the PMR and SMR is derived from the differential mathematical properties of the two models—the PMR design and the cohort (SMR) design. These properties lead to different results, even if one analyzes data from the same deaths, because the cohort study additionally includes data on living persons and on deceased persons during the years before they died. This component can be measured by comparing the PMR_{ALL} based on all deaths versus the RSMR, based on the same deaths. Kupper et al. (1978) have shown mathematically that confidence intervals (CIs) can be calculated, and one can predict the magnitude of the difference between the PMR_{ALL} and the RSMR.

Table 1

Components of Difference Between a PMR Based on Employee Benefits Program Deaths (PMR_{EBP}) and an SMR Based on Cohort Follow-up

Component	Measure
1. Total force of mortality	RSMR - SMR
2. Differential mathematical properties	PMR_{All} - RSMR
3. Biased ascertainment by cause	PMR_{EBP} - PMR_{All}

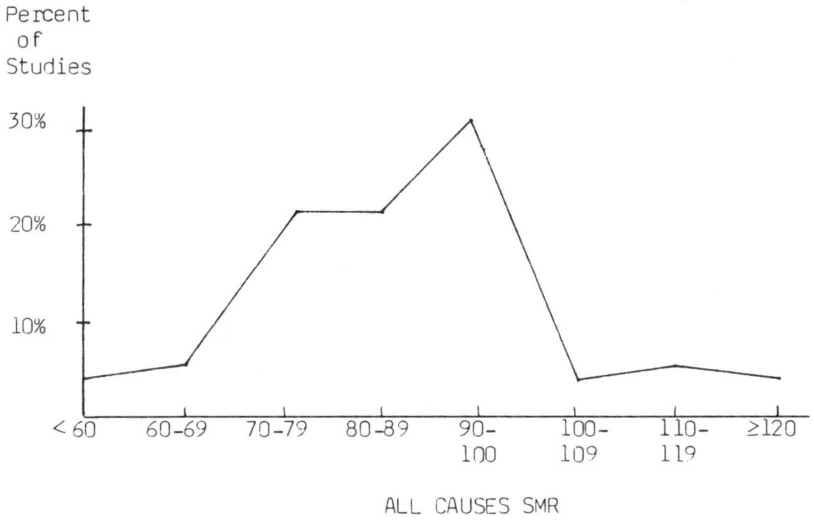

Figure 1
Distribution of all-causes SMRs for 50 occupational cohort studies

The third component is biased ascertainment by cause. It can be measured by the difference between a PMR based on readily available death certificates—in this case, through those known to an employee benefits program; and a PMR based on all deaths, subsequent to total follow-up of the cohort. By adding these three components together, the total difference can be measured between an SMR based on complete cohort follow-up and a PMR, based on records readily available at a company.

METHODS AND RESULTS

The magnitude of the first component (SMR - RSMR) is determined by the inverse of the all-causes SMR. To quantify how large this difference is likely to be, we reviewed 50 occupational cohort studies in the *Journal of Occupational Medicine* and *Annals of the New York Academy of Sciences*. The distribution of the all-causes SMR, based usually on U.S. expected rates, for these studies had a median of 89 (Fig. 1), but more importantly, the 10th percentile was 69 and the 90th percentile was 101. Thus, the all-causes SMRs for 80% of these published occupational cohort studies fell between 69 and 101. Because a cause-specific RSMR equals the cause-specific SMR divided by the all-cause SMR, in 80% of these studies the RSMR would lie between 99% (1/1.01) and 145% (1/.69) of its corresponding cause-specific SMR. Thus, based on 50 studies, 90% of the time the first component would be expected to account for less than a 45% increase between an SMR and the measure eventually being sought, a PMR_{EBP}. A slightly smaller effect would be expected for all malignant neoplasms which had a median SMR 9 points higher than the all-causes SMR for these same studies.

For the rest of the presentation, a specific occupational retrospective cohort study is considered. In this ongoing study a cohort of white males employed between 1950-1977 at a large plant was followed through 1977 using routine follow-up sources such as the Social Security Administration, Internal Revenue Service, and Bureau of Motor Vehicles. Observed and expected deaths and SMRs based on U.S. expected rates for white males, adjusted by age and calendar period, were calculated separately for person-years at risk both below and above 15 years duration of employment (Table 2). Separation at 15 years of employment was made because employees working more than 15 years would be expected to be vested in the employee benefit program sponsored by the company. Below 15 years employment the all-causes SMR was 83, thus, the cause-specific RSMRs could be calculated by multiplying the cause-specific SMRs by 100/83 or 1.21. Thus, in this study the low total force of mortality will cause the eventual PMR's to be 21% greater than the corresponding SMRs. For the group employed longer, the inflation is 100/71, or 40%.

The effect of the second component, differential mathematical properties, is measured by comparing the RSMR with the PMR, the latter being calculated from the same observed deaths as the RSMR (Table 3). In this study, this factor accounted for differences of less than 4% with one exception—for accidental deaths the PMR was 15-20% greater than the RSMR.

In 4 other studies (Kupper et al. 1978; Beaumont 1979 and pers. comm.), only one cause of death out of 53 examined had greater than a 5% difference

Table 2
Comparison of SMR and RSMR by Duration Employed at Study Plant

	<15 Years			≥15 Years		
	SMR		RSMR	SMR		RSMR
All causes (multiple factor)	83	(1.21)	100	71	(1.4)	100
All malignant neoplasms	76		92	81		112
Pancreas	75		92	169		236
Respiratory	79		96	64		90
Kidney	0		0	202		282
Stroke	74		90	85		119
Cardiovascular disease	89		108	71		99
Nonmalignant Respiratory disease	81		98	32		45
Accidents	89		108	68		95

Table 3
Comparison of RSMR and PMR_{ALL} by Duration Employed at Study Plant

	<15 Years		≥15 Years	
	RSMR	PMR_{ALL}	RSMR	PMR_{ALL}
All causes	100	100	100	100
All malignant neoplasms	92	92	112	113
Pancreas	92	90	236	238
Respiratory	96	93	90	91
Kidney	0	0	282	285
Stroke	90	88	119	115
Cardiovascular disease	108	107	99	100
Nonmalignant Respiratory disease	98	97	45	44
Accidents	108	**128**	95	**108**

between the RSMR and the PMR based on the same deaths. Therefore, this component usually is insignificant in causing differences between an SMR and PMR. Furthermore, its magnitude can always be predicted based on a formula derived by Kupper (1978).

The third component is biased ascertainment of deaths by cause. In this study, among persons dying before 15 years of employment, the company knew about 35% of the deaths through administration of their employee benefits program (Table 4). Among persons dying after 15 years of employment, the company knew of 90%. This difference is due to two phenomena:

1. Regardless of duration employed, death ascertainment is good among active employees, retirees, and disabled employees, because the company is paying these people on a regular basis.
2. Regardless of duration employed, death ascertainment is poor among persons who were laid off or who quit voluntarily (terminated employees). The large number of these employees who terminated with less than 15 years of employment substantially decreases the ascertainment percentage for the entire group of those who died before 15 years employment. On the other hand, among those having worked <15 years, few people terminated prior to retirement. Less than 10% of the deaths in this latter group occurred among terminators. Thus, the overall ascertainment rate remains high–90% in these long term workers.

Although the ultimate goal is to assess cause-specific differences in ascertainment, it is obvious that such biases have a much greater probability of arising in the group employed less than 15 years because of the low rate of overall death ascertainment. The 90% ascertainment in the greater-than-15 group leaves little room for cause-specific biased ascertainment.

Table 4
Completeness of Death Ascertainment through An Employee Benefits Program by Employee Status

	Duration employed					
	<15 Years			≥15 Years		
Employee status at death	known to EBP[a]	total deaths	(%)	known to EBP[a]	total deaths	(%)
All causes	92	265	35	222	246	90
Actives	73	75	97	107	108	99
Retirees	8	12	67	62	64	97
Disabled	6	11	54	39	44	89
Terminated	5	161	3	8	20	40
Transferred	0	6	0	2	8	25
Unknown	0	0	0	1	2	50

[a]Employee benefits program.

Table 5
Comparison of PMR_{ALL} and PMR_{EBP} by Duration Employed at Study Plant

	<15 Years		≥15 Years	
	PMR_{ALL}	PMR_{EBP}	PMR_{ALL}	PMR_{EBP}
All causes	100	100	100	100
All malignant neoplasms	92	**123**	113	116
Pancreas	90	**149**	238	226
Respiratory	93	83	91	90
Kidney	0	0	285	317
Stroke	88	72	115	111
Cardiovascular disease	107	117	100	102
Nonmalignant Respiratory disease	97	**60**	44	40
Accidents	128	120	108	112

Table 5, which compares the PMR based on total follow-up and the PMR based on deaths known through the employee benefits program, quantifies the effect of cause-specific death ascertainment biases. For those with less than 15 years duration, substantial differences occur for all malignant neoplasms, pancreatic malignant neoplasms, and nonmalignant respiratory disease. In the greater than 15 years group, only trivial differences occur.

It is easier to see the relative effects of these three components by examining the differences measured as a percentage of the SMR, and represented

Table 6
Relative Contribution of Major Factors to Differences (Δ) between SMR and PMR_{EBP}

	<15 Years duration employed			
	SMR – RSMR	RSMR – PMR_{ALL}	PMR_{ALL} – PMR_{EBP}	
	Δ_a (%)	Δ_b (%)	Δ_c (%)	Δ total (%)
All causes	21	0	0	21
All malignant neoplasms	↓	0	40	62
Pancreas		-1	79	99
Respiratory		-4	-13	5
Kidney		—	—	—
Stroke		-3	-22	-3
Cardiovascular disease		-1	11	31
Nonmalignant Respiratory disease		-1	-46	-26
Accident	↓	22	-9	35

by Δ in Table 6. Among those employed less than 15 years, the Δ_c due to cause-specific death ascertainment bias fluctuates wildly and can easily overwhelm the effect of the other two components. In this example, the company knew about a much higher percentage of deaths due to malignant neoplasms than about deaths due to stroke or nonmalignant respiratory disease (NMRD). In the right hand column, the total Δ, or total difference between the PMR_{EBP} and SMR, as a percent of the SMR varies from +99% to -26%. This clearly makes the PMR an unacceptable surrogate measure of the SMR for workers employed less than 15 years in the particular population studied here.

Among those employed longer than 15 years (Table 7), there is a larger Δ_a, (40%) due to the very low total force of mortality. The cause-specific Δ_b values representing the differential mathematical properties, remain small. The Δ_c values, representing cause-specific death ascertainment biases, are also minor–just as predicted from the 90% ascertainment of deaths described in Table 4. Thus, while the total Δ values are sizeable, their distribution by cause is over a fairly narrow range, 25-65%, and for cause-specific malignancies, between 34-57%. On average the cause-specific PMR_{EBP} are roughly 40% greater than the corresponding SMRs, as was true for the RSMRs. Since RSMRs depend upon the all-causes SMR, which is clearly a function of the comparison population chosen, this raises a crucial concept–what is an appropriate control group. If one argues that United States mortality rates are appropriate, and thus SMRs based on them are valid, then based on the cumulative experience of other studies we could make an appropriately estimated adjustment across the board

Table 7
Relative Contribution of Major Factors to Differences (Δ) between SMR and PMR_{EBP}

	>15 Years duration employed			
	SMR — RSMR Δ_a (%)	RSMR — PMR_{ALL} Δ_b (%)	PMR_{ALL} — PMR_{EBP} Δ_c (%)	Δ total (%)
All causes	40	0	0	40
All malignant neoplasms	↓	1	4	43
Pancreas	↓	1	-7	34
Respiratory	↓	1	-1	40
Kidney	↓	1	16	57
Stroke	↓	-5	-5	31
Cardiovascular disease	↓	1	3	44
Nonmalignant Respiratory disease	↓	-3	-13	25
Accident	↓	19	6	65

to every cause-specific PMR. These PMRs would then fairly accurately predict the SMRs.

On the other hand, if the ideal comparison group is not the U.S. general population, but a much healthier "employed" population, then perhaps the RSMR rather than the SMR is a better parameter to assess occupational health problems. This single study indicates that PMRs based on deaths ascertained through an employee benefits program among long term employees are closer to the RSMRs than are the SMRs. Furthermore, PMR studies based on readily available death certificates are less expensive than cohort studies. Thus, the PMRs may be better parameters for occupational mortality surveillance than the SMRs. A fear of false positives may deter some investigators from proceeding with PMR studies based on data from employee benefit programs. But, in order to confirm or refute the suggested excesses, positive results should be followed with inexpensive in-plant case-control studies and subsequently, if need be, with cohort studies of selected subpopulations within the plant.

REFERENCES

Beaumont, J. 1979. *Mortality of Welders, Shipfitters, and Other Metal Trades Workers in Boilermakers Local No. 104, AFL-CIO.* Ph.D. Dissertation University of Washington.

Kupper, L.L., A.J. McMichael, M.J. Symons, and B.M. Most. 1978. On the utility of proportional mortality analyses. *J. Chrom. Dis.* **31**:15.

COMMENTS

AXELSON: I wonder if there is any need at all at this time for using the PMR concept. If you take out the cases under study from the denominator, the PMR study goes over into the case-control, case-referent, study of the incidence density type. Then one can use all the ideas and tools that have been developed around the case-control study during the 1970s, particularly by Olli Miettinen, Harvard School of Public Health.

WAXWEILER: I disagree with you. One of the most important components, I think, is biased ascertainment of deaths. If you are talking about a PMR study, you have to talk about the study design and the analysis. It is very important to include in the design how those deaths are ascertained. The theoretical argument that you should take out the cause of interest and compare your cause of interest only versus all other causes of death is important only if the cause of death in which you are interested accounts for a substantial proportion of deaths. The only time that I can think of where that occurs is if you are looking at all malignant neoplasms or looking at coronary heart disease—something like that. But for a site-specific cancer, I think it is totally inconsequential, and I think you could go through calculations to show that.

AXELSON: I think it is useless to argue in more detail right now, but I would like to refer those of you who are interested in these methodological aspects to Axelson (1979).

RADFORD: I would just like to point out that there is another use that is commonly overlooked for looking at proportions of deaths. Whether you are doing an SMR, a classic cohort analysis, or not, it is important to look within the causes of death for the linked causes. For example, we have heard a lot about cigarette-induced disease. The ratio of particular causes to which we have high attributable risks ought to be in proportion, because if they are cigarette-induced, then larynx, lung, and chronic respiratory disease ought to be proportionately similar. If they are not, then it may very well flag an important difference. In Sam Milham's study of the carpenters and joiners, if you look at the ratio of SMRs for lung cancer to those of laryngeal or buccal cancer and to those of chronic respiratory disease, they don't fit at all with the idea that the lung cancer is purely cigarette related. It led me to conclude that there was a lung cancer excess with an SMR of 106.

I agree with the argument you are presenting, but I just wanted to emphasize that you can look at these proportions in many ways. Alcohol-related diseases should track together—automobile accidents, cirrhosis, and so forth.

WAXWEILER: I think that is true in SMR studies, too.

RADFORD: Yes.

SARACCI: You presented these three components as if they are, in a sense, things that you can add up. Is that correct?

WAXWEILER: Yes, very definitely, they are additive.

SARACCI: Have you looked at the actual SMRs at the two ends of the chain?

WAXWEILER: Yes, I have compared the SMRs in Table 2 and the $PMRs_{EBP}$ in tables.

PADDLE: Just a comment, then a question. While I am doing a case-control study, I like to have a piece of paper in a drawer that rationalizes the argument that the finding is random. But my question is: Do you think from your experience that perhaps this finding of terminated employees with nonmalignant respiratory disease might be typical of the chemical industry? This could be a good reason for terminating employment in that industry.

WAXWEILER: I think it is very possible. Again, as I said, I think this model is important. Dr. Milham has compared SMR studies and PMR studies, where we have two different data sets–for example, comparing a PMR for aluminum workers in the State of Washington with an SMR of a cohort of aluminum workers–and has shown they they come out the same, I think it is incredible encouragement for continuing with statewide mortality studies of PMRs. But it is just as important to identify to what these differences are due, given you have the same data set, and given you are going into a plant. There are so many plants around this country that have employee benefits programs with death certificates, and they aren't even close to an ongoing surveillance project of mortality of terminated employees.

WEN: There is a dilemma in conducting PMR analysis, and that is once you have positive results–and you do not have a way of ascertaining whether these are biased or unbiased death certificates that you have–the next step that you jump into is the case-control study, which is going to confuse the issue rather than clarify it, whether it is a false positive or a positive. The next step after PMR to clarify whether the cancer is indeed increased or not should be SMR, rather than case-control.

WAXWEILER: Well, I would disagree with you. I think if we took every positive PMR and tried to do a cohort study on it, we would run out of money very quickly. I think that the case-control study is a lot less expensive.

WEN: But it won't give you the answer to whether it has increased or not.

WAXWEILER: No, it won't give you the answer to whether it has increased or not, but if you go into a plant, especially some of these large chemical facilities with lots of different chemicals at hand, departments, and so forth, and you can take a kidney cancer excess and identify that a particular job or department is at high risk, then that would be the time, I would propose, that we would start then studying that one particular group in a cohort study. An example is some of the cohort studies that Otto Wong was showing of dibromochloropropane (see Wong, this volume), or something like that. I don't think this country can afford to study every chemical. We need a surveillance mechanism.

WEN: Well, you also cannot afford, when you have incomplete ascertainment of cases, to do a control study where the result would be inefficient and inaccurate.

WAXWEILER: But what I am saying is that I don't think that argument holds water. I think that once you get beyond 10 years of employment, you have close to complete ascertainment of deaths.

Although that probably is a fairly generalizable statement, it is negotiable. There are going to be some companies that have horrible employee benefits programs and you can't do this at all.

REFERENCES

Axelson, O. 1979. The case-referent (case-control) study in occupational health epidemiology. *Scand. J. Work Environ. Health* 5:91.

Occupational Data Sets Appropriate for Proportionate Mortality Ratio Analysis

JAMES J. BEAUMONT, TERRY L. LEET, AND ANDREA H. OKUN
Industrywide Studies Branch
Division of Surveillance, Hazard Evaluations, and Field Studies
National Institute for Occupational Safety and Health
Cincinnati, Ohio 45226

The reason deaths are known in an occupational mortality data set may determine how appropriate the data are for proportionate mortality (PMR) analysis. The reason is important because it can influence which causes of death are known. If certain causes are over- or underrepresented in a data set, then the PMR results may be biased. For example, if most deaths are known from lawsuits filed because of deceased workers' exposure to a suspect carcinogen, then the data set probably contains an unusually high proportion of cancer deaths. The PMR for cancer would, therefore, show an excess that may or may not be real.

There are many reasons why a company or union would know about deaths among its workers, but there are four situations that epidemiologists commonly encounter (these are summarized in Table 1).

1. Financial. There is a life insurance plan or pension death benefit plan that covers all active workers and terminated workers who have worked long enough to be "vested" (commonly a minimum of 10 to 20 years). Therefore, there is a financial incentive for survivors to report deaths that have occurred.
2. Nonfinancial. Deaths among actively employed workers are known and deaths among former workers are known because of obituary reports in newspapers, inquiries about death benefits, or because of the popularity of the former worker.
3. Combined. Deaths are known for both financial and nonfinancial reasons. This situation is actually a combination of situations 1 and 2.
4. Active Only. In some cases, the only record of death is in the personnel or dues record, where death has been written down as the reason the person is no longer employed.

Given that there are several types of data sets that epidemiologists encounter at unions and companies, which type is likely to give the least biased, and therefore, the most accurate PMRs? To address this question, we analyzed data in which all four of the above data set types could be approximated, yet

Table 1
Deaths Known to a Union or Company: Four Common Situations Encountered by Epidemiologists

Situation	Workers included
1. Financial	active, vested nonactive
2. Nonfinancial	active, miscellaneous nonactive
3. Combined	active, vested nonactive, miscellaneous nonactive
4. Active only	active

for which follow-up to ascertain vital status had been done previously and standardized mortality ratio (SMR) results produced. Therefore, we could determine which data set would have best represented the various causes of death, and would have yielded PMRs most similar to the SMRs. Most previous reports that have compared PMRs and SMRs have used PMRs based upon all deaths that actually occurred (Redmond and Breslin 1975; Kupper et al. 1978; Decoufle et al. 1980). The present analysis examines PMRs based upon just the deaths known without complete follow-up, a more realistic condition. We are aware of only one previously published report that has taken a similar approach (Decoufle and Thomas 1979).

METHODS

The deaths were from a long-term mortality study of 3247 welders identified through a union in Seattle, Washington (Beaumont and Weiss 1980). The welders were members of the union for at least 3 years and were employed some time between 1950 and 1973. Their vital status as of January 1, 1977, was ascertained via union records and the Social Security Administration. Vital status ascertainment was 91% complete, and 95% of the death certificates were obtained.

Because most of the deaths that actually occurred among the welders were known (from the previous vital status ascertainment for the SMR study), it was possible to compare how well the various causes of death would have been represented if a PMR approach had been taken instead of an SMR. Each of the four PMR situations could be approximated because, at the time of initial data collection, deaths that were known to the union were noted, and the reason they were known (death benefit, etc.) was also noted.

There were a number of reasons why this union knew of deaths. A life insurance program, which existed from 1941 to 1970, covered all active members, and nonactive members who achieved 20 years of continuous membership (vested). Although the program ended in 1970, those individuals who achieved 20 years by 1970 remain eligible to this day. A union pension death benefit program was started in 1962 and it is still in existence. It covered all active members, and former members who had been members for at least 10 years (vested). The union also knew of deaths for miscellaneous nonfinancial reasons: Its clerks read the obituary columns of the local newspapers, it received inquiries about benefits from ineligible survivors, and it recorded deaths learned of via word-of-mouth (usually deaths of former members who had been friendly to the union).

Table 2 gives a breakdown of the welders by their status with the union at the time of death. The first column in Table 2, the maximum number of deaths that could have occurred in each employment status category, had to be estimated because the union had not classified all of the deaths, it had only classified deaths that it was aware of. The number of active member deaths was estimated by counting deaths where the year most recently worked was the same as the year of death, and the nonactive number was the remainder. The nonactive were further classified as to their benefit eligibility by applying the general rules described in the preceeding paragraph. Of the total of 529 deaths that occurred, little more than half (58%) were known to the union at the time of data collection for the SMR study. For the various status categories the percent known to the union varied considerably, from 40% for the benefit ineligible to 78% for the active members. While these percentages were not precise because of the estimation that was required (the number of possible benefit eligible deaths in particular was likely to be overestimated because we only knew of gaps in employment of 6 months or greater), it was evident that union knowledge of deaths was greatest for those actively employed, and among the nonactives knowledge was greatest for those who were benefit eligible.

Because deaths were known for both financial and nonfinancial reasons, the situation that actually existed at this union was the "combined" situation (Table 1). Situation 1, "financial," was approximated by the 124 active deaths

Table 2
Deaths Among the Welders According to Their Status with the Union at the Time of Death

Status	Number possible[a]	Number reported to union	Percent reported to union
Active ($)	158	124	78%
Nonactive			
Benefit Eligible ($)	211	118	56%
Benefit Ineligible	160	64	40%
Total	529	306	58%

[a]Estimated numbers.

and the 118 vested deaths (these have dollar signs in Table 2). Similarly, situation 2, "nonfinancial," was approximated by the 124 active deaths and the 64 miscellaneous deaths. There would probably have been more than 64 miscellaneous deaths had there not been vesting programs, i.e., it is likely that some of the deaths in the vested category would have been known for miscellaneous reasons if no death benefits had been available. Finally, situation 4 was approximated by the 124 deaths where the death year and the last year of membership were the same.

RESULTS

Representation of the Various Causes of Death

The first phase of the analysis was to see how well the various causes of death would have been represented in each of the four situations. Figures 1 through 4 demonstrate the results graphically. In each figure the horizontal axis presents five major death categories and the vertical axis presents the percentages of deaths known to the union (out of those that actually occurred) in each cause-of-death category.

Figure 1, for example, shows how the financial situation (active and vested workers) would have represented the various causes of death. The dotted line at 46% indicates that, overall, 46% of the 529 deaths would have been known if this situation (financial deaths only) had existed at the union. If each cause of death were represented equally, then 46% would have been the result for each death category. It can be seen that this is not what was found: diseases of the circulatory system were overrepresented and external causes were underrepresented. Circulatory system deaths probably were overrepresented because of the large proportion (51%) of this data set's deaths having been among active members. This is discussed in greater detail in the Situation 4 (active only) discussion. The external causes may have been underrepresented because people who worked long enough to be vested (10-20 years) might have been relatively stable individuals and, therefore, less likely to have died from external causes (motor vehicle accidents, homicide, suicide, etc.).

If there had been no death benefit program, the union would have known about most of the 124 active deaths and the 64 miscellaneous deaths. These 188 deaths constituted 36% of the 529 deaths that actually occurred, as denoted by the dotted line in Figure 2. It can be seen in Figure 2 that cancer would have been underrepresented relative to other causes of death if the nonfinancial situation had existed. This may be because active deaths were a large proportion of the total deaths in this situation, and among the active deaths, cancers were underrepresented. Cancers were expected to be underrepresented among the actives because cancer often has a long degenerative period that causes employees to quite working long before death. Conversely, acute causes of

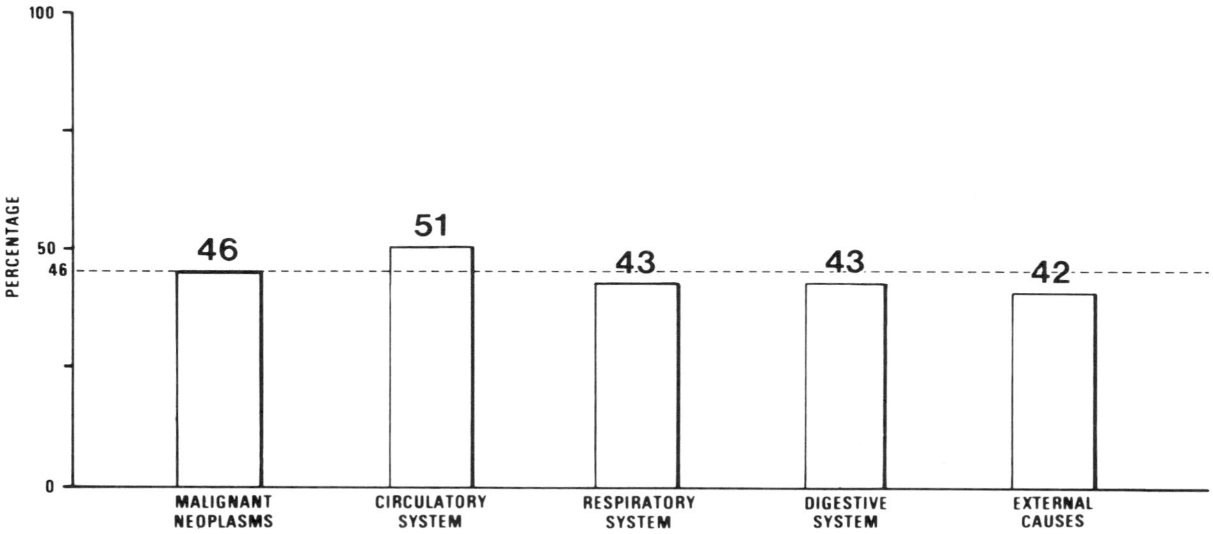

Figure 1
Representation of causes if deaths were known only for financial reasons (life insurance or other death benefits)

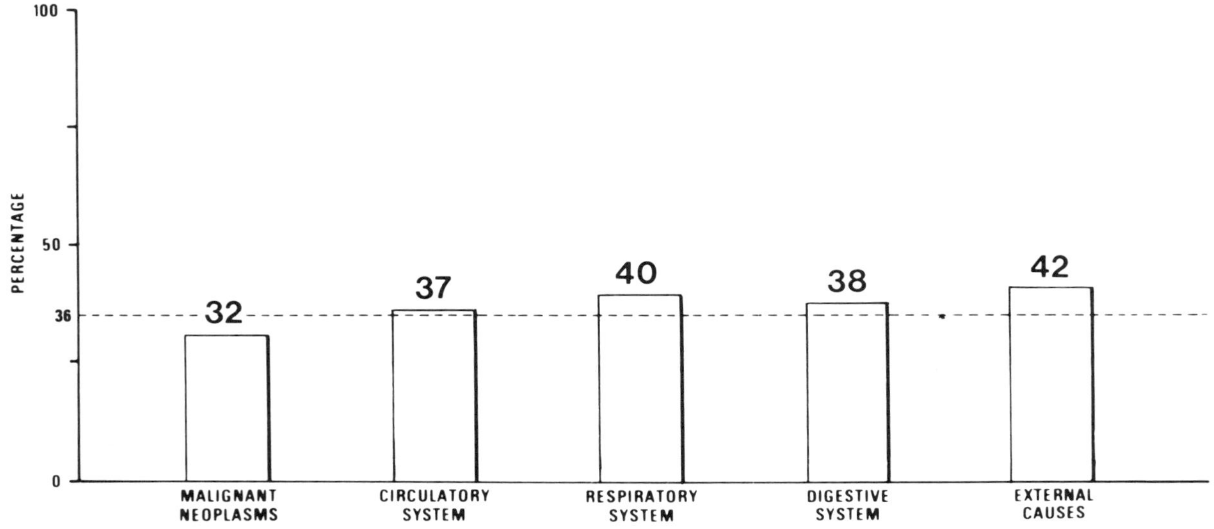

Figure 2
Representation of causes if deaths were known only for nonfinancial reasons (actively employed or miscellaneous)

death such as heart attacks were expected to be overrepresented among workers who were actively employed at the time of their deaths. Although not acute, nonmalignant respiratory deaths were represented more than any other deaths. This overrepresentation may be due to the union's concern about respiratory exposures and, therefore, these deaths may have been reported relatively often.

Figure 3 shows the situation that actually existed at the union, where deaths were known for both financial and nonfinancial reasons (the combined situation). This was all of the deaths known to the union, including active, vested and miscellaneous deaths. It can be seen in Figure 3 that the union knew of 58% of the deaths, and that cancer and external causes were somewhat underrepresented relative to the other causes of death. The underrepresentation of cancer and external causes was a reflection of the two types of data previously examined: financial, where external causes were underrepresented (Figure 1), and nonfinancial, where cancer was underrepresented (Figure 2).

Finally, if deaths were known only among the active union members, the data set would have been that shown in Figure 4. Just 23% of the total deaths would have been known. Cardiovascular deaths would have been represented to a far greater extent than the other causes of death, probaby due to the acute nature of many deaths in the cardiovascular category (stroke, myocardial infarction, etc.). In contrast to the nonfinancial situation (Fig. 2), respiratory system and external-cause deaths were underrepresented. This shows that the overrepresentation of respiratory and external-cause deaths seen in Figure 2 was a result of the deaths known for miscellaneous reasons.

Accuracy of the PMRs

The second phase of the analysis was to determine which situation gave PMRs that most closely approximated SMRs from the follow-up study. The SMRs were considered to be the standard in this comparison, i.e., the correct figures to which the PMRs aspired. It was expected that the representation problems just discussed would influence the accuracy of the PMRs.

Figures 5-11 compare PMRs and SMRs for the various situations (the SMRs are the same in each figure). Whereas the horizontal axes in these figures present cause-of-death categories as before, the vertical axes are now mortality ratios, with a dotted line at 100 to indicate the division between an excess and deficit of deaths relative to the U.S. population. The primary focus here is the height of the PMR and SMR bars for each death category. If the PMR gives an accurate estimate of the SMR, the PMR and SMR bars within each death category will be the same height. It is not expected that the various death categories should have bars of the same height (as it was in Figures 1-4), only that the SMR and PMR be similar within each cause-of-death category.

Figure 5 compares SMRs and PMRs where the PMRs were based upon all deaths that actually occurred. This is not one of the four situations being

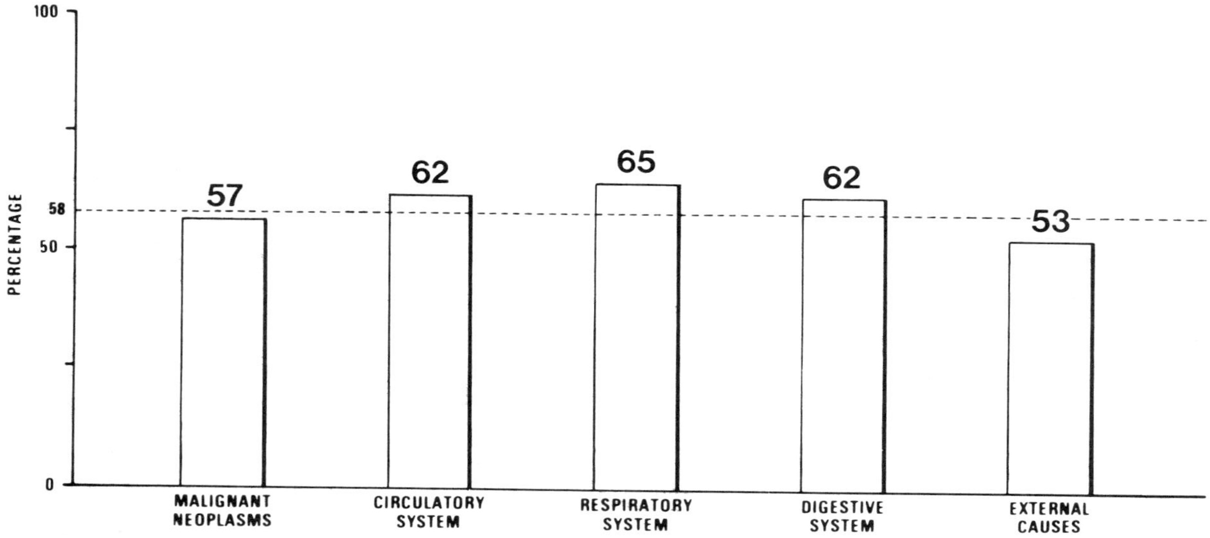

Figure 3
Representation of causes if deaths were known for both financial and nonfinancial reasons combined

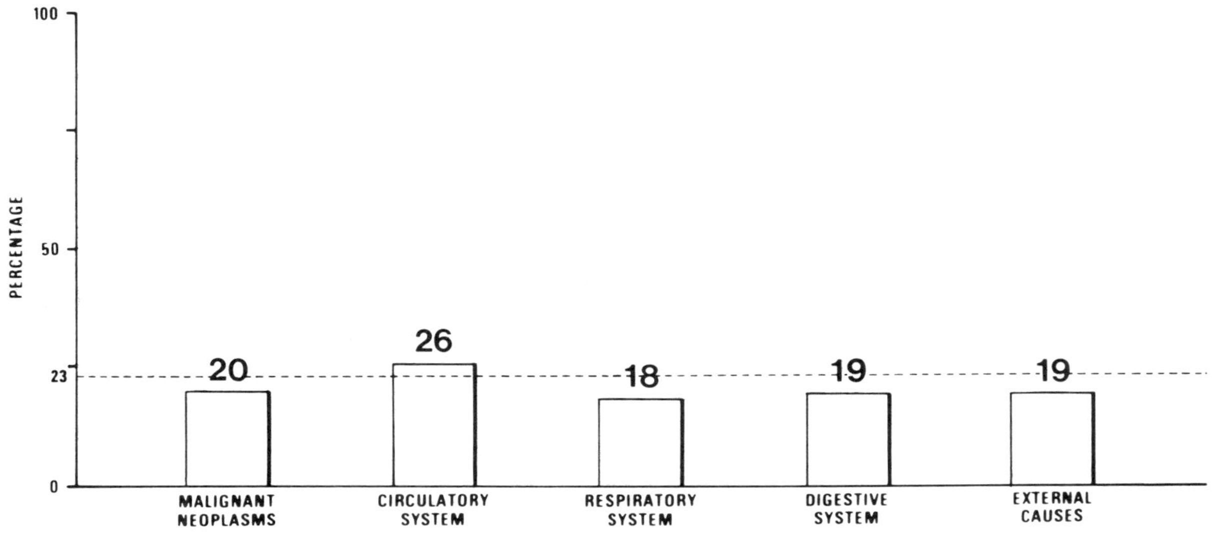

Figure 4
Representation of causes if deaths were known for actively employed workers only

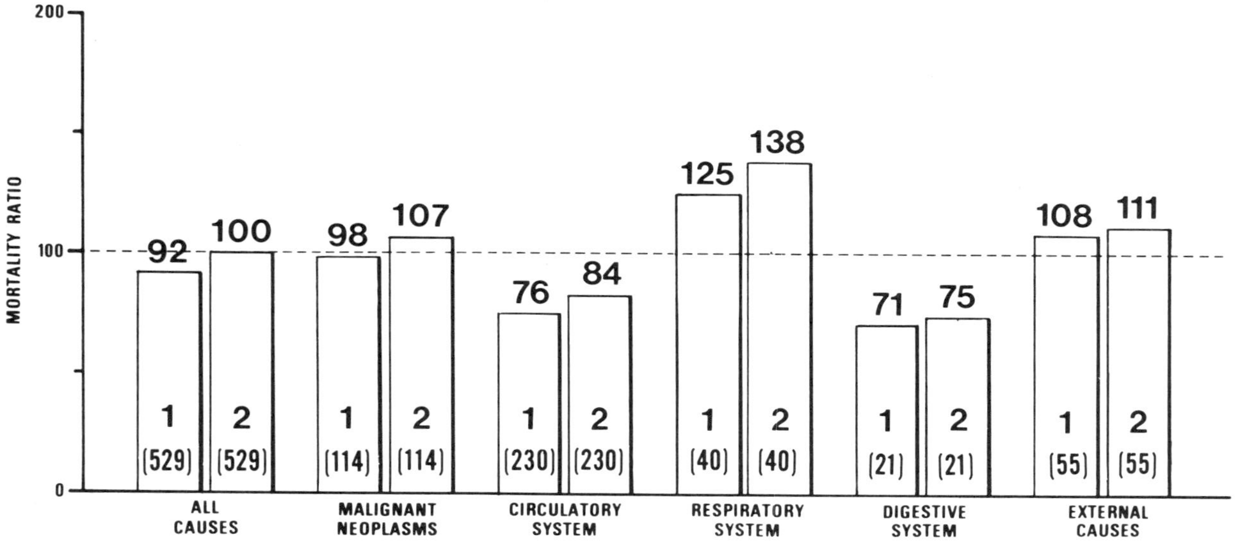

Figure 5
Comparability of SMRs and PMRs where the PMRs are based upon all 529 deaths ([1]) SMR; ([2]) PMR.

discussed because it is very unrealistic: The only way to obtain all of the deaths is to do a cohort study with follow-up of all study members, and if that were done, SMRs would be calculated in preference to PMRs. Figure 5 is presented to illustrate the following statistical feature of the PMR method: The overall force of mortality in a PMR study is assumed to be equal to the comparison population, and if that is not true, the PMRs for each cause of death will be off by a factor relating to the overall difference. Here the overall SMR was 92, whereas the overall PMR, by definition, was assumed to be 100. This difference, about 8%, caused the PMR for each cause of death category to be high by about that same amount. The PMR-SMR differences that follow are, therefore, a function of this statistical problem as well as the unequal representation of cause-of-death categories.

The financial situation is presented in Figure 6. It can be seen that the PMRs and SMRs were very similar. The slight overrepresentation of circulatory system deaths and underrepresentation of external causes visibly affected the PMRs for those categories, but not so much that different conclusions would have been reached as to excesses and deficits.

Figure 7 presents the nonfinancial situation. The most striking feature here was the large differences between the PMR and SMR for nonmalignant diseases of the respiratory system. It was seen in Figure 2 that these deaths were known more often than other deaths, and in conjunction with the 8% methodologic difference, the total difference was substantial. Although cancer was shown to be underrepresented in this situation (Fig. 2), the PMR and SMR statistics were very similar, because the underrepresentation and the 8% methodologic increase cancelled out one another. In general, the PMRs and SMRs in this situation would have led to similar conclusions, although the numerical size of the statistics varied considerably.

The actual situation at the union, deaths being known for both financial and nonfinancial reasons (the combined situation), is presented in Figure 8. It was observed that the circulatory and respiratory PMRs were higher than their respective SMRs, and the external causes PMR was lower than its SMR. These PMRs were generally more accurate than nonfinancial PMRs, but less accurate than the financial PMRs. They were, therefore, adversely affected by the deaths known for miscellaneous reasons from the nonfinancial situation.

The last situation, deaths among active workers only, is presented in Figure 9. As expected, the overrepresentation of circulatory system deaths caused the PMR for that category to be substantially higher than the SMR, and the PMRs for the other causes were either lower than or equal to their respective SMRs, rather than 8% higher. These PMRs would have led generally to the same conclusions as the SMRs, except for the circulatory system diseases, for which a substantial deficit (in comparison to the U.S.) would have been missed totally.

The last analysis was to see whether a PMR study would have led to the same major findings as the previously published SMR study (Beaumont and

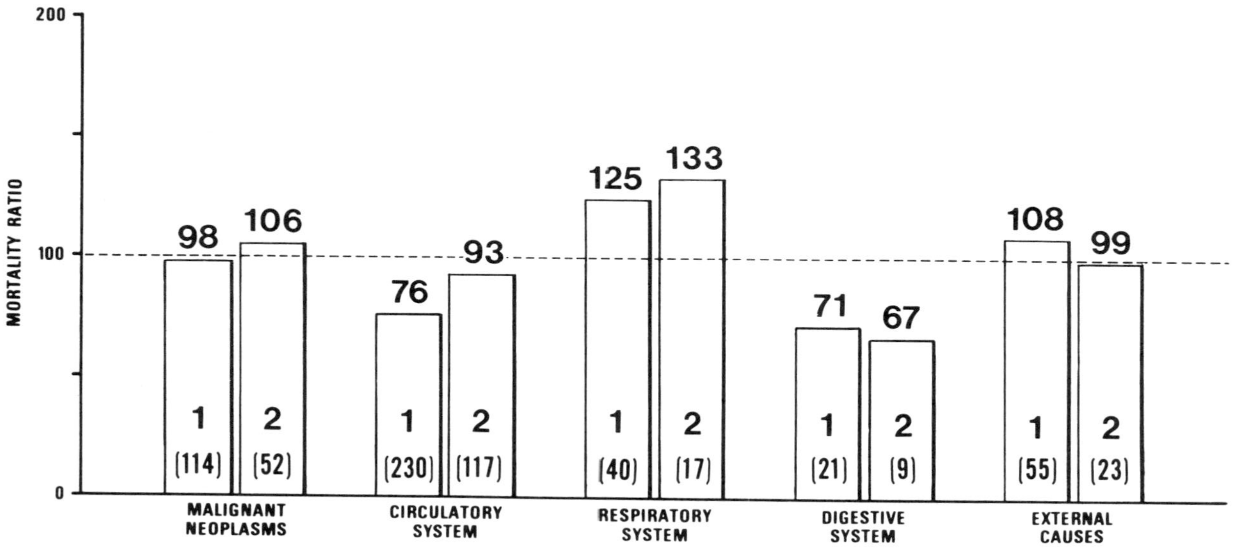

Figure 6
Comparability of SMRs and PMRs where the PMRs are based upon deaths from the financial situation (1) SMR; (2) PMR.

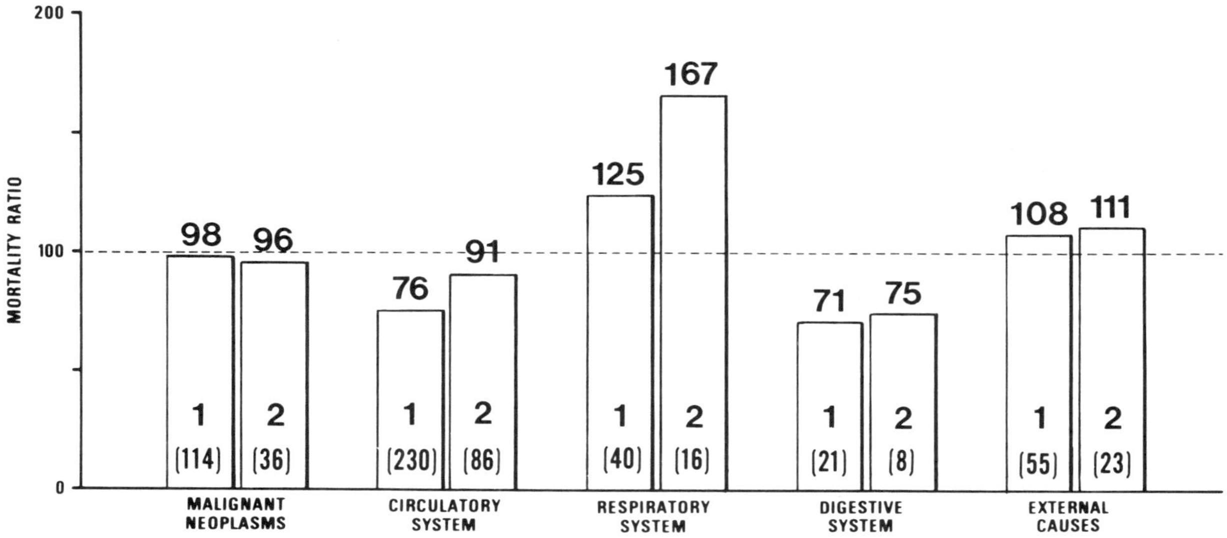

Figure 7
Comparability of SMRs and PMRs where the PMRs are based upon deaths from the nonfinancial situation ([1]) SMR; ([2]) PMR.

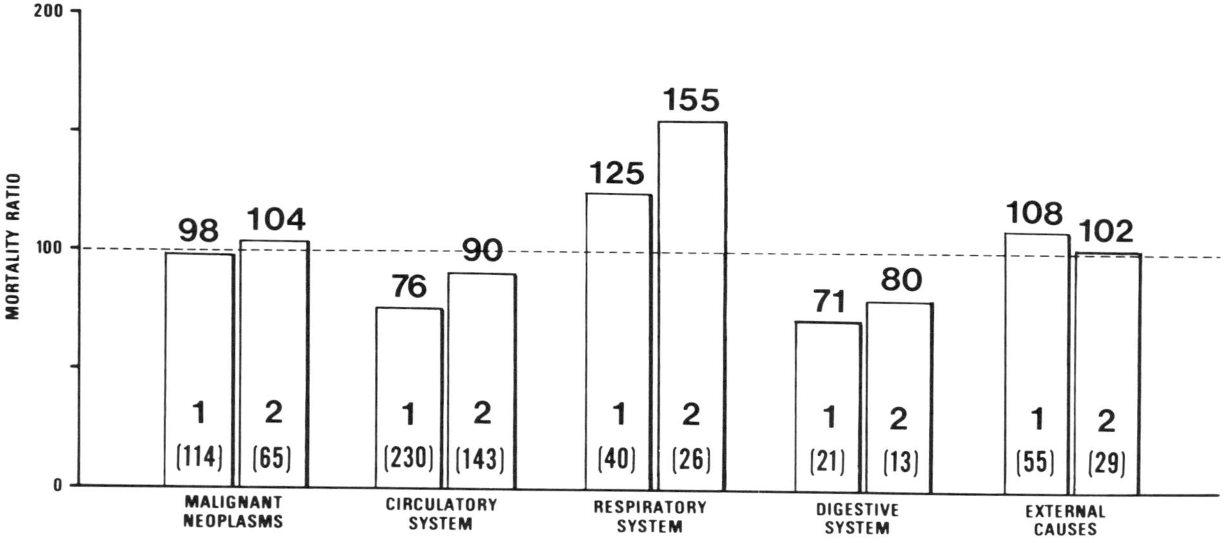

Figure 8
Comparability of SMRs and PMRs where the PMRs are based upon deaths from the combined situation (1) SMR; (2) PMR.

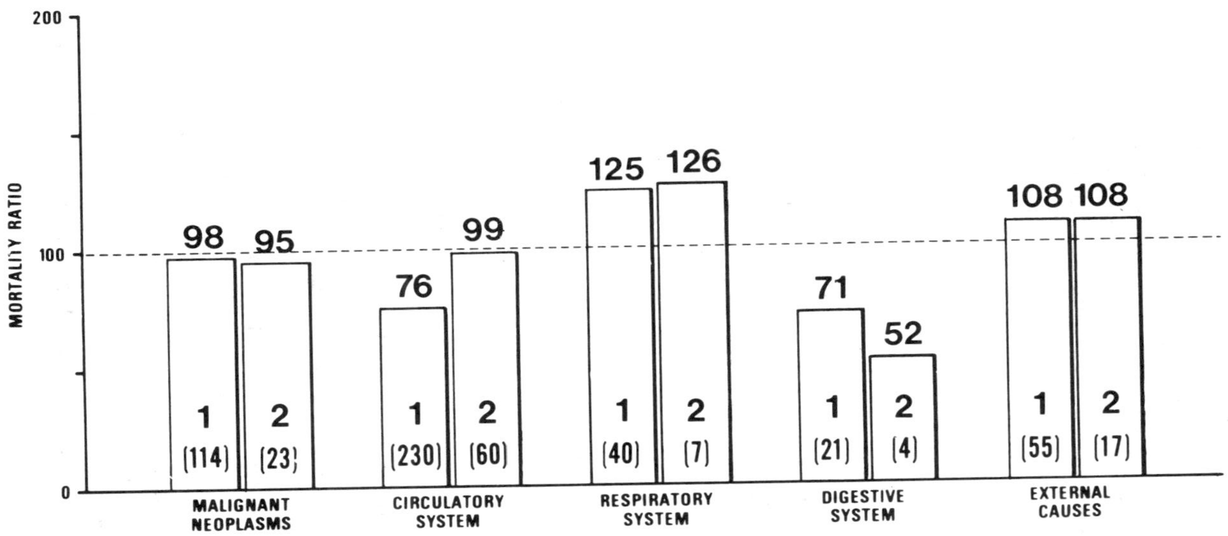

Figure 9
Comparability of SMRs and PMRs where the PMRs are based upon deaths from the active-only situation (1) SMR; (2) PMR.

Weiss 1980). They were that respiratory cancer was in excess by 31%, increasing to 69% ($p < 0.01$) after 20 years latency, and that other diseases of the respiratory system were high by 25%, increasing to 61% ($p < 0.01$) after 20 years latency. Figure 10 shows what the results would have been without consideration of latency. It can be seen that the excesses would have been noted by a PMR study, regardless of the situation, although the exact accuracy of the PMRs would depend on the situation. Figure 11 shows the results when only the deaths occurring 20 years after first employment were considered. The PMRs for cancer of the respiratory system were all relatively accurate. For other diseases of the respiratory system, the accuracy varied considerably for the various situations, although all situations would have documented the excess of deaths.

DISCUSSION

The PMR, now well established as a method for assessing occupational mortality, has developed a reputation that has both positive and negative aspects. On the positive side, PMR studies tend to be quick and inexpensive relative to their chief alternative, SMR studies. This is because, for a PMR analysis, only deceased workers are needed; it is not necessary to establish the complete population at risk. It is also not necessary to do any follow-up of the workers to ascertain every death, as long as the deaths that are known are representative of all deaths (disregarding sample size considerations).

This leads to a negative aspect of PMRs which can bias results: If all the deaths are not known, and among the deaths that are known, some causes of death are represented more than others, then the causes that are overrepresented will appear to be in excess. For example, if accidental deaths are known more often than chronic disease deaths, then accident mortality will appear to be in excess.

Another source of bias than can occur with PMR studies is the "seesaw effect," caused by the mathematical necessity that the cause-specific PMRs balance out to an overall PMR of 1.00 (the all causes PMR is always 1.00, by definition) (Decoufle et al. 1980). Thus, if one cause of death is higher or lower than 1.00 (in reality or due to the unequal representation problem discussed above), then the other causes will have PMRs generally in the opposite direction, so that the all causes PMR can equal 1.00. The seesaw effect results from the fact that the all causes PMR is not allowed to fluctuate up or down, to reflect the influence of the individual death categories. Instead, it is a fixed pivot around which the death categories must balance. The result is a multiplicative bias where each cause of death is inflated or deflated equally. For example, if one cause of death is low (e.g., circulatory deaths because of the "healthy-worker effect") and the others are normal, then the all causes PMR should ideally be below 1.00 and the other causes PMRs should ideally be

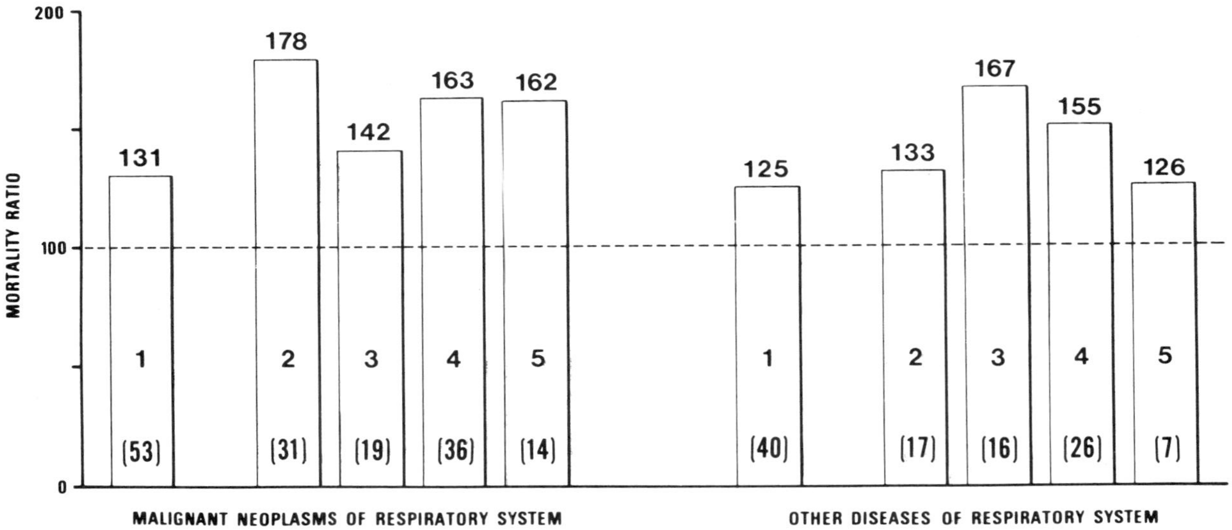

Figure 10
Reproducibility of the main findings of the SMR study with PMRs (1) SMR; (2) PMR (if financial situation); (3) PMR (if nonfinancial situation); (4) PMR (if combined situation); (5) PMR (if active-only situation).

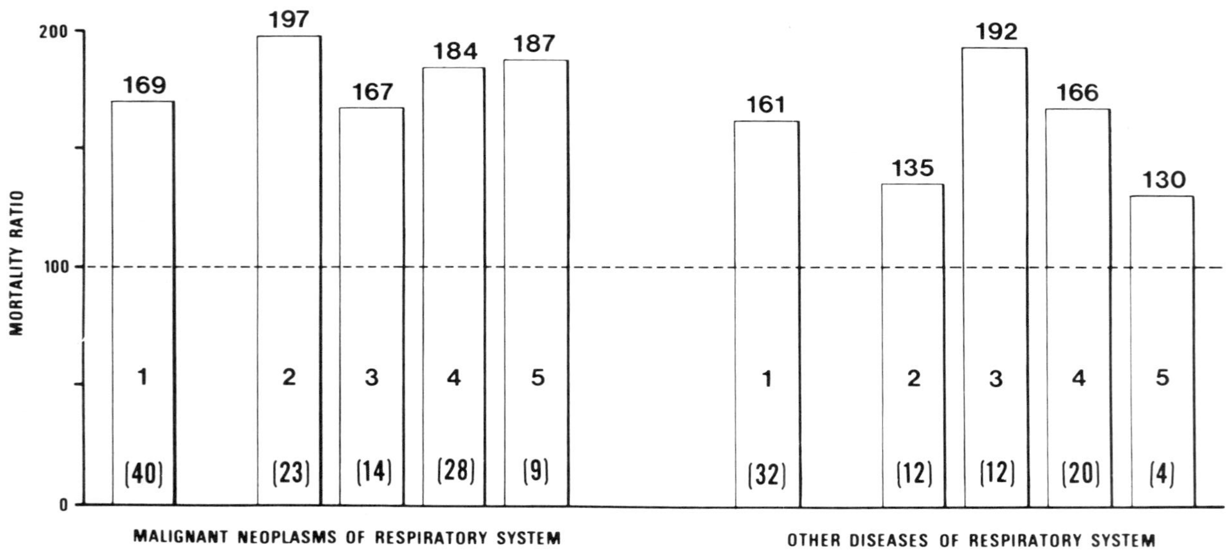

Figure 11
Reproducibility of the main findings of the SMR study with PMRs, considering only the deaths after 20 years from first employment (1) SMR; (2) PMR (if financial situation); (3) PMR if nonfinancial situation); (4) PMR (if combined situation); (5) PMR (if active-only situation).

unaffected. But because the overall PMR is fixed at 1.00, every individual death category, including the one that was low to begin with, is inflated by the percentage that the all causes PMR should have been decreased. This multiplicative effect was empirically demonstrated in Figure 5. The factor by which the results are influenced has previously been shown to be approximately the inverse of the overall SMR (Butler et al. 1980).

We can do little about this last source of bias, the seesaw effect, except to exclude causes of death that are not of interest. An example of this is calculation of proportionate *cancer* mortality ratios (PCMRs), which exclude all noncancer deaths. We can do more about the other bias source, unequal representation of the different causes of death in a data set, in that we can judge whether a data set is likely to represent all causes equally before embarking on an analysis. Of the four common types of PMR data sets defined in this report–financial, nonfinancial, combined, and active–the financial best represented the various causes of death and yielded PMRs most similar to the SMRs. Visual inspection of Figures 1-9 gives this impression, and comparability scores, calculated by summing the percentage differences between the SMRs and PMRs for each of the five major death categories, substantiate the impression quantitatively (Table 3). The all deaths data set, as might be expected, gave the lowest score (39), but of the data sets known to the union, financial was the lowest with a score of 52, nonfinancial was second lowest with 64, combined was third lowest with 67, and active was highest with 71.

The actual situation at the union was combined, in that deaths were known for both financial and miscellaneous nonfinancial reasons. It can now be seen, with the advantage of hindsight, that a PMR study at that union would have been most accurate if the deaths known for miscellaneous nonfinancial reasons had been ignored. Respiratory disease deaths were substantially overrepresented among these miscellaneous deaths, possibly because of concern about respiratory exposures.

In assessing whether the PMRs agreed with the SMRs, one consideration was whether or not the directions of the ratios agreed. There was generally good

Table 3
Comparability Scores for the PMR Data Sets, Calculated by Summing the Percentage Differences Between the SMRs and PMRs for the Five Major Death Categories

Data set	Comparability score
All deaths	39
Financial	52
Nonfinancial	64
Combined	67
Active only	71

agreement as to excesses and deficits for all data set types, with one important qualification: statistical testing results would not be expected to agree because in all PMR data sets the number of deaths was much smaller than the number in the SMR study. In other words, PMRs have relatively low statistical power in comparison to SMRs because they are not based upon complete data, and hypothesis testing results would be expected to be different even when the ratios were exactly the same. For this reason no hypothesis testing was performed.

There are several issues that limit our ability to generalize these findings. One is that pension plans and life insurance programs differ greatly among companies and unions in terms of eligibility requirements and history of coverage. Another is that policies vary regarding the notation of miscellaneous deaths, e.g., whether obituary column reports are noted. Third, there is variability in the degree of reporting within the active, vested, and miscellaneous nonactive categories. This is important because a low degree of reporting leaves considerable room for cause-of-death ascertainment bias. Fourth, our nonfinancial data set approximation probably underestimated the number of deaths known for miscellaneous reasons (this was discussed in the methods section). The effect of the underestimation is not known. Finally, the sizes of the data sets analyzed were not large, thus chance variability may have come into play. The results presented within this paper, therefore, are to some degree specific to these data.

Generalizations are best made when several studies show the same result, and in this case, there are only a few other studies that have approached the problem. Decoufle and Thomas (1979) compared active only PMRs and active and retiree PMRs to all deaths PMRs, a comparison which is similar to the present investigation because, as seen in Figure 5, all deaths PMRs are related to SMRs via a multiplicative factor. They found, as did we, that the PMRs varied by data set. Of the two data sets they examined, active only and active and retired, comparability scores showed their active and retired data set to be superior with a score of 21 (versus 40 for active only). (In computing the scores, the tuberculosis and "other causes" categories were not included in order to make the scores comparable to those from the present study.) We showed in our data that the active only data set was the most biased (score = 70), and that active and vested (roughly equivalent to their active and retired) was least biased (score = 52), thus there was agreement that financial data sets appear to be more appropriate for PMR analysis than active only data sets. Their results for specific causes of death did not always agree with ours, however. For example, circulatory system deaths were just slightly overrepresented in their active only data set, as opposed to substantial overrepresentation in ours.

Data from a 9-year follow-up study of steelworkers showed that the proportion of deaths known to the employer varied considerably by cause (Redmond et al. 1969). For example, 79% of the circulatory system deaths were known, while just 55% of cancer deaths were known (71% of the deaths were known overall). Because the follow-up period was short (9 years), a relatively high percentage of the deaths occurred among the actively employed. The overrepresentation of circulatory system deaths among the deaths known to the steel companies agreed with our findings for those actively employed.

In conclusion, the PMRs for the welders were similar to the SMRs, in that there was general agreement as to excesses and deficits. However, the exact numerical sizes of the mortality ratios were sometimes very different. The financial data set gave the closest numerical agreement between the SMRs and PMRs as judged by a comparability score. For these data it appears, therefore, that the best PMR data set resulted from a financial incentive for survivors to report deaths among inactive workers. Life insurance and pension death benefit programs that allowed workers to become vested (eligible for benefits after termination of employment) provided this incentive.

ACKNOWLEDGMENTS

The authors wish to thank William E. Halperin, David P. Brown, Robert A. Rinsky, William J. Butler, Pierre Decoufle, and Carol K. Redmond for their advice during the preparation of this manuscript.

REFERENCES

Beaumont, J.J., and N.E. Weiss. 1980. Mortality of welders, shipfitters, and other metal trades workers in Boilermakers Local No. 104, AFL-CIO. *Am. J. Epidemiol.* **112**:775.

Butler, W.J., N.J. St. Clair, R.G. Cornell, R.L. Farrell, J.M. Becker, D. Finkelstein and L. Howard. 1980. *Assessment of proportionate analysis methods: Preliminary investigation.* Vector Research, Incorporated, Ann Arbor, Michigan.

Decoufle, P., and T.L. Thomas. 1979. A methodological investigation of fatal disease risks in a large industrial cohort. *J. Occup. Med.* **21**:107.

Decoufle, P., T.L. Thomas, and L.W. Pickle. 1980. Comparison of the proportionate mortality ratio and standardized mortality ratio risk measures. *Am. J. Epidemiol.* **111**:263.

Kupper, L.L., A.J. McMichael, M.J. Symons, and B.M. Most. 1978. On the utility of proportionate mortality analysis. *J. Chronic Dis.* **31**:15.

Redmond, C.K., E.M. Smith, J.W. Lloyd, and H.W. Rush. 1969. Long-term mortality study of steelworkers. III Follow-up. *J. Occup. Med.* **11**:513.

Redmond, C.K., and P.P. Breslin. 1975. Comparison of methods for assessing occupational hazards. *J. Occup. Med.* **17**:313.

A Population-based Cohort Study of Brain Tumor Mortality Among Oil Refinery Workers with a Discussion of Methodological Issues of SMR and PMR

CHI PANG WEN, SHAN POU TSAI, NANCY S. WEISS,
WILLIAM A. McCLELLAN, AND ROY L. GIBSON
Gulf Oil Corporation
Houston, Texas 77001

Several epidemiological studies have examined the association of cancer risk and employment in oil refineries (Tabershaw/Cooper Associates 1974; Hanis et al. 1979; Theriault and Goulet 1979; Rushton and Alderson 1980; Thomas et al. 1980a). This interest is highlighted by a recent workshop sponsored by the New York Academy of Sciences (NAS) on Brain Tumors in the Chemical Industry (October 27-29, 1980) in which several papers discussed such a risk among refinery workers.

The reported results from the workshop presentations and other published papers have been inconsistent as to the risk of brain tumor mortality (Alexander et al. 1980; Cook et al. 1980; Reeve et al. 1980; Rushton and Alderson 1980; Thomas et al. 1980b; Wen et al. 1980). At the NAS workshop, results from the largest cohort study of refinery workers ever conducted in North America were presented by Wen et al. (1980). These results showed no significant increase in mortality from brain tumor among male refinery workers, as compared to the U.S. male experience. This finding differed from that reported by a National Cancer Institute (NCI) study of union workers by use of the proportionate mortality ratio (PMR) method (Thomas et al. 1980b). Despite the fact that almost five times as many death certificates were collected in Wen's study as in the NCI study, one criticism made during the workshop was that this study included both white- and blue-collar workers and, thus, its results could have been affected by inclusion of the white-collar workers. The purpose of this paper is to examine further the previous findings in more detail and present results that may provide an explanation for the apparent difference reported.

MATERIALS AND METHODS

The refinery cohort consists of all employees who worked at the Texas refinery between June 15, 1935, and January 1, 1978, regardless of the length of their employment, i.e., anyone ever employed for 1 day or more was included. (This provides the flexibility of evaluating the experience of workers with different lengths of employment time.) Demographic information and the work history of each cohort member were reconstructed from reviews of personnel records, verified, and supplemented by other corporate records, such as annuitant records, insurance benefit records, seniority lists, medical records, and mortality records. The pay status of all workers was determined from entries on the work history and each worker was then classified according to the duration of employment (expressed as percentages of total employment) that was spent on an hourly or salaried basis. All of the essential data elements were computerized. The vital status of employees as of January 1, 1978, was determined from several sources: Corporate and local personnel benefit records, searches by the Social Security Administration and the Motor Vehicle Bureaus of Texas and Louisiana, and verifiable information available locally. The person-years of those lost to follow-up prior to the common closing date were calculated up to the last known date, commonly the date of separation from employment.

Death certificates for the deceased individuals identified from these follow-up investigations were collected and the underlying cause of death was classified by a trained nosologist according to the rules of the International Classification of Diseases (ICD) revision in effect at the time of death and then recoded to the ICDA 8th revision for analysis.

For analytical purposes, standardized mortality ratios (SMRs) were calculated utilizing a computer program that compares age-sex-race-year-specific mortality rates with those comparable rates of the U.S. general population (Monson 1974). Those rates that were not available from Monson's program, such as the benign or nature-unspecified brain tumor rates, were generated from data available from the National Center for Health Statistics (NCHS) and the National Institute for Occupational Safety and Health (NIOSH), computerized, and then incorporated into Monson's program. Significance testing of SMRs was based on the assumption of a Poisson distribution for the observed deaths, utilizing a two-sided test of significance (Bailar and Ederer 1964). In addition, PMRs have been calculated for reference and discussion (Monson 1974).

RESULTS

Characteristics of the cohort are described in Table 1. Out of the total 17,350 workers studied, 75% were white males, 15% were nonwhite males, and 10% were females. A total of 406,659 person-years of survival were observed and 78% of these were contributed by white males. The cohort has an average year of entry of 1948 at an average age of 28.6 and was observed and followed for an average of 23.4 years. It should be noted that 10% of the male cohort

Table 1
Cohort Characteristics—June 15, 1935, to January 1, 1978

	Male[a]				
	white	nonwhite	subtotal	Female	Total
Number of employees	12,960	2,596	15,556	1,794	17,350
(% of total)	(75%)	(15%)	(90%)	(10%)	
Years of survival	315,167	59,035	374,202	32,457	406,659
(% of total)	(78%)	(15%)	(92%)	(8%)	
Average survival	24.3	22.7	24.0	18.1	23.4
Average age of entry	28.9	30.0	29.1	24.1	28.6
Average year of entry	1948.7	1946.1	1948.3	1948.2	1948.3
Average year of death	1964.0	1963.8	1964.0	1967.3	1964.3
Lost to follow-up	1,216	335	1,551	634	2,185
(% lost to follow-up)	(9%)	(13%)	(10%)	(35%)	(13%)
Number of observed deaths	3,494	842	4,336	98	4,434
Death certificates unascertained	299	72	371	11	382
(% unascertained)	(8.5%)	(8.5%)	(8.5%)	(11.2%)	(8.6%)
Number of expected deaths	3,969.8	1,117.2	5,087.0	129	5,216.0
Observed death/expected death	0.88	0.75	0.85	0.76	0.85

[a]Male employees whose race is unknown (1.8%) are included in the "white" category.

Table 2
Length of Employment of Male Employees

	White		Nonwhite		Total		
Years of service	number	percent	number	percent	number	percent	
Less than 1	3,304	25.5	504	19.4	3,808	24.5	
1-4	2,181	16.8	542	20.9	2,723	17.5	
5-9	1,210	9.3	244	9.4	1,454	9.3	
10-14	632	4.9	128	4.9	760	4.9	
15-19	545	4.2	116	4.5	661	4.2	
20-24	839	6.5	193	7.4	1,032	6.6	40% (20 years or more)
25-29	1,131	8.7	170	6.6	1,301	8.4	
30-34	1,225	9.5	271	10.4	1,496	9.6	
35-39	1,148	8.9	233	9.0	1,381	8.9	
40-44	579	4.5	135	5.2	714	4.6	
45-49	152	1.2	59	2.3	211	1.4	
50 or more	14	0.1	1	0.0	15	0.1	
Total	12,960		2,596		15,556		

(1551) were lost to follow-up, and that 8.5% of the male deaths (371) were without known causes of death.

The follow-up of the female cohort was only 65% successful. This large percentage of women lost to follow-up (35%) probably was due to the fact that many women changed their last names as the result of marriages, thus making the tracing of them very difficult, if not impossible. Also, in view of the fact that female employees contributed only 8% of the total person-years of the cohort, the following results and discussion will be limited to only male refinery workers.

Table 2 shows the distribution of length of employment of male employees by race. The stability of workers in this refinery is reflected by the fact that almost 40% of them worked 20 years or more. The distribution for white and nonwhite employees in terms of length of employment was quite similar.

The distribution of year of hire of male employees, as seen in Table 3, showed that over one-third were hired prior to 1940 and another one-third in the 1940-1949 interval. Thus, over 70% of the male employees in the cohort began employment before 1950.

Table 4 shows the distribution of employees according to pay status. It was found that 82% of white males and 85% of the total male cohort worked exclusively as hourly, blue-collar workers. These blue-collar workers represented at least six different unions. Approximately 11% of the total could be classified as "salaried" with 75% or more of their employment being in a salaried capacity.

Table 3
Year of Hire of Male Employees

	White		Nonwhite		Total		
Year of hire	number	percent	number	percent	number	percent	
1900-1909	80	0.6	7	0.3	87	0.6	36%
1910-1919	735	5.7	165	6.4	900	5.8	
1920-1929	2,090	16.1	574	22.1	2,664	17.1	
1930-1939	1,645	12.7	275	10.6	1,920	12.3	
1940-1949	4,486	34.6	954	36.8	5,440	35.0	
1950-1959	2,143	16.5	190	7.3	2,333	15.0	
1960-1969	581	4.5	51	2.0	632	4.1	
1970-1978	1,200	9.3	380	14.6	1,580	10.2	
Total	12,960		2,596		15,556		

Table 4
Distribution of Male Employees by Pay Status

Percentage of employment[a]		White		Nonwhite		Total		
salaried	hourly	number	percent	number	percent	number	percent	
0%	100%	10,627	82.0	2,540	97.8	13,167	84.6	
25%	75%	301	2.3	8	0.3	309	2.0	
50%	50%	280	2.2	6	0.2	286	1.8	
75%	25%	198	1.5	1	0.0	199	1.3	11%
90%	10%	254	2.0	2	0.1	256	1.6	
100%	0%	1,249	9.6	27	1.0	1,276	8.2	
Unknown		51	0.4	12	0.5	63	0.4	

[a]Based on the percentage of employment rounded to the nearest percentage category.

Table 5 shows mortality results of the male cohort. All causes of death showed a deficit of 751 deaths with an SMR of 0.85. The SMR for the nonwhites, 0.75, was lower than the SMR for the whites, 0.88. All of these SMRs were decreased significantly. A total of 822 deaths due to cancer were observed whereas 873 deaths were expected, resulting in an SMR of 0.94.

In the examination of brain tumor mortality, 28 deaths were observed among the male cohort and 30.39 deaths were expected, yielding an SMR of 0.92. For the white males, where nearly a twofold increase was shown by the NCI study which used the PMR method (Thomas et al. 1980b), the SMR was 0.86.

Table 5
SMRs for Male Cohort (1935-1978)

	White			Nonwhite			Total		
Cause of death	O	E	SMR	O	E	SMR	O	E	SMR
All causes	3494	3970	0.88[a]	842	1117	0.75[a]	4336	5087	0.85[a]
All malignant neoplasms	666	705	0.94	156	168	0.93	822	873	0.94
Brain cancer									
Malignant (ICD–191,192)	15	19.69	0.76	3	1.93	–	18	21.62	0.83
Benign or nature unspecified (ICD–225,238)	8	7.19	1.11	2	1.59	–	10	8.78	1.14
Total brain	23	26.88	0.86	5	3.52	1.43	28	30.39	0.92

SMRs were not calculated for observed deaths less than 5.
[a] $p < 0.01$.

Table 6 shows the mortality results of workers on an hourly or salaried payroll basis during refinery employment. Note that pay status was classified either as hourly (100% of employment on an hourly basis) or salaried (75% or more of employment on a salaried basis). Some salaried workers first started as hourly employees and then were promoted to salaried rankings. For the hourly workers, the SMR for all causes was 0.88, and for all cancer, 0.95. There were 25 deaths from brain tumors among the hourly employees with 25.64 expected. The resultant SMR was 0.97. Although nonwhite hourly workers showed an excess of brain tumor mortality (SMR = 1.44), the observed number was small ($N = 5$) and showed no statistical significance ($p > 0.4$). The observed number of brain tumor deaths among the salaried workers was too small to be conclusive. Nevertheless, there was no trend of increased risk observed.

In relationship to brain tumor risk, latency (defined as the period of time from the first exposure to the time of death from brain tumor) has been examined and tabulated in Table 7. No significant increased risk of brain tumor was noticed after a latency period of 20 years or more. SMRs were 1.14 and 1.10 for hourly and total males, respectively. Increasing the latency period to 35 years or more the brain tumor risk was still unremarkable (SMR = 1.04 and 1.27 for hourly and total males, respectively).

The increase shown by nonwhite males but not white males with 35 years or more of latency is based on three cases[1] and is not statistically significant. Nevertheless, further steps are currently being undertaken to verify this finding. Such a racial difference has not been reported in the literature.

Brain tumor mortality and length of employment were examined in Table 8. Although SMRs for those who worked over 20 years are greater than those who worked less than 20 years, none of the increases in the SMRs reached statistical significance (SMR = 1.40 and 1.35 for the hourly and total males with length of employment 20 years or more, respectively).

Based on the finding that a large number of employees lost to follow-up were either employed for only a short period of time (e.g., less than 6 months) or terminated employment prior to the inception of the social security system (making follow-up next to impossible), a subgroup of the cohort was selected for analysis. This cohort, hereafter referred to as the 1940 cohort, consists of those employees hired on or after January 1, 1940, and with a minimum of 6 months employment.

Table 9 shows the characteristics of this 1940 cohort. Those employees lost to follow-up and the number of unascertained deaths in this 1940 cohort were both reduced to 4%, from approximately 10%. In other words, 96% of the 1940 cohort were successfully traced.

[1] The immediate cause of death of one of the three cases was listed as cerebral vascular accident on the death certificate with possible brain tumor and Parkinsonism. The person had suffered from Parkinsonism for more than 20 years and sought early retirement due to paralysis agitans. Possibility of brain tumor was mentioned with no substantiative evidence (i.e., no autopsy data available).

Table 6
SMRs by Pay Status for Male Cohort (1935-1978)

	Hourly			Salaried		
Cause of death	white	nonwhite	subtotal	white	nonwhite	subtotal
All causes						
O	3015	833	3848	297	2	299
E	3262	1103	4365	430.33	2.23	432
SMR	0.92[a]	0.76[a]	0.88[a]	0.69[a]	–	0.69[a]
All cancer						
O	559	152	711	61	0	61
E	581	167	748	74.39	0.20	74.59
SMR	0.96	0.91	0.95	0.82	–	0.82
Brain cancer (ICD–191,192,225,238)						
O	20	5	25	2	0	2
E	22.16	3.48	25.64	2.91	0.00	2.91
SMR	0.90	1.44	0.97	–	–	–

[a] $p < 0.01$.

Table 7
SMRs of Brain Tumor by Latency (Males)

Latency	White			Nonwhite			Total		
	O	E	SMR	O	E	SMR	O	E	SMR
< 20 Years									
Hourly	4	7.08	–	1	1.05	–	5	8.13	0.62
Total	4	8.45	–	1	1.06	–	5	9.51	0.53
⩾ 20 Years									
Hourly	16	15.07	1.06	4	2.43	–	20	17.50	1.14
Total	19	18.39	1.03	4	2.45	–	23	20.84	1.10
⩾ 35 Years									
Hourly	3	4.98	–	3	0.78	–	6	5.76	1.04
Total	6	6.32	0.95	3	0.79	–	9	7.11	1.27

Latency is defined as the period of time from the first exposure (or employment) to the time of death from brain tumor.

The next two tables (Tables 10 and 11) present the results of this 1940 cohort. The SMRs for all causes and all cancer are similar to those of the original cohort with the former being significantly decreased. SMRs of brain tumor in the 1940 cohort for male workers (0.98) or specifically for hourly workers (1.04) are not much different from those calculated for the entire 1935 cohort. It would seem, therefore, that those lost to follow-up or those unascertained deaths have not significantly affected the results of the 1935 cohort.

Table 8
SMRs of Brain Tumor by Length of Employment (Males)

Length of employment	White			Nonwhite			Total		
	O	E	SMR	O	E	SMR	O	E	SMR
< 20 Years									
Hourly	9	13.05	0.69	1	1.95	–	10	15.00	0.67
Total	9	15.13	0.59	1	1.96	–	10	17.09	0.59
⩾ 20 Years									
Hourly	11	9.17	1.20	4	1.53	–	15	10.70	1.40
Total	14	11.78	1.19	4	1.55	–	18	13.33	1.35

Table 9
1940 Cohort Characteristics—January 1, 1940, to January 1, 1978

	Male[a]				
	white	nonwhite	subtotal	Female[a]	Total
Number of employees	9,511	2,015	11,526	1,097	12,623
(% of total)	(75%)	(16%)	(91%)	(9%)	
Years of survival	230,164	45,621	275,785	20,329	296,114
(% of total)	(78%)	(15%)	(93%)	(7%)	
Average survival	24.2	22.6	23.9	18.5	23.5
Average age of entry	30.9	32.2	31.1	25.3	30.6
Average year of entry	1949.1	1948.8	1949.0	1950.9	1949.2
Average year of death	1964.6	1964.7	1964.6	1966.9	1964.8
Lost to follow-up	360	130	490	298	788
(% lost to follow-up)	(3.8%)	(6.5%)	(4.3%)	(27.2%)	(6.2%)
Number of observed deaths	2,667	707	3,374	71	3,445
Death certificates unascertained	97	38	135	6	141
(% unascertained)	(3.6%)	(5.4%)	(4.0%)	(8.4%)	(4.1%)
Number of expected deaths	3155.2	909.7	4064.9	89.1	4154.0
Observed death/expected death	0.85	0.78	0.83	0.80	0.83

[a]Limited to those with minimum employment of 6 months.

Table 10
SMRs for Male 1940 Cohort (1940-1978) (Males)

	White			Nonwhite			Total		
	O	E	SMR	O	E	SMR	O	E	SMR
All causes	2667	3155	0.85	707	910	0.78	3374	4065	0.83
All cancer	540	567	0.95	135	143	0.94	675	710	0.95
Brain									
Malignant (ICD–191,192)	10	15.26	0.66	3	1.59	–	13	16.85	0.77
Benign or nature unspecified (ICD–225,238)	8	5.43	1.47	2	1.28	–	10	6.71	1.49
Total brain	18	20.69	0.87	5	2.87	1.74	23	23.56	0.98

Table 11
SMRs by Pay Status for 1940 Cohort (1940-1978) (Males)

	Hourly			Salaried		
	white	nonwhite	subtotal	white	nonwhite	subtotal
All causes						
O	2217	698	2915	277	2	279
E	2515	897	3412	378.59	1.86	380.45
SMR	0.88[a]	0.78[a]	0.85[a]	0.73[a]	–	0.73[a]
All cancer						
O	439	131	570	57	0	57
E	453	141	594	66.30	0.18	66.48
SMR	0.97	0.93	0.96	0.86	–	0.86
Total brain cancer (ICD–191,192,225,238)						
O	15	5	20	2	0	2
E	16.43	2.83	19.26	0.67	0.00	0.67
SMR	0.91	1.77	1.04	–	–	–

[a] $p < 0.01$.

DISCUSSION

Our previous results showed a lack of evidence of an increased brain tumor mortality risk among all male refinery workers at this Texas refinery. Further analysis of the results presented in this paper showed that the inclusion of salaried (white collar) workers had minimal effect on the results. Workers on either an hourly (represented by at least 6 unions) or salaried payroll did not show a brain tumor risk significantly different from that of the U.S. population. These results are consistent with those conclusions reached by Tabershaw/Cooper Associates (1974), Hanis et al. (1979), and Rushton and Alderson (1980). On the other hand, the results do not support the findings of Thomas et al. (1980b) and Theriault and Goulet (1979).

The sample size of this study, as discussed in the previous paper (Wen et al. 1980), is sufficiently large to detect an SMR of brain tumor in the males as small as 1.75 with Type I error, (α) = 0.05, and Type II error, (β) = 0.2 (Walter 1977). In other words, the power of the test is more than capable of detecting a twofold risk, if such a risk did indeed exist.

To pursue further the differences observed between the NCI study and this study, PMRs of this study were calculated as shown in Table 12. The PMR results of brain tumor for total and hourly white males were both 0.97 (20 observed and 20.6 expected based on 3015 deaths, for the hourly males). This is in contrast to the reported PMR of 1.90 (10 observed and 5.3 expected based on 729 deaths) for the white male workers at the same plant as reported by the NCI study.

Thus, the observed difference might seem to be attributable to the differing sizes of data bases rather than to the different methodologies, i.e., PMR vs SMR. However, the problem does not appear to be unique in this particular case. In conducting PMR analyses, it must be assumed that the number of unascertained deaths is small and inconsequential or those deaths not studied have a proportionate mortality pattern similar to those studied. Unfortunately, the validity of such an assumption has been tested rarely and incomplete data have been analyzed frequently by the PMR method. Thus, the very nature of PMR methodology can lead to conclusions with false positive (or more rarely, false negative) results unrecognized by investigators.

There seems to be an apparent excess of brain tumor risk for those who worked 20 years or more (SMR = 1.20) when compared with those who worked less than 20 years (SMR = 0.69). However, it is well known that summary SMRs, being an indirect standardization statistic, cannot be compared if the age structure of the two subgroups is not similar (C.P. Wen and S.P. Tsai, in prep.). This is indeed true as shown in Table 13, where the person-year distribution of the two subgroups is shown to be quite different and those employed more than 20 years are much older. Thus, an adjustment is necessary before the two SMRs can be compared. By using the distribution of the sum of

Table 12
PMRs for White Male Cohort (1935-1978)

	Hourly			Total			NCI	
	PMR	(number observed)	SMR	PMR	(number observed)	SMR	PMR	(number observed)
All causes	1.00	(3015)	0.92	1.00	(3494)	0.88	1.00	(729)
All cancer	1.07	(559)	0.96	1.04	(666)	0.94	1.22	(166)
Brain cancer								
Malignant (ICD–191,192)	0.98	(15)	0.92	0.87	(15)	0.76	–	–
Benign or nature unspecified (ICD–225,238)	0.91	(5)	0.84	1.26	(8)	1.11	–	–
Total brain	0.97	(20)	0.90	0.97	(23)	0.86	1.90	(10)

Table 13
Person-year Distribution by Age and Length of Employment for White Male Hourly Workers

Age	< 20 years		≥ 20 years	
< 25	15,297 (8%)		0 (–)	
25-29	22,851 (12%)		4 (0%)	
30-34	27,929 (15%)		12 (0%)	
35-39	30,731 (16%)		1,187 (2%)	
40-44	27,497 (15%)		6,443 (9%)	
45-49	21,340 (11%)		11,044 (16%)	
50-54	16,257 (9%)		12,563 (18%)	
55-59	11,244 (6%)		11,472 (17%)	
60-64	7,301 (4%)		9,592 (14%)	
65-69	4,139 (2%)	22% (ages 50–85+)	7,444 (11%)	74% (ages 50–85+)
70-74	1,956 (1%)		5,060 (7%)	
75-79	750 (0%)		2,839 (4%)	
80-84	219 (0%)		1,205 (2%)	
85+	89 (0%)		481 (1%)	
Total	187,600 (99%)		69,346 (101%)	

expected deaths from the two subgroups as the weighting factor (as shown in the Appendix), it appears that the SMRs for those 20 years or more and less than 20 years of service have changed from 1.20 and 0.69 to 0.93 and 0.67, respectively (Table 14). The resultant ratio of these two adjusted SMRs is 1.39 (0.93/0.67) in contrast to 1.74 (1.20/0.69), which is derived from a direct comparison of the two unadjusted SMRs.

Another approach has been taken by calculating the relative risk based on the Mantel-Haenszel method (Mantel and Haenszel 1959) by use of a computer program (Schoenbach 1979). The result of such an approach yields

Table 14
RR by Length of Employment (White Hourly Males)

	≥ 20 years	< 20 years	Ratio (≥ 20 yrs/< 20 yrs)
SMR	1.20	0.69	1.74
Adjusted SMR[a]	0.93	0.67	1.39
RR (Mantel-Haenszel)			1.38[b]

[a]Adjustment based on the average expected deaths of the two subgroups.
[b]Based on Mantel-Haenszel chi-square test with one degree of freedom ($\chi^2 = 0.35$, $p > 0.28$).

an age and calendar-year-adjusted relative risk (RR) of 1.38 ($\chi^2 = 0.35$, $p > 0.28$). Thus, the RR and the ratio of the adjusted SMRs indicate that the mortality rates of the two subgroups are comparable. The need for such an adjustment of SMRs is obvious and is particularly important in cases where workers with different lengths of employment or latency periods are to be compared, for they usually show different age distributions.

The diagnoses of the brain tumor deaths as they appeared on the death certificates are listed in Table 15. One half of the diagnoses were listed only as "brain tumor" or "carcinoma of brain," with no specific cell types indicated. Another 15% included the word "metastatic" or it was implied from the cell types mentioned. Only 29% (8) were glioblastoma and 7% (2) astrocytoma. Misclassification of brain cancer on death certificates has been well documented by Percy et al. (1981). It would seem not only desirable but essential to review these brain tumor deaths clinically and (or) histopathologically to establish their true classification. Results from further in-depth studies of brain tumor mortality short of such an effort need to be interpreted with caution.

It should be noted that of all the refinery workers' deaths, only 0.6% of them could be attributed to brain tumor. Based on the current results, this cohort study has failed to show that the workers at this Texas refinery experienced an increased mortality risk of cancer as a whole (SMR = 0.94) or specifically of brain tumor (SMR = 0.92). The risks are not statistically different from those of the comparable U.S. population. Study of this cohort will be continued and future mortality information will be incorporated and any new findings reported. Furthermore, a case-control study already in progress will be continued for the purpose of exploring the relationship between specific work exposure and the risk of brain tumor mortality.

Table 15
Diagnoses of Brain Tumor for the Male Cohort

	White	Nonwhite	Total	(%)	
Glioblastoma	7	1	8	29	36%
Astrocytoma	2	–	2	7	
Carcinoma of brain	1	2	3	11	50%
Brain tumor	9	2	11	39	
Metastatic carcinoma of brain	2	–	2	7	
Metastatic neuroblastoma	1	–	1	4	
Malignant melanoma	1	–	1	4	
Total	23	5	28		

Diagnoses as they appeared on the death certificates as the underlying cause of death.

REFERENCES

Alexander, V., S.S. Leffingwell, J.W. Lloyd, R.J. Waxweiler, and R.L. Miller. 1980. Brain cancer in petrochemical workers—a case series report. Paper presented at the New York Academy of Sciences Workshop on Brain Tumors in the Chemical Industry, October 27-29.

Bailar, J.C. III and F. Ederer. 1964. Significance factors for the ratio of a Poisson variable to its expectation. *Biometrics* **20**:639.

Cook, R.R., G.G. Bond, R.J. Shellabarger, R.L. Daniel, and W.A. Fishbeck. 1980. Case-control study of brain tumor deaths among employees at a chemical manufacturing plant. Paper presented at the New York Academy of Sciences Workshop on Brain Tumors in the Chemical Industry, October 27-29.

Hanis, N.M., K.M. Stavraky, and J.L. Fowler. 1979. Cancer mortality in oil refinery workers. *J. Occup. Med.* **21**:167.

Mantel, N. and W. Haenszel. 1959. Statistical aspects of the analysis of data from retrospective studies of disease. *J. Natl. Cancer Inst.* **32**:719.

Monson, R.R. 1974. Analysis of relative survival and proportional mortality. *Comput. Biomed. Res.* **7**:325.

Percy, C., E. Stanek, and L. Glockler. 1981. Accuracy of cancer death certificates and its effect on cancer mortality statistics. *Am. J. Pub. Health* **71**:242.

Reeve, G.R., J.W. Lloyd, V. Alexander, S.F. Leffingwell, R.J. Waxweiler, H. Bell, and W.E. Halperin. 1980. A progress report: The investigation of brain tumors at the Texas division of Dow Chemical. Paper presented at the New York Academy of Sciences Workshop on Brain Tumors in the Chemical Industry, October 27-29.

Rushton, L. and M.R. Alderson. 1980. "An epidemiological survey of eight oil refineries in the U.K." Final report prepared for the Institute of Petroleum.

Schoenbach, V.J. 1979. *Stratification analysis macro for use with the Statistical Analysis System (SAS).* The University of North Carolina at Chapel Hill.

Tabershaw/Cooper Associates. 1974. *A mortality study of petroleum refinery workers.* Project OH-1 prepared for the American Petroleum Institute, Washington, D.C.

Theriault, G. and L. Goulet. 1979. A mortality study of oil refinery workers. *J. Occup. Med.* **21**:367.

Thomas, T.L., P. Decoufle, and R. Moure-Eraso. 1980a. Mortality among workers employed in petroleum refining and petrochemical plants. *J. Occup. Med.* **22**:97.

Thomas, T.L., R.J. Waxweiler, M. Crandall, D.W. White, R. Moure-Eraso, S. Itaya, and J.F. Fraumeni, Jr. 1980b. Brain cancer among OCAW members in three Texas oil refineries. Paper presented at the New York Academy of Sciences Workshop on Brain Tumors in the Chemical Industry, October 27-29.

Walter, S.D. 1977. Determination of significant relative risks and optimal sampling procedures in prospective and retrospective comparative studies of various sizes. *Am. J. Epidemiol.* **105**:387.

Wen, C.P., S.P. Tsai, and R.L. Gibson. 1980. A report on brain tumor from a retrospective cohort study of refinery workers. Paper presented at the New York Academy of Sciences Workshop on Brain Tumors in the Chemical Industry, October 27-29.

APPENDIX—COMPARISON OF SMRs

SMR calculations are based on indirect standardization. Thus comparison of two summary SMRs is valid only if it can be shown that the age structure of these groups does not differ significantly (Liddell 1960; Kilpatrick 1963). Otherwise, appropriate adjustment must be made. According to Miettinen (1972), the SMR estimates for different subgroups are "internally standardized but not mutually comparable." The summary SMR can be written:

$$\begin{aligned} \text{SMR} &= \frac{\text{total observed deaths}}{\text{total expected deaths}} \\ &= \frac{\Sigma\, O_i}{\Sigma\, E_i} \\ &= \frac{\Sigma\, (O_i/E_i) \cdot E_i}{\Sigma\, E_i} \\ &= \frac{\Sigma\, \text{SMR}_i \cdot E_i}{\Sigma\, E_i} \end{aligned} \tag{1}$$

where O_i = observed death of age group i; E_i = expected death of age group i; and SMR_i = age specific mortality ratio (O_i/E_i).

The SMR expressed in the above formula is a weighted average of SMR_i. The weights are the expected deaths in the particular subgroup.

If the distributions of expected deaths or person-years are significantly different between two subgroups, the two SMRs should not be compared directly and an adjustment is necessary. If comparison is to be done, SMR_i can be weighted by the sum of the expected deaths of the two subgroups. The equations for adjustment are:

$$\text{adjusted SMR}_1 = \frac{\Sigma\, \text{SMR}_{1i}\, (E_{1i} + E_{2i})}{\Sigma\, (E_{1i} + E_{2i})} \tag{2}$$

$$\text{adjusted SMR}_2 = \frac{\Sigma\, \text{SMR}_{2i}\, (E_{1i} + E_{2i})}{\Sigma\, (E_{1i} + E_{2i})} \tag{3}$$

where E_{1i} and E_{2i} are the expected deaths of age group; for the subgroups 1 and 2, respectively. Thus, from Table A, the adjusted SMR for less than 20 years of service is:

$$\text{adjusted SMR}_{<20} = \frac{0.722 \times (1.386 + 0.052) + \ldots + 1.455 \times (1.375 + 1.699)}{13.050 + 9.169} \quad (4)$$

$$= 0.665$$

and for 20 years or more the adjusted SMR is:

$$\text{adjusted SMR}_{\geqslant 20} = \frac{1.997 \times (1.952 + 1.502) + \ldots + 2.278 \times (0.139 + 0.439)}{13.050 + 9.169} \quad (5)$$

$$= 0.933$$

Table A
Observed and Expected Deaths of Brain Tumor by Age and Length of Employment

	< 20 yrs			⩾ 20 yrs		
Age	O_i	E_i	$O_i/E_i(SMR_i)$	O_i	E_i	$O_i/E_i(SMR_i)$
< 25	–	0.264	–	–	–	–
25-29	–	0.516	–	–	0.000	–
30-34	–	0.893	–	–	0.000	–
35-39	1	1.386	0.722	–	0.052	–
40-44	2	1.643	1.217	–	0.385	–
45-49	2	1.839	1.088	–	0.947	–
50-54	1	1.952	0.512	3	1.502	1.997
55-59	1	1.767	0.566	2	1.764	1.134
60-64	2	1.375	1.455	3	1.699	1.766
65-69	–	0.846	–	1	1.347	0.742
70-74	–	0.396	–	1	0.866	1.155
75-79	–	0.139	–	1	0.439	2.278
80-84	–	0.027	–	–	0.131	–
85+	–	0.007	–	–	0.037	–
Total	9	13.050	0.692	11	9.169	1.200

Observed and expected deaths of brain tumor based on white male hourly worker.

References

Liddell, F.D.K. 1960. The measurement of occupational mortality. *Brit. J. Industr. Med.* **17**:228.

Kilpatrick, S.J. 1963. Mortality comparisons in socioeconomic groups. *Appl. Stat.* **12**:65.

Miettinen, O.S. 1972. Standardization of risk ratios. *Am. J. Epidemiol.* **96**: 383.

SESSION 6: Methodology

Indicators of Exposure Trends

FRED D. HOERGER
Regulatory and Legislative Issues
Health and Environmental Sciences
The Dow Chemical Company
Midland, Michigan 48640

Most of us tend to think of risk as the probability of the occurrence of an adverse event. In discussing carcinogenicity, risk is a function of both the toxicity and the degree of exposure. It follows then that exposure trends are important for two reasons: (1) to predict future cancer burdens and (2) to target our resources for epidemiology, health surveillance, and risk management programs.

Quantification of exposure trends is difficult because of the gaps and uncertainties in the data base. The experience and perspective of colleagues from several disciplines (industrial hygiene, chemistry, biology, environmental science, and process development) were relied upon in preparation of this paper to compensate for gaps in direct data or past exposure.

This presentation considers exposure trends from several perspectives. Trends in the concentrations of ambient air pollutants and ubiquitous contaminants will be examined along with trends in chemical production volumes as gross surrogates of exposure. Numbers of employees exposed to chemicals on an industry-wide basis and in terms of specific substances will be examined, and numerous examples of monitoring data on specific substances collected from 1950 to the present will be presented. Finally, many of the risk-management practices available today will be compared qualitatively with the practices of the past.

Wherever possible, data and information were collected to characterize exposure conditions circa 1950, 1970, and the present. Although it has been necessary to rely upon indirect information and fragments of data, I believe that the aggregation of this information and the consistency of the data give a realistic indication of exposure trends.

GROSS SURROGATES OF EXPOSURE

Criteria and Ubiquitous Pollutants

Data are available on the background level of several ambient and ubiquitous pollutants. The Environmental Protection Agency (EPA) reports that general air

Table 1
Improvement in the Air Quality Index

	Total number of days in 23 cities		
	1974	1978	percent change
Unhealthful	1405	1264	-10
Very unhealthful	514	343	-33
Hazardous	33	15	-55

Data from Environmental Quality (1980).

quality has improved during the 1970s. As an example, EPA maintains a composite index of air quality for 23 cities reflecting the numbers of days in the combined cities in which one or more of the criteria pollutants exceeds the national emission standards. Table 1 shows that the index has improved for the three levels of severity of general pollution. Table 2 shows that the gross tonnage of total suspended particulate emissions decreased significantly between 1970 and 1978. Other criteria pollutants—SO_2, NO_2, volatile organics, and carbon monoxide—have remained relatively constant. Levels of benzo[*a*]pyrene have fallen some 85% between 1966 and 1977 (from 4.5 ng/m^3 to 0.5 ng/m^3). (Environmental Quality 1980).

Data on the concentrations of several ubiquitous pollutants (DDT, polychlorinated biphenyls [PCBs], dieldrin, methyl chloride, and chloroform) are shown in Table 3. Concentrations in milk, adipose tissue, and fish meal prepared from Chesapeake Bay fish are all at relatively low levels and are declining. Methyl chloride and chloroform originate from natural sources as well as industrial sources; thus, their concentrations are relatively constant at the fractional ppb level.

The data presented here support a general conclusion that the absolute concentrations of the criteria and ubiqutious pollutants are low in relation to

Table 2
National Emissions Estimates

	Millions of metric tons/year				
Year	TSP[a]	SO_2	NO_2	volatile organics	CO
1970	23	30	20	28	103
1978	12	27	23	28	102
Change (%)	-46	-10	+17	—	-1

Data from EPA (1980).
[a]Total suspended particulate.

Table 3
Some Background Levels of "Ubiquitous" Substances

Material	Substrate	Concentration	Year	Trend
DDT[a]	human milk	1.6 ppm	1977	D[e]
Dieldrin[a]		0.03 ppm	1977	D
PCBs[a]		0.09 ppm	1977	D
DDT[b]	human fat	5 ppm	1974	D
Methyl chloride[c]	atmosphere	0.7 ppb	1975	S[f]
Chloroform[c]		0.02 ppb	1975	S
DDT[d]	fish meal	0.02 ppm	1975	D
PCBs[d]		0.02 ppm	1975	D

[a]Currie et al. (1979).
[b]Kutz et al. (1977).
[c]National Academy of Sciences (1978).
[d]Hardin (1980).
[e]Decreasing.
[f]Stable.

occupational exposures and that most are relatively stable or decreasing. It follows that the general backyard pollution need not be considered in analyzing occupational exposure trends.

PRODUCTION VOLUMES

Frequently, production volumes are used as gross surrogates of exposure. Table 4 shows production volumes for several mining-related activities. It can be seen that arsenic trioxide production has dropped by about 20% in the 1964-1973 period. Iron ore production has remained relatively constant over the last three

Table 4
Production of Selected Mining-related Commodities in the United States

Commodity	Period	Change (%)
Arsenic trioxide[a,b]	1964-1973	-20
Iron ore[a,b]	1950-1979	none[d]
Nickel[a,b]	1965-1979	+30
Copper (primary)[a,b]	1950-1979	+50
Coal[c]	1950-1978	+18

[a]Bureau of Mines (1975).
[b]Bureau of Mines (1981).
[c]Department of Commerce (1979).
[d]Considerable year-to-year fluctuation.

Table 5
Production of Selected Agricultural Commodities in the United States

Commodity	Period	Change (%)
Peanuts	1965-1979	+67
Corn	1950-1979	+150
Beef	1950-1979	+150

Data from Department of Agriculture (1980); Historical statistics of the United States

decades while copper, nickel, and coal production have shown increases up to 50%. Production of agricultural commodities has increased more significantly as shown in Table 5. Corn and beef production are up 150% in the past three decades.

Increases in the production of synthetic organic chemicals are more dramatic, rising from 4 billion pounds in 1940 to 22 billion pounds in 1950 to 228 billion pounds in 1979 as shown in Figure 1. Another indicator of chemical

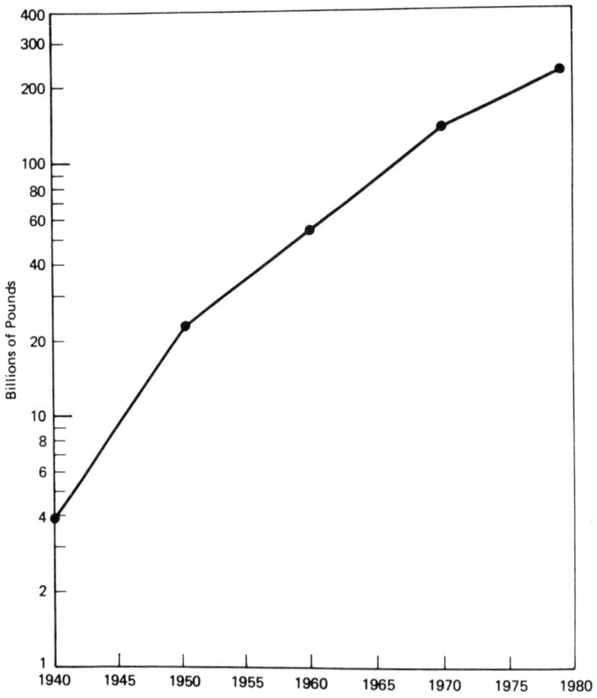

Figure 1
U.S. Production of synthetic organic chemicals 1940-1979 in billions of pounds

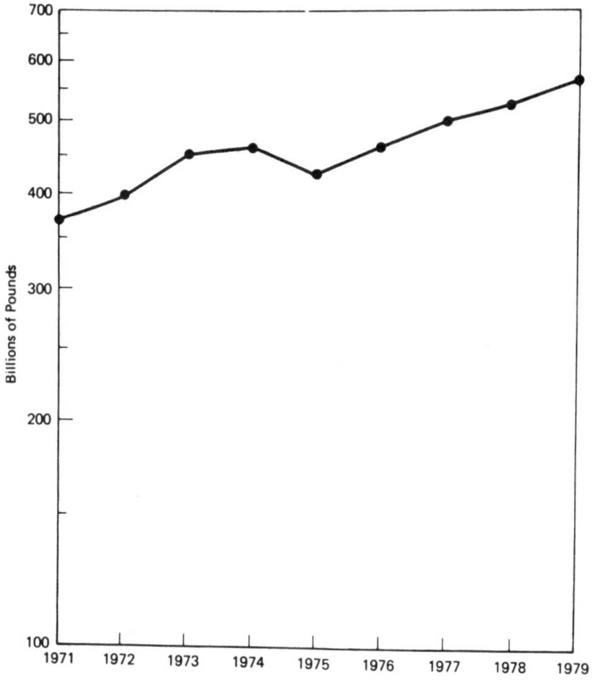

Figure 2
Production volume The top 50 U.S. chemicals in billions of pounds 1971-1979

production is shown in Figure 2, a plot of the increase in the "top 50." These are the 50 largest-volume chemicals produced in the United States. Sulfuric acid, at 84 billion pounds per year, is the largest-volume chemical. Ethyl alcohol, regarded by some as a "friendly" chemical, is the 50th largest chemical, at a production volume of about 1.3 billion pounds (synthetic grade). It should be pointed out that the top 50 include about half organic materials and half inorganic substances.

Another profile of the chemical industry is provided by a look at the distribution of the approximately 55,000 chemical substances in commerical production. Data from the EPA inventory of chemicals collected under the Toxic Substances Control Act (TSCA) in 1977 (OTS 1979) show that 70% of the commercial chemicals are produced in annual volumes of less than 100,000 pounds and that some 30% are at less than 1000 pounds per year (Table 6). Expressed another way, less than 2% of the commercial chemicals represent more than 80% of the production tonnage (Table 7).

During the past few years there has been much speculation about the potential risks that might be posed by the many new chemicals introduced into

Table 6
Volumes of Production Reported for TSCA Inventory, September 1979

Percent	Lb/yr
70	<100,000
50	< 10,000
30	< 1,000

Data from OTS (1979).

commerce each year. In my view, this speculation is overplayed. Almost every new chemical starts as a small-volume chemical. Most never grow beyond the small-volume stage of a few thousand to 100,000 pounds. Those few that do grow to significant volumes do so only over a relatively long period of time, from one to several decades. Based on the assumption of continued innovation of new chemicals and optimistic growth trends for these chemicals, I have estimated the 1990 annual production for all new chemicals developed during the entire decade of the 1980s. This optimistic estimate is 0.5 billion pounds. It is a relatively trivial volume compared to the 565 billion pounds of production for the "top 50" in 1980 and an estimated 900 billion pounds for the "top 50" in the year 1990. It seems reasonable to conclude that the majority of our exposure potentials are associated with a relatively small number of chemicals, perhaps only a few hundred.

THE NUMBER OF EMPLOYEES EXPOSED TO CHEMICALS

The number of employees exposed to potentially toxic substances is a crude indicator of the magnitude of any potential public health problem. Since 1950, population, general employment, and employment in the private sector have all increased, but at relatively modest rates (Table 8). Within the general increase in employment however, the mining industry and general manufacturing have

Table 7
Inventory Breakdown

Production volume, (10^6 lbs/yr)	Percent of total number produced	Percent of estimated annual tonnage
<1	87	3
1-10	7	2
10-100	4	15
100-1000	1	46
>1000	<1	34

Data from OTS (1979).

Table 8
U.S. Population and Work Force (10^6 people)

Year	Population	Number employed	Private sector production, or nonsupervisory
1950	152	–	34
1960	180	66	39
1970	204	87	48
1979	221	96	60
1960-1979 change (%)	23	45	55

Data from Bureau of Labor Statistics (1980).

Table 9
Production or Nonsupervisory Workers on Private Payrolls (employment $\times 10^6$)

Year	Mining	Manufacturing	Construction
1950	0.8	13	2.1
1960	0.6	13	2.5
1970	0.5	14	3.0
1979	0.7	15	3.7
Change (%)	-10	+15	+75

Data from Bureau of Labor Statistics (1980).

Table 10
Total Employees in Chemicals and Allied Products

Year	10^6 employees
1950	0.6
1960	0.8
1970	1.0
1979	1.1

Data from Bureau of Labor Statistics (1980).

shown little growth. Employment in both the construction industry and in the chemical and allied products industries has increased about 75-80% between 1950 and the present (Tables 9 and 10).

Employment in the chemical and allied products industry, however, has been at a much slower rate than the growth in production volume (80% vs 1000%). This contrast is due to process technology and automation advances

Table 11
Plant Size vs Labor Force (general estimate same technology)

Plant capacity factor	Capital factor	Labor factor	Engineering estimate
$2X$	$1.6X$	$1.2X$	capital = $X^{.7}$
$10X$	$5.0X$	$1.6X$	labor = $X^{.2}$
$100X$	$25X$	$2.5X$	

Data from K. L. Burgess and J. E. Tollar et al. (unpubl. results); SRI International (unpubl. results).

and to increased efficiency as a result of larger plants. For example, reports from the Stanford Research Institute (unpubl. results) contain estimates that an economic plant for a commodity chemical such as styrene utilized 35% less labor in 1977 than a smaller plant built in 1967. Production volume for the recent plant design was 500% more than the earlier design. Table 11 represents a generalized engineering estimate for plant size in relation to labor and capital investment requirements.

In the early 1970s, National Institute for Occupational Safety and Health (NIOSH) conducted what became known as the National Occupational Hazard Survey (NOHS). This survey attempted to estimate the number of employees exposed to specific chemical substances. The methodology of the survey was relatively simple, which proved to be a major pitfall. Substances were inventoried by plant along with the number of employees in the plant. These values for individual plants were then summed up and factored to relate to broader industry segments. Little or no attempt was made to determine whether a specific employee in a given plant worked with the substance being inventoried.

Recently, to rectify misinformation from the NOHS data, several contractors have surveyed specific substances. These contractor approaches involve identification of all the manufacturers, processors, and users. Employees in each plant handling the specific substance were then inventoried. In addition, exposure profiles for various subsets of employees were obtained.

Comparison of the NOHS results and contractor surveys are shown in Tables 12 and 13. It can be seen that the NOHS estimates overstated the employment census for monochlorobenzene, *ortho*-dichlorobenzene, and *para*-dichlorobenzene by roughly a factor of 400. In the case of vinylidene chloride, employment was overestimated by factors of 2 to 20.

Table 12
Comparison of NOHS and Contractor Studies—The Chlorobenzenes

Substance	Number of employees exposed	
	NOHS estimate	contractor estimate[a]
Monochlorobenzene	1,097,000	3150
ortho-Dichlorobenzene	1,977,000	3240
para-Dichlorobenzene	544,000	820

[a]Data from Hull and Company (1980).

Table 13
Comparison of NOHS and Contractor Studies—Vinylidene Chloride

	Number of employees exposed
NOHS estimate	
Definites	6,500
Probable	58,000
Contractor estimate[a]	2,975-3,200

[a]Data from Sittenfield and Associates (1979).

MONITORING DATA ON SPECIFIC SUBSTANCES

The Occupational Safety and Health Administration (OSHA) adopted permissible exposure levels for some 400 substances in 1972. These standards were derived from a list developed over the years by the American Conference of Governmental Industrial Hygienists (ACGIH) and published in 1968. Since that time, the ACGIH has revised many of its recommendations while OSHA has issued additional standards for a few carcinogens. It has been possible to make a comparison of 22 substances of carcinogenic concern which currently are listed by both ACGIH and OSHA. Of these 22 materials, the ACGIH standard is lower than the OSHA standard in 13 instances, the same as OSHA in 7 instances, and greater in 2 instances. In general, professional industrial hygienists follow the ACGIH guideline if it is lower than the OSHA standard. To some degree then, the industry targets for carcinogen exposure levels are today somewhat lower than the OSHA standard.

To gain a more accurate and representative picture of trends in occupational exposure, a number of case examples are presented here. They are believed to be typical of trends occurring over the last 30 years and to be representative of profile differences between various subgroups of employees associated with a given substance. Exposure data on a number of noncarcinogenic substances are presented to scrutinize a larger data base for

Table 14
Exposure Profile: Chlorobenzenes (employee exposure by time)

Hours of exposure per week	Number of people exposed MCB	ODCB	PDCB
1	328	415	113
1-8	377	427	129
9-20	305	210	61
20	2136	259	518
Total	3146	1311	821
		+1930[a]	
		3241	

Data from Hull and Company (1980).
[a]Total estimated number exposed to ODCB after resale.

Table 15
Exposure Profile: Vinylidene Chloride

	Number surveyed	Range of exposure[a] (8-hr TWA[b])
Manufacturers	523	0.2-2.4 ppm
Processors	803-813	0.1-2.8 ppm
Converters	1649-1860	N.D.-0.18 ppm

Data from Sittenfeld and Associates (1979).
[a]Of the approximately 3000 people in survey, about 1700 (more than half) are exposed to 0.2 ppm (8-hr TWA).
[b]Time-weighted average.

Table 16
Caustic Dust

Dates	Developments	Exposure
1930	production start up	
1951-1958	area samples	0-7.7 mg/m^3
	evaporator operators	0.5-2 mg/m^3 (TWA)[a]
	finishing operators	0.5 mg/m^3 (TWA)
1959-1960	closed finishing system installed	
1970	flaking operation discontinued	
1975	packaging was automated	
1980	operators	0.1 mg/m^3 or less

Data from Ott et al. (1977).
[a]Time-weighted average.

Table 17
Styrene Monomer

	Exposure
Monomer production	
1942	24 ppm (area samples)
1945	1.4 ppm (area samples)
1972	0.1-6.0, average 1.0 (TWA[a])
1973	0.2-5.4, average 1.0 (TWA)
1980	0.01-3.3, average 0.4 (TWA)
Polymer production	
1955	<200 ppm (area samples)
1963	97 ppm (area samples)
1973	<0.1-19 ppm (10 TWAs)
1975-76	0.1-1.2 ppm (42 TWAs)
1980	0.03-0.2 ppm (19 TWAs)

Data from Dow (unpubl. results).
[a]Time-weighted average.

trends. All data are believed to be typical of a broad range of industry programs and illustrate that risk management practices extend beyond the field of carcinogens.

The contractor studies on chlorobenzene and vinylidene chloride in Tables 14 and 15 illustrate rather markedly the differences in exposure for various subgroups of employees. Significant differences in both the frequency of exposure and in the level of exposure dependent upon manufacturing industry are illustrated in these profiles. Over the years, significant improvements have been made in the manufacturing process for caustic dust. Table 16 shows that a 5- to 20-fold reduction in exposure was accomplished over a 20-year period. Tables 17, 18, and 19 show that similar exposure reductions were accomplished with styrene, acrylonitrile, and benzene exposure over the last three decades.

Table 18
Benzene: Use as a Manufacturing Solvent

	TWA[a] ppm					
	1952-1953	1961	1965	1973	1974	1978
Manufacturing area[b]	17-36	–	5-17	3.8-4.0	–	0.03-1.3
Lab technician	–	16	–	–	4.0	–
Fabrication area	35	–	11-32	–	–	–

Data from Ott et al. (1978).
[a]Time-weighted average.
[b]Eight job classifications.

Table 19
Acrylonitrile: Plastic Production

		TWA ppm	
Year	Area samples (ppm)	range	number sampled
1955	13	–	–
1959	4	–	–
1965	17	–	–
1973	–	0.2-19	6
1973	3	2.3-2.5	2
1975-1976	–	0.1-4.5	37
1980	–	0.02-0.9	19

Data from Dow (unpubl. results).

Significant reduction in arsenic levels in the workplace environment was achieved by ASARCO over several decades by instituting engineering controls. Data are shown in Table 20. Imposition of personal hygiene practices also was responsible for reductions in actual personal exposure as indicated by monitoring of urinary concentrations of arsenic as shown in Figure 3.

Table 20
Average Airborne Arsenic in the Arsenic-producing Part of the Plant

Year	Average arsenic concentration (mg/m^3)	Number of samples
1947	15.29	49
1948	39.87	8
1950	21.82	23
1951	2.67	15
1952	2.08	10
1953	5.22	8
1954	0.63	95
1955	1.65	51
1956	1.54	48
1957	0.153	144
1960	1.66	74
1963	0.17	15
1968	0.715	21
1971	0.17	97
1973	0.639	44
1974	0.612	80

Data from S. F. Bundy (pers. comm.).

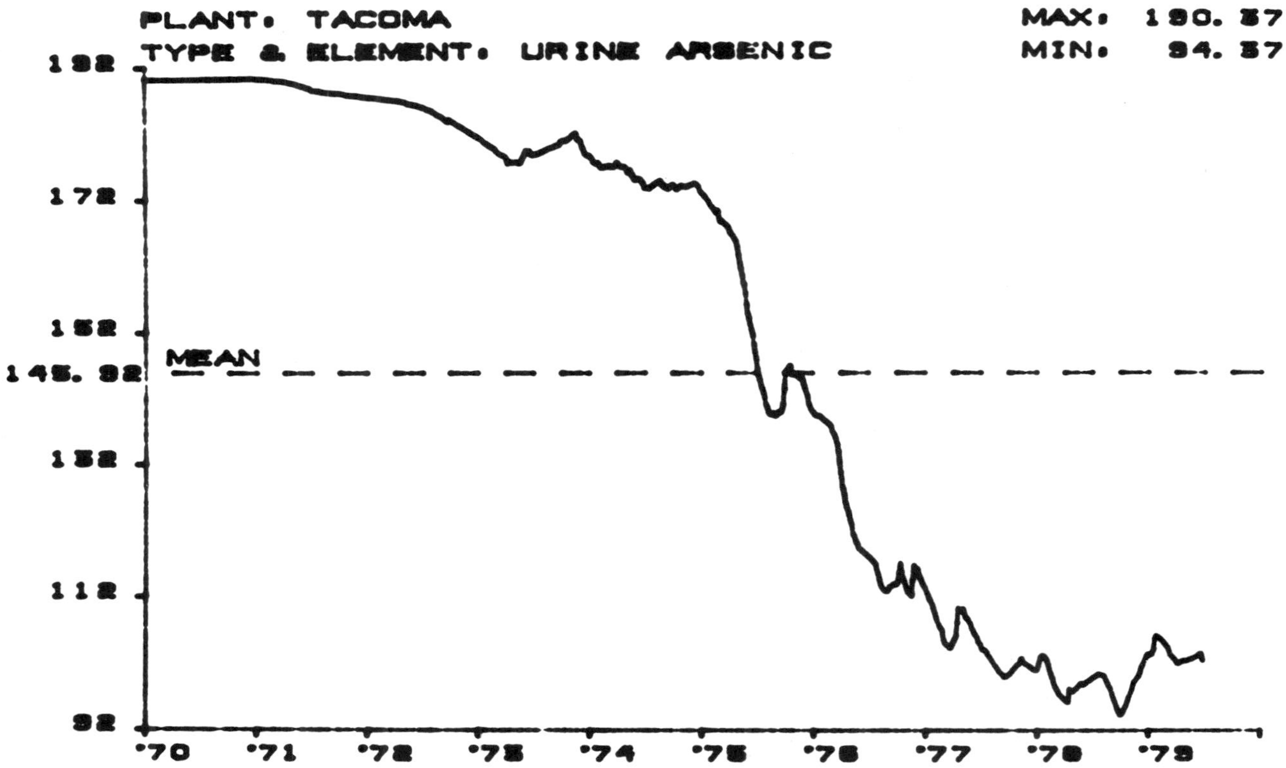

Figure 3
ASARCO Inc. 10-Year plant average (Nelson 1981)

Table 21
Vinyl Chloride Monomer: Copolymer Production Operations

	TWA ppm			
	1950-1959	1960-1963	1975	1979
Unit I				
Dry end	5-10	5	–	0.7
Wet end	10-385	10-80	–	0.8
Unit II	5-825	5-240	10	1.0

Data from Ott et al. (1975).

In the late 1970s, Dupont toxicologists identified hexamethylphosphoric-triamide as a very potent animal carcinogen. Upon this finding, Dupont initiated an extensive retrofitting of their production and handling facilities (Karrh 1977). Exposures were reduced from 100 ppb to 0.5 ppb over a 1- or 2-year period. Analytical methods were developed and an extensive monitoring program was established. Protective equipment, administrative controls, and engineering controls constituted part of the risk-management program.

Vinyl chloride represents perhaps the classic example of exposure reduction by a relatively broad segment of industry. Data from a Dow polymerization production plant are presented in Table 21. Recently, J. Stafford (unpubl. results) in England has estimated vinyl chloride exposure levels, on a generalized basis, for the industry. These are shown in Table 22 and indicate that peak levels on the order of 1000 or more ppm were believed to be prevalent in the industry in the 1950s.

Table 22
Estimated Exposures of Vinyl Chloride in Polyvinylchloride Plants

	ppm
1945-1955	1000
1955-1960	400-500
1960-1970	300-400
mid-1973	150
1980	<1-10

Polymerization > monomer production > fabrication > fence line

Data from J. Stafford (unpubl. results).

Table 23
Clustering of Liver Angiosarcoma Cases in Vinyl Chloride Monomer Plants

	Number of cases cluster/total	Number of factories in clustered cases
Western Europe	35 of 43	10
North America	31 of 36	4[a]
Rest of world	8 of 8	3

Data from J. Stafford (unpubl. results).
[a]43 of 49 factories have had no cases.

It seems significant that the cases of angiosarcoma of the liver associated with vinyl chloride have been clustered in relatively few plants (Table 23). For example, of the 36 cases of angiosarcoma identified in North America, 31 of the cases have been clustered in 4 plants; 43 of 49 plants have never had cases of angiosarcoma (J. Stafford, unpubl. results).

TRENDS IN RISK MANAGEMENT PRACTICES

Qualitatively, and with considerable confidence, it can be stated that risk-management practices designed to control exposure levels are at a very advanced state, compared with as recently as 1970. Communication of new findings of carcinogenicity is now a relatively well-established practice in the industry. Generally, manufacturers communicate new findings of carcinogenicity or other chronic health effects directly to employees through safety meetings, special meetings, "tailgate" sessions, memos, or physician conferences. Manufacturers communicate information to processors and converters who in turn inform employees. Government agencies and labor unions also frequently receive communications describing new findings and may transmit them to various sectors. Technical information brochures include sections on health hazards and management practices. Education and training programs run a variety of formats. Many aspects of risk reduction and control are built into standard operating instructions.

Monitoring for employee exposure is more prevalent and more frequent today than ever before. New analytical methods are being developed continually. Sophisticated instrumental methods for continuously monitoring work areas are in place in many processing areas. It can be said that industrial hygiene practices now provide an awareness of the usual and the basis for detecting the unusual exposure.

Engineering technology has been applied to improving old plants and in the design of new plants. Protective equipment and improved ventilation have been the cornerstones of activity for many years, but new types of pumps and mechanical seals have contributed extensively to the control of fugitive emission. In recent years, it has been recognized that sampling operations for volatile liquids often resulted in significant employee exposure. This has been a targeted area for corrective action. Much attention on a case-by-case basis has been given to exposure possibilities in the handling of waste streams and in maintenance operations. World-scale plants, conversion of batch to continuous processes, containment strategies, and automation are now parts of plant design considerations.

CONCLUSIONS

The following conclusions can be drawn from the data presented:

1. Background levels of criteria and ubiquitous pollutants were constant or declining in the 1970s. Their concentrations seem minor or trivial so far as occupational relevancy.
2. Employment increases have trended with population growth; general manufacturing employment has lagged. Employment in the chemical industry has increased only 80% while organic chemical production has increased nearly 1000% in the past three decades.
3. General estimates of employee exposure frequently overstate the number of employees exposed to a substance and frequently do not profile either frequency or level of exposure.
4. Examples of monitoring data support a conclusion of significant reductions in workplace exposure over the past 10-30 years.
5. Numerous positive indicators illustrate greatly improved risk-management practices compared to the 1950-1970 period.
6. As a generalization, control of carcinogenic agents today is at least an order of magnitude greater than in the 1950-1970 era.
7. The occupational component of total cancer will be significantly less in the year 2000 than it is today (assuming other etiological and environmental factors remain relatively constant).

ACKNOWLEDGMENTS

The author gratefully acknowledges the contributions of W. H. Beamer, S. Bundy, K. L. Burgess, J. W. Conder, L. Hampton, E. E. Kenaga, and D. E. Rapp in discussing potential indications of trends and in retrieving data from varied and obscure sources.

REFERENCES

Bureau of Labor Statistics. 1980. *Handbook of labor statistics, bulletin 2070.* U.S. Department of Labor, Washington, D.C.

Bureau of Mines. 1975. *Mineral Facts and Problems.* U.S. Department of Interior, Washington, D.C.

_____. 1981. *Mineral commodities summary.* U.S. Department of Interior, Washington, D.C.

Currie, R.A., V.W. Kadis, W.E. Breitkreitz, G.B. Cunningham, and G.W. Bruns. 1979. Pesticide residues in human milk, Alberta–1966-1970, 1977-1978. *Pestic. Monit. J.* **13**:52.

Department of Agriculture. 1980. *Agricultural statistics.* USDA, Washington, D.C.

Department of Commerce. 1975. *Historical facts of the United States, colonial times to 1970,* part 1. U.S. Department of Commerce, Washington, D.C.

_____. 1979. *Statistical abstracts of the United States.* U.S. Department of Commerce, Washington, D.C.

Environmental Protection Agency (EPA). 1980. *National air pollutant emission estimates, 1970-1978,* p. 2. EPA-450/4-80-002, Washington, D.C.

Environmental Quality. 1980. *The Eleventh Annual Report of the Council on Environmental Quality.*

Hardin, J. 1980. "Summary of present knowledge of pesticides in fisheries products." Paper read at Seminar and Workshop on Agrichemicals and Estuarine Productivity. Duke University Marine Laboratory, Beaufort, North Carolina.

Hull and Company. 1980. Survey prepared for the Society of Organic Chemicals Manufacturers, April 14.

Karrh, B. 1977. Record comments on the OSHA carcinogen proposal. 42 *Fed. Reg.* **192**:54197.

Kutz, F.W., A.R. Yobs, S.C. Strassman, and J.F. Viar, Jr. 1977. Effects of reducing DDT usage on total DDT storage in humans. *Pest. Monit. J.* **11**:61.

National Academy of Sciences. 1978. *Chloroform, carbon tetrachloride, and other halomethanes: An environmental assessment.* National Academy of Sciences, Washington, D.C.

Nelson, K.W. 1981. *Symposium, RSEN, 3.* Spirdnelenent. Karl Marx University, Leipzig. u. Freidr.-Schuller University, 3 Jena.

Office of Toxic Substances (OTS). 1979. *Toxic Substances Control Act (TSCA) Chemical Substances Inventory, 1979.* OTS, Washington, D.C.

Ott, M.G., R.R. Langner, and B.B. Holder. 1975. Vinyl chloride exposure in a controlled industrial environment. *Arch. Environ. Health* **30**:333.

Ott, M.G., H.F. Gordon, and E.J. Schneider. 1977. Mortality among employees chronically exposed to caustic dust. *J. Occup. Med.* **19**:813.

Ott, M.G., J. Townsend, W. Fishbeck, and R.R. Langner. 1978. Mortality among individuals occupationally exposed to benzene. *Arch. Environ. Health* **33**:3.

Sittenfield and Associates. 1979. Survey prepared for The Dow Chemical Company, August 31.

COMMENTS

ACHESON: I was interested in the material but wondered whether it was a shade complacent to use the final conclusion as a working hypothesis. If I understood the final conclusion, it was that in the year 2000 the proportion of occupationally or industrially related cancer would be less than today. Now, that may be correct. But I think it would be mistaken to use that as a working basis on which to distribute research funds today. We know far too little about dose/response relationships, and about the effects of exposures that have occurred in the last 10-15 years.

HOERGER: I would comment only this. I think that the resources we have in this area of occupational carcinogenicity, occupational health are needed, and we must continue them. But I do think that it is important to keep in mind that, if we saw major increases, then we would want to push a lot more resources into it. You know, if you listen to a weather forecast and we are going to get one-inch of rain tomorrow, you are going to do certain things. If a 20-inch downpour, deluge, or monsoon is forecasted, you are going to do things a heck of a lot differently. I think this is one of the perspectives we are trying to sort out here. But there is a one-inch rain out there that is going to continue in the year 2000. I, in no way, want to say forget about resources in this area. I don't want to be interpreted that way at all.

DAVIS: Fred, perhaps we can hook up our data. One thing that occurred to me—this could be benzene or it could be PVC resins, both of which are in the IARC Class I and II carcinogens. My figures are shown in Figure 3 (Davis et al., this volume).

I was quite pleased, as I am sure Eula Bingham would be, to note that Dow workers have been exposed to 1 ppm benzene for the past few years. This is the level that OSHA recommended and which the American Petroleum Institute (API) prevented OSHA from applying.

Your data indicate, Dow, along with, Arco that I know of has been meeting the proposed OSHA standard for some time.

Now, the question is, what does this mean about exposure. I don't know, but it seems to me that, if we could link this sort of information and get it out more for public discussion, then it would be possible for people to use it to come up with better estimates. But my position still is that, in light of the fact that there are a number of IARC Class I carcinogens that follow this pattern of production, in light of the improved treatments and the improved therapy outcomes for many kinds of cancers, I would say that it is premature to draw conclusions about the burden of all of this to occupational cancer.

HOERGER: I suggest that we are emphasizing the volume and exposure trends quite differently. It is clear that synthetic organic chemical production was increasing dramatically in the 1940s and 1950s (Figure 1) so, using production volume as a crude surrogate of exposure, the potential for increases in occupational cancer would have been manifested by this past decade. Your selected data failed to emphasize the much earlier production increases.

Epidemiology and Occupational Classification Systems

SHELIA K. HOAR
Environmental Epidemiology Branch
National Cancer Institute
Bethesda, Maryland 20205

To quantify risks associated with occupational exposures, epidemiologists would like to identify and record chemical and physical agents encountered by the study subjects. Although specific workplace measurements rarely exist, job titles and industry affiliations commonly are available. To use these data effectively, it is essential to group job titles and industries according to exposure. Crude or inappropriate classification systems may create occupational groupings with dissimilar exposures, thereby reducing or obscuring associations between occupational exposures and disease. Today, I will discuss general considerations when making the critical choice of an occupational coding system, the advantages and disadvantages of some commonly used codes, and some recent and possible future developments in occupational classification systems.

GENERAL CONSIDERATIONS

Occupation can be an indicator of socioeconomic status, educational level, task, chemical exposure, or other aspects of occupation. The first consideration when choosing an occupational coding system is the facet of occupation under study. The appropriate coding system should group occupations according to the aspect of interest.

The degree of refinement in the study hypothesis also affects the choice of the occupational classification system. If the hypothesis is specific and restricted to a few jobs, the classification system can be simple. The code can be as brief as the dichotomy: (1) the occupation of interest, (2) all other jobs. If there is no a priori suspect occupation or if there are many a priori suspect occupations, the classification system needs to encompass most imaginable jobs.

Related to the specificity of the study hypothesis is the level of detail of the occupational data and the coding system. The code should preserve the specificity of the occupational data if the study hypothesis and the quality of the raw data justify it. A code less detailed than the data will lose potentially valuable information. For example, a manufacturer's personnel code may have unique job titles and codes for occupations that would be grouped into one category by a comprehensive government classification system. An overly-detailed system will dictate that many broadly described jobs will be arbitrarily assigned codes that suggest a level of detail not in the original data. For example, if the classification system contains codes for every engineering speciality but lacks a general "engineer" category, then "engineer" cannot be assigned a code or will be inappropriately assigned a specialty code.

Critical to the level of detail issue is the presence of "not otherwise specified" and "not elsewhere classified" categories. "Not otherwise specified" categories are used for general titles that do not indicate specialty or subgroup, such as "engineer." "Not elsewhere classified" categories usually represent a collection of miscellaneous specialty or subgroup titles and are not used for general titles. In the former case, there is no specialty or subgroup data. In the latter case, the specialty or subgroup is known but is not included in other categories of the coding scheme. Both "not otherwise specified" and "not elsewhere classified" categories are needed to complete any coding scheme, regardless of the level of detail in the code.

Even if a code scheme captures the facet of occupation under study and makes the distinctions that the hypothesis requires and the dataset permits, it can be worthless if the coders cannot use it easily. Ideally, different coders will assign the same code to a particular job, a property called reliability. Thus, the ease in locating the correct code should also influence selection of an occupational classification system. Alphabetical cross-indices of occupations and codes are useful. Definitions of job titles and industries ensure that the appropriate code has been located. The absence of definitions might discourage use of a system if the coders were inexperienced.

A final consideration is whether the study data needs to be compatible with other data based on a particular classification system. For example, if the occupational data were to be linked to information from the Bureau of the Census surveys, then the Census industrial and occupational codes probably should be used.

The occupational epidemiologist must consider the purposes and the quality of the data for each study and choose the coding system accordingly.

ADVANTAGES AND DISADVANTAGES OF THREE CODING SYSTEMS

There are three government occupational classification systems that commonly are used by epidemiologists: the Bureau of the Census Index of Industries and Occupations (Bureau of the Census 1971), the Department of Labor Dictionary of Occupational Titles (DOT) (Department of Labor 1977), and the Office of Management and Budget Standard Industrial (SIC) and Occupational Classification (SOC) Systems (Office of Management and

Budget 1972, 1977a, b). None were designed for epidemiologic purposes; consequently, each system has advantages and disadvantages. In general, they do not capture data in a scheme that is ideal for the hypotheses we test, but, they are tested, developed, and documented schemes that give reproducible results. Also, they exist.

Bureau of the Census

The Bureau of the Census Index of Industries and Occupations (Bureau of the Census 1971) contains 417 and 215 unique codes representing approximately 23,000 occupational and 19,000 industrial titles, respectively. The occupation and industry codes are arranged into 12 major groups each. This is the code scheme for the decennial census.

The Bureau of the Census system has several positive features: The alphabetic listing of multiple alternative job titles and industry names allows suitable codes to be located quickly, the general "not otherwise specified" categories allow undetailed data to be assigned codes, and the code has been used in many government surveys that an epidemiologist may want to link to the study occupational data.

The Census code has some deficiencies that stem from the differences in the basic purpose of the Census and epidemiology. The Census is organized according to socioeconomic status, instead of by commonality of exposure, the variable usually of interest to the occupational epidemiologist. Also, the index makes some distinctions that are irrelevant to epidemiologists. These include differentiating persons who are self-employed from persons doing identical work for an employer, trainees and apprentices from experienced persons in the same trades, and persons in the military or government service from persons performing the same function in the private sector.

The Census code also has operational problems. It is not highly reliable; conceivably, several different codes can be assigned to one job title. This problem results, in part, from the lack of detailed definitions of the titles, and, in part, from the code's repetitious nature.

Dictionary of Occupational Titles

The U.S. Department of Labor devised a code scheme called DOT (Department of Labor 1977) to provide job descriptions that would aid career guidance, training, and placement. The DOT contains definitions for approximately 20,000 jobs represented by 559 occupational codes in 9 major groups. The DOT does not contain code numbers for industries, per se; however, the occupational codes frequently distinguish a job in one industry and the same job title in a different industry. The detailed job definitions in DOT make it possible to assign unique, reliable codes and also are an excellent reference regardless of coding system used. The DOT contains many categories for occupations "not elsewhere classified" and "not otherwise specified." Thus, the detailed code can "collapse" for crude data.

The major disadvantage of the DOT is the time required to locate the appropriate code. Selecting possible codes and reviewing the descriptions can use large amounts of time and money.

Standard Occupational Classification and Standard Industrial Classification Systems

The Office of Management and Budget developed the SOC (Office of Management and Budget 1977a, b) and SIC (Office of Management and Budget 1972) systems in an attempt to reconcile the Census and the DOT systems. SIC and SOC are considerably more complex than the other codes. The SOC has 662 codes in 22 major groups for approximately 13,000 job titles. The SIC has 552 codes in 11 divisions and 84 major groups for approximately 18,000 industrial titles. Both SIC and SOC provide alphabetic indices. Also, SIC has excellent descriptions of the activities and materials produced in each industry and its subcategories. SOC does not contain job descriptions; it refers users to the DOT.

Although the SIC and SOC are extremely detailed coding systems, and include "not elsewhere classified" categories, they lack the "not otherwise specified" classifications necessary for coding less detailed occupational data. The epidemiologist must supplement the system and establish coding rules for these situations.

Despite this limitation, the SIC and SOC, which were "designed for use in statistical analysis and presentation of data about occupations," are becoming a popular choice for epidemiologic studies.

AN EXPOSURE-LINKED SYSTEM

The major problem with the systems I have just described is that they classify occupation according to industry or job title, whereas we are interested in grouping occupations according to the chemicals or other agents to which exposure occurred. Persons in the same industries, or performing similar tasks in different industries, may be grouped even if exposures are dissimilar. This misclassification reduces and obscures associations between disease and exposures. As epidemiologists try to identify causal agents to quantify low-level risks from occupational exposures, it is critical to minimize such misclassification (Cole and Merletti 1980). Also, elevated risks in persons with a rare exposure will be missed if those persons are grouped with nonexposed persons.

In response to this problem, I and colleagues at Harvard School of Public Health recently developed an occupation and exposure linkage system (Hoar et al. 1980). Occupations were classified by industry and task within industry.

Table 1
Industrial Categories and Code Numbers Used in the Occupation and Exposure Linkage System

Industry	Code number
Agriculture, forestry, fishing	01
Mining	02
Construction	03
Processors, producers, and users of products made from	
Paper and wood	04
Glass, clay, and stone	05
Metal	06
Machinery	07
Shipbuilding, motor vehicles, aircraft, and other transportation methods	08
Food and tobacco	09
Textiles	10
Chemicals, drugs, and paints	11
Rubber, plastics, and synthetics	12
Fuel	13
Leather	14
Medicine and science	15
Entertainment and recreation	16
Art	17
Occupations with few chemical exposures (business, law, communications, sales, etc.)	99

Lists of suspect carcinogens were assembled and each suspect carcinogen was linked to industries and tasks in which it has been used. These links make it possible to place in the same category all study subjects whose employment history suggests contact with a particular agent. Epidemiologic analysis then can be based on chemical and physical exposures, rather than on industries or tasks. We designed the system to allow the addition of links as knowledge of relevant exposures increased.

The occupation code is composed of approximately 500 five-digit sequences. The first two digits comprise an industry code. The final three digits designate task or process and are based, with modification, on the occupational title number from the DOT. The industry-title categories reflect the readily available information regarding chemical or physical exposure in particular processes. Jobs and corresponding exposures have been well described for some industries while for others description is very limited. The list of 18 industrial categories is shown in Table 1 and detailed occupational titles for the textile industry (industrial category:10), as an example, are shown in Table 2. The

Table 2
Occupational Titles and Code Numbers for the Textile Industry

Title	Code number (industry-task)
Industrial engineer	10-012
Managers and officials (including accountant, buyer)	10-183
Office work, nonmanagerial, nonprofessional, NOS[a] (includes secretary, office, and errand boys)	10-209
Production clerk (includes warehouseman and storekeeper mainly concerned with paperwork, timekeeping, etc., as opposed to handling stock)	10-229
Sales: Textiles and textile products	10-263
Processing:	
Shaping, blocking, stretching, and tentering	10-580
Separating, filtering, and drying fibers (includes spinner, winder, weaver, piecer, slubber, doffer, tuber, doubler, beamer, carder)	10-581
Washing, steaming, and saturating fibers and textiles (includes dyer, bleaching machine operator, crabber)	10-582
Ironing, pressing, glazing, staking, calendering, embossing	10-583
Mercerizing, coating, and laminating	10-584
Singeing, cutting, shearing, shaving, and napping	10-585
Filtering and fulling	10-586
Brushing and shrinking	10-587
NOS (includes inspector, examiner)	10-589
Machine and equipment mechanics and repair (includes roller coverer, millwright)	10-628
Model maker, patternmaker (machine trade) (includes designer, display card maker)	10-693
Upholstering, fabrication, and repair of mattresses and bedspreads	10-780
Fur working occupations	10-783
Hat, cap, and glove fabrication and repair	10-784
Sewers, embroiderers, knitters, seamstresses, and tailors	10-789
Laundering, domestic	10-302
Laundering, dry cleaning, pressing	10-363
Dyeing finished textile products (includes person mixing dyes for textile printing)	10-364
Apparel and furnishings service occupations, NOS	10-369
Mechanic and maintenance occupations	10-899
Packaging and materials handling occupations (includes warehouseman, storekeeper, leader, fork lifter)	10-929
Occupation known, cannot classify	10-998
Occupation unknown	10-999

[a]Not otherwise specified.

occupational code has the desirable "not otherwise specified" and "not elsewhere classified" categories for coding crude data.

To construct the agent list, a review was made of several comprehensive sources to identify chemical hazards and the processes and industrial environments where these exposures occur (Clayson 1962; Hueper and Conway 1964; Grady 1971; IARC 1972-1976; Cole and Goldman 1975; Key et al. 1977; Maugh 1977; Schottenfeld and Haas 1979). The agent list includes primarily known or suspect chemical carcinogens, but has been expanded to include some chemicals with other chronic or acute effects. Approximately 400 agents were assigned four-digit code numbers. A list of the 24 major categories of agents included in the code, and, as an example, a list of specific substances included as "aromatic amines," are presented in Table 3.

Each five-digit industry-task designation was linked to all related four-digit agent numbers. Whenever possible, a fifth digit (1, 2, or 3) was added to each occupation-agent link to characterize crudely the degree of exposure to the agent which the specific task entails. A "3" was assigned to jobs that appeared to involve a heavy degree of exposure to the agent, or that were classified by Hueper and Conway (1964) as hazardous because of that exposure; "2" was assigned to processing occupations in the same industry as other jobs that appeared to entail heavy exposure to the agent, and to occupations classified by Hueper and Conway (1964) as suspected of being hazardous; and "1" was assigned to engineers, managers, officials, salespersons, production clerks, or professionals in the same industry as other jobs considered to entail heavy exposure.

The links between occupations and agents exist as a computer file of 15,000 pairs of occupation codes and agent numbers, accompanied by the degree-of-exposure designator when available. Linkage can be made in either direction with respect to occupations and agents. As examples, Table 4 gives a list of agents to which carpenters in the construction industry (occupation code 03-860) are considered to be exposed and Table 5 gives a list of occupations which are linked to asbestos exposure (agent code 6505). The linkage of carpenter in the construction industry to asbestos (degree of exposure: moderate) is indicated by the box in both tables. Carpenters in the construction industry also are linked to coal tar and pitch, creosote, petroleum, coke tar and pitch, etc. (Table 4). Other occupations linked to asbestos include those in the mining, construction, shipbuilding, and paper and wood industries (Table 5).

The exposure linkage makes reliability of code assignments a moot issue: Alternative job codes would most likely be linked to the same exposures. For example, one coder may assign a "carpenter" the occupational code 03-860 from the construction industry while a second coder may assign the code 04-860 from the paper and wood industry. Both codes are linked to almost identical lists of agents, which would then be the basis for analysis. The slight degree of unreliability in the occupational code has no effect.

Table 3
Agent list: Major Exposure Categories with Detailed Listing of Aromatic Amines

Category	Code number
Organic compounds	
Aromatic hydrocarbons	
Aromatic amino Compounds	
2-Acetylaminofluorene	1005
4-Aminodiphenyl	1010
para-Aminophenol	1015
Aniline	1020
Auramine	1025
Benzidine	1030
4-Dimethylaminoazobenzene	1035
Dye intermediates	1040
Dyes, NOS[a]	1045
8-Hydroxyquinoline	1050
Magenta	1055
4-4′-Methylenebis (2-chloroanilene)	1060
Methyl-*para*-aminophenolsulfate	1065
α-Napthylamine	1070
β-Napthylamine	1075
4-Nitrodiphenyl	1080
Paints	1085
Paraphenylenediamines	1090
Pigments	1095
Aromatic nitro compounds	
Aromatic halogens	
Aromatic azo compounds	
Phenols	
Aromatic hydrocarbons, NOS[a]	
Alicyclic hydrocarbons	
Alicyclic halogens	
Alicyclic hydrocarbons, NOS	
Alkylating agents	
Aliphatic hydrocarbons	
Aliphatic halogens	
Aliphatic nitro compounds	
Alcohols, glycols, acids, and derivatives	
Aldehydes, ketones, ethers, and derivatives	
Esters	
Aliphatic hydrocarbons, NOS	
Other organic compounds NOS	
Inorganic compounds	
Metals, metalloids, and their compounds	
Minerals	
Inorganic halogens	
Inorganic compounds, NOS	
Physical agents	
Nonionizing radiation	
Ionizing radiation	
Dusts	
Other physical agents	

[a]Not otherwise specified.

Table 4
Agents Linked to Employment As A Carpenter in the Construction Industry (carpenter, construction industry (industry-task code: 03-860))

Agent	Degree of exposure
Azo compounds	
1350. Oil orange SS	2. moderate
Phenols	
1420. Creosote	2. moderate
Aromatic hydrocarbons	
1560. Coal tar and pitch	2. moderate
1640. Petroleum, coke tar and pitch	2. moderate
Aliphatic compounds	
4910. Water insoluble carbon polymers	1. light
4870. Polysiloxanes	1. light
Metals	
6140. Chromium	3. heavy
Minerals	
6505. Asbestos [a]	2. moderate
Physical agents	
9300. Wood dust	3. heavy
8250. UV radiation	2. moderate

[a]Linkage of carpenter in the construction industry to asbestos exposure is indicated by boxes in Tables 4 and 5.

It is important to remember that the linkages only suggest exposures that are likely to have occurred. The data provided by the system could be viewed as an initial list to be corroborated and added to by interviews with the study subjects, industrial hygiene data, or other sources.

Developments that could improve this epidemiologic tool include: Addition of job titles, exposures, and linkages; refinement of the degree of exposure variable; provision of conversion tables for the other commonly used coding systems; and inclusion of route of exposure and calendar years of use in the workplace. Scientific and commercial manufacturing and marketing data bases could provide almost unlimited information for expansion of the system. If such data were available, susceptible ages, sensitization or acclimatization periods, and latency periods for specific diseases could also be added.

The occupation-exposure linkage system could be used in conjunction with other proposed developments in occupational epidemiology, for example, the Experience Transformation Algorithm, suggested by Spirtas (1976). The occupation-exposure information could be used to create the job groupings that are entered into the algorithm.

Table 5
Occupations Linked to Asbestos Exposure (asbestos (agent code:5510))

Industry	Task	Degree of exposure
02. Mining	professional and clerical work[a]	1. light
	extraction of minerals occupations[a]	3. heavy
03. Construction [b]	829. electrician	2. moderate
	860. carpenter [b]	2. moderate
	861. brick and stone mason	2. moderate
	863. asbestos and insulation workers	3. heavy
04. Paper and wood	860. carpenter	2. moderate
05. Glass, clay, and stone	861. brick and stone masons	2. moderate
06. Metal	515. ore refining, crushing, grinding	2. moderate
07. Machinery	729. electrical equipment assembly and repair	2. moderate
	829. structural work, assembly, and repair	2. moderate
08. Shipbuilding, motor vehicles, aircraft, and other transportation methods	729. electrical equipment assembly and repair	2. moderate
	900. drivers, chauffers, truckers, and pilots	2. moderate
	905. boilermakers	3. heavy
	999. shipbuilding and motor vehicle manufacturing	3. heavy
10. Textiles	589. textiles processing, NOS[c]	2. moderate
13. Fuel	959. boilermakers, utilities production and distribution occupations, NOS[c]	3. heavy
17. Art	textile processing, machinery fabrication and repair[a]	2. moderate

[a]Title represents several tasks condensed for presentation in the table.
[b]Linkage of carpenter in the construction industry to asbestos exposure is indicated by boxes in Tables 4 and 5.
[c]Not otherwise specified.

CONCLUSION

To quantify occupational cancer, epidemiologists need to code occupational and exposure data. The most detailed occupational and exposure information is useless if it cannot be manipulated and analyzed. An appropriate coding system is essential for wise stewardship of money, time, and data. I have reviewed some commonly used coding schemes and described a recently developed occupational code and its companion linkages to suspect carcinogens. I hope that the material presented today will be of practical benefit for people pondering coding and linkage systems for occupational epidemiologic studies.

REFERENCES

Bureau of the Census. 1971. *1970 census of population alphabetic index of industries and occupations.* Government Printing Office, Washington, D.C.

Clayson, D.B. 1962. *Chemical carcinogenesis.* Little, Brown and Company, Boston.

Cole, P. and M.B. Goldman. 1975. Occupation. In *Persons at high risk of cancer: An approach to cancer etiology and control* (ed. J.F. Fraumeni, Jr.), p. 167. Academic Press, New York.

Cole, P. and F. Merletti. 1980. Chemical agents and occupational cancer. *J. Environ. Pathol. Toxicol.* **3**:399.

Department of Labor. 1977. *Dictionary of occupational titles, fourth edition.* Government Printing Office, Washington, D.C.

Grady, G.S. 1971. *Materials handbook, tenth edition,* McGraw-Hill, New York.

Hoar, S.K., A.S. Morrison, P. Cole, and D.T. Silverman. 1980. An occupation and exposure linkage system for the study of occupational carcinogenesis. *J. Occup. Med.* **22**:722.

Hueper, W.C. and W.D. Conway. 1964. *Chemical carcinogenesis and cancers.* Charles C. Thomas, Springfield.

International Agency for Research on Cancer (IARC). 1972-1976. *Evaluation of carcinogenesis risk of chemicals to man, monographs 2-10.* International Agency for Research on Cancer, Lyon.

Key, M.N., A.F. Henschel, J. Butler, R.N. Ligo, and I.R. Tabershaw. 1977. *Occupational diseases: A guide to their recognition* (ed. M.N. Key et al.), publication no. 77-181. Government Printing Office, Washington, D.C.

Maugh, T.H. 1977. Carcinogens in the workplace: Where to start cleaning up. *Science* **197**:1268.

Office of Management and Budget. 1972. *Standard industrial classification manual.* Government Printing Office, Washington, D.C.

______. 1977a. *Standard occupational classification manual.* Government Printing Office, Washington, D.C.

______. 1977b. *Index: Standard occupational classification manual.* Government Printing Office, Washington, D.C.

Schottenfeld, D. and J.F. Haas. 1979. Carcinogens in the workplace. *CA-A Cancer J. Clin.* **20**:144.

Spirtas, R. 1976. An algorithm for transforming work histories in occupational health studies. In *Compstat, Proceedings in Computation Statistics,* (ed. J. Gordesch and P. Naeve) p. 475. Physica-Verlag-Wurzburg-Wien, West Berlin.

COMMENTS

MILHAM: Have you used your system?

HOAR: Yes. When we developed the system, we used it to reanalyze data from Dr. Philip Cole's bladder cancer case-control study. The original analysis was based on a priori "suspect" industries involving exposure to aromatic amines. We used the linkage system to convert the industry and occupational titles into a variable indicating exposure to aromatic amines. Our analysis yielded higher risk estimates than the original analysis.

The reason for the difference in the risk estimates was that the linkage system, presumably accurately, classified as "nonexposed" some persons who had had production jobs in the suspect industries, but who were not exposed to aromatic amines. There are several other groups who are now using the system. Their analyses have not been completed.

BEEBE: It seems to me that this is a very important beginning on something that is very much needed. But I am wondering, who is the keeper of this system? Are you going to invest your life, or much of it, in the maintenance, improvement, and extension of this system? Or is it going to be adopted, or has it been, by the Harvard School of Public Health, the National Cancer Institute (NCI), or some other group? If not, each of us is going to be making changes ad hoc. Standardization will fall and the general improvement in its usefulness will not be realized.

HOAR: Currently, a group at NCI is evaluating the feasibility of systematically updating the system. The present linkage file should be viewed as a pilot file; it was never considered to represent a comprehensive review of the literature. However, the structure of the system allows infinite addition of links. If feasible and of sufficient interest to warrant the resources, a contract may be offered for this task.

SCHNEIDERMAN: Dr. Rosenberg talked to us yesterday about the National Center for Health Statistics (NCHS) plans to code occupation on death certificates. Are you in communication with him? Or are they using another system?

HOAR: They are probably planning to use the SIC and SOC system. I intend to contact him.

TULINIUS: I had two questions. First, what coding system would you advise Dr. Rosenberg to use? And second, have you considered the International Labor Office (ILO) code? How does it compare with your system?

HOAR: With regard to the first question, I would probably advise Dr. Rosenberg to use the SIC and SOC system. I might develop a conversion table between our codes and the SIC and SOC codes. Incidentally, the SIC code was published after we began this project or we might have utilized it in some way.

Your second question asked about the ILO code. Originally we designed the system for use in a tumor registry located in the Boston area and did not anticipate international applications. However, one group used the code for a study in three countries and had some difficulties. Codes for certain occupations and industries were missing. In Japan, we needed codes for rice washers, which had not been a popular job in the Boston area.

PADDLE: I enjoyed your remark that you would get higher relative risks, rather than better ones. Have you thought of using the Chemical Abstracts (CAS) numbers for your chemicals? You would then be able to make contact with a great many other systems and you might lose contact if you don't do this.

HOAR: That is a good point. Use of CAS numbers would make the system compatible with many other data bases, but would not allow the easy grouping of agents by class which our numbers facilitate. We could add the CAS numbers to the agent dictionary or the linkage pairs.

ACHESON: Two points. First, is the classification published or is it available for colleagues?

HOAR: Yes, it is (Hoar et al. 1980). This article refers people to Dr. Alan Morrison at Harvard School of Public Health, who is in charge of distributing copies of the file.

ACHESON: Second, I noticed that you indicated on your list that the carpenters in the construction industry are heavily exposed to wood. That may sound obvious, but so far as I know, there is no evidence that carpenters in the construction industry are exposed to respirable wood particles. Furniture workers in furniture factories are, but I don't think there is any evidence that carpenters are exposed. I think it is an example of an assumption. One has to be careful about making assumptions without measurements.

HOAR: We have two categories–wood and wood dust. So we could make that distinction in the code.

SARACCI: One could think of extending the code to cover other countries, but probably there are problems that are specific to each country. International Agency for Research on Cancer (IARC) is interested in exploring the possibility of expanding such a system and discussing this problem.

My question is related. I think you said that this is a classification for case-control studies. It seems to me that an industry-based study would require a different tactic. I would like your comment.

HOAR: I agree. I don't think this system can contribute to cohort studies within a particular industry. I think that the company or union under study can supply much better exposure information and job title information than this system. It wasn't meant to be used in that setting.

HOERGER: Are you giving any thought to continual maintenance of the product mix to which a worker is exposed as technology changes? The carpenter used glue in 1960, but today probably uses an epoxy resin. The insulator used asbestos in 1960, but today may be using glass fibers. Is there any plan for technology updating?

HOAR: One of the possible future developments that I mentioned was the addition of a third axis to the linkage pairs—the calendar years of the agent's use in the work place. A subject would be considered exposed to an agent only if he or she held the critical job during the years in which the agent was used. The same job during different years would be considered unexposed. Presently, there is no information of this type in the system, but it might be added if the maintenance contract is offered.

SILVERSTEIN: How does your scheme take into account, if at all, the fact that the same job in different types of plants can involve vastly different sets of chemical exposures, for example, the job of pipefitter in an iron foundry vs in a machine workshop.

HOAR: The occupational code and exposure linkages make a distinction between industries. However, within one industry persons with the same job title, regardless of plant, are grouped together. This system reduces some misclassification of exposure in comparison to analyzing job title or industry alone, but not all.

SCHNEIDERMAN: It appears as if this classification system would require the kinds of developments that the ICD system required. There may be a need for an international organization, corresponding to the World Health Organization, to take on the responsibility for creating such a system, monitoring it, and keeping it current. I think we are just at the birth of a new era of some rather difficult developments. Disease classification have under revision for a long time and we are still having troubles with them. So I don't anticipate that we will get any simple answers to occupational coding. Diseases apparently change a little more slowly than do occupations.

References

Hoar, S.K., A.S. Morrison, P. Cole, and D.T. Silverman. 1980. An occupation and exposure linkage system for the study of occupational carcinogenesis. *J. Occup. Med.* **22**:722.

Exposure-based Case Control Approach to Discovering Occupational Carcinogens: Preliminary Findings

JACK SIÈMIATYCKI
Centre de Recherche en Épidémiologie et Médecine Préventive
Institut Armand-Frappier
Laval-des-Rapides, Québec H7V 1B7
and Department of Epidemiology and Health
McGill University
Montréal, Québec

MICHEL GÉRIN
Département de Médecine du Travail et d'hygiène du milieu
Faculté de Médecine
Université de Montréal
Montréal, Québec H3C 3T7

JOSEPH HUBERT
Département de Chimie
Université de Montréal
Montréal, Québec H3C 3J7

Chemical and physical agents encountered in the occupational environment may be an important class of human carcinogens, not only because of the disease produced among workers but also because many occupational exposures find their way into the general environment. The determination of which occupational exposures may be carcinogenic is one of the main public health problems of our era. However, of the tens of thousands of chemicals in common use, only a few have been evaluated in terms of human carcinogenic potential. Although somewhat larger numbers have been evaluated in terms of experimental carcinogenesis, there is as yet no consensus as to the applicability of animal experimental and mutagenicity evidence to humans. (McCann and Ames 1977; Berenblum 1979; Gehring et al. 1979; Rall 1979; Shubik 1979; Tomatis 1979; Purchase 1980). A major deficiency in our ability to evaluate such proxies is the lack of human evidence with which to correlate experimental evidence. Thus the rapid accumulation of human evidence concerning chemical carcinogenicity is important not only for its intrinsic implications, but also to tell us more about the applicability of experimental systems to the problem of human risk assessment.

Those discoveries on which our current knowledge is based were largely the result of serendipitous observation on the part of astute clinicians (Doll 1975). Because such discoveries required the conjunction of several coincidences, it may be assumed that only the tip of an iceberg of occupational carcinogens has been identified. The rather recent widespread acceptance of the importance of physical-chemical environment in human carcinogenisis has led to demands for a more systematic approach to discovering human carcinogens. The problem we have been concerned with is how to uncover a larger part of the iceberg of occupational carcinogens, which have contributed to today's cancer burden.

Among epidemiologic approaches used in the past to scan the occupational spectrum, studies based on geographic correlations between cancer rates and industrial patterns or on jobs noted in death certificates are subject to serious biases and lack of statistical sensitivity (Siemiatycki et al. 1981). Record linkage between death records and census records or other sources of information on occupation may attenuate some of the disadvantages (Acheson 1979). Apart from imprecision and biases resulting from inaccurate, recorded job titles and even causes of death, such approaches do not permit control of potential confounders. Case-control or cohort studies of one or a few exposures at a time, while avoiding some of these difficulties, cannot satisfy our need to scan the gamut of occupational environments.

Some investigators have adapted the case-control approach from its usual hypothesis-testing function to a "fishing expedition" or monitoring system by requesting complete job histories of persons diagnosed with any of several types of cancer and computing relative risks for all occupation-site combinations (Williams et al. 1977). By collecting data on lifetime job histories and other personal characteristics directly from cases and controls (or their close proxies), many problems related to other methods can be avoided. However this approach still suffers from the inadequacy of job titles as descriptions of occupational exposures for the following reasons:

1. If an elevated risk is detected for a broad occupational category, it is usually impossible to infer which of many chemical exposures may be responsible for elevated risks.
2. Even within a company there may be considerable variation in occupational exposures of different people who have the same job title. The heterogeneity is magnified when persons having a common job title are grouped across industries and across decades. A risk may go undetected because only a subset of a category was exposed to a carcinogen and the dilution blurred the association.
3. Because many materials are used by subsets of several occupation categories, there is considerable loss in statistical power if persons with common exposure but different job titles are not pooled.

EXPOSURE-BASED APPROACH

If the working histories of each case and control can be translated into an exposure history, i.e., into a list of compounds to which the person was exposed, then the data base would be available for analyses which avoid the three major deficiencies of an occupation title-based system. Hoar et al. (1980) developed a methodology whereby a correspondence system links jobs to exposures. Thus, a person employed in a given job is automatically attributed exposure to each of a number of substances. The exposure axis of the job-exposure matrix is potentially unlimited but for practical purposes has been limited to a list of known and suspect carcinogens. Thus, this system as presently defined will be capable of elucidating the effects of known or suspected carcinogens. Once the jobs of each person have been translated into exposure histories, a case-control type statistical analysis can be carried out for each site-exposure combination. The job histories can be obtained by interview or from routine record sources such as death certificates. However, analyses based on death certificate or tumor registry occupation information will be subject to the errors inherent in such sources. The authors have shown the statistical power of this approach by reanalyzing data from an occupation title-based study and finding that the exposure-based analyses highlight relationships more clearly than did the original analysis.

Our line of development has differed. On the one hand, we wanted a system that would be capable of raising the alarm on unsuspected carcinogens and, on the other hand, we were impressed with the considerable variation in working environments among persons having common job titles. The Hoar et al. system, by mechanistically translating jobs into exposures, still does a fair amount of aggregating of persons who may have had quite different work environments. Our approach was to try to individualize our exposure information by obtaining the best possible exposure histories from cases and controls, and to do this irrespective of our prior knowledge of the carcinogenicity of the exposures.

Although the patient may not be able to identify chemical compounds to which he was exposed, he usually can provide detailed descriptions of the activities of firms with which he worked, the industrial processes in which he was involved, and his specific duties. From this description, experts in engineering and chemistry can with appropriate research and consultation, establish a list of chemicals to which the patient may have been exposed in each of his past jobs. This is not a simple task, nor can it be done with precision.

To be successful, the system requires the following characteristics: (1) access to a population-based register of patients; (2) an efficient case-ascertainment procedure which permits access to newly diagnosed cancer patients while they can still be interviewed; (3) probing interviews with cases and controls to obtain a detailed description of each job as well as information on potential confounders; (4) review of each job description by chemists and (or) engineers for the purpose of inferring possible chemical exposures. As much of the latter involves jobs of bygone eras, there is considerable detective work in attempting to describe such chemical environments. The list of chemicals thus inferred becomes part of the person's data file and the basis of subsequent statistical analyses. In essence, the analysis consists of examining the exposure lists of patients with a common tumor to determine whether any chemicals appear in an unusually high proportion of cases. Statistical analyses are carried out not only on physical-chemical exposures but also on job titles and industries to detect significant associations.

For each site series, controls can be selected in the general population, in a noncancer hospital series, or among other cancer sites. Each approach has advantages and disadvantages. Interviewing only cancer patients and using for each site all others as a source of controls, provides a self-contained data collection system that minimizes cost and risk of interview bias. However, carcinogens that are equally potent at several different sites would not be detectable. Statistical sensitivity of the approach depends on several factors, including size of population catchment area, study duration, proportion of population exposed to a carcinogen, and potency of the carcinogen. It is more likely to detect unsuspected carcinogens than any method previously attempted (Siemiatycki et al. 1981).

PILOT STUDY

A pilot study of this methodology has been underway in Montreal since late 1979 and we will present some preliminary methodologic findings. For the purpose of the pilot study, target subjects were incident cases of cancer of any of 10 sites (esophagus, stomach, colon, pancreas, lung, melanoma of skin, prostate, bladder, kidney, lymphoid tissue) among males aged 35-70, residing in the Montreal area. Controls for each site were to be selected, at the time of statistical analysis, among patients with the other 9 sites of cancer. The 17 largest hospitals in the Montreal area, accounting for the vast majority of nonskin cancer reported to the provincial tumor registry, agreed to collaborate. Because an interview with the subject is an important component of the data collection process and because several sites included have less than 50% 1-year survival rates, it was considered desirable to attempt to interview the patient as soon as possible after initial pathological diagnosis. An active case ascertainment procedure was set up in each hospital whereby an employee of the pathology department telephoned us whenever a patient fitting our inclusion criteria was diagnosed. An interviewer was then dispatched to the hospital or, to the home if the patient had been discharged or was diagnosed on an outpatient basis. Regular monthly checks of medical records in each hospital serve to pick up cases missed by the active case-finding procedure. In the first 8 months of

Table 1
Response Rate in First 8 Months of Fieldwork

Outcome	Number	Percent
Complete	452	69.8
Refused	67	10.3
Dead	68	10.5
Psychiatric or too ill	20	3.1
As yet unable to contact	41	6.3
Total eligible cases	648	

fieldwork some 834 cases were recorded. Because permission to interview came late in three hospitals and because of lack of sufficient interviewing staff, attempts to interview were made in 648 cases. Table 1 describes the outcome of these attempts. The relatively high nonresponse rate is due to our reluctance to persuade unwilling patients, who for the most part were quite ill and had just been informed of the diagnosis. Although no special attempt was made to obtain information from proxy responses in the case of deceased patients, this procedure will be instituted in the future.

Obtaining Job Histories

Job histories are obtained in two steps: (1) a brief, self-administered questionnaire delivered to the patient as soon as he is identified, and (2) a lengthier interview. The former helps in preparing for the latter. Whereas the section of the interview questionnaire on potential confounders is structured, the occupational section is semistructured. Different questions may be asked of teachers and welders, for example, and the project chemist-engineer may be called upon to advise the interviewer as to important questions to ask. We have found patients to be more than willing to discuss and describe their job histories. Of course, neither the chemist-engineer nor the interviewer know the patient's disease status. (The term "chemist-engineer" will be used generically to convey the type of expertise required. As no single person is trained to be able to infer the chemical exposures that may be present in different jobs, a team of chemists and engineers with complementary areas of expertise is ideal.)

To evaluate the quality of job information given by patients, the most important question is whether they report all of their jobs. To get a handle on this problem, we needed some routinely recorded source of employment status of each person with which to correlate his responses. The best, though not ideal, such source was the Quebec Pension Plan (QPP), which since its inception in 1966 has annual records of the name of employer for most residents of the Province of Quebec. Reported job histories were compared with histories recorded since 1966 by the QPP for 321 respondents. To call it a validation of job histories is something of a misnomer because it is really a validation of the names of employers. The names of employers as reported by a respondent may differ from that recorded by the QPP without this reflecting a substantial error. For instance if a company name changed during a worker's period of employment, he would be recorded as having worked at two companies. If he only reported one of the names, we would incorrectly infer respondent error for part of the period. Similarly a person may report that he was a night guard at a university whereas his actual employer was a company that contracts out night watchmen. For these reasons, the extent of discrepancy in employer names exaggerates discrepancy in jobs. On the other hand, the respondent who reported the employer correctly but the job title incorrectly would be coded as an agreement. The reported and recorded employers were compared in each year from 1967 to 1979. As explained above, this underestimates the validity of reporting of job histories. Report and record agreed in over 82% of person-years compared.

Translating Job Histories into Histories of Occupational Exposures

After the interview is carried out, the next and crucial stage concerns the inference of exposures. Besides drawing upon their own knowledge and experience, the chemist-engineers have access to libraries, technical documentation, and consultants in local industries. A cross-filing system permits rapid access to the research done on previous patients in the same job category. The computerized data entry system is set up so that information on patient's files can be updated. In the course of the study, we learn more and more about jobs that recur. It is important that new knowledge can be applied to correct coding of files that were evaluated previously. The research and coding of exposures in each job can be carried out as a checklist procedure or as an open-ended question. We have established a checklist of 172 chemical and physical agents for systematic evaluation in each job (i.e., present or absent with some indication of presumed degree of exposure) and also attempt to list what other exposures may have been present. The products on the checklist, some of which are proper chemicals (e.g., acetamide, benzene) and some of which are general categories (e.g., solvents, wood dust), were selected with the following criteria—some should be presumed carcinogens and some presumed noncarcinogens, as a type of control for the system as a whole; some of the most common occupational exposures should be included; the total number should not be inordinate. There is no need, nor is it desirable, for the categories of exposures to be mutually exclusive. Although the amount of time spent by the project chemist-engineer researching each job history is potentially unlimited, we have found that about 4 person-hours per case on average permits what seems like a reasonable, albeit crude, estimate of possible job exposures.

We have taken three approaches to the evaluation of this activity. The major drawback of the job title-based case-control approach is that job titles are too nonspecific as descriptions of occupational exposures and that a given job title can cover a wide variety of different environments. If the chemist-engineer routinely attributed the same exposures to patients having a common job title, it would raise doubts about the value of the extra work of inferring exposures. On the other hand, if we find that subsets of job title categories are distinguished on the basis of exposures and that workers in different job categories are allocated to common exposure categories, then we may consider that the exposures are not simply proxies for job titles, and on the face of it at least, the major justification for an exposure-based system would be satisfied. With 452 cases processed and computerized, there already is such evidence, which will be illustrated by the following typical examples:

1. Twenty-two jobs have been coded as "welding and flame cutting occupations." However this covers workers in different activities and different eras. When examined individually, 22 were assigned exposure to welding emissions, 17 to carbon monoxide, 15 to ozone, 15 to acetylene, 10 to lead, 5 to copper, 9 to asbestos, 4 to glass fiber, and subsets to 27 other categories of exposure.
2. Thirty-one jobs have been coded as "motor vehicle mechanics and repairmen." When examined individually, 31 were assigned exposure to lead and its compounds, 31 to carbon monoxide, 31 to lubricating oil, 14 to welding emissions, 25 to lubricating oil, 11 to paints, 5 to glues, 7 to asbestos, and subsets to 32 other categories of exposure.
3. The exposure "welding emissions" was attributed to 128 jobs. Of these only 22 were welders. The rest were spread among subsets of 53 different job codes including some machinists, equipment installing occupations and so on.
4. The exposure "asbestos" was attributed to 94 jobs. Of these only 4 were insulation workers. The rest were spread among subsets of 40 different job codes.

The second type of evaluation of the chemist activity consists of interobserver comparisons. That is, do different chemist-engineers agree with each other in their coding of exposures and do they agree with experts in the specific industry? Comparisons of independent readings among the three chemist-engineers who have worked on the project have thus far served to iron out inconsistencies in interpretation. Thus, a set of guidelines has been developed that provide rules on how to carry out the function. Initial testing with the new set of guidelines indicates considerable agreement among these chemist-engineers. A "validation" of their ratings against those of technical experts in specific industries is being organized.

The third approach is the "proof is in the pudding" approach. What kind of substantive findings are generated above and beyond what would be found

Table 2
Significant Associations between Site and Job (52 categories) and between Site and Exposure (209 categories)

	Site and job associations
Esophagus	salesmen
Stomach	fabricating, repairing—textile, fur, leather; auto mechanics and repairmen
Colon	salesmen
Lung	excavating, grading, paving occupations; railway transport occupations and water transport occupations
Prostate	metal shaping and forming occupations excluding machinist; fabricating and assembling metal products; stationary engine and utilities equipment operating
Bladder	natural scientists and engineers; auto mechanics and repairmen
	Site and exposure associations
Stomach	leather
	gasoline
Colon	carbon monoxide
	lead
	fire smoke
Lung	extreme noise
	gold and compounds
Prostate	metal dust
Bladder & Kidney[1]	silver and compounds
	iron oxides
Skin melanoma	engine emissions
Lymphoid tissue	cotton dust

These associations are presented for their methodological implications. We are not considering here their substantive meaning.

This table only lists significant associations where there were at least 4 exposed cases.

[1] These two sites were combined because it was noted that each was significantly associated with the two exposures, but there were only 3 cases of each site.

using a job title-based methodology? Although the small number of cases interviewed in the pilot study afford little statistical power in substantive analyses, and consequently those associations that are statistically significant may very well be due to chance, the pattern of significant associations illustrates the potential value of the methodology. Analyses were carried out for each combination of site by job and site by exposure. For each site, controls consisted of patients in all other site groupings. To obtain sufficient numbers in each job category, the 290 distinct four-digit job titles coded among the first 452 patients were regrouped into 52 mutually exclusive categories. A person was considered "exposed" if he worked at least 3 years in the job and had first worked in it more than 10 years before diagnosis. Mantel-Haenzsel analyses were carried out, stratifying on age (35-54 and 55-69) and on smoking (0-9 per day and 10+). We excluded from analysis those job-site combinations where there were fewer than 4 exposed cases. A similar process was repeated for chemical exposures. The 209 distinct exposures were analyzed in relation to each of the 10 sites, excluding combinations with fewer than four exposed cases. Table 2 presents associations that were significant at the .05 level. Given the low statistical power in such small series of cases and the fact that the exposure information is based on our initial evaluation of these dossiers and is presently being corrected, we believe that most if not all of the significant associations are due to chance. Nevertheless, they illustrate an important methodologic point. Some associations from job-based analyses can predict some from exposure-based analyses and vice versa. Others, however, are not predictable from one type of analysis to the other. These findings illustrate the potential value of an approach that permits both types of analysis.

DISCUSSION

Animal testing and mutagenicity screening programs eventually may prove to be most useful components of a cancer prevention strategy. Until precise laws permitting generalization from one biological system to another are determined, epidemiologic evidence will be necessary both in its own right as a guide to cancer control and as a crucial data base for determining the predictive value of experimental carcinogenicity and mutagenicity testing.

The experience of the pilot study, although not yet complete, encourages us that the various practical aspects of this approach—cooperation from hospitals, efficient case ascertainment, accurate job histories, and meaningful translation of job histories into exposure histories—are feasible. The last item is perhaps the most problematical especially with regard to reproducibility of translations. It is unlikely that two teams of chemist-engineer would develop identical procedures and translations. It is likely that two teams would come up with different results. So long as their evaluations are blind with regard to the patients' conditions, both sets of results would be unbiased. Each team might identify different carcinogens. The fact that no team and indeed no approach can be expected to identify all carcinogens does not detract from the value of one team's results. From a cost-benefit point of view, the methodology described costs about 25% more than would a job title-based case-control system.

Hundreds and perhaps thousands of statistical tests will be carried out and false alarms will inevitably be rung. However, the need to identify rapidly real carcinogens outweighs the inconvenience of dealing with false alarms. Furthermore, it is not widely realized that the ordinary mechanisms by which suspicions of excess risk are raised—namely case reports and epidemiologic observations—also arise from a multiple testing context. That is, in a clinician's or pathologist's practice or in any of the one-at-a-time epidemiologic studies carried out in the world there is a chance that coincidence will bring together a cluster of cases in some occupation. Those which are noticed may be published. We may, thus, be certain that some unknown proportion of all reported suspicions in the literature are simply due to chance. But we have no statistical context in which to judge all of these suspicious leads. In fact, we believe it is a strength of the systematic multiple testing approach that it provides a statistical context for evaluating the number of significant associations. Having such a context may not simplify decisions but it sheds some light on what is going on. Since this is admittedly a "fishing expedition," any alarms would have to be cautious ones. Each association observed must be evaluated for internal consistency (insofar as the data permit, is there dose-response relation?), biologic plausibility, and prior knowledge even before suggesting that leads be followed up by additional research. As the sample sizes increase, the ratio of true associations to spurious ones will also increase. If there are more occupational carcinogens than the thirty-odd thus far identified, an exposure-based case-control approach may be the most powerful epidemiologic method to discover them. Further analyses of our pilot study are in progress.

ACKNOWLEDGMENTS

We benefitted from the advice of Drs. Graham Gibbs, Peter Nicoll, Fred Knelman, and Norman Cooke. Fieldwork was run by Lesley Richardson and chemical evaluations were carried out, in part, by Howard Kemper. Interviewers were Denise Bourbonnais, Yves Céré, Lucie Felicissimo, and Hélène Sheppard. Comparison of job histories reported and recorded by the QPP was carried out by Mona Baumgarten. We appreciate the cooperation of the QPP. This study would not be possible without the cooperation of the following clinicians and pathologists, and their respective hospital authorities: Drs. R. Vauclair and Y. Méthot, Hôpital Notre-Dame; Dr. L. Stutzman, Royal Victoria Hospital; Drs. C. Lachance and H. Frank, Sir Mortimer B. Davis Jewish General Hospital; Drs. W.P. Duguid and J. MacFarlane, Montreal General Hospital; Drs. S. Tange and D. Munro, Montreal Chest Hospital; Drs. F. Gomes and F. Wiegand, Queen Elizabeth Hospital; Drs. B. Artenian and G. Pearl, Reddy Memorial Hospital; Drs. D. Kahn and C. Pick, St. Mary's Hospital; Dr. C. Piché, Hôpital Ste-Jeanne d'Arc; Drs. P. Bluteau and G. Arjane, Centre Hospitalier de Verdun; Drs. Yves McKay and A. Bachand, Hôpital du Sacré-Coeur; Drs. A. Neaga and A. Reeves,

Hôpital Jean-Talon; Drs. Yvan Boivin and M. Cadotte, Hôtel-Dieu de Montréal; Dr. A. Iorizzo, Hôpital Santa Cabrini; Dr. André Bonin, Hôpital Fleury; Drs. J. Lamarche and G. Lachance, Hôpital Maisonneuve-Rosemont; Drs. G. Gariépy and S. Legault-Poisson, Hôpital St-Luc. We also thank the pathology department and tumor registry staff of above-mentioned hospitals who notify us of new cases. This research was supported by grants from the Conseil de la recherche en santé du Québec and the National Cancer Institute of Canada.

REFERENCES

Acheson, E.D. 1979. Record linkage and the identification of long-term environmental hazards. *Proc. R. Soc. Lond. B.* **205**:165.

Berenblum, I. 1979. Carcinogenicity testing for control of environmental tumor development in man. *Isr. J. Med. Sci.* **15**:473.

Doll, R. 1975. Pott and the prospects for prevention. *Br. J. Cancer* **32**:263.

Gehring, P.J., P.G. Watanabe, and G.E. Blau. 1979. Risk assessment of environmental carcinogens utilizing pharmacokinetic parameters. *Ann. N.Y. Acad. Sci.* **239**:137.

Hoar, S.K., A.S. Morrison, P. Cole, and D.T. Silverman. 1980. An occupation and exposure linkage system for the study of occupational carcinogenesis. *J. Occup. Med.* **22**:722.

McCann, J. and B.N. Ames. 1977. The salmonella/microsome mutagenicity test: Predictive value for animal carcinogenicity. *Cold Spring Harbor Conf. Cell Proliferation* **4**:1431.

Purchase, I.F.H. 1980. Procedures for screening chemicals for carcinogenicity. *Br. J. Ind. Med.* **37**:1.

Rall, D.P. 1979. Validity of extrapolation of results of animal studies to man. *Ann. N.Y. Acad. Sci.* **239**:85.

Shubik, P. 1979. Identification of environmental carcinogens: Animal test models. In *Carcinogens: Identification and mechanisms of action*. (ed. A.C. Griffin and C.R. Shaw), p. 37, Raven Press, New York.

Siemiatycki, J., N.E. Day, J. Fabry, and J.A. Cooper. 1981. Discovering carcinogens in the occupational environment: A novel epidemiologic approach. *J. Natl. Cancer Inst.* **66**:217.

Tomatis, L. 1979. The predictive value of rodent carcinogenicity tests in the evaluation of human risks. *Annu. Rev. Pharmacol. Toxicol.* **19**:511.

Williams, R.R., N.L. Stegens, and J.R. Goldsmith. 1977. Associations of cancer site and type with occupation and industry from the Third National Cancer Survey Interview. *J. Natl. Cancer Inst.* **59**:1147.

COMMENTS

BEEBE: Can you tell us something about cost?

SIEMIATYCKI: Our paid staff consists of a fieldwork organizer, four interviewers, two chemists, a secretary, and a nurse to check diagnoses. We also pay consultants and pathology department secretaries who report cases to us. The costs including supplies, services, and travel, is approximately $200,000 per year. We estimate that the chemist function comprises about 25% of the overall cost. In other words, a purely job title-based case-control study without the translation of job histories into exposure histories would cost 25% less.

AXELSON: You indicated some difficulties in getting into the hospitals, delays and so on. Could you expand a little on that?

SIEMIATYCKI: I was referring to the diplomatic activity in persuading 17 sets of hospital directors, pathology departments, surgery departments, departments of medicine, and so on. In three hospitals the process took longer than in others, for reasons having to do with local politics. We tried to establish contact with one prominent person in the hospital initially to introduce us. Sometimes we chose the wrong person. In general, however, our clinical colleagues have been very receptive and encouraging.

R. PETO: What is the extra cost, over and above a more brief questionnaire, of the extra time spent on questioning and the extra time spent on coding it into the computer?

SIEMIATYCKI: Very little, 5%-maybe less. The cost of getting to the patient dwarfs the cost of the actual interview and data management. Since we try to interview the patient soon after diagnosis, he is often too ill or depressed the first time the interviewer visits.

ACHESON: There is another question, and that is whether the additional costs of the interview are worthwhile as compared with the self-administered questionnaire approach. We are hoping to cast some light on this question by a validation study in the following way, very briefly: We are descending upon one of the hospitals in Southampton on visiting day without warning. In fact, this is being done this week. We are asking the patients and their nearest visiting relative, to complete an occupational questionnaire about the patient, separately, without collusion.

This means that it will be possible to determine what, for example, a widow knows about her husband's occupations, without collusion. I think I know what the result is, but we had better wait.

SILVERSTEIN: Have you made any attempt to validate the information that you get off of the questionnaires with more objective forms of personnel records?

SIEMIATYCKI: As I indicated, we did a validation check against records of the QPP. We have been very reluctant to go back to employers of patients for the purpose of validating histories, because this would, in our view, be an infringement. I think many people would be reluctant to allow us to go back to their employer. Some of them are still working and don't want their employer to know they are sick. We have stayed away from that.

Guiding Experiences on the Etiology of Acute Myeloid Leukemia

OLAV AXELSON, ULF FLODIN, CARL-GÖRAN ANJOU, AND OLLE VIKROT
Departments of Occupational Medicine, Medical Informatics, and Internal Medicine
Linköping University
S-581 85 Linköping, Sweden

Genetic, environmental, and infectious factors seem to be involved in the etiology of leukemia. Relatively frequent contacts with cats, poultry, and cattle among cases of leukemia suggest a viral etiology (Heath et al. 1975; Gallo 1978), but a familial aggregation also tends to occur (MacMahon and Levy 1964; Gunz 1974). Exposure to different solvents might be of etiological importance (Brandt et al. 1978), and interest has been focused especially on benzene (Vigliani 1976; Infante et al. 1977). Ionizing radiation is another relatively well-recognized risk factor for leukemias of all types except the chronic lymphatic type (Lewis 1963; Court Brown and Doll 1965).

To delineate somewhat the relative importance of various potential risk factors for acute myeloid leukemia (AML) in Sweden and to obtain experience about the methodological aspects involved in the evaluation of multiple risk factors and the possible effect of background radiation, a pilot study of the case-referent (case-control) design was undertaken with the utilization of all dead cases above the age of 20 in the register of the Linköping University Hospital during the years 1972-1978. It is the intention to present the study in some more detail elsewhere, but for the purpose of indicating some methodological features, a description of the general outline is given here together with a brief summary of the results.

SUBJECTS

A total of 46 cases was available, out of which 1 newly deceased individual was directly excluded for ethical reasons. The remaining cases were identified in the parish registers of deaths and burials, and 6 referents (controls) were chosen for each case from this source. These referents were taken as those individuals of the same gender and age (±7 years) who were without a cancer diagnosis and who had entered the parish register of causes of deaths in the three nearest positions before and after each case. Due to problems of finding referents fulfilling the selection criteria, the final number of cases and referents amounted

Table 1
Status or Exposure among Cases and Referents along with Estimates of Crude Risk Ratios and Etiologic Fractions

Status or exposure	Number of exposed individuals among: cases (n=42)	referents (n=244)	Crude rate ratio	Etiologic fraction (%)
Male gender	23	121	1.1	–
Rural domicile	11	59	1.1	–
Smoking	19	117	0.9	–
Pesticides	3	6	3.1	5
X-ray treatment	4	20	1.2	2
X-ray examination	12	68	1.1	3
Animal contacts	16	79	1.3	9
Cat	14	62	1.5	11
Poultry	8	36	1.4	5
Cattle	10	43	1.5	8
Solvent exposure	11	13	6.3	22
Background radiation category				
I	12	110	(1.0, reference)	
II	9	49	1.7	9
III	21	85	2.3	28

to 44 and 260, respectively. Out of the 44 cases, 1 was found to have lived abroad for a very long time and another had primarily suffered from a multiple myeloma and had been treated with cytotoxic agents; therefore, these 2 individuals were excluded from the study.

EXPOSURE

Information about various types of exposure among the cases and referents was obtained through a nine-page questionnaire, preceeded by an introductory letter and sent out by mail to the next of kin. The questionnaire encompassed 30 main questions; 15 concerned occupational exposures, and some of them were subspecified further with regard to specific details. Four questions were devoted to medical care, e.g., use of drugs, X-ray examinations, and treatments. Aspects about residency were covered in six main questions and another four questions were given in reference to various environmental aspects, leisure time activities, etc., as well as information about urban or rural domicile during the lifetime of the individual. The shortfall turned out to encompass 16 referent individuals; 5 due to refusal to participate and the others for various "technical" reasons, usually that the next of kin could not be found or was unable to answer the questions; 2 referents had died recently and their next of kin therefore were not disturbed with questionnaires for ethical reasons. In all, information was obtained for 42 cases and 244 referents, with the analyses encompassing 286 individuals.

Exposure to various factors was read from the questionnaires and crudely weighted with regard to intensity and duration, requiring a minimum of 1 year of exposure or, for X-ray exposure, at least five examination episodes or one series of treatment 5 or more years prior to death (see Table 1). Various leisure-time exposures were disregarded as well as all exposures beyond 20 years prior to death.

Considerable interest was devoted to background radiation in this study as influenced by outdoor or indoor work, leisure time being spent outside or inside, and type of residency and workplace with regard to building material. Thus, an exposure index was created by estimating the background radiation and the time spent in various situations during a "time window" encompassing the period from 5 to 25 years prior to death (truncated at birth for the youngest). Finally, the subjects were allocated to one of three exposure categories according to their estimated background exposure, with those in the highest exposure category probably being exposed to at least double the exposure of those in the lowest category and the second category roughly corresponding to the average of the two others.

RESULTS

A number of crude-rate ratio (odds ratio) analyses were undertaken according to Table 1 showing somewhat increased rate ratios with regard to contacts with animals, exposure to solvents, and pesticides. Furthermore, there was a positive relationship to background radiation. The calculated etiologic fractions (Miettinen 1974) crudely indicate the relative importance of various exposures, although there is considerable uncertainty due to random variation in the small numbers involved.

A rather complex and interesting pattern of confounding appeared in the study, as illustrated in Table 2, e.g., there was a negative relationship between degree of background radiation, contacts with animals, and pesticide exposure, whereas a positive relationship was obtained between background radiation and X-ray treatment. Solvent exposure was somewhat more frequent in the second category of background radiation than in the other categories.

To evaluate more precisely the effects of solvent exposure, the material was restricted through the exclusion of individuals with exposure to pesticides and X-ray treatment. These exclusions homogenized the material with regard to animal contacts as well. The effect from solvent exposure, as reflected in Table 3, corresponded to a crude rate ratio of 6.0, the Mantel-Haenszel rate ratio by stratification on age and background radiation being 5.5 (Mantel and Haenszel

Table 2
Relationship in Terms of an Odds Ratio between Various Risk Factors (according to evaluation in Table 1) and Background Radiation Categories as Indirectly also Reflecting Interrelationships of the Different Exposures

Risk factor	Background radiation category	Referents exposed	Referents nonexposed	Odds ratio
Pesticides	I	6	104	(1.0)
	II	0	49	–
	III	0	85	–
X-ray treatment	I	8	102	(1.0)
	II	5	44	1.5
	III	7	78	1.1
Animal contacts	I	62	48	(1.0)
	II	14	35	0.3
	III	3	82	0.3
Solvent exposure	I	5	105	(1.0)
	II	5	44	2.4
	III	3	82	0.8

1959) with a 95% approximative confidence interval (CI) 2.1-14.4 (Miettinen 1976). From Table 3, it appears as if there were a rather strong effect from the combination of solvent exposure and a situation of high background radiation. Unfortunately, it was not possible to obtain any detailed information through the mailed questionnaires about the type of solvents to which the subjects were exposed, but both chlorinated and nonhalogenated hydrocarbons seemed to be involved and some of them might have contained benzene.

DISCUSSION AND CONCLUSION

This study indicates a complex interrelationship of various risk factors with regard to confounding and effect modification that requires due consideration in the design and analyses of future studies. However, a particular problem is involved in assessing the individual exposure to a generally occurring phenomenon like background radiation. First, there is the need of getting some general idea about the magnitude of radiation in various situations like outside, inside, and with regard to building materials, etc. Luckily, relatively good information exists (in Sweden) at this time (Hultqvist 1956; Swedjemark 1979), but the difficulty of estimating the degree of the individual exposure remains. For this purpose, a gamma radiation index, GEI, was created. By denoting the

Table 3
Distribution of Cases of AML and Referents with Regard to Age, Background Radiation, and Exposure to Solvents

Ages	Background radiation category	Case/ referent	Solvent exposure present	Solvent exposure absent	Stratum specific rate ratio
20-49	I	C	0	1	<6.5
		R	2	13	
	II	C	1	1	>7.0
		R	0	7	
	III	C	3	4	>14.0
		R	0	19	
50-69	I	C	0	0	–
		R	0	29	
	II	C	1	3	2.7
		R	2	16	
	III	C	3	6	19.5
		R	1	39	
70+	I	C	0	7	<2.4
		R	3	50	
	II	C	1	2	4.3
		R	2	17	
	III	C	0	2	<4.3
		R	2	17	
All	I	C	0	8	<2.3
		R	5	92	
	II	C	3	6	5.0
		R	4	40	
	III	C	6	12	12.5
		R	3	75	
Crude rate ratio			6.0	(1.0)	
Mantel-Haenszel rate ratio					
point estimate			5.5	(1.0)	
95% CI (approximate)			2.1-14.4		

Subjects with exposure to pesticides and X-ray treatment are excluded, including 2 cases and 1 referent with solvent exposure (compare numbers in Table 1).

estimated background radiation dose in the various situations by r, exposure time in years by t, and the total of the considered time period by T (i.e., the "time window" of 5-25 years prior to death), one obtains

$$\text{GEI} = \sum_i \sum_j rt/T \tag{1}$$

with summation over three main activities, i (time of work, leisure, and sleeping), and over the years, j. The background radiation, r, was taken as 2 for stone houses (e.g., alum shale and other concrete), 1 for wooden houses, and 1.5 for "mixed" types of houses (e.g., plastered and (or) brick houses) in a relative scale. The minimum score amount to 3 points and the maximum score to 6 points; in the tables, the exposure information was reduced into three categories, however, with category II encompassing individuals with a score from 4 to less than 5 points, and the other categories having higher and lower scores, respectively. Obviously, it is necessary to classify the individuals blindly with regard to their status of a case or a referent, because subjective judgments are involved in this procedure. In an earlier study concerning possible lung cancer effects of exposure to radon and radon daughters in dwellings, we used a somewhat similar classification with regard to wooden houses and stone houses, allowing for a category of "mixed houses" in between (Axelson et al. 1979; Axelson and Edling 1980).

Exposure categorization of this type might well be criticized from various viewpoints, but in principle it is unlikely that there will be any better possibilities to account for generally occurring exposures with modifying effects, as seems possible for background radiation. Correlation studies of regional incidence rates and background radiation or, say, air pollution, are not likely to be sensitive and (or) valid enough to assess convincingly, or even indicate, an existing causal connection, especially as various other risk factors might be distributed in such a way that they tend to obscure the effect of a particular factor under study.

Based on prior knowledge, and in the light of the results of the study, it seems as if a good deal of the myeloid leukemia mortality might be prevented by reducing (unnecessary and easily avoidable) solvent exposure. It might also turn out to be important to use building materials with a low content of radioactivity, but apparently further epidemiologic evaluations are needed on this point. Diminished animal contacts might be suggested, especially to cats, but again further confirmation is needed. These various suggestions are certainly not justified on the basis of this study per se but merely on the agreement between these findings and experiences from other studies. It might also be recalled in this context, that among Japanese A-bomb survivors, there seemed to be an especially high incidence of leukemia when exposure to benzene had taken place (Ishimaru et al. 1971).

In conclusion, it seems worthwhile to study larger populations, although the rather complex relationships of various potential risk factors must be borne in mind and allowed for in collecting and analyzing data on AML and perhaps also other malignancies.

ACKNOWLEDGMENTS

We are indebted to Ms. Gunilla Desai for typing and editing and to Mr. Lennart Andersson and Mr. Hans Kling for technical assistance.

REFERENCES

Axelson, O. and C. Edling. 1980. Health hazards from radon daughters in dwellings in Sweden. In *Health implications of new energy technologies* (ed. W.N. Rom and V.E. Archer), p. 79. Ann Arbor Science Publishers, Ann Arbor, Michigan.

Axelson, O., C. Edling, and H. Kling. 1979. Lung cancer and residency—A case referent study on a possible impact of exposure to radon and its daughters in dwellings. *Scand. J. Work Environ. Health* **5**:10.

Brandt, L., P.G. Nilsson, and F. Mitelman. 1978. Occupational exposure to petroleum products in men with acute nonlymphatocytic leukaemia. *Br. Med. J.* **4**:553.

Court Brown, W.M. and R. Doll. 1965. Mortality from cancer and other causes after radiotherapy for ankylosing spondylitis. *Br. Med. J.* **4**:1327.

Gallo, R.C. 1978. Leukaemia, environmental factors, and viruses. In *Viruses and environment* (ed. E. Kurstack and K. Maramorosch), p. 43. Academic Press, New York.

Gunz, F.V. 1974. Genetics of human leukaemia. *Series of Haematology* **7**:164.

Heath, C.W., Jr., G.G. Caldwell, and P.C. Feorino. 1975. Viruses and other microbes. In *Persons at high risk of cancer* (ed. J.F. Fraumeni, Jr.), p. 241. Academic Press, New York.

Hultqvist, B. 1956. Studies on naturally occurring ionizing radiations, with special reference to radiation doses in Swedish houses of various types. In *Kungl. Svenska Vetenskapsakademins samlingar, fjärde serien,* band 6, no. 3. Almkvist & Wicksell Boktryckeri AB, Stockholm.

Infante, P.F., J.K. Wagoner, R.A. Rinsky, and R.J. Young. 1977. Leukaemia in benzene workers. *Lancet* **ii**:76.

Ishimaru, T., H. Okada, T. Tomiyasu, T. Tsuchimothoshino, and M. Ishimaru. 1971. Occupational factors in the epidemiology of leukaemia in Hiroshima and Nagasaki. *Am. J. Epidemiol.* **93**:157.

Lewis, E.B. 1963. Leukaemia, multiple myeloma and aplastic anaemia in American radiologists. *Science* **142**:1492.

MacMahon, B. and A. Levy. 1964. Prenatal origin of childhood leukaemia. Evidence from twins. *N. Engl. J. Med.* **270**:1082.

Mantel, N. and W. Haenszel. 1959. Statistical aspects of the analysis of data from retrospective studies of disease. *J. Natl. Cancer Inst.* **23**:719.

Miettinen, O.S. 1974. Proportion of disease caused or prevented by a given exposure, trait or intervention. *Am. J. Epidemiol.* **99**:325.

_____. 1976. Estimability and estimation in case-referent studies. *Am. J. Epidemiol.* **103**:226.

Swedjemark, G.A. 1979. *In-door measurements of natural radioactivity in Sweden.* SSI: 1979/026. Arbetsdokument SSI, Box 6024, 104 01 Stockholm.

Vigliani, E.C. 1976. Leukemia associated with benzene exposure. *Ann. N.Y. Acad. Sci.* **271**:143.

COMMENTS

R. PETO: What were you assessing with solvent exposure?

AXELSON: We did not have very detailed information regarding this. Most of these people had been painters, varnishers, lacquerers, degreasers—that sort of thing. They were required to have had an exposure of more than 1 year and the exposure had to have been of a professional type that took place more than 5 years prior to death. So, there is some latency time taken in; otherwise, it wasn't considered an exposure.

PADDLE: If this relative risk of 6 is correct, then one really ought to be seeing this in other populations. I don't think this is found generally.

AXELSON: This is the second study in Sweden showing a risk of about 5-6 for nonlymphatic leukemia and solvent exposure. The other one is published from the University of Lund in southern Sweden (Brandt et al. 1978).

GAFFEY: Do you have any plans to do a large study? This one seems to be interesting, but very small. Can you multiply this by 10 or 20?

AXELSON: Yes, that is what we intend to do. We are trying to set up a prospective study for leukemia. However, the problem is that although our hospital is one of the seven big regional hospitals in Sweden, the number of cases per year is not very large. Perhaps we should try to set up a multicenter study to get cases from the whole of southeastern Sweden or even try to do something in common for all of Sweden. There is probably one more study going on that is focusing somewhat on these aspects, so we might obtain some more information fairly soon. However, it is difficult to get large numbers in a small country.

DAVIS: Your model did not seem to take into account ground exposure to radiation. Sometimes deposits occur very close to the surface. Isn't that a problem in the area?

AXELSON: It doesn't take care of ground exposure very well. I would say there is a general ground exposure that is roughly about the same all over the area from which the cases were taken. So you might add another point to the exposure score for everyone irrespective of what type of house they are living in, just moving upwards on a relative scale.

DAVIS: Then it wouldn't be necessary to include it. I wondered if you had any rough estimates of the amount of time people spent indoors in their homes. There is growing interest in this country in the problem of indoor air pollution. Increasing insulation also would increase the burden of exposure to indoor air pollutants, ranging from radon daughters to, perhaps, formaldehyde, carbon monoxide, and other by-products of cooking.

AXELSON: There have been such estimates. I don't recall the exact figures, but I think the estimates have been about 85% of the time indoors for an urban population. In this specific context, we had a rather primitive model. We took one-third as leisure time, another one-third as sleeping time, and the remaining one-third as working time.

DAVIS: I understand that there has been some work on ventilation rates that may also enter into it.

AXELSON: Ventilation rates are a concern with regard to radon, but they don't affect the gamma radiation. The radon matter is a big problem in Sweden. There were measurements made by Hultqvist (1956), and there have been new measurements made during the last 2 years. They indicate about an 2.5-fold increase in indoor radon in Sweden over the past 2 decades, which is probably rather serious. Average radon concentrations increased from 23 Bq/m^3 (0.6 pCi/e) to 57 Bq/m^3 (1.5 pCi/e) on an average in those monitored buildings from the 1950s that still existed in 1975 (Swedjemark 1979).

SARACCI: Are the types of houses—stone, wood, etc.—distributed differently among different people by social class and occupation.

AXELSON: No, I wouldn't say so, at least not to any great extent. If you look at the modern homes today, they are what we classify as a mixed type. There is some brick material, some concrete in the basement, and the rest is wood. The old traditional Swedish house was of wood, built without a basement. The big apartment houses that are being built in the cities now are, of course, stone houses. But there is no social gradient. If there were, I would even wonder if one should take that into account since, first of all, there should be a difference with regard to the incidence of leukemia in various social classes. If so, then one might ask what it might depend on, and maybe it would depend just on differences in background radiation.

BEAUMONT: This is very interesting from a biological standpoint. Here we have a single disease being caused possibly by a virus, a chemical, and radiation. I don't know if there are any other cancers quite like that.

R. PETO: I'd like to ask you about the statistical significance in various of your findings. For example, it seems that the effect on cats would be nonsignificant.

AXELSON: Yes, the effect is not significant in this respect, just indicated in an elevated rate ratio.

R. PETO: The relationship with radiation seems to be of marginal statistical significance. I make it to be about 2 S.D. Could you give us the *p* values for these things?

AXELSON: Yes, exactly. If the gamma radiation categories are taken as the exposure and the Mantel extension is applied, you will get a *p* value at the 2% level, which is not very strong but is rather suggestive.

AUSTIN: Could you explain how you selected the controls?

AXELSON: The controls were taken as those from the parish registers that were similar in age, which is ± 7 years. They had to be of the same sex and appear next to the case, either before or after, in the parish registers of deaths. These registers are books in which the causes of deaths are entered sequentially, just individual by individual. So it is a sort of a matching, if you wish, although we didn't maintain the matching in the analysis.

AUSTIN: Could it have included other cancer deaths?

AXELSON: No. That is an important point. We didn't take other cancer deaths, because if there should be a general effect of background radiation, it would have been inappropriate to take in the other cancer deaths, because then the controls or referents would not have reflected the exposure of the source population for the cases.

J. PETO: Are there any long-lived radon daughters or isotopes with half-lives of years that could be assayed in human tissue?

AXELSON: Yes, lead-210, which stays very long.

J. PETO: Would it be possible to do autopsy studies?

AXELSON: Yes, there is a discussion that we should do that, actually take bone samples from lung cancer cases and controls. Perhaps it should be done with leukemias, as well, to see if there is a difference in the content of lead-210 in the skeleton, as there is a reasonable correlation, probably, between gamma radiation exposure and radon daughter exposure.

EPSTEIN: That isotope is also a bone seeker, so that one needs to consider there the marrow exposure.

RADFORD: You can also do lead-210 assays by whole-body counting. You don't have to get bone samples; you can also do it in vivo. It is interesting to note that the only positive finding of the 800 people who were assayed at Three Mile Island were elevated lead-210 burdens in about 10.

ACHESON: You expressed a concern that you had, and others shared, about the effect of radon in dwellings in Sweden. Is there other evidence to back this concern?

AXELSON: Yes, there is a study (Axelson et al. 1979) in which we looked at lung cancer in the most rural areas, which didn't give us many lung cancers. But if you cover areas large enough, you might find some cases, and we did. It turned out that there was about a fivefold risk for lung cancer for those living in stone houses in the extremely rural areas of Sweden as compared to those living in wooden houses. I know there can be misclassifications and all sorts of problems in here, but it is easy to single out the classical Swedish wooden house from the rest. If you do that comparison, it is about a doubled risk for living in all sorts of houses in comparison to the traditional wooden houses. But, again, the figures are small. We are continuing a couple of studies in Sweden now to see whether or not we can confirm these preliminary findings.

References

Axelson, O., C. Edling, and H. Kling. 1979. Lung cancer and residency–A case referent study on a possible impact of exposure to radon and its daughters in dwellings. *Scand. J. Work Environ. Health* 5:10.

Brandt, L., P.G. Nilsson, and F. Mitelman. 1978. Occupational exposure to petroleum products in men with acute nonlymphatocytic leukaemia. *Br. Med. J.* 4:553.

Hultqvist, B. 1956. Studies on naturally occurring ionizing radiations, with special reference to radiation doses in Swedish houses of various types. In *Kungl. Svenska Vetenskapsakademins samlingar fjärde serien,* band 6, no. 3. Almkvist & Wicksell Boktryckeri AB, Stockholm.

Swedjemark, G.A. 1979. *In-door measurements of natural radioactivity in Sweden.* SSI: 1979/026. Arbetsdokument SSI, Box 6024, 104 01 Stockholm.

The International Context of Carcinogen Regulation: Benzidine

SHELDON W. SAMUELS
Industrial Union Department, AFL-CIO
Washington, D.C. 20006

Benzidine is the focus of this study since there is relatively little disagreement by labor or management or government or academia on its effects. The relatively long history of its regulation provides us with some basis for international regulation. A number of countries already have set regulations. If a morally consistent method of international regulation can succeed, the best chance of demonstration appears to be the control of benzidine.

The regulatory concept that evolved from this study is National Stewardship. The essence of National Stewardship is not technological or legalistic, it is based on taking responsibility for our own actions. This concept is applied not only to the import of chemicals, but also to the export of standards and concepts that assist the creation of microcosmic hell in countries throughout the world.

THE EXPORT OF STANDARDS AND DECEPTIVE CONCEPTS

After April 28, 1971, the first effective date of the Occupational Safety and Health Act, the American Conference of Governmental Industrial Hygienists (ACGIH) and similar organizations were replaced as a source of voluntary and mandated official standards by the then newly-created National Institute for Occupational Safety and Health (NIOSH). Prior to that date, ACGIH efforts were praiseworthy as voluntary private acts by government officials, acting as individuals in alliance with management specialists, to control acute effects prior to the passage of the act. Review of the documentation of ACGIH values (ACGIH 1971) indicates that little attention was given to chronic effects. The selected studies were, at best, sources of data critical in the selection of exposure limits which when exceeded meant that most workers would experience acute effects that would disrupt production. That sad chapter of American labor history ended with the passage of the Occupational Safety and Health Act, but the current chapter is only less sad. Presently, the ACGIH Threshold Limit Values (TLV) committee exists almost solely for the purpose of exporting environmental values (they are not full standards) to other countries less stringent than those of the United States. This is being done with the knowledge and consent of government and management specialists in the recipient countries, but without the knowledge of most of their legislative or rule-making bodies. As a consequence of the warnings of many in the international labor movement and in academia, Scandinavia and West Germany and other European countries recently have abandoned dependence on ACGIH.

Aside from the implied interference by United Nations (U.N.) agencies in a dispute within a member nation, the attention given ACGIH values in U.N. publications hinders the dialogue in the international community from reflecting the redefinition of the concept "standard" that occurred in the United States with the passage of the Occupational Safety and Health Act.

A "standard" in U.S. law is a total system of use and enforcement: An environmental value or work practice or process containment or personal protection—or any combination of these—in concert with a system of employer-employee education, monitoring, medical surveillance, warning devices, record-keeping, protection for the complaining or medically-removable worker, and the right of both the worker and manager to participate in the interpretation of data and compliance. The asbestos standard is a case in point. Therefore, the American standard is not simply an environmental or biological number. It is an expression of scientific, technical, and economic values in a matrix of social values.

Without question, similar systems of control (mandated or voluntary) exist in other countries where the term "standard" simply is used in a more narrow sense. In these countries other portions of the enabling legislation or body of law and tradition provide the balance of the system. Even when there is a strong consensual determination of a cancer risk, the official international response is far from being uniform or satisfactory. In the United States, proposals vary from banning and prohibitions to exposure, to stringent work practices (as is the case for benzidine). There are also proposals for what is, in effect, massive human experimentation in search of a "threshold" (Weill 1976). Internationally, the response is similar, (Montesano and Tomatis 1977) with some notable additions.

USE OF LATENCY

Gadian (1975), medical officer for Lankro Chemicals, notes one of the precautions taken in Great Britain to control exposure to industrial carcinogens: "In general, older men—usually over the age of 40—are employed as dichlorobenzidine workers. This is a legacy of the days when betanaphthylamine and benzidine were used, and the possibility of a tumour developing was much higher. It was reasoned that if a man did become affected, he would at least have a fairly long life before becoming so, as the latent period is so long."

According to Gadian, that long latency period "average(s) 18 years for occupational bladder tumors." The felicific calculus: 40 years of age + 18 years of latency = 58 years of age at death or management's decision as to what a worker's fairly long life should be. This administrative practice, apparently accepted in Russia International Labor Organization ([ILO] 1977) has been proposed in India out of despair and in the face of almost total official inaction (Lobo-Mendoca 1977). To be fair, it is important to note that in neither of these cases is this the only method of control proposed. The danger arises from reliance on a Kafkaesque rationalization.

Even if we assume the effect described by Druckrey (1977), that is, decreasing the dose of a carcinogen increases the time to tumor, and if we assume that exposure could be reduced to the point when tumors would be expected beyond the limited life span of an individual, and that this carcinogen would be the only one to which the individual was exposed, we cannot tolerate the massive human experiment that would be required to estimate such a point. Moreover, even if retrospective population studies were possible, we could not determine a no-effect level for any single individual lifetime.

THE THRESHOLD CONCEPT

The concept of a "real threshold" accepted on theoretical grounds by a WHO technical report (WHO 1974) on this subject, contrary to wide acceptance on mathematical and biological grounds of the absence of no-effect doses in populations, is a morally repugnant basis for control in the workplace. This concept is widely rejected by the international labor movement because of its use in determining deceptive "safe" levels of exposure.

Until recently the public position of ACGIH was that "safe limits of exposure . . . for a working lifetime and even thereafter" could be determined (Stokinger 1974). We now learn from one of the retired industrial participants in the ACGIH TLV committee that "the numbers in the TLV list were never meant to be guaranteed safe levels of exposure for all exposed workers under all conditions" (Zapp 1977). The current lists add that precaution.

The consensus is overwhelming that even with qualification, this concept is a statistically and biologically meaningless concept (NAS 1975). Yet, it still appears in current western regulatory literature (Health and Safety Commission 1979) and is the basis for setting the maximum allowable concentration (MAC) in Russia (Holmberg and Winell 1977). At best, it is a commonly misunderstood term. At worst, it is a conscious deception that masks the actual basis for the selection of an environmental value or permissible exposure limit.

Other Deceptive Methods

The assumption of a threshold and (or) the allegation of data supporting a threshold is not the only deceptive method of setting standards. Providing the impression, but not the substance, of science, is the proposal often made in the United States to reduce environmental exposures to levels "not detectable by the recommended method" (NIOSH 1974). In Russia, an analogous practice is reported: reduction of exposure below a level that "will not cause disease or disorders from a normal state of health *detectable* [emphasis added] by current methods of investigation . . ." (WHO 1975). In both cases, detectable has meant detection by older methods that can change, may be arbitrary, and often are not the increasingly sensitive analytic methods at the leading edge of science.

Another deceptive method of setting standards is common in the control of ionizing radiation: cumulative whole-body doses over time. The apparently precise calculation of permissible exposure limits by adding units of exposure over time masks the fact that the limits are based on imprecise nonscientific data relating to an arbitrarily selected socially "acceptable" level of specific organ damage (ICRP 1977).

Equally arbitrary is the selection of one disease entity rather than another as the basis of control. In the United States prior to passage of the Occupational Safety and Health Act this has meant the selection of acute rather than chronic diseases. Since that time the emphasis has been on chronic effects, but with little attention to intergenerational effects. In the USSR, the emphasis appears to be on neurological phenomena (Holmberg and Winell 1977).

The asbestos experience in the United States and in Great Britain provides us with an additional example (Lane et al. 1968). In that case the United States was very much influenced by British pioneering. The 2f/cc of air permissible exposure limit and its rationalization by the British Occupational Health Society (BOHS), who helped their government set the value, describes very clearly that they were not considering a limit that would protect workers against cancer, even though cancer was the most important cause of death among asbestos workers! Presumably because of feasibility considerations, description of the supporting data by BOHS appears to mean that they chose on nonbiological grounds environmental values associated with one set of biological effects, asbestosis, against which they wished to protect the worker. The BOHS acknowledged that protection against cancer would have meant the choice of more stringent values. Health was only one consideration. The fact that the British were able to achieve the number without adversely affecting the asbestos industry was the deciding factor in the U.S. decision to adopt (roughly) the British value. The U.S. government, in justifying its action through comparison with the British action, neglected to point out that a permissible exposure limit in Great Britain is not a license to unnecessarily pollute the workroom to the prescribed level (as it is in the United States). Therefore, the values were not commensurate.

THE HISTORY OF BENZIDINE REGULATION

The ILO published a report in 1921 associating benzidine and betanapthylamine as the most common causes of occupationally attributable bladder cancer, reflecting scientific evidence accumulated since 1895.

In the United States, until 1971, regulation was potentially vested in the States. In 1957 and 1961, New York and Pennsylvania, respectively, and probably one or two other states, took steps to reduce employee exposures. The response of industry was to either move or continue production in states that did not take action. Thus by 1929 Dupont had confirmed cases of bladder tumors, but continued benzidine production in New Jersey for another four decades.

In 1967, the Carcinogenic Substances Regulation in the United Kingdom permitted manufacture of benzidine and mixtures with more than 1% benzidine only in "closed apparatus . . . specifically authorized by the Chief Inspector of Factories." This was followed by similar action in Sweden and Switzerland. Production and use is reported to have ended in Japan in 1971 (ILO 1977).

Following a 1967 resolution, in June 1974, the General Conference of the ILO adopted Convention 139 which called for the control of occupational carcinogens by law or by "any other method consistent with national practice." "Guides" established by ILO (1977) are to be considered in the implementation of Convention 139. The guide for the prevention and control of occupational cancer includes benzidine in its list of carcinogens warranting the highest level of control (ILO 1977).

By January 1980, the ILO office in Washington reported that 16 countries ratified Convention 139 (see Table 1). Benzidine regulation, however, has proceeded in a significant number of nonratifying countries. In a survey of standards in 18 countries, the ILO found official standards in only 12 countries (Table 2). Two countries not designated as having official standards in the master table of the ILO report are shown elsewhere in the report to have "prohibited" above the 1% level (Japan) or "discontinued" (USSR) the production of benzidine.

In 1973, after petition from the Oil, Chemical and Atomic Workers, the Occupational Safety and Health Administration (OSHA) issued an emergency temporary standard for benzidine and 13 other carcinogens. In 1974, this was followed by a permanent standard including compounds with more than 0.1% benzidine. The implementation of the U.S. standard excluded dyes derived from benzidine. Pressure from industrial unions triggered the publication of Current Intelligence Bulletin 24, jointly issued by the National Institute for Occupational Safety and Health (NIOSH) and the National Cancer Institute (NCI) on April 17, 1978. The warning, which covered three benzidine-based

Table 1
Ratification of Occupational Cancer Convention, 1974, by Country

Afghanistan
Argentina
Denmark
Ecuador
Finland
Federal Republic Germany
Guinea
Hungary
Iraq
Japan
Norway
Peru
Sweden
Switzerland
Syria
Yugoslavia

Data from ILO 1980.

Table 2
Benzidine Regulation in Selected Countries

Countries with official standards	Countries without official standards
Australia	Bulgaria
Belgium	Czechoslovakia
Finland	Hungary
GDR	Italy
Federal Republic Germany	Japan
Netherlands	USSR
Poland	
Romania	
Sweden	
Switzerland	
United States	
Yugoslavia	

Data from ILO 1977.

dyes: direct blue 6, direct black 38, and direct brown 95, essentially requested that these dyes be handled as if they were benzidine. A month later five industrial unions petitioned for an amendment to the benzidine standard to include these dyes. In response to the unions' petition, on February 22, 1980, OSHA issued a compliance directive calling for regulation of the dyes covered by the NIOSH/NCI alert under the General Duty provision of the Occupational Safety and Health Act, which enables control of generally recognized hazards likely to cause death or serious physical harm.

In most western countries, concern about occupational injury and disease—especially occupational cancer—accelerated after World War II concomitant with accelerated development in the chemical industry and accompanying evidence of disease (Vigliani 1977). Increased government regulation parallels this development (Montesano and Tomatis 1977).

The preOSHA health standards covered only a small portion of the workforce and were primarily set by ACGIH through the American National Standards Institute (ANSI) and other industry associations. They were adopted as an interim measure in 1971. At that time the government began to establish more stringent permanent standards. However, the serious promulgation of U.S. standards did not begin until 1975 and their enforcement prior to that time had been uneven. Prior to 1975, new standards and their effective enforcement took place only after massive legal, political, and public pressure applied by industrial unions (U.S. House of Representatives 1976). In 1975 the United States as a nation began to develop world-wide leadership, and in 1976 the commitment to effective control became government policy at the highest levels. That commitment ended in February 1981 with the orders for massive "deregulation" transmitted to OSHA and other agencies by the current administration.

Progress in other western countries, with the striking exception of the nordic nations, until recently had not kept pace with the United States. While all western and most other countries make liberal use of U.S. preOSHA industry-derived (interim) standards, only Scandinavia is influenced significantly by U.S. adoption of more stringent permanent standards. Nevertheless, movement away from the preexisting ACGIH TLV is taking place in the west. Russia has a separate and noncommensurate system of standards. Its satellites use a mixture of U.S. interim and USSR values. This regulatory history reflects the underlying economics of regulation and, to a lesser extent, other factors. Data is scant, however.

ECONOMIC IMPACT

The biological, economic, and social impacts of regulation have been rather well defined for the protection of whales, but not for our species. Assessments of the impact on humans of internationally uneven occupational and environmental health and safety regulation are limited in number and quality. There are some data emanating from our economic agencies.

The Organization for Economic Cooperation and Development (OECD 1979) reports that in general environmental regulation has resulted in a short-run net increase in employment and minimal inflationary impact which is now the problem

(0.2-0.3% annually). However, the data indicate a trade off between the stimulation of economic growth and the protection of the environment of the worker and his community. Market demands for changes in our industrial structure, such as emphasis on the development of the chemical industry (OECD 1978), create additional pressure to sacrifice the worker's environment, but only when the design and introduction of a technology does not or cannot fully take the human factor into account. Indeed, we are entering a stage of global industrial change when the construction of new plants to utilize new technologies could incorporate into their designs the most advanced controls.

At the same time, the result could well be to locate older uncontrollable technologies, or new technologies stripped of their controls, in countries where health-related values and regulatory policies are least selective. In these countries, the sacrifice of human life will take place unnecessarily and, because of market demands, partially in response to the lack of humane selection, in the import policies of the western nations.

The concern for the welfare of rare birds, reptiles, and furry mammals—as reflected in the import policies of the United States—has not been extended to the workers of the exporting countries.

The impact of U.S. workplace and environmental health and safety regulations on the international distribution of economic activity—and of worker exposures—is poorly documented. Partial studies of some key regulated industries, however, indicate that the expected pattern does indeed prevail: regulated production processes with (potentially) increased compliance costs result in a shift toward offshore production at unregulated sites from which the product can be economically imported back into the regulated market. Evidence of this shift is seen in Table 3.

Domestic production of direct black 38 in 1971 exceeded five million pounds, 64% of the benzidine-derived dyes produced in that year. By 1975, the year after benzidine regulation, production dropped to about 42%. By 1978, production was about 15% of the 1971 level. Currently, production appears to have ceased altogether. Imports have become a significant source, but do not fully compensate for the drop in domestic production.

It is significant that, based on voluntary company reports, the Economics Department of McGraw-Hill reported that the only substantial investment by U.S. industry in Eastern Europe was by the chemical industry. They invested 65 million dollars in 1976 and planned an additional 158 million dollars through 1979 (McGraw-Hill 1977-79).

Table 4 summarizes U.S. International Trade Commission (USITC) data for a group of benzenoid products that include benzidine-based dyes. In 1974, the year in which benzidine was regulated in this country, imports of these products from Mexico increased about five times over the previous year. Imports from all countries dropped in that year, although the long-term trend has shown a steady increase. But what is most notable about these trends is the increased number and the developmental status of newly exporting countries.

Table 3
U.S. Production, Domestic Production Value and Imports of Direct Dye Black 38

	1968	1969	1970	1971	1972	1973	1974	1975	1976	1977	1978
Production											
millions of pounds	6.3	6.1	4.1	5.3	6.7	6.7	NR[a]	2.2	3.8	NA[b]	0.8
Imports											
millions of pounds	NA	NA	NA	NA	NA	NA	NA	NA	.07	.05	0.2
Domestic value U.S. production											
millions of dollars	4.9	3.9	3.3	3.4	4.6	5.6	NR	NR	6.2	NA	NA

Data compiled from annual reports of the USITC.
[a]Not reported.
[b]Not available.

Table 4
General Imports of Colors, Dyes and Stains, Except Toners, from Benzenoid Products (5310030)

	1968	1969	1970	1971	1972	1973	1974	1975	1976	1977	1978	1979
Mexico												
Thousands of Pounds	5.2	<1	1.1	6.0	1.0	26.6	131.0	12.3	73.9	32.3	NA	30.1
All Countries												
Millions of Pounds	13.5	16.3	17.2	24.3	27.1	24.7	19.8	11.5	18.7	21.6	24.6	23.6
Value												
Millions of Dollars	–	46.9										>139
New Exporting Countries (Selected)												
Thousands of Pounds		NL							India			625.5
									Phillipines			16.5
									Rep. of Korea			49.0
									Egypt			133.2
									Mauritania			29.1

Data supplied from annual reports of USITC.

In 1969, India, Phillipines, Republic of Korea, Egypt, and Mauritania were not listed by USITC as exporters of these products to the United States. They were listed 10 years later and have now become significant exporters to the United States. This is especially true of India (625,500 pounds in 1979).

In an unusual comment in a statistical report, the staff of the USITC reports a reaction in other industrial countries similar to the export of capital and hazardous technology by American firms: "... Some European and Japanese companies are constructing dye plants in several developing countries where low labor and minimal pollution controls now exist" (USITC 1977).

On the other hand, where international transportation costs or trade barriers are prohibitively high, where compliance technologies are efficient, or where locational factors such as high and long-lasting capital costs or access to a highly skilled labor supply predominate, potentially hazardous production is likely to remain in the regulated country with necessary steps being taken to bring worker exposures down to the regulated levels.

The effect of the 1974 benzidine regulation in the United States radically reduced domestic production of this highly carcinogenic product. The decline (as seen in Table 3) was accompanied by an increase in imports of benzidine-based dyes, from 1974-1979 (Table 5). Quantities of imports appear to have stabilized at a lower level than pre1974 use of these dyes would have warranted. This suggests that domestic users of benzidine dyes may have begun to end benzidine dependence and now use substitutes. Nevertheless, as we have seen, national policy encourages the import of dyes (and dye-bearing goods) produced abroad, often under conditions inferior to those prevailing in the United States and possibly financed by the export of capital.

Table 5

Benzidine-based Dyes Imported to U.S., 1974-79

Selected country of origin	Quantity in pounds 1974	1976	1979
India	16,193	23,149	47,733
Egypt	None	None	86,641
Poland	3,910	32,684	21,714
Romania	None	79,365	11,023
France	250	17,750	220,018
Canada	None	440	2,205
Total	20,353	153,388	389,334[a]

Data supplied by USITC in 1977 and 1980 to A. Maguire, pers. comm.

[a]The total quantity reported for 1979, including imports from the Benelux countries, is 469,917 pounds.

The economic effect of possible capital export and related import of carcinogenic dyes does not appear to be significant to our economy. This is illustrated by considering the imported quantities of the most widely used benzidine-based dye relative to domestic production.

Direct black 38 is a benzidine-derived dye used for textiles such as cotton, silk, wool, nylon, and acetate and also has commercial use in leather goods, in printing inks, as a biological stain, in plastics, wood stains, wood flour, and hair dyes.

Domestic production of benzidine-derived dyes was approximately 35 million pounds (25% of all dyes domestically manufactured) in 1948. When the OSHAct went into effect in 1971 production dropped to 11.4 million pounds. In 1971 5.3 million pounds of direct black 38 were produced. No production is recorded by USITC in 1974 (the year in which the benzidine regulation went into effect) but rose to 2.2 million pounds in 1975 after adjusting to the OSHA requirements and rose further to 3.8 million pounds in 1976. In that year, 70,753 pounds of direct black, 38 were imported. Imports more than doubled (to 170,442 pounds) by 1978, while domestic production fell (Table 3).

The import of these dyes does not appear to be an economic issue of great significance in the United States. When production of direct black 38—the most economically important such dye—peaked in 1973, the value of its U.S. production was less than 6 million dollars. In 1976, the value of 3.8 million pounds of domestically produced direct black 38 was little more than 6 million dollars. In that year less than 71,000 pounds were imported. Relative to actual and potentially lost domestic production of all dyes, the imported portion of domestically-used dyes remains small. The import of these dyes is a moral issue that manifests itself in the action both of American importers and of foreign exporters of the dyes and products using the dyes.

BARRIERS TO INTERNATIONAL STANDARDS

There are many barriers to achieving identical health standards in every country. Indeed, given the differences in health status, physical environment (Noweir 1975), control over the direction and dissemination of technology, the availability of technical resources and trained personnel compounded by differences in value systems—even a perfectly empowered and politically unfettered United Nations would have difficulty in promulgating and enforcing identical standards in every country. Nevertheless, greater consistency of conditions and greater protection in the work environment are worthwhile but difficult goals to achieve.

ILO's record of accomplishment for the control of carcinogens is no less than that of any member country. Convention 139 and its supporting documents, if implemented, could provide a basis of control: It could become a minimum international labor standard for benzidine and other carcinogenic chemicals. But, as we have seen, it has not been widely adopted. Its guiding document has been diluted by compromise and supporting publications are marred by inaccuracy.

The ILO (1977) compares ". . . the stringent USSR concept of maximum allowable concentration (MAC), which in no case should produce biological or functional changes, and the more elastic approach of the ACGIH of the USA, whose threshold limit values (TLV) make allowance for reversible clinical changes."

The work of ACGIH, a private sector society, was incommensurate with the work of the USSR before, but especially after, April 28, 1971 for several reasons.

The information available to us is that generally the methods of monitoring (air sampling-laboratory analysis) may never have been and are not now the same in the United States and in Russia. While we prefer personal sampling in the breathing zone of the worker, the USSR practice is to use area sampling (Roschin and Timofeevskaya 1975). If this is correct, without adequate theoretical and empirical studies U.S. and USSR values cannot be comparatively assessed. The USSR values, contrary to the illusion created by the comparison of unqualified numbers, may often be much less stringent by several orders of magnitude.

Contrary to misinformation often disseminated that in the United States "proposed permissible levels are based solely on health considerations" (El Battawi 1977), the OSHAct adds the clear qualification "to the extent feasible" (P.L. 91-596) to every standard. There is no bifurcation between so-called "official" standards and actual practice. U.S. standards are not goals, but are enforceable, mandated prescriptions. Comparison with standards of countries in which the term is synonomous with goal or guideline is not possible without taking this fact into consideration.

Comparison becomes possible if we are able to compare standards as systems of control, the broad meaning U.S. law gives the term "standard." Within this definition, some mode of feasibility becomes apparent as the basis for every standard in every country.

There are no workplace health standards, as defined by any country, based solely on empirical biological data. That is, there are no environmental values based on empirical dose-effects information from which a simple deduction or calculation was made. Assumptions of thresholds, arbitrary "safety factors," selection of methods of agent detection or analysis, mouse-to-man relationships, choice of diseases to be prevented and other methodological devices have always been used in the standard-setting process. Such devices may have heuristic meaning and become deceptive when they are given other meanings.

A NATIONAL APPROACH TO INTERNATIONAL STANDARDS

Benzidine has been recognized as a human carcinogen for 85 years, producing a cancer that is commonly fatal after much suffering. This carcinogenicity is not seriously disputed, yet benzidine's use is still widespread despite a demonstrated lack of social or even industrial necessity. Its control is uneven internationally and even in advanced countries it is often not regulated. Industrial convenience and custom have taken precedence over human need and welfare, as a pliant and often unconcerned governmental bureaucracy stood by.

Research provides little more than a few clues to assessing adequately the stringency of control for the purpose of international comparison. No international on-site inspection system exists on the basis of which objective comparison can be made.

It appears that regulation in the United States is at least as stringent as in any country other than Sweden. Japan and the United Kingdom (ILO 1977) regulate mixtures containing 1% or more by weight of benzidine. United States regulates mixtures at 0.1% by weight but, unlike the British regulation, does not require a production permit (despite the entreaties of the Industrial Union Department in the rule-making process).

Stringent carcinogen regulation in any country, as suggested by the ILO guide, appears to be determined not by taking prudent action on the basis of convincing animal data, but only on the basis of available human evidence, i.e. a body count. Regardless of their meaning, it is significant that the terms "prohibit" or "discontinue" have been applied to benzidine. The bodies have been counted.

We found no evidence of significant adverse economic effects of regulating benzidine in any country, either because of the cost of control or import competition. It is apparent that companies and state enterprises in some countries are making or perceive some level of profit through consciously creating havens for polluters. Economic advantages to the countries themselves, except for the obvious immediate effect of marginally increased employment, net exports and relatively small amounts of imported capital, are not clearly established.

Since the evidence of carcinogenicity of benzidine and many benzidine-related chemicals has justified regulation, and since the production or import of these chemicals is not crucial to the economic, social or biological well-being being of any country, the nature of the issue is clear. Failure to regulate is a moral failure in a large number of both advanced and underdeveloped countries.

In those countries that attempt to control these compounds–through regulation or social pressures of some sort–the bases of regulation show wide variation and none are uniformly applied. These bases–biological, analytical, technological, administrative, legal, economic, work practices–cannot be uniformly formulated in each country.

ILO Convention 139 plus its guide is an international standard for benzidine that approaches in comprehension the American concept of a standard. The convention, however, is not widely ratified and, indeed, encourages irregular application. This does not mean that international standards that can be uniformly applied are not possible. What it does mean is that international standards must be more than mirror images of national standards. The goal of such a standard can be uniform or constant: a state of health. That goal is difficult to achieve uniformly because the real bases of regulation–other-than-health criteria such as measurement of environmental levels, substitution, assessment of engineering controls, use of work practices–must also vary. Nevertheless, despite their variations, examples of achievement can be uniformly disseminated.

An "example of achievement" that can be uniformly disseminated is itself exemplified by a recent paper by Holmberg and Westlin (1979) describing vinyl chloride and polyvinyl chloride production standards in Sweden "as low as technologically feasible," resulting in levels of worker exposure "around 0.5 ppm or lower" achieved "by applying known technology only."

Such examples can become the critical element in an international system of standards enforced by National Stewardship.

ACKNOWLEDGMENT

The author is grateful for the support and stimulus of Howard D. Samuel, President of the department, and Brian Turner, Assistant to the President.

REFERENCES

American Conference of Governmental Industrial Hygienists (ACGIH). 1971. *Documentation of Threshold Limit Values* (Third Edition). American Conference of Governmental Industrial Hygienists, Cincinnati.

Druckrey, H., Jr. 1967. Potential carcinogens' hazards. *UICC Monogr. Ser.* **7**.

El Battawi, M.A. 1977. Testimony. Transcript OSHA lead hearing. *Also*: WHO Technical Report Series, No. 601.

Gadian, T. 1975. Carcinogens in industry. *Chem. Ind.* **4**(19):821.

Health and Safety Commission. 1979. Man-made mineral fibres. Report of a Working Party. Health and Safety Commission. Her Majesty's Stationery Office, London.

Holmberg, B. and A. Westlin. 1979. Considerations in the decision of the Swedish occupational health standard for CVM. *Ann. N.Y. Acad. Sci.* **328**:201.

Holmberg, B. and M. Winell. 1977. Occupational health standards. *Scand. J. Work Environ. Health* **3**:8.

International Commission on Radiation Protection (ICRP). 1977. Review of a standard for ionizing radiation. *ICRP Publication Number 26*, Pergamon Press, Oxford.

International Labor Organization (ILO). 1977. *Occupational Cancer-Prevention and Control.* OSH Series 39, p. 24, ILO, Geneva.

———. 1977. Occupational Exposure Limits for Airborne Toxic Substances. OSH Series 37, p. 3, 279, ILO, Geneva.

———. 1977. Working Document IV. Meeting of Experts on Limits of Exposure to Dangerous Airborne Substances, p. 2, ILO, Geneva.

Lane, R.E., J.M. Barnes, D.E. Hickish, J.G. Jones, S.A. Roach, and E. King. 1968. Hygiene standard for chrysotile asbestos dust. *Ann. Occ. Hyg.* **11**:47.

Lobo-Mendoca, R. 1977. Letter. *Ind. J. Occ. Hlth*XX(9):172.

McGraw-Hill. 1977-1979. Overseas operations of U.S. industrial companies. Report of McGraw-Hill. Economics Department, p. 14.

Montesano, R. and L. Tomatis. 1977. Legislation concerning chemical carcinogens in several industrialized countries. *Cancer Res.* **37**:310.

National Academy of Sciences (NAS). 1975. Principles for evaluating Chemicals, p. 83. NAS, Washington, D.C.

National Institute for Occupational Safety and Health (NIOSH). 1974. Recommended Occupational Health Standard for the Manufacturing of Synthetic Polymer from Vinyl Chloride. Memorandum. March 11, 1974.

Noweir, M.H. 1975. Safe level criteria for air contaminants for developing countries. Bulletin of the High Institute of Public Health of Alexandria. Vol. V. No. 1.

Organization for Economic Cooperation and Development (OECD). 1978. Future industrial structures: Report on the evolution of industrial structures. Paris. 13 March 1978.

———. 1979. Environmental policies and prospects for the 1980's. Paris. 11 April 1979.

Roschin, A. and V. Timofeevskaya. 1975. Chemical substances in the work environment: Some comparative aspects of USSR and U.S. hygienic standards. Ambio V. No. 1. Royal Swedish Academy of Sciences, Stockholm.

Stokinger, H. 1974. In *Behavioral Toxicology* (ed. Xintaras et al.). DHEW publication number (NIOSH) 74-126.

U.S. House of Representatives, Committee on Government Operations. 1976. *Chemical Dangers in the Workplace.* House Report No. 94-1688.

U.S. International Trade Commission (USITC). 1977. Synthetic Organic Chemicals. U.S. Production and Sales. USITC p. 90. Publication number 90.

Vigliani, E. (ed.). 1977. *Methods used in western european countries for establishing maximum permissible levels of harmful agents in the workplace.* Fondazione Carlo Erba, Milano.

Weill, H. 1976. *Submission of the Asbestos Information Association on Proposed Revision of the OSHA Asbestos Standard.* Docket No. H-033. Docket Office, OSHA. 8 April, p. 24.

World Health Organization (WHO). 1974. *Assessment of carcinogenicity and mutagenicity.* WHO Technical Report Series Number 546, Geneva.

———. 1975. Methods used in the USSR for establishing biologically safe levels of toxic substances. World Health Organization, Geneva.

Zapp, J.A., Jr. 1977. An acceptable level of exposure. The Herbert E. Stokinger Lecture. ACGIH, New Orleans.

P.L. 91-596, §66(5) (Ninety-First Congress)

Proportion of Cancer Due to Occupation in Washington State

SAMUEL MILHAM, JR.
Epidemiology Section
Washington State Department of Social and Health Services
Olympia, Washington 98504

I have developed a data set in Washington State that can address the question of proportion of cancer due to occupational exposure. The file contains death certificate information for all male resident deaths, age 20+, that occurred in the years 1950-1979 (438,000). Recently, 80,000 female deaths, 1974-1979, have also been added. The death record occupational statements have been abstracted, coded, and keyed into the existing death record. A computer program was written and run on the data to perform an age and year of death standardized proportionate mortality ratio (PMR) analysis.

In 1976, National Institute for Occupational Safety and Health (NIOSH) published this information in a monograph that included PMR tables (Milham 1976). For each of 195 occupational groups, observed and expected deaths and a PMR were computed for 158 cause-of-death groups. This study covered the years 1950-1971 (300,000 male deaths) and was able to demonstrate intuitive, previously reported, and new occupational mortality associations that have been substantiated in population-based studies (Milham 1979). Many other occupational mortality associations remain to be pursued.

The strength of this data set is that it includes all resident male deaths age 20+ for a 30-year period. Expected deaths are based on the proportionate mortality experience of about 440,000 men, standardized for year of death and age at death.

RESULTS

Table 1 shows total cancer mortality and respiratory cancer mortality by major Census Bureau occupational groups. Total observed and expected deaths are slightly different because the computer program rounds expected frequencies. These occupational group totals were developed by summing the individual occupational rubric results. As some rubrics containing only a few deaths were not run, the grand total of 430,287 deaths is slightly less than the total file size. Managers, officials, and proprietors have a 7% excess of total cancers

Table 1
Mortality by Major Census Occupational Groups for All Malignant Neoplasms and Malignant Neoplasms of Respiratory System, Washington State (males age 20+, 1950-1979)

Major census occupational groups	Total deaths	7th ICD 140-204, all malignant neoplasms			7th ICD 160-165, malignant neoplasms of respiratory system		
		O	E	PMR[a]	O	E	PMR[a]
Professional and technical	31,902	5,763	5,528	104	1,295	1,587	82
Farmers	58,069	8,820	9,356	94	1,893	2,233	85
Managers, officials, proprietors	25,138	4,778	4,485	107	1,231	1,286	96
Clerical workers	16,074	3,016	2,881	105	769	846	91
Sales workers	18,906	3,557	3,416	104	951	1,010	94
Craftsmen, kindred workers	122,647	23,304	22,059	106	7,286	6,501	112
Operatives	48,710	8,954	8,789	102	2,897	2,613	111
Service workers	34,686	6,350	6,279	101	1,916	1,842	104
Laborers	63,274	9,621	10,870	89	2,772	2,971	93
Institutionalized and unknown	10,881	1,283	1,762	73	291	443	66
Total	430,287	75,446	75,425	100	21,301	21,332	100

[a]PMR = O/E × 100.

(PMR = 107) and a 4% deficit of respiratory cancers (PMR = 96). Because these men are not ordinarily exposed to carcinogens at work, I would assume that the all-cancer excess was due to life-style variables. Professional and technical workers have a 4% total cancer excess in spite of an 18% respiratory cancer deficit.

Craftsmen and kindred workers have a 6% excess of total cancers (PMR = 106) due primarily to a 12% excess of respiratory cancers (PMR = 112). Operatives have an 11% respiratory cancer excess. Many of these men work in jobs with known carcinogenic exposures.

Table 2 presents the 20 occupational groups (of 200) with the highest PMRs due to all malignant neoplasms. Asbestos-insulation workers have an 82% excess of all cancers. None of the other occupational classes has more than a

Table 2
"Top 20" Occupations—Total mortality due to malignant neoplasms (7th ICD 140-204) Washington State (males age 20+, 1950-1979)

			Deaths		
Rank	Occupation	Code[a]	O	E	PMR[b]
1.	Asbestos and insulation workers	630	76	42	182
2.	Foresters	103	54	42	129
3.	Glaziers	434	68	54	126
4.	Manufacturing workers	462	85	68	125
5.	Bankers	305	308	251	123
6.	Fruit warehouse workers	975	97	79	123
7.	Brewery workers	818	101	83	122
8.	Plasterers	505	160	132	121
9.	Interior decorators	420	49	41	120
10.	Credit men	253	80	67	119
11.	Surveyors	181	67	57	118
12.	Insurance adjusters	321	87	74	118
13.	Brick masons	405	314	266	118
14.	Foremen (not elsewhere classified)	430	144	122	118
15.	Aluminum workers	526	297	253	117
16.	Milk-route men	656	80	68	117
17.	Porters	241	49	42	117
18.	Labor union officials	275	172	149	116
19.	Purchasing agents	285	227	199	114
20.	Paperhangers	501	165	145	114
	Total		2680	2234	120

[a]Modified U.S. Census Bureau Code (see Milham 1976).

[b]$PMR = \frac{\text{Observed Deaths}}{\text{Expected Deaths}} \times 100.$

30% excess. Occupational exposures almost certainly do not account for the presence on the list of bankers, credit men, surveyors, insurance adjusters, porters, milk-route men, labor union officials, or purchasing agents. These 20 occupations account for only 3.5% of all the malignant neoplasms in the file. The overall PMR for the group is 120.

Table 3 repeats the process for respiratory neoplasms. Only newspaper editors, hospital attendants, and railroad conductors do not fit the concept of exposure to known or suspected inhaled carcinogens. The 1787 respiratory cancers in these occupations represent 8.3% of all respiratory cancer deaths in the file. The overall PMR for this selected group is 136.

Table 4 presents what I consider to be a "worst case" scenario. These are the 12 occupations that I believed offered the worst possible inhalation

Table 3
"Top 20" Occupations—Respiratory cancer mortality (7th ICD 160-165) Washington State (males age 20+, 1950-1979)

			Deaths		
Rank	Occupation	Code[a]	O	E	PMR[b]
1.	Asbestos and insulation workers	630	44	14	326
2.	Copper smelter workers	435	107	63	169
3.	Roofers	514	66	40	165
4.	Oilers	692	28	18	159
5.	Plasterers	505	51	34	149
6.	Boilermakers	403	114	82	140
7.	Brick masons	405	99	71	139
8.	Paperhangers	501	56	41	137
9.	Newspaper editors	76	32	24	133
10.	Boatbuilders	407	26	20	132
11.	Miners	685	201	154	130
12.	Inspectors (NEC)	450	38	29	129
13.	Plumbers	510	307	239	128
14.	Tinsmith	525	154	121	128
15.	Tool and die maker	530	35	27	128
16.	Hospital attendant	810	40	31	128
17.	Railroad conductors	252	56	44	127
18.	Metal moulders	492	28	22	126
19.	Pressmen, printers	512	126	100	126
20.	Welders	721	179	144	125
	Total		1787	1318	136

[a]Modified U.S. Census Bureau Code (see Milham 1976).

[b]$PMR = \frac{\text{Observed Deaths}}{\text{Expected Deaths}} \times 100.$

Table 4
Worst-case Example: Occupations Selected for Inhalation Exposure to Known or Suspected Carcinogens. Mortality Due to All Malignancies and Malignancy of Respiratory System Washington State (males age 20+, 1950-1979)

	Deaths, 7th ICD 140-204 all malignant neoplasms			Deaths, 7th ICD 160-165 MN of respiratory system		
Occupation	O	E	PMR	O	E	PMR
Blacksmiths	189	194	97	37	38	98
Boilermakers	306	285	107	114	82	140
Pavers, excavators	926	886	104	332	280	119
Copper smelter workers	240	214	112	107	63	169
Metal moulders	93	86	86	28	22	126
Paper and pulp mill workers	696	706	99	214	224	96
Roofers	134	128	105	66	40	165
Aluminum workers	297	253	117	98	88	112
Asbestos and insulation workers	76	42	182	44	14	326
Laundry and dry cleaner workers	268	243	110	73	71	103
Miners	670	665	101	201	154	130
Welders	439	423	104	179	144	125
Total	4334	4125	105	1493	1220	122

exposures to known or suspected carcinogens. I reasoned that if occupational exposures were causing a large proportion of cancers in any group of workers, it would have to show in this group. Ten of the twelve occupations did show respiratory cancer PMRs over 100; however, the overall total malignant neoplasm PMR in these 12 occupations was only 105, and the respiratory cancer PMR was 122.

DISCUSSION

A number of findings in this study indicate that occupational exposures can only account for a small part of the cancer burden.

1. Only 1 of 200 occupational rubrics shows a cancer excess greater than 30%.
2. Occupations selected in advance for known or suspected respiratory cancer hazards showed only a 22% respiratory cancer excess.
3. The all-cancer excess for the 20 occupations (of 200) with the highest cancer PMRs is 20%.

4. The respiratory cancer excess for the 20 occupations (of 200) with the highest respiratory cancer PMRs is 36%.

Because the rubrics craftsmen, kindred workers, and operatives contain most of the occupational groups with carcinogenic exposures, the PMR results for total cancers and respiratory cancers in these groups can provide upper-limit estimates for the proportion of cancers due to occupational exposures. These are 5% for total cancers and 12% for respiratory cancers. This agrees well with data from the United Kingdom and with estimates published recently by the International Agency for Cancer Research (IARC) (Higginson 1980).

REFERENCES

Higginson, J. 1980. Proportion of cancers due to occupation. *Prev. Med.* **9**: 180.

Milham, S. 1976. *Occupational mortality in Washington state.* DHEW Publication No. (NIOSH) 76-175-A. Government Printing Office, Washington, D.C.

———. 1979. *Experience in using death certificate occupational information.* DHEW Publication No. (PHS) 79-1214, p. 419. Government Printing Office, Washington, D.C.

COMMENTS

DAVIS: With respect to recorded occupations, you said that you cross-validated the occupations pretty well. Are you fairly confident?

MILHAM: Yes, we interviewed about 1000 widows as to their husbands' occupations. Other validation is provided by the fact that, in a study of copper smelter workers, county death records alone were able to ascertain 24 of 25 lung cancers. The one case we missed died out of state.

DAVIS: What are the out- and in-migration patterns in your state?

MILHAM: It is basically in from California.

DAVIS: I noticed in your data that managers seemed to have the highest rate of cancer. Is that right?

MILHAM: Yes, for life-style reasons, obviously.

DAVIS: Well, perhaps. But a lot of people who end up being managers, even in the last 10 or 15 years of their lives, start out working in factories doing other sorts of jobs. It really becomes important, I think, to try to link the hypothesis that may come from your work to the work that Jack [Siemiatycki] and Shelia [Hoar] are suggesting with respect to exposure histories, before we can draw any conclusions about the relative role that occupational factors play.

MILHAM: Well, this study is a fishing expedition. What I wanted to do was identify factories that had worker exposure and occupational mortality problems. I picked out the aluminum mills, paper mills, and plywood mills.

DAVIS: I understand that, but I would like to suggest that, while you did that for those people who may have spent 15, 20, or 25 years in the factory and ended up dying with that listed as their occupation, the effect may be diluted by the fact that some small percentage of those people then go on and do other things, having had that exposure, which these data will never evidence.

MILHAM: No data set is perfect. I think that within the limitations of the death record, we have learned a lot. Nobody has done this sort of study before in the United States. People said it couldn't be done.

BINGHAM: Do you have chemical workers?

MILHAM: No, we don't have much of a chemical industry in the State. But we did show that men who were identified on the death record as chemists did show an increase of pancreatic cancer. I don't know where they worked or what they did.

However, I am convinced that if you did this study in a big industrialized state, you would really put your finger on a number of industries. My recommendation is that, if anybody is going to start this type of study today, he should do occupational and industrial coding, because the rubrics that were of most interest to me were those I added—the industrial codes.

ACHESON: Sam [Milham], do you think the Registrar General would do better not to try to do SMRs, but just do PMRs?

MILHAM: I think so.

ACHESON: A lot of his problems occur because his denominators are inappropriate.

MILHAM: I spent 2 hours with him last month and he agreed to do industrial classification and PMR analysis, which I think will really put the finger on problem industries.

DARBY: One of the question marks, in my mind, with the Hanford data is just how good they were at finding dead bodies. But if you look at the observed over expected for people more than 20 years after they started work, it is only 0.84. Now, do you think that your data would provide a means of verifying how good they were at finding dead bodies?

MILHAM: Well, I have done that for them. I give every death I get to them on an ongoing basis. Each month, when we code the death certificates, I make a copy of all Hanford deaths. I also do that for the Bremerton shipyard workers' deaths.

We did the overlap studies with the Hanford workers' deaths comparing ascertainment through death records with employer records. The death record does a very good job of ascertaining deaths in Hanford workers resident in the State.

EPSTEIN: In the major industrial groups that you studied, do you have any idea at all of the relationship between occupation at death and occupation of the major duration of employment?

MILHAM: You can get that from the California record, because they ask both, but I can't in my state. The Washington State death record asks only for usual occupation.

EPSTEIN: Well, as a corollary to that, on the basis of experience in other states, such as California, how legitimate is it to attempt to develop inferences from occupation at death vis-a-vis occupational exposure during lifetime?

MILHAM: I think you have to do it on an occupation-by-occupation basis. Once a physician, always a physician. But with the laboring trades, a worker may get promoted or, as he gets old and infirm, he will become a janitor or a watchman.

If that was the case with my data, I wouldn't have done the study initially. I am glad we asked the question that way. California gets it both ways, and they ask duration in employment. So, by looking at their data, they could answer your question.

GAFFEY: One of the worries about going national with this approach has been the quality of the occupational and industrial statements. From your work with validation, it sounds as if Washington looks pretty good. Now, you also worked with Utah and I think maybe with California.

MILHAM: And New York.

GAFFEY: Do you think you are exceptional or do you think the other states have data that are equally good?

MILHAM: Well, I didn't work a complete New York State data set but I got the feeling in the New York Hodgkin's disease study that the death record was pretty good. I did a large carpenters union study nationally, in which I got deaths from every state. When I got the death records back, I was amazed at how many of them said carpenter or some trade that was covered by the union. This was a national study and said that carpenters dying in every state were properly identified on death certificates. Actually, I could answer that question by going back to the carpenters' data. I think it is good enough.

MILHAM: Limiting occupational mortality analysis to men dying under age 60 is another area in which I think that the Registrar General and Guralnick erred. If you are interested in occupational cancer, you have a very long latent phase. Therefore, if you limit analysis to deaths before age 60, you lose most of your deaths. I would say you have to look at deaths at all ages.

RADFORD: Sam, do you want to say anything briefly about the paper-wood relationship that you have been interested in?

MILHAM: Well, NIOSH has a cohort study under way, but they are waiting for the death certificates. But I have seen a continuing excess of aplastic anemia, Hodgkin's disease, lymphatic and hematopoietic cancers, and cardiovascular disease in Washington State paper workers.

WAXWEILER: There is already in existence in the United States a data file that would help you out tremendously. The Social Security Administration has entire work histories on everybody by quarter. The only question is getting access to the data; that will take a change in the laws of the country. But access to such data would provide total detailed work histories and allow anyone to go in on a county basis, even for case-control studies such as Shelia [Hoar] and Jack [Siemiatycki] are talking about, to validate those histories and substantially cut down on the cost, too.

MILHAM: Tom Mancuso has written extensively and made use of that system, but I don't think we have done enough with it.

Cancer Incidence and Occupations in an Area of Low Air Pollution

HRAFN TULINIUS AND HELGI SIGVALDASON
Icelandic Cancer Registry
121 Reykjavik, Iceland

In the background paper for this meeting, it was stated that the intention was to review cancer incidence attributable to occupations, both from exposure of workers in the workplace, and from exposure of persons dwelling in the vicinity of industrial facilities. This presentation first will discuss the absence of heavy industry and meteorological conditions that result in low air pollution in Iceland. The incidence pattern of neoplastic diseases in males will then be compared with that in an area of high air pollution.

To look for the effect of exposure of workers in the workplace, there is no direct information available; however, stated occupations are registered in the Cancer Registry. This information has been used to estimate the expected number of cases occurring at each of 15 sites within each of 8 groups of occupations, assuming that the site distribution of neoplastic diseases is the same in each group as it is in all groups.

AIR POLLUTION IN ICELAND

Iceland is an island situated in the north Atlantic, reaching the Arctic Circle. Its closest neighbor is Greenland, 280 km away. The distance to Scotland is 700 km and to Norway nearly 1000 km.

The predominant feature of the weather is rain and wind. From 1931 to 1960, the average yearly number of days with wind force 9 Beaufort or more was 13.5 in Reykjavik, the capital, and 70.7 in the Westman Islands of the south shore.

The country is sparsely populated, with a total area of 103,000 km^2 (40,000 mi^2) and a population of 228,785 on December 1, 1980, giving a population density of 2.2/km^2 (5.7/mi^2).

About 80% of houses are heated with geothermal water or electricity (mainly thermal water); industries utilize electricity for power. Petrochemicals are used almost solely for transport.

Heavy industry is new in the country with an aluminium refinery, which started about 10 years ago, and a recently established ferrosilicate smelting plant. These conditions, therefore, favor an atmosphere of low pollution.

One measureable index of atmospheric pollution is the pH value of rain water. The monthly averages of pH of rainfall remained constant from 1955 to 1972 at between 5.5 and 5.6, but since then the average has fallen to about 5.0. It is the opinion of meteorologists that this is due to global changes rather than changes in the local production.

Very occasionally—less than once a year—air pollution becomes visible to the public. One such period occurred in July 1980. Due to stationary high pressure over the British Isles, air masses were moved to Iceland. In this period, the highest daily measurement of sulfate (SO_4) reached about 12 $\mu g/m^3$ air, but on an ordinary day this is around 1 or 2 $\mu g/m^3$. In Scandinavia, measurements of around 14 $\mu g/m^3$ are not unusual in an area of low air pollution; on a bad day in a heavily polluted area measurements can go above 150 $\mu g/m^3$ (Eliasen et al. 1973). In Birmingham in 1963, the extreme daily value was 273 $\mu g/m^3$ air in an industrial area, and 119 $\mu g/m^3$ in a residential area. Since 1963, a great change has taken place in Birmingham because in a smoke-zoned area a comparable extreme value for 1977 was 48 $\mu g/m^3$ air (78 $\mu g/m^3$ air in an area not completely smoke zoned) (J. A. H. Waterhouse, pers. comm.).

COMPARING WITH BIRMINGHAM

To compare the incidence pattern of malignant diseases in Iceland, an area of low atmospheric pollution, with another area of high atmospheric pollution. The Birmingham Cancer Registry in central England was chosen. The figures are from Waterhouse (1970).

Table 1 shows those organs where the incidence is higher in Iceland and where incidence is higher in Birmingham. If atmospheric pollution is contributing substantially to the incidence at certain sites, these sites should show up in the right hand column. The most substantial difference is found in the rates for lung, a difference of 56.1/100,000 per annum. That site alone does more than make up the difference in the total rates, Birmingham 254.5 and Iceland 212.9 or 41.6/100,000. Larynx behaves like the lungs. Next in magnitude is the Birmingham excess in skin tumors, but this could be largely explained by possible difference in the coding of skin tumors. There is a large difference in the rates for rectum and less in the rates for colon, but for all the other gastrointestinal sites, the rates for Iceland are higher. Birmingham has higher rates for tongue, and the oral and the pharyngeal regions except for nasopharynx and lip. The last should be considered together with the previously mentioned observation that skin, other than melanoma, is higher in Birmingham. Urinary bladder and penis are higher in Birmingham; the other urinary organs are higher in Iceland. Finally, lymphomas are higher in Birmingham, but Hodgkin's disease, multiple myeloma and leukemias are higher in Iceland.

Table 1
Cancer Incidence in Iceland, 1955-79, and Birmingham, 1963-66, Inclusive, Males

		I[a] >	B[b]	I <	B
140	Lip	5.5	1.6		
141	Tongue			0.4	1.3
142	Salivary glands			0.5	1.2
143-4	Oral cavity			0.6	1.4
145+7+8	Pharynx, excluding nasopharynx			0.6	1.9
146	Nasopharynx	1.4	0.5		
150	Esophagus	5.9	4.7		
151	Stomach	48.5	25.2		
152	Duodenum, small intestine	1.4	0.7		
153	Colon			12.0	15.3
154	Rectum			6.4	15.8
155	Liver	4.0	2.4		
157	Pancreas	7.9	7.2		
160	Nasal cavity and paranasal sinuses	1.1	0.7		
161	Larynx			2.4	3.8
162	Lung			17.2	73.3
177	Prostate	26.2	18.4		
178	Testis	2.4	2.1		
179	Penis and other urinary organs			0.6	1.0
180	Kidney	11.1	4.0		
181	Bladder and urethra			9.9	11.5
190	Malignant melanoma of skin	1.7	1.1		
191	Skin, melanomas excluded			5.1	27.9
192	Eye	1.2	0.5		
193	Nervous system	8.6		5.9	
194	Thyroid gland	4.3	0.6		
195	Other endocrine glands	0.7	0.5		
196	Bone	1.7	0.9		
197	Connective tissue and muscle	2.4	1.4		
200	Lymphosarcoma and reticulosarcoma			3.4	3.5
201	Hodgkin's disease	3.1	2.7		
202	Other lymphomas			0.1	0.8
203	Multiple myeloma and plasmocytoma	2.3	1.3		
204	Leukemia	7.7	5.3		
140-204	All sites			212.9	254.5

(standardized to world population.)
[a]Iceland.
[b]Birmingham.

Table 2
Cancer Incidence in Iceland, 1955-79, Birmingham, 1963-66, and Norway, 1964-66, Males

	Iceland	Birmingham[a]		Norway[a]	
		region	center	rural	urban
162 Lung	17.2	73.3	96.9	10.5	25.2
161 Larynx	2.4	3.8	4.7	1.3	3.1
191 Skin, excluding melanoma	5.1	27.9	32.6		
154 Rectum	6.4	15.8	17.1	6.0	8.0

Standardized to world population per 100,000 per annum.
[a]Birmingham center is subset of Birmingham region, whereas the population of Norway is divided into rural and urban.

Table 2 shows incidence rates for the most relevant sites for the Birmingham County borough, kindly supplied by Dr. Waterhouse of the Birmingham Cancer Registry (J. A. H. Waterhouse, pers. comm.), and for rural and urban Norway for a comparable period (Pedersen 1970).

This comparison has shown that the most strikingly higher rates in Birmingham are for cancer of the lung, but in general those sites with higher rates in Birmingham are those to which atmospheric air has access, i.e., lung, larynx, skin, penis, mouth, tongue, sinuses, and pharynx. Nonexposed organs with higher rates in Birmingham are rectum, colon, urinary bladder, and lymphoma.

CLASSIFICATION OF OCCUPATIONS IN THE CANCER REGISTRY

The classification has been used in the Registry since it started in 1954, but is not used by the Bureau of Statistics; 26 rubrics have been used. The information classified comes from the doctors, hospitals, or laboratories that have sent the information to be registered. Some verification has been done, but not in a systematic way. For the purpose of this presentation, we have arranged the rubrics into 10 groups, which will be used here. Groups 1, 2, and 3 contain educated and managerial professions; group 5, farmers; and group 6 seamen and people in aviation. Groups 4 and 8 are mixtures of laboring professions and industry. Group 7 is for housewives and does not appear in the following tables, which are prepared for males only. Finally, Table 3 shows two more columns, i.e., one for occupation otherwise specified, and another for occupation not specified.

Table 3
Malignant Neoplasms in Iceland in Males 1955-1979 Inclusive

	All groups		1.			2.			3.			4.			5.			6.			8.			Other			NS			Total
Site (code)	N	percent	rank	N	percent	rank	N	percent	rank	N	percent	rank	N	percent	rank	N	percent	rank	N	percent	rank	N	percent	rank	N	percent	rank	N	percent	(%)
All sites	5488	100		125	2.3		80	1.5		596	10.9		900	16.4		839	15.3		452	8.2		989	18.0		168	3.1		1339	24.4	100.1
1. Stomach (151)	1251	22.8	**3.**	12	1.0	**1.**	17	1.4	**1.**	124	9.9	**1.**	215	17.2	**1.**	261	20.9	**1.**	119	9.5	**1.**	274	21.9	**1.**	45	3.6	**2.**	183	14.6	100.0
2. Prostate (177)	731	13.3	**2.**	14	1.9	**2.**	16	2.2	**2.**	72	9.8	**3.**	90	12.3	**2.**	136	18.6	**3.**	48	6.6	**2.**	106	14.5	**2.**	22	3.0	**1.**	227	31.1	100.0
3. Bronchus (162)	423	7.7	**4.**	10	2.4	**7.**	3	0.7	**3.**	58	13.7	**2.**	109	25.8	**7.**	30	7.1	**2.**	51	12.1	**3.**	77	18.2	**3.**	13	3.1	**6-7.**	72	17.0	100.0
4. Colon (153)	317	5.8	**1.**	17	5.4	**5-6.**	4	1.3	**4.**	54	17.0	**5.**	48	15.1	**4.**	36	11.4	**4.**	28	8.8	**4.**	47	14.8	**4.**	9	2.8	**5.**	74	23.3	99.9
5. Kidney (186)	278	5.1	**5-6.**	8	2.9	**8-12.**	2	0.7	**5.**	41	14.7	**4.**	52	18.7	**3.**	41	14.7	**6.**	19	6.8	**7.**	38	13.7	**10-12.**	5	1.8	**6-7.**	72	25.9	99.9
6. Urinary bladder (181)	252	4.6	**10.**	5	2.0		1	0.4	**6.**	33	13.1	**7.**	40	15.9	**6.**	33	13.1	**10-12.**	11	4.4	**5.**	46	18.3	**5.**	8	3.2	**4.**	75	29.8	100.2
7. Brain (193)	210	3.8	**5-6.**	8	3.8	**3-4.**	5	2.4	**10.**	18	8.6	**9.**	30	14.3	**8-9.**	29	13.8	**8-9.**	12	5.7	**8.**	37	17.6	**8-9.**	6	2.9	**8.**	65	31.0	100.1
8. Pancreas (157)	209	3.8	**11.**	4	1.9	**3-4.**	5	2.4	**8.**	22	10.5	**6.**	44	21.1	**8-9.**	29	13.9	**5.**	21	10.0	**6.**	40	19.1	**6-7.**	7	3.3	**11.**	37	17.7	99.9
9. Leukemia (204)	200	3.6	**8-9.**	6	3.0	**8-12.**	2	1.0	**9.**	21	10.5	**11.**	22	11.0	**12.**	24	12.0	**8-9.**	12	6.0	**11.**	23	11.5	**6-7.**	7	3.5	**3.**	83	41.5	100.0
10. Rectum (154)	174	3.2	**7.**	7	4.0	**8-12.**	4	2.3	**7.**	25	14.4	**8.**	37	21.3		20	11.5		7	4.0	**10.**	32	18.4	**8-9.**	6	3.4	**12.**	36	20.7	100.0
11. Esophagus (150)	146	2.7	**8-9.**	6	4.1		2	1.4	**11.**	14	9.6	**10.**	29	19.9	**10-11.**	25	17.1	**7.**	14	9.6	**9.**	35	24.0		3	2.1		18	12.3	100.1
12. Lip (140)	146	2.7		0			2	1.4		4	2.7		11	7.5	**5.**	34	23.2		9	6.2	**10.**	33	22.6	**10-12.**	4	2.7	**10.**	49	33.6	99.9
13. Skin, excluding melanoma (191)	132	2.4		2	1.5		1	0.8		9	6.8		13	9.8	**10-11.**	25	18.9	**10-12.**	11	8.3		16	12.1		1	0.8	**9.**	54	40.9	99.9
14. Thyroid (194)	104	1.9		1	1.0		1	1.0		12	11.5	**12.**	18	17.3		12	11.5	**10-12.**	11	10.6		14	13.5		3	2.9		32	30.8	100.1
15. Liver and biliary tract (155)	101	1.8	**12.**	3	3.0		0		**12.**	13	12.9		13	12.9		14	13.9		8	7.9		14	13.9	**10-12.**	4	4.0		32	31.7	100.2
16. Lymphoma, excluding Hodgkin's (200 & 202)	90	1.6		2	2.2	**8-12.**	2	2.2		8	8.9		12	13.3		11	12.2		6	6.7	**12.**	19	21.1		2	2.2		28	31.1	99.9
17. Hodgkin's (201)	78	1.4		2	2.6		1	1.3		10	12.8		14	17.9		8	10.3		7	9.0		16	20.5		3	3.8		17	21.8	100.0
18. Larynx (161)	59	1.1		2	3.4		1	1.7		12	20.3		10	16.9		2	3.4		10	16.9		10	16.9		3	5.1		9	15.3	99.9

METHODS

Table 3 contains all the information on 18 sites for these occupational groups, and the rank order of each cancer site for each profession. All ages of cancer incidence have been used in Table 3, whereas in Tables 4-12, ages 0-19 inclusive have been removed.

We do not know the distribution of persons according to occupational groups in the general population as it is registered for the cancer cases. Therefore, we cannot compute incidence rates for each occupational group to see if there is a significant deviation in incidence for a specific group for cancer in general or for specific sites. On the other hand, it is possible to see whether there are deviations in the relative frequency for sites within an occupational group or for occupational groups within a site. We have used the first approach in Tables 4-12.

Expected numbers of cases for the most frequent sites for each occupational group have been computed. As the age distribution of persons differs from one group to another and cancer incidence varies differently with age for different sites, we have computed expected numbers in the following way: Cases of age less than 20 years have been excluded.

Let N_{ijk} be the observed number of cases for age group i (5-year groups), occupational group j, and site k. Let $N_{ij\cdot}$ be the sum of observed cases for age group i and occupational group j and other sums denoted in the same manner. The expected number of cases X_{jk} is then computed as

$$X_{jk} = \sum_i N_{i\cdot k} \times N_{ij\cdot}/N_{i\cdot\cdot} \qquad (1)$$

Deviations of observed numbers from expected ones are tested using chi square with Yates correction. In the tables, those observations showing significant deviation at 1% level are marked by footnote[a] and significance at 5% level by footnote[b].

COMPARING OCCUPATIONAL GROUPS

Table 4 shows that for the group of academic professions, there is a significant excess of observed cancer of the colon–17 observed when 7.9 were expected. Cancer of the stomach is significantly below expectation.

Table 5 shows occupational group 2, which is too small, only 79 men, to show any significant deviation from expected. Table 6 shows occupational group 3. In this group of mainly white-collar workers, cancer of the colon is in excess of expected–53 cases when 33.6 were expected. In this group, the small number (4) of cancer of the lip is significant compared with 16.1 expected.

Table 7 shows another mixed group of professions, but probably of somewhat lower social class. Here the cancer of the lung is in excess of what was expected, but lip is below the expected number.

Table 4
Occupational Group 1, Excluding Ages 0-19

		N	Expected	Percent	All groups rank	All groups percent
1.	Colon (153)	17[a]	7.9	13.6	4.	5.9
2.	Prostate (171)	14	16.8	11.2	2.	13.7
3.	Stomach (151)	12[a]	29.1	9.6	1.	23.4
4.	Bronchus (162)	10	10.0	8.0	3.	7.9
5-6.	Kidney (180)	8	6.4	6.4	5.	5.1
5-6.	Brain (193)	8	4.5	6.4	8.	3.4
7.	Rectum (154)	7	4.1	5.6	9.	3.2
8-9.	Leukemia (204)	6	3.5	4.8	12.	2.7
8-9.	Esophagus (150)	6	3.2	4.8	10-11.	2.7
10.	Urinary bladder (181)	5	6.0	4.0	6.	4.7
11.	Pancreas (157)	4	5.0	3.2	7.	3.9
12.	Liver and biliary tract (155)	3	2.4	2.4	15.	1.6
	Lip (140)	0	3.5		10-11.	2.7
Other sites		21		16.8		
Site not known (199)		4		3.2		
Group 1 total		125		100.0		

Professors, scientists, engineers, architects, medical doctors, veterinarians, judges, barristers, clergy.
[a]Significant at 1% level.

Table 5
Occupational Group 2, Excluding Ages 0-19

					All groups	
		N	Expected	Percent	rank	percent
1.	Stomach (151)	17	17.4	21.5	1.	23.4
2.	Prostate (177)	16	9.7	20.3	2.	13.7
3-4.	Brain (193)	5	2.7	6.3	8.	3.4
3-4.	Pancreas (157)	5	2.9	6.3	7.	3.9
5-6.	Colon (153)	4	4.4	5.0	4.	5.9
5-6.	Rectum (154)	4	2.6	5.0	9.	3.2
7.	Bronchus (162)	3	6.2	3.8	3.	7.9
8-12.	Kidney (180)	2	3.9	2.5	5.	5.1
8-12.	Leukemia (204)	2	2.6	2.5	12.	2.7
8-12.	Esophagus (150)	2	1.9	2.5	10-11.	2.7
8-12.	Lip (140)	2	2.0	2.5	10-11.	2.7
8-12.	Lymphoma, excluding Hodgkin's (200 + 202)	2	1.4	2.5	16.	1.6
Other sites		15		20.0		
Site not known (199)		0				
Group 2 total		79		100.0		

Agronimists, technicians, teachers, nurses, nuns, technologists.

Table 6
Occupational Group 3, Excluding Ages 0-19

					All groups	
		N	Expected	Percent	rank	percent
1.	Stomach (151)	124	139.6	21.1	1.	23.4
2.	Prostate (177)	72	71.1	12.2	2.	13.7
3.	Bronchus (162)	58	52.0	9.9	3.	7.9
4.	Colon (153)	53[a]	33.6	9.0	4.	5.9
5.	Kidney (180)	41	30.9	7.0	5.	5.1
6.	Urinary bladder (181)	33	28.7	5.6	6.	4.7
7.	Rectum (154)	25	19.1	4.3	9.	3.2
8.	Pancreas (157)	22	22.5	3.7	7.	3.9
9.	Leukemia (204)	19	16.2	3.2	12.	2.7
10.	Brain (193)	18	22.0	3.1	8.	3.4
11.	Esophagus (150)	14	14.7	2.4	10-11.	2.7
12.	Liver and biliary tract (155)	13	10.8	2.2	15.	1.6
20-21.	Lip (140)	4[a]	16.1	0.7	10-11.	2.7
Other sites		87		14.8		
Site not known		5		0.9		
Group 3 total		588		100.1		

Directors, managers, owners of small firms, shipowners, merchants, auditors, representatives, cashiers, librarians. Salesmen, clerical workers, telephonists, telegraphists, students.

[a]Significant at 1% level.

Table 7
Occupational Group 4, Excluding Ages 0-19

					All groups	
		N	Expected	Percent	rank	percent
1.	Stomach (151)	215	211.5	23.9	1.	23.4
2.	Bronchus (162)	109[a]	80.5	12.1	3.	7.9
3.	Prostate (177)	90	102.5	10.0	2.	13.7
4.	Kidney (180)	52	48.4	5.8	5.	5.1
5.	Colon (153)	48	51.2	5.3	4.	5.9
6.	Pancreas (157)	44	33.8	4.9	7.	3.9
7.	Urinary bladder (181)	40	43.6	4.4	6.	4.7
8.	Rectum (154)	37	28.8	4.1	9.	3.4
9.	Brain (193)	30	36.7	3.3	8.	3.8
10.	Esophagus (150)	29	21.8	3.2	10-11.	2.7
11.	Leukemia (204)	21	25.2	2.3	12.	2.7
13-14.	Liver and biliary tract (155)	13	15.8	1.4	15.	1.6
13-14.	Skin, excluding melanoma (191)	13	21.0	1.4	13.	2.4
15-16.	Lip (140)	11[a]	24.4	1.2	10-11.	2.7
Other sites		135		15.0		
Site not known		12		1.3		
Group 4 total		899		99.6		

Senior skilled laborers, skilled foremen, mechanics, printers, bookbinders, seamstresses, surveyors, bankers, drivers, policemen, inspectors, gardeners, fishmongers.

[a]Significant at 1% level.

Table 8 shows occupational group 5, which is probably the "purest" group, composed solely of farmers. Here the significant deviations from expected are an excess of cancer of the stomach (261 against 197.4 expected) and a lack of cancer of the lung (30 cases when 57.9 were expected) and cancer of the colon (36 cases and 52.6 expected).

Table 9 shows the group of seamen and pilots. Here the excess is in cancer of the lung (51 against 35.5 expected), but the significantly low observed is for urinary bladder–11 when 21 were expected. Recent information from Iceland (Olafsson 1981) indicates, that seamen as a group, smoke cigarettes heavily and in greater numbers than other groups. If that explains their lung cancer experience, the observation on urinary bladder is interesting.

Table 10 shows occupational group 8, which again is somewhat mixed, but consists mainly of laboring professions. Here stomach cancer is higher than expected, and cancer of the prostate is lower.

Table 11 shows occupations otherwise specified, a small group with no significant changes, and Table 12 the relatively large group where the information on occupation was missing. In that group two urinary sites, prostate and bladder, and two exposed sites, skin and lip, show numbers significantly in excess of expected, and two upper gastrointestinal sites, stomach and esophagus, show a deficit. It is hard to postulate any explanation of this, and it indicates that further work is needed to clarify the occupational history of these men.

CONCLUSIONS

Regarding the distribution of cancer within the broad occupational groups, significant differences are found in a greater number than would be explained by random if age-standardized expected incidence rates are compared with observed. By selecting the occupation one makes a contribution to the choice of an organ in which to get a malignant disease, if one gets one. This method opens some interesting questions, but cannot be used to follow up these clues, other methods are needed for example, a record linkage approach to forming cohorts for prospective studies.

As far as the effect of atmospheric air pollution on incidence rates of malignant diseases, as observed by comparing Birmingham in England and Iceland, is concerned, the following points can be made. Birmingham was chosen as a population dwelling in the vicinity of industrial carcinogens. Perhaps the most interesting observation is that most of the sites that are in excess in Birmingham as compared to Iceland are, in fact, sites to which the atmospheric air has access.

But the problem remains if the 5.6-fold difference in the rates of lung carcinoma can be explained by differences in smoking habits. If they are going to explain it all, then there is nothing left for the industry.

Table 8
Occupational Group 5, Excluding Ages 0-19

		N	Expected	Percent	All groups rank	All groups percent
1.	Stomach (151)	261[a]	197.4	31.1	1.	23.4
2.	Prostate (177)	136	136.3	16.2	2.	13.7
3.	Kidney (180)	41	39.9	4.9	5.	5.1
4.	Colon (153)	36[b]	52.6	4.3	4.	5.9
5.	Lip (140)	34	23.4	4.1	10-11.	2.7
6.	Urinary bladder (181)	33	38.5	3.9	6.	4.7
7.	Bronchus (162)	30[a]	57.9	3.6	3.	7.9
8-9.	Brain (193)	29	22.0	3.5	8.	3.4
8-9.	Pancreas (157)	29	34.6	3.5	7.	3.9
10-11.	Esophagus (150)	25	26.0	3.0	10-11.	2.7
10-11.	Skin, excluding melanoma (191)	25	22.0	3.0	13.	2.4
12.	Leukemia (204)	24	25.7	2.9	12.	2.7
Other sites		120		14.3		
Site not known		16		1.9		
Group 5 total		839		100.2		

Farmers.
[a]Significant at 1% level.
[b]Significant at 5% level.

Table 9
Occupational Group 6, Excluding Ages 0-19

		N	Expected	Percent	All groups	
					rank	percent
1.	Stomach (151)	119	102.8	26.7	1.	23.4
2.	Bronchus (162)	51[a]	35.5	11.4	3.	7.9
3.	Prostate (177)	48	58.6	10.8	2.	13.7
4.	Colon (153)	28	26.0	6.3	4.	5.9
5.	Pancreas (157)	21	16.9	4.7	7.	3.9
6.	Kidney (180)	19	22.7	4.3	5.	5.1
7.	Esophagus (150)	14	12.3	3.1	10-11.	2.7
8.	Brain (193)	12	16.3	2.7	8.	3.4
9-10.	Urinary bladder (181)	11[b]	21.0	2.5	6.	4.7
9-10.	Leukemia (204)	11	12.5	2.5	12.	2.7
11-12.	Skin, excluding melanoma (191)	10	11.3	2.2	13.	2.4
11-12.	Thyroid (194)	10	8.4	2.2	14.	1.9
16-17.	Rectum (154)	7	14.6	1.6	9.	3.2
Other sites		78		17.5		
Site not known		7		1.6		
Group 6 total		446		100.1		

Captains, pilots, mates, machinists, stewards, airplane mechanics, fishermen, deckhands, stokers.
[a]Significant at 1% level.
[b]Significant at 5% level.

Table 10
Occupational Group 8, Excluding Ages 0-19

	N	Expected	Percent	All groups rank	All groups percent
1. Stomach (151)	274[a]	236.0	27.8	1.	23.4
2. Prostate (177)	106[a]	133.2	10.8	2.	13.7
3. Bronchus (162)	77	81.3	7.8	3.	7.9
4. Colon (153)	47	58.4	4.8	4.	5.9
5. Urinary bladder (181)	46	46.8	4.7	6.	4.7
6. Pancreas (157)	40	39.2	4.1	7.	3.9
7. Kidney (180)	38	49.9	3.9	5.	5.1
8. Brain (193)	36	31.4	3.7	8.	3.4
9. Esophagus (150)	35	26.4	3.6	10-11.	2.7
10. Rectum (154)	32	32.3	3.2	9.	3.2
11. Leukemia (204)	23	26.0	2.3	12.	2.7
12. Lymphoma, excluding Hodgkin's (200 + 202)	19	13.1	1.9	16.	1.5
Other sites	197		20.0		
Site not known	15		1.5		
Group 8 total	985		100.1		

Laborers, watchmen, caretakers, mailmen, bill collectors. Farm hands, skilled laborers.
[a]Significant at 1% level.

Table 11
Other Specified Occupational Groups, Excluding Ages 0-19

					All groups	
		N	Expected	Percent	rank	percent
1.	Stomach (151)	45	37.0	27.4	1.	23.4
2.	Prostate (177)	22	20.3	13.4	2.	13.7
3.	Bronchus (162)	13	12.8	7.9	3.	7.9
4.	Colon (153)	9	9.1	5.5	4.	5.9
5.	Urinary bladder (181)	8	7.4	4.9	6.	4.7
6.	Pancreas (157)	7	6.0	4.3	7.	3.9
7-8.	Rectum (154)	6	5.2	3.7	9.	3.2
7-8.	Leukemia (204)	6	4.9	3.7	12.	2.7
9.	Kidney (180)	5	8.3	3.0	5.	5.1
10-12.	Brain (193)	4	8.6	2.4	8.	3.4
10-12.	Lip (140)	4	4.2	2.4	10-11.	2.7
10-12.	Liver and biliary tract (155)	4	3.0	2.4	15.	1.6
Other sites		28		17.1		
Site not known		3		1.8		
Total other specified occupational groups		164		99.9		

Table 12
Occupational Group Not Specified, Excluding Ages 0-19

					All groups	
		N	Expected	Percent	rank	percent
1.	Prostate (177)	227[a]	182.6	18.8	2.	13.7
2.	Stomach (151)	183[a]	279.0	15.1	1.	23.6
3-4.	Urinary bladder (181)	74[a]	55.6	6.1	6.	4.7
3-4.	Colon (153)	74	73.2	6.1	4.	5.9
5.	Bronchus (162)	72	86.7	6.0	3.	7.9
6.	Kidney (180)	64	59.7	5.3	5.	5.1
7.	Skin, excluding melanoma (191)	53[a]	30.7	4.4	13.	2.4
8.	Lip (140)	49[a]	33.1	4.1	10-11.	2.7
9.	Brain (193)	38	37.0	3.1	8.	3.4
10.	Pancreas (157)	37	48.0	3.1	7.	3.9
11.	Rectum (154)	36	39.6	3.0	9.	3.2
12.	Leukemia (204)	33	33.3	2.7	12.	2.7
14.	Esophagus (150)	18[a]	35.4	1.5	10-11.	2.7
Other site		224		18.5		
Site not known		26		2.2		
Total occupational group not specified		1208		100.0		

[a]Significant at 1% level.

Table 13
Number of Cigarettes Sold Per Adult Per Annum

	1935	1950	1960	1973
United Kingdom	1590	2180	2680	3230
Iceland	480	1490	1840	2030
I/U.K. (%)	30	68	69	63

Data from WHO Expert Committee on Smoking Control (1979).

In Table 13 is shown the number of cigarettes sold per annum in Iceland and in the United Kingdom. In 1935, that is, 20 years before our observation begins, the difference was very substantial. The rates of sale in Iceland were only 30% of those in the United Kingdom. In 1950, this rose to 68%; it was 69% in 1965, and 63% in 1973.

Are differences in smoking rates a sufficient explanation of differences in incidence rates of lung cancer? If they are, then there is no deleterious effect of fairly strong differences in atmospheric air pollution as caused by industrial processes. If, however, differences in smoking rates are not enough to explain all of the difference then the explanation is most likely to be in poisoning coming somehow from industry.

These figures do not quantify occupational cancer, they create new questions. We need to corroborate information on smokers and nonsmokers (such as Mormon and Adventists cohorts in the western United States) and study them again and again, as Doll (1978) did, to try to reconcile these two observations. In Iceland, we can produce rates by smoking standards, and perhaps that will be of some help.

Urban vs rural in Birmingham vs Iceland certainly covers more things than just the difference in air pollution. The effects of population density and many other effects are hidden in this urbanization, but certainly air pollution is one measurable part of it.

REFERENCES

Doll, R. 1978. Atmospheric pollution and lung cancer. *Environ. Health Perspect.* 22:23.

Eliasen, O., O. Jensen, J. Nordö and J. Saltbones. 1973. Transport Computations Covering a Stagnant Weather Situation Primo October 1972. In *Long range transport of air pollutants. A cooperative OECD program.* Norwegian Institute for Air Research, Kjeller, Norway.

Olafsson, O. 1981. Nokkrar niôurstöôur ûr hôprannsôkn Hjartaverndar, Skŷrsla C XXI. In *Raôstefna* um rânnsôknir i laeknadeild Hâskôla Îslands, p. 35, March 7.

Pedersen, E. 1970. Cancer incidence in Norway 1964 to 1966. In *UICI:*

Cancer incidence in five continents, volume II (ed. R. Doll, C.C. Muir, and J.A.H. Waterhouse). UICC, Geneva.

Waterhouse, J.A.H. 1970. Cancer incidence in U.K. England, Birmingham Region 1963 to 1966. In *UICC: Cancer incidence in five continents,* volume II. (ed. R. Doll, C.C. Muir, and J.A.H. Waterhouse.) UICC, Geneva.

WHO Expert Committee on Smoking Control. 1979. *Controlling the smoking epidemic.* World Health Organization Technical Report Series 636, Geneva.

COMMENTS

J. PETO: It seems that you would expect a difference of about that magnitude given the difference in cigarette smoking. You have 30% in 1935, and presumably it was 20% in 1925. I assume that the graph went on down. As the comparison is dominated by lung cancer deaths taking place at the age of 60 or over, these are people who would have started to smoke quite a long time ago. There is a reasonable quantitative relationship between the difference you are seeing and the difference in cigarette smoking. Recent cigarette smoking, which is mainly the effect of recruitment among young people, is not going to affect itself in total lung cancer rates. You haven't got lung cancer rates among young people, have you? I suppose the numbers are too small, but if you were to observe the age group 35-40 in recent years, you will see a very much smaller difference than you saw in the overall standardization.

R. PETO: I actually did this for Iceland. In fact, I looked at the death rates among young people in the 1970s in Iceland from lung cancer and tried to relate it to cigarette smoking habits earlier on. It was exactly on the line suggested by many other countries. In fact, there is a relationship between cigarette smoking in early adult life and lung cancer mortality in early middle age. Iceland happens to lie right on that graph, although I, in fact, left it off the graph, because I wanted to have cases in only those countries that have at least 25 cases of lung cancer. But, for what it is worth, the Icelandic data lay right on that graph, when you plot smoking habits when people are young against lung cancer among that generation as they enter middle age.

So it is possible that, as Julian [Peto] says, differences in smoking habits right back in 1915 and 1920 could be determining the differences in lung cancer rates over the period 1955 to 1975 or so that you are studying.

TULINIUS: If that is the consensus, then this comparison between Birmingham and Iceland would indicate that it has very little effect on your likelihood of developing neoplastic disease, whether you have got clean air or not.

Hepatic Angiosarcoma Registries: Implications for Rare-tumor Studies

HENRY FALK AND PETER J. BAXTER*
Chronic Diseases Division
Centers for Disease Control
Atlanta, Georgia 30333

In this paper we describe the nationwide case-finding efforts for hepatic angiosarcoma (HAS) in the United States for the years 1964-1974 (conducted by the Centers for Disease Control [CDC]) and in the United Kingdom for the years 1963-1977 (conducted by the Employment Medical Advisory Service [EMAS]). A summary of our results is included, along with a discussion of the role of rare-tumor registries, the methodologic difficulties involved, and possible future approaches.

BACKGROUND

The stimulus for starting these studies was the discovery by Creech and Johnson in early 1974 that polyvinyl chloride (PVC) polymerization workers exposed to vinyl chloride monomer (VCM) appeared to have a markedly increased relative risk for the development of the rare HAS (Creech and Johnson 1974). The HAS registries were intended to complement the retrospective occupational cohort studies that were initiated at about the same time and to identify any other modes of exposure to VCM leading to HAS (e.g., PVC fabrication, where exposures had been much lower than in PVC polymerization plants). Furthermore, because HAS at that time was considered to have three apparent causative agents with widely differing chemical and physical properties (VCM, Thorotrast, and inorganic arsenic) (Roth 1957; Horta et al. 1974), it was thought that additional causative agents might be related to the development of HAS. Additional reasons for establishing the registries were to obtain precise incidence data, to study the pathogenesis of HAS in greater detail, and to compare the VCM-induced cases with those of unknown etiology. Underlying our thinking for studying this marker tumor was the concern that other illnesses

*On leave of absence from: Health and Safety Executive, Employment Advisory Service, London NW1 5DT, England

(such as other tumor types and nonmalignant hepatic disease) were probably much more common than HAS in populations exposed to these causative agents.

METHODS

Detailed reviews of both the British and American studies have been published (Baxter et al. 1980a; Falk et al. 1981c). The methods are summarized here to compare the main features of the studies.

In the United States, information relating to cases of HAS occurring from 1964 through 1974 was solicited in a variety of ways, including: (1) announcements in medical journals; (2) a single mailing to all pathologists in the country; (3) additional mailings to tumor registries, tumor referral centers, and state epidemiologists; (4) a review of cases on file at the Armed Forces Institute of Pathology (AFIP); and (5) a review of death certificates in code 197.8 (liver tumors, unspecified primary or secondary), International Classification of Diseases (ICD), eighth revision, for 1966-1973. For each identified case, appropriate pathologic specimens were requested for review and were obtained in about 95% of the cases. After confirmation of the diagnosis, and with permission of the local physician, the next of kin was identified and contacted. Consent was obtained to review medical records, and a questionnaire was administered by telephone to obtain detailed occupational, residential, and chemical exposure histories. A total of 168 confirmed deaths from HAS was identified during this 11-year period (mean = 15.3/yr).

The approach in Britain was slightly different. The EMAS of the Health and Safety Executive, in cooperation with the Office for Population Censuses and Surveys (England and Wales) and the General Register Office (Scotland), reviewed death certificates for all hepatic neoplasm-related codes (including eighth revision ICD Nos. 155.0, 155.1, 197.7, 197.8, 211.5, 227 and 230.5) for the 15-year period, 1963-1977. It should be noted that in the United States it would have been prohibitively expensive and impractical to obtain death certificates for all liver neoplasm codes from all 50 states. Other sources of identification of cases (such as hospital pathologists, tumor registries, factory medical departments, and published reports) were also used in the United Kingdom. The U.K. pathology review process also included control cases of liver neoplasms certified as other than angiosarcoma. After pathologic confirmation of the diagnosis, full medical records were sought. Interviews of next of kin for exposure information were conducted in person by an employment medical or nursing advisor using a standardized questionnaire. In all, 35 confirmed cases were identified (mean = 2.3/yr).

RESULTS

A major feature of both the American and British studies was the difficulty in finding cases. There is no ICD code for HAS, and as a result, even when

Table 1
Classification by Pathology Review Panels of Cases Identified Through Death Certificate Search with Recorded Diagnosis of HAS (1964-1974 in U.S.; 1963-1977 in U.K.)

	United States	United Kingdom
Confirmed HAS	31 (42%)	18 (26%)
Confirmed not HAS	37 (50%)	27 (40%)
No pathology available	6 (8%)	15 (22%)
Doubtful or unclassifiable	–	8 (12%)
Total	74	68

cases were identified as HAS or one of its commonly used synonyms (e.g., malignant hemangioendothelioma or Kupffer cell sarcoma), they were distributed over a number of ICD codes, the most common being 197.8 (Baxter et al. 1980a). (In the U.S., only code 197.8 was reviewed in the death certificate search.)

Because of the rarity of the tumor, and because many cases were diagnosed only at autopsy, it had been anticipated that the death certificate review would miss a large number of cases. About 50% of the cases in Britain and about 80% of the cases in the United States were identified by sources other than the death certificate search. What was not so readily anticipated was that even when a death certificate recorded HAS, the diagnosis agreed upon by the pathology review panel was not HAS in the majority of cases where specimens were available for review (Table 1). The pathologic review in the British study had an obvious effect on conclusions regarding time trends of this rare disease (Baxter et al. 1980a).

In the United States, the best source of case material was the single mailing to all pathologists; the second best was the large case series already in the files of the AFIP. The utility of collections such as the latter in epidemiologic studies should always be kept in mind, as for example in the large case-control study of benign hepatic adenoma and oral contraceptive use (Rooks et al. 1979).

On the basis of the U.S. death certificate review, we were also able to note a number of differences between HAS and other sarcomas of the liver. HAS has a striking preponderance in males (4:1 in the U.K. and 3:1 in the U.S.) that persists even when cases of known etiology are excluded (Table 2); this is not seen in the other hepatic sarcomas (leiomyosarcoma, fibrosarcoma, undifferentiated sarcoma, and miscellaneous sarcomas). Further, HAS appears to occur at an earlier age than do other sarcomas of the liver (Falk et al. 1981c).

In the United Kingdom, the incidence of HAS may well be increasing, although the numbers are very small. In the United States, time trends for HAS occurrence were not striking, but were particularly revealing when looked at in terms of causative agents. Four main causative agents were identified and

Table 2
Sex Ratios for Confirmed HAS Cases by Etiologic Categories (1964-1974 in U.S.; 1963-1977 in U.K.)

	Male	Female	Ratio
United States			
VCM	12	0	12:0
Thorotrast	15	5	3:1
Arsenic	4	2	2:1
Androgenic-anabolic steroids	3	1	3:1
Idiopathic	93	33	2.8:1
Total	127	41	3.1:1
United Kingdom			
VCM	2	0	2:0
Thorotrast	7	1	7:1
Idiopathic	19	6	3.2:1
Total	28	7	4:1
Combined			
VCM	14	0	14:0
Thorotrast	22	6	3.7:1
Arsenic	4	2	2:1
Androgenic-anabolic steroids	3	1	3:1
Idiopathic	112	39	2.9:1
Total	155	48	3.2:1

they have been discussed in detail for both the British and American studies (Berk et al. 1976; Baxter et al. 1977, 1980a, b; Falk et al. 1979a, b, 1981a, b, c). VCM, Thorotrast, and arsenic had been reported previously; androgenic-anabolic steroids were implicated as a fourth cause of HAS (Table 2). In the United States, the distribution of cases occurring during the 11-year period 1964-1974 reflects the patterns of use of these causative agents. Arsenic-associated cases occurred primarily in the early years of the study, since the use of Fowler's solution (potassium arsenite) for therapeutic purposes was discontinued in the 1940s and early 1950s. VCM- and androgenic-anabolic steroid-associated cases occurred primarily in the second half of the study period, due to the relatively recent introduction and use of these substances.

Most surprising was the recent increase in the numbers of Thorotrast cases that was prominent in both studies. This increase appears to be related to the increasing cumulative dose in the dwindling population of survivors. The Thorotrast data in the United States also suggest that the most recent cases had relatively low-dose exposures compared with the earlier cases; a longer latent period in recent cases also was noted (Falk et al. 1979). The latent period as calculated from the earliest cases lengthened as the cohort matured. Therefore, one should not discount the possibility of increased numbers of VCM-associated HAS cases in the future in individuals with low exposure from occupational or environmental sources.

Geographic clusters of cases in rare-tumor studies are readily identifiable because of the low background rates. In the United States, clusters of VCM-associated cases were seen near some of the PVC polymerization plants and Thorotrast cases clustered in the northeastern cities (e.g., Philadelphia, New York, and Washington, D.C.) where Thorotrast was first introduced. A particularly good example is the cluster of six Thorotrast-induced cases seen in and around Edinburgh, where Thorotrast was first and most widely used in the United Kingdom (Baxter et al. 1980b).

DISCUSSION

Completeness of case finding is particularly important in a rare-tumor registry such as this, where even a few cases might identify an affected plant, a different means of exposure, or a new causative agent. Because of diagnostic and classification limitations (and despite an intensive search), it is likely that a sizeable fraction of cases was missed, particularly in the United States. These studies confirmed that death certificate reviews alone clearly are inadequate for the study of rare tumors and that rigorous pathologic review is needed.

In addition to the four causative agents discussed above, individual cases related to a variety of factors, including chloroprene, radiotherapy, radium implants, acrylonitrile, hemochromatosis, diethylstilbestrol, echinococcosis, copper, phenelzine, and urethane chemotherapy, were seen in these studies or have been reported elsewhere (Ross 1932; Baghirzade et al. 1971; Sussman et al. 1974; Pimentel and Menezes 1977; Hoch-Ligeti 1978; Daneshmend et al. 1979; Pollice 1979). A number of experimental carcinogens (in addition to VCM and some of its structural analogs) also are known to cause HAS; these include nitrosamines, urethane, hydrazines, azoxymethane, and lasiocarpine (Deringer 1962; Herrold 1967; Toth 1972, 1973; Maltoni and Lefemine 1974; Narisawa et al. 1976; Rao and Reddy 1978; Infante and Marlow 1980). The pathology panels were not able to distinguish morphologically between idiopathic HAS and the cases related to the various causative agents (Popper et al. 1978). It appears that the agents that cause HAS differ from traditional hepatocarcinogens in that they affect both hepatocellular and sinusoidal cell lines in the liver and represent, in a sense, a new class of hepatotoxins capable of causing both angiosarcoma and other liver lesions (Falk et al. 1979a). It would not be surprising, therefore, for other causative agents to be identified in the future, and time trends will continue to reflect the introduction, use, and discontinuation of the various causative agents. The potential to identify a new causative agent, even with only a handful of cases, makes the rare-tumor registry an attractive option.

The major limitations of these studies included: (1) the long start-up time and the considerable effort required to find and confirm cases; (2) the difficulty of getting detailed, accurate information from the widely dispersed family members in this retrospective setting; (3) the lack of adequate control groups in the United States (although the small number of cases limited the usefulness of control groups in the U.K.); and (4) the absence or limitations of past occupational exposure records.

A number of other rare marker tumors have been identified and studied in great detail. In addition to HAS, these include mesothelioma (related to asbestos), osteosarcoma (radium), vaginal adenocarcinoma (diethylstilbestrol), and hepatic adenoma (oral contraceptives). For these tumors, the associations with known causative agents and the concern about other agents that may be identified in the future (e.g., other fibers in mesothelioma, a variety of other halogenated hydrocarbons in HAS, and other internal alpha-emitters such as thorium or plutonium in osteosarcoma) make continuation of rare-tumor registries valuable. Registries covering a prolonged period of time may also be useful in evaluating dose-response relationships and latent periods.

Perhaps the most economical use of limited resources would be to develop the means of canvassing pathologists and others in a more systematic way for a variety of these tumors, either by computerizing and consolidating pathology (biopsy and autopsy) records or by querying pathologists from a centralized source at a single time for information on a variety of tumor types.

In addition to studying the above known marker tumors, a systematic approach also would allow study of other rare tumors that are of interest because of epidemiologic or experimental data. HAS, for example, would have been of interest even before the association with VCM was known for the following reasons: (1) the higher male:female ratio and earlier age of appearance than that for all other hepatic sarcomas; (2) the previously noted human causative agents (Thorotrast and arsenic); and (3) the large number of experimental chemicals that induce HAS in animals.

One must also be very specific when considering rare tumors. Epidemiologically, HAS is very different from angiosarcoma of the breast, limb, skin, and other sites (McBride et al. 1969; Girard et al. 1970; Chen et al. 1979, 1980), although, experimentally, some nonhepatic angiosarcomas also are induced by VCM, and their possible appearance in humans cannot be dismissed (Maltoni and Lefemine 1974). Recent reports have suggested an increased risk of soft-tissue sarcomas in groups exposed to chlorophenols and phenoxy acetic acids (Hardell and Sandstrom 1979); our experience suggests that it would be very important to consider carefully the various histologic types and sites that might be involved when addressing this issue.

In summary, although the absolute numbers of cases are small, registries for rare marker tumors provide unique opportunities for epidemiologic and pathogenetic studies of occupational and environmental carcinogens. A systematic or centralized approach to case finding would greatly facilitate such studies.

ACKNOWLEDGMENTS

Dr. Peter Baxter worked on the British angiosarcoma registry while with EMAS in the United Kingdom. We are both greatly indebted to the highly skilled and motivated pathologists (H. Popper, K.G. Ishak, L.B. Thomas, P.P. Anthony, R.N.M. MacSween, and P.J. Scheuer) who worked with us on the U.S. and British studies. We also thank all the individuals who worked on and supported these studies.

Use of trade names is for identification only and does not constitute endorsement by the Public Health Service or by the U.S. Department of Health and Human Services.

REFERENCES

Baghirzade, M.F., E.U. Hertel, and P. Schumacher. 1971. Hamangioendotheliom (reticulosarcoma angioplasticum) der leber und alte echinokokkusinfektion. *Acta Hepato-splenologica* **18**:224.

Baxter, P.J., P.P. Anthony, R.N.M. MacSween, and P.J. Scheuer. 1977. Angiosarcoma of the liver in Great Britain, 1963-73. *Br. Med. J.* **2**:919.

______. 1980a. Angiosarcoma of the liver: annual occurrence and aetiology in Great Britain. *Br. J. Ind. Med.* **37**:213.

Baxter, P.J., A.O. Langlands, P.P. Anthony, R.N.M. MacSween, and P.J. Scheuer. 1980b. Angiosarcoma of the liver: A marker tumour for the late effects of Thorotrast in Great Britain. *Br. J. Cancer* **41**:446.

Berk, P.D., J.F. Martin, R.S. Young, J. Creech, I.J. Selikoff, H. Falk, P. Watanabe, H. Popper, and L. Thomas. 1976. Vinyl chloride-associated liver disease. *Ann. Intern. Med.* **84**:717.

Chen, K.T.K., J.C. Bolles, and E.F. Gilbert. 1979. Angiosarcoma of the spleen—A report of two cases and review of the literature. *Arch. Pathol. Lab. Med.* **103**:122.

Chen, K.T.K., D.D. Kirkegaard, and J.J. Bocian. 1980. Angiosarcoma of the breast. *Cancer* **46**:368.

Creech, J.L. Jr. and M.N. Johnson. 1974. Angiosarcoma of liver in the manufacture of polyvinyl chloride. *J. Occup. Med.* **16**:150.

Daneshmend, T.K., G.L. Scott, and J.W.B. Bradfield. 1979. Angiosarcoma of liver associated with phenelzine. *Br. Med. J.* **1**:1679.

Deringer, M.K. 1962. Response of strain HR/De mice to painting with urethan. *J. Natl. Cancer Inst.* **29**:1107.

Falk, H., L.B. Thomas, H. Popper, and K.G. Ishak. 1979a. Hepatic angiosarcoma associated with androgenic-anabolic steroids. *Lancet* **ii**:1120.

Falk, H., G.G. Caldwell, K.G. Ishak, L.B. Thomas, and H. Popper. 1981a. Arsenic-related hepatic angiosarcoma. *Am. J. Ind. Med.* (in press).

Falk, H., N.C. Telles, K.G. Ishak, L.B. Thomas, and H. Popper. 1979b. Epidemiology of Thorotrast-induced hepatic angiosarcoma in the United States. *Environ. Res.* **18**:65.

Falk, H., J.T. Herbert, L. Edmonds, C.W. Heath, Jr., L.B. Thomas, and H. Popper. 1981b. Review of four cases of childhood hepatic angiosarcoma–Elevated environmental arsenic exposure in one case. *Cancer* **47**: 382.

Falk, H., J.T. Herbert, S. Crowley, K.G. Ishak, L.B. Thomas, H. Popper, and G.G. Caldwell. 1981c. Epidemiology of hepatic angiosarcoma in the United States 1964-1974. *Environ. Health Perspect.* (in press).

Girard, C., W.C. Johnson, and J. H. Graham. 1970. Cutaneous angiosarcoma. *Cancer* **26**:868.

Hardell, L., and A. Sandstrom. 1979. Case-control study: Soft-tissue sarcomas and exposure to phenoxyacetic acids or chlorophenols. *Br. J. Cancer* **39**:711.

Herrold, K.M. 1967. Histogenesis of malignant liver tumors induced by dimethylnitrosamine. An experimental study in Syrian hamsters. *J. Natl. Cancer Inst.* **39**:1099.

Hoch-Ligeti, C. 1978. Angiosarcoma of the liver associated with diethylstilbestrol. *J. Am. Med. Assoc.* **240**:1510.

Horta, J. Da Silva, L.C. Da Motta, and M.H. Tavares. 1974. Thorium dioxide effects in man–epidemiological, clinical, and pathological studies (experience in Portugal). *Environ. Res.* **8**:131.

Infante, P.F. and P.B. Marlow. 1980. Evidence for carcinogenicity of selected halogenated hydrocarbons including ethylene dichloride. *Banbury Rep.* **5**:287.

Maltoni, C. and G. Lefemine. 1974. Carcinogenicity bioassays of vinyl chloride. 1. Research plan and early results. *Environ. Res.* **7**:387.

McBride, C.M., J.W. Reeder, and J.L. Smith. 1969. Angiosarcoma in the lymphedematous limb. *South Med. J.* **62**:378.

Narisawa, T., C.Q. Wong, and J.H. Weisburger. 1976. Azoxymethane-induced liver hemangiosarcomas in inbred strain-2 guinea pigs. *J. Natl. Cancer Inst.* **56**:653.

Pimental, J.C. and A.P. Menezes. 1977. Liver disease in vineyard sprayers. *Gastroenterology* **72**:275.

Pollice, L. 1979. Primary vascular tumors of the liver. *Pathol. Res. Pract.* **165**:145.

Popper, H., L.B. Thomas, N.C. Telles, H. Falk, and I.J. Selikoff. 1978. Development of hepatic angiosarcoma in man induced by vinyl chloride, Thorotrast, and arsenic–Comparison with cases of unknown etiology. *Am. J. Pathol.* **92**:349.

Rao, M.S. and J.K. Reddy. 1978. Malignant neoplasms in rats fed lasiocarpine. *Br. J. Cancer* **37**:289.

Rooks, J.B., H. W. Ory, K.G. Ishak, L.T. Strauss, J.R. Greenspan, A.P. Hill, and C.W. Tyler, Jr. 1979. Epidemiology of hepatocellular adenoma–the role of oral contraceptive use. *J. Am. Med. Assoc.* **242**:644.

Ross, J.M. 1932. A case illustrating the effects of prolonged action of radium. *J. Pathol.* **35**:898.

Roth, F. 1957. Arsen leber tumoren (hemangioendotheliom). *Z. Krebsforsch.* **61**:468.

Sussman, E.B., I. Nydick, and G.F. Gray. 1974. Hemangioendothelial sarcoma of the liver and hemochromatosis. *Arch. Pathol.* **97**:39.

Toth, B. 1972. Morphological studies of angiosarcomas induced by 1,2-dimethylhydrazine dihydrochloride in Syrian golden hamsters. *Cancer Res.* **32**:2818.

______. 1973. 1,1-dimethylhydrazine (unsymmetrical) carcinogenesis in mice. Light microscopic and ultrastructural studies on neoplastic blood vessels. *J. Natl. Cancer Inst.* **50**:181.

COMMENTS

EPSTEIN: I have two brief questions. First, could you comment on the most interesting case of angiosarcoma of the penis in association with angioma of the liver in a VC worker (Mnaxmneh and Gonzalez 1981)?

The second question relates to this problem of so-called idiopathic angiosarcoma of the liver. To what extent do you think the idiopathic angiosarcomas reported in the literature should be reviewed with a view specifically to examining the possibility of an exposure to such agents as anabolic steroids, and in particular, proximity of residence to VC-PVC industry? You may recall that there are now about 6 or 7 cases of angiosarcoma of the liver reported in individuals living within approximately a 2-mile radius of industries in this country and in England (Table A).

FALK: To take your first question, the case that was recently reported of a man who worked in a plastics fabricating plant was really very unusual. The man had a primary angiosarcoma of the penis and also had

Table A
Angiosarcomas of the Liver in Residents Near VC/PVC Plants

Date of diagnosis or death[a]	Age/sex	Distance from plant (miles)	Reference	Comments
1967	73/male	2	Christine et al. (1974)	both PVC fabricating plants with in-plant cases also
1973	83/female	0.5	Christine et al. (1974)	
1970	61/male	<0.5	Baxter et al. (1977)	6-year resident; 1 in plant case also
1965	40/female	0.8	Brady et al. (1977)	–
1970	45/female	0.8	Brady et al. (1977)	–
1972	31/female	0.3	Brady et al. (1977)	8-year resident
1973	62/female	0.3	Brady et al. (1977)	–
1974	31/female	0.2	Brady et al. (1977)	–

Community cases of brain tumors also noted in 2 other reports (Infante 1976; Iturra 1976).

[a]None of these 8 cases had a history of occupational exposure to VC, or any history of exposure to or treatment with arsenicals or thorium dioxide.

angiosarcoma within what were thought to be previously existing cavernous hemangiomas in the liver. It did not appear that the tumor had developed de novo in the liver, so it was interpreted as primary penile angiosarcoma.

It is fascinating. I don't know what more to say about that. Our pathology review panel struggled at times when considering whether angiosarcomas that appeared to be widespread in the body were primary in the liver or not. They looked for whether or not the characteristic precursor lesion of the progression to HAS was apparent. In the penile angiosarcoma case, it was believed that such precursor lesions were not apparent in the liver, so it was not considered as primary in the liver.

With regard to the second question about individuals with lower exposure, I know at least that almost all of the cases in our registry (there were a few for which we didn't get adequate residential histories) did not live near any of the PVC polymerization plants. I think more instructive, perhaps, than going back over all of those cases would be to continue the registry forward in time, from, say, 1975. One will then see whether cases with relatively low environmental or occupational exposure occur in larger numbers or not.

MILHAM: If you went back and restricted your analysis just to the death certificate-ascertained cases, would you have missed anything significant?

FALK: There are a few things we would have missed. We would have missed the apparent clustering of arsenic cases with a single treatment clinic in Mississippi. There have been 5 case reports in the literature of Fowler's solution- or arsenic-associated HAS, in addition to one autopsy survey. We found 7 more. I think 12 such cases really begins to build up, in terms of numbers. So perhaps we strengthened the relationship between arsenic and hemangiosarcoma.

We would also have missed the association with androgenic-anabolic steroids. The androgenic-anabolic steroids are really fascinating, because they appear to cause four rare liver diseases: benign adenomas, reversible carcinomas, peliosis (which are dilated sinusoids), and angiosarcoma. They, in a sense, appear to cause the entire spectrum of both hepatocellular and sinusoidal cell lesions in the liver.

In addition, the much larger number of cases strengthened the ability to study the morphologic features and pathogenesis of the disease.

BEEBE: How did you actually assign cause? Was it simply on the basis of any association to these four known agents? And if so, how did you then come to the steroids?

FALK: For the three causative agents that were known, we included cases with known and accepted relationships. The VC cases that I listed were all in polymerization workers. The Thorotrast cases all have Thorotrast readily seen within their bodies. The arsenic cases that I have included are basically all Fowler's solution cases who took very large amounts of arsenic by ingestion; that is the association with arsenic that has been reported in the literature. The steroid association is based on skimpy data from the FDA suggesting that far fewer than one person in our case population would have been likely to have been taking androgenic-anabolic steroids for a prolonged period of time. So it is four versus something considerably less than one. How much considerably less than one, I couldn't say. But there are also theoretical reasons for thinking that this association is real.

SARACCI: You said before that you didn't have any control series. But what about the sort of implicit controls that are presented by your non-angiomatous sarcomas? What are the patterns of exposure of those?

FALK: What we actually did, in a sense after the fact, was to take the 22,000 or so death certificates in the unspecified code, 197.8, and choose matched controls (up to 4 per case) for each of the angiosarcoma cases; we then looked at occupation as recorded on the death certificate for both groups. The reasoning behind this is that code 197.8 (unspecified liver) largely represents a variety of metastatic lesions with uncertain primaries and is unlikely to be totally weighted towards any one category.

What we found, in looking at occupation by death certificate, was a striking increase for PVC polymerization workers, and also a small increase, not statistically significant, for people who worked in a group of laboring categories, including machinists and sheet metal workers. But the numbers were very small and there was no clustering in any one particular plant or category. So it is no more than suggestive that there is an increased risk in these categories.

Many of the cases in these categories could conceivably have had any one of a number of exposures, such as to nitrosamines or arsenic, in the past.

ACHESON: Can you please tell me what the sex ratio was in the residual? When you had got your four causes and you had the remainder, what was the sex ratio?

FALK: This, again, surprised me. The VC workers were all males. The Thorotrast HAS cases were almost three to one males, but I don't have the sex ratio of all Thorotrast recipients in the United States to compare to the ones who have angiosarcoma. The idiopathic cases were also approximately three to one.

ACHESON: Three men to one woman?

FALK: That is right. This was different than the sex ratio for other sarcomas of the liver, but is perhaps consistent with what one sees in primary liver cancer. The high sex ratio is one reason for my thinking that there still are other causative factors to be teased out of the idiopathic group. The age distribution of the cases with known etiologic factors was younger than that for the idiopathic cases, however.

References

Baxter, P.J., P.P. Anthony, R.N.M. MacSween, and P.J. Scheuer. 1977. Angiosarcoma of the liver in Great Britain, 1963-73. *Br. Med. J.* **2**:919.

Brady, J.S., F. Liberatore, P. Harper, P. Greenwald, W. Burnett, J.N. Davies, M. Bishop, A. Polan, and N. Viann. 1977. Angiosarcoma of the liver: An epidemiologic survey. *J. Natl. Cancer Inst.* **59**:1383.

Christine, B.W., H.S. Barrett, and D.S. Lloyd. Angiosarcoma of the liver—Connecticut. *Morbidity and Mortality Weekly Report* **23**:210.

Infante, P. 1976. Oncogenic and mutagenic risks in communities with polyvinyl chloride production facilities. *Ann. N. Y. Acad. Sci.* **271**:49.

Iturra, H. 1976. *Proceedings toxic substances in the air environment: Specialty conference,* p. 96. Air Pollution Control Association, Pittsburgh, Pennsylvania.

Mnaxmneh, L.G. and L.G. Gonzalez. 1981. Angiosarcoma of the penis with hepatic angioma in a patient with vinyl chloride exposure. *Cancer* **47**: 1318.

SESSION 7: Broad Approaches to Occupational Cancer Quantification

Problems in Assessing Risk from Occupational and Environmental Exposure to Carcinogens

JOEL B. SWARTZ AND SAMUEL S. EPSTEIN
School of Public Health
University of Illinois Medical Center
Chicago, Illinois 60680

The contribution to cancer from occupational exposures to chemicals and radiation is substantial and accounts for a major proportion of all cancers. Although this contribution appears to be increasing, there are major difficulties, which will be discussed here, in quantifying the effect.

One problem in assessing the effects of occupational exposure to carcinogens arises from inherent methodological limitations. We will summarize some of these limitations, suggest possible ways of resolving them, and refer to some work we are doing in attempts to overcome them.

Another problem is caused by various mythologies that have appeared in the scientific and lay literature with such regularity and that have been quoted with such frequency and apparent authority as to encourage their acceptance as dogma, even though they have little or no scientific basis. Generally, these mythologies have been proposed by those who advocate the life-style theory of cancer causation to the virtual exclusion of occupational and environmental exposures. One result is a general misconception that occupational exposures induce only a small proportion of all cancers. Another result is that proper and adequate research has not been performed, suggestive leads have not been followed up on occupational cancers, and proper regulations have not been promulgated to protect workers from such involuntary exposures.

METHODOLOGICAL LIMITATIONS

A number of methodological limitations have built a series of biases and defects into numerous published studies, which thus result in major underestimates of the importance of occupational exposures in inducing cancers. These limitations include:

1. Improper consideration of the latent period or, more properly, the tumor induction period.
2. The effect of cessation of exposure.
3. The age effect.

4. Competing risks.
5. The healthy-worker effect.

A major limitation in performing epidemiologic studies to assess the effects of occupational exposures to carcinogens is taking proper account of factors such as time since initial exposure, age at initial exposure, and cessation of exposure. These factors can play a crucial role in making qualitative and quantitative estimates of the effects of such exposures (Pasternack and Shore 1977; Whittemore 1977). Improper consideration of these factors has led to gross underestimation of the carcinogenic role of occupational exposures. For example, a study on vinyl chloride-exposed workers (Waxweiler et al. 1976) found significant excess cancer rates at a number of organ sites while, in a similar study on a similar population, an industrial consulting group found no such excesses (Tabershaw and Gaffey 1974). The reason for this difference is that the former study characterized the exposed workers by time since initial exposure, while the latter grouped all workers together, irrespective of exposure duration. Because cancer generally has a long latent period, failure to take this into account can and does result in gross underestimates of cancer rates and risks attributable to occupational exposures.

The effect of cessation of exposure to a carcinogen varies greatly with the type of carcinogen and the organ affected (Whittemore 1977; Day and Brown 1980). In some cases, cessation of exposure has little effect on cancer rates, whereas in others cessation resulted in a rapid reduction in cancer incidence down to rates similar to those for unexposed persons. For instance, within a few years of stopping smoking, there is a big drop in mortality rates of lung cancer (Table 1); after 20 years, the mortality rates for exsmokers are very close to those of nonsmokers (Day and Brown 1980).

In a recent experiment (EDO-1) using inbred mice with 2-acetylamino-fluorene, bladder cancer showed a similar pattern of reduction in incidence following cessation of carcinogen administration (Littlefield et al. 1979). If the

Table 1
Effect of Smoking Cessation on Lung Cancer Mortality

Years after stopping smoking	Per cent of lung cancer mortality rate at time of stopping: nonsmokers	exsmokers[a]	continuing smokers[a]
0	9	100	100
3	10	60	200
8	25	65	370
13	42	75	600
20	80	200	1000

[a]Includes persons who smoked 5 or more years, standardized for amount smoked and age at stopping smoking. (Based on Day and Brown 1980).

exposure was stopped, the incidence of bladder cancer quickly approached that of the controls; cessation of exposure had little effect on the induction of liver tumors, however.

Most occupational epidemiologic studies include many subjects for whom exposure has already stopped, either because of retirement or change of job. In no cases of which we are aware has the possibility of an important effect of exposure termination been considered in the analysis of the data. This could very easily result in an underestimate of the effect of exposure, by including subjects for whom exposure has ceased.

A number of observers have pointed out that susceptibility to carcinogenesis varies with age at first exposure, at least in certain cases (Mancuso et al. 1977; Pasternack and Shore 1977; Whittemore 1977; and Selikoff et al. 1978). Although these authors note the importance of considering the age effect, this is never done except when computing mortality rates by broad categories.

We suggest that by fitting modifications of the multistage model that include the exposure cessation effect and the age of effect, and by building in the effect of the induction period so as to eliminate consideration of the problem of whether or not to consider people who worked for 5, 10, or 15 years, it is possible to improve greatly the power and accuracy of occupational cancer epidemiological studies; this is likely to result in the findings of much greater cancer risk.

In preliminary calculations performed to test these methods and techniques, a simulated study population of 3000 persons was created and followed for 30 years. Life-table data for U.S. white males were used to estimate the background probabilities of dying from each cause of death, and various relative risks (RR) were assigned to the cancer deaths (J. B. Swartz et al., in prep.).

Both the life-table method and the technique involving the multistage model were used to assess the RR. Although the results are still preliminary, it appears that, in general, the technique of the multistage model produced higher and more accurate RRs than the life-table method; and variances in lifetime probability of developing cancer and in the mean times to tumor induction were much reduced using multistage modeling (J. B. Swartz et al., in prep.).

Thus, correction of such various methodological limitations should make a substantial contribution to correcting the biases resulting in underestimation of the effects of exposure to occupational carcinogens.

MYTHOLOGIES

The following are some major mythologies in occupational cancer risk assessment that appear to act as a major deterrent to performing appropriate studies and serve to create the erroneous impression of low risk.

Extrapolation From High to Lower Doses

The first mythology states that it is possible to extrapolate from a high to a lower dose by a straight line through the origin, and, moreover, that such extrapolation gives an upper limit on the effect of low-dose exposures to carcinogens. This method has been used to trivialize the effects of ambient air pollution and also to trivialize the effects of low-dose exposure to carcinogens.

One example of this mythology is the following concept (Doll 1978):

> "General knowledge of carcinogenesis suggests that at low doses carcinogenic effect is likely to be linearly proportional to the dose received. It should, therefore, be assumed that the small amounts (of polyaromatic hydrocarbons and heavy metals) contribute to the causation of some cases of lung cancer that occur in clinical practice. Extrapolation from occupational studies suggests that this effect is unlikely to be large."

Another example occurs in an extrapolation by Pike, in which it is estimated that there will be only approximately 0.3 excess lung cancer cases per 100,000 per year per benzo[*a*]pyrene unit (Pike et al. 1975). However, numerous epidemiological studies, not involving high-low dose extrapolations, have produced risk estimates 10-30 times higher (Carnow 1978). It must be remembered that the epidemiological studies very likely underestimate the effect because of confounding variables–populations are mobile and individuals do not remain stationary in any one location even over daily periods.

So what then is wrong with the argument of linear extrapolation from high to low doses? Simply, we have just completed examining a large number of carcinogenic bioassays, and have found that the curve is not linear at all through the origin. A typical bioassay on vinyl chloride is shown in Figure 1 (Maltoni 1975). As can be seen, an increase in exposure level, from 250 ppm to 2500 ppm, increases the percent responders from 17% to 54%. However, a further 200-fold increase brought about no change. The slope of the dose-response curve tends to flatten as the response increases, sometimes sharply by a factor of 10 to 100. As this begins, percent response is in the neighborhood of 10%.

Calculations on what error would occur by doing this estimate from the high-dose exposure demonstrates in almost all cases that it was at least a factor of 10, but sometimes it was in the hundreds or even thousands (Swartz et al. 1981).

Evidence from experimental and epidemiological studies on carcinogenesis indicate that in the measurable regions, i.e., where incidences range from a few percent on up to 80%, the curve is in no way linear. It flattens out very sharply. Any attempt to make a linear extrapolation through the origin will thus result in an underestimate of the effect at low doses, sometimes by a factor of 100 or 1000.

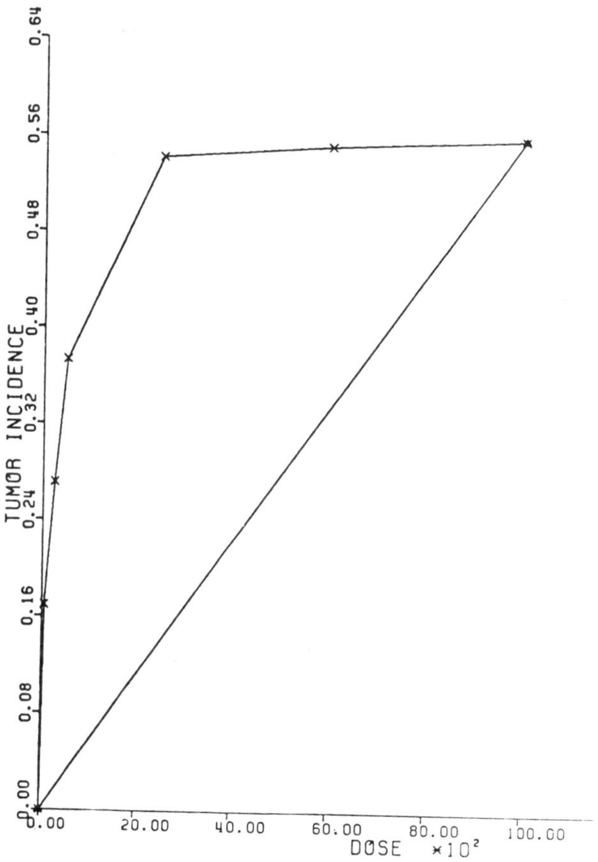

Figure 1

Comparison of tumor incidence predicted by linear extrapolation through origin from highest dose with actual incidence. Point A is highest measured dose; point B is actual measured incidence at low dose; point C is incidence predicted by linear extrapolation. Data are from a vinyl chloride bioassay by Maltoni (1975).

Low-dose Radiation is Only a Minor Cause of Occupational Cancer

Radiation has been discussed in great detail at this meeting (see Darby; Mancuso et al.; Radford; all this volume). The mythology is based on the use of the BEIR report (BEIR 1972) for making estimates on the effect of radiation. Contrastingly, estimates of the risk not based on this report put the effect at from 10 to 100 times higher (Goffman et al. 1972; Kneale et al. 1978). The findings of the BEIR report rely mainly on questionable analysis of two sets of data:

1. The atomic bomb data. This event produced a single major radiation dose (BEIR 1972). Examination of carcinogenesis bioassay data, however,

demonstrated that the tumorigenic response is greatly increased by fractionating a dose, keeping the same total dose (Saffiotti and Shubik 1956; Druckrey 1967; Shimkin et al. 1967).
2. Spondylitis data. Spondylitis is a debilitating disease and many of the patients died early from competing risks of pneumonia or other diseases (Morgan 1980). As a result, they cannot be used for an accurate estimate of the effect of radiation.

Smoking Is Responsible For the Overwhelming Majority of Lung Cancer in Workers and Recent Increases in Lung Cancer Rates are Due Largely to Smoking

There are several problems with this point of view.

1. Smoking rates in the United States are declining for men. The percent of male smokers declined from 50% in 1955 to 37% in 1978; and the rates have been declining in the number of smokers, the number of people who smoke large numbers of cigarettes, and the number of people who smoke fewer cigarettes (Moss 1979).
2. The data presented in Table 1 indicate that we already should have seen an effect from this decline in smoking. In 5 years, the lung cancer rate will be 68% for those who continued smoking, but after 15 years it is down to 11% of those who continued smoking (Day and Brown 1980). So it would seem reasonable to infer that the number of lung cancers due to smoking should be going down, not up.
3. Various estimates have placed the percent of male lung cancers in the United States among nonsmokers in the range of about 20% (Schneiderman 1978; Enstrom 1979). Data from a recent study (Enstrom 1979) indicated that this rate in nonsmokers doubled between 1958 and 1969.
4. The role of occupation was not considered in most classical studies on lung cancer (Sterling 1979, 1980; Epstein and Swartz 1981). Frequently, smoking is confounded with occupation. Also we see an increase in the numbers of adenocarcinomas, as opposed to squamous and oat cell carcinomas, in many occupational groups (Epstein and Swartz 1981), and these have not been shown to be related to smoking.
5. For many occupational groups, the overall lifetime incidence of lung cancer for smokers is not substantially different than for nonsmokers. This has been reported in uranium miners, zinc lead miners, mustard gas workers, and copper smelter workers (Epstein and Swartz 1981). Although the induction period is sometimes lower for smokers, the lifetime risk is not substantially altered.
6. There are in the literature high RR figures for the carcinogenic effects of smoking that are not borne out or are contradicted by other carefully documented studies. For example, some studies state that the lung cancer

RR for smokers is 15 for men (Doll and Peto 1976), while others say 8 (Doll 1977). The last study that was published in *The New England Journal of Medicine* found no significant excess risk for pancreatic cancer for smokers (MacMahon et al. 1981), although a number of previously published studies found RRs of the order of 2 or 3 (Doll 1977).

7. Finally, smoking cannot reasonably account for the disproportionately sharp increase in lung cancer among blacks. Twenty years ago, the lung cancer rate among the black population in the United States was lower than among whites; now, it is about 25% higher and is increasing about twice as fast as for whites. There is substantial evidence, however, that the black population is disproportionately represented in the most hazardous occupations, besides residing in the most highly polluted urban areas, often in close proximity to polluting industries (Devesa and Silverman 1978; Mancuso 1979; Mancuso and Sterling 1979).

Elimination of People or Statistics From Data

The fourth mythology is based on the assumption that cancer mortality trends can be analyzed in spite of the arbitrary elimination of certain population groups or statistics from occupational cancer data. Many times, data on the nonwhite U.S. population merely are rejected without any reasonable explanation. For example, Peto tries to rationalize such exclusion with the claim that "previously poor people, especially blacks" have been specifically affected by recent improvements in medical care and "cancer counting" (Peto 1980). He claims that these trends have caused upward biases in cancer mortality rates that most particularly affect blacks, poor people, and old people. Peto demands that we restrict our attention to rates and trends among middle-aged whites, where these supposed upward biases might be expected to be least prominent. No evidence is presented to support these categorical assertions.

In fact, there is no validity to any of these assertions. Blacks in the United States could hardly be categorized as formerly poor. Living standards for the general U.S. population have declined sharply in the past 4 years and have returned to 1960 levels. The decline for the U.S. black population is even sharper. Furthermore, the past few years have seen the closing of many public hospitals and other institutions that treat medically indigent people. Despite this, the mortality rates from lung cancer and cancer of other sites are still higher and continue to rise faster for the black than white populations in the U.S.

An equally disturbing and scientifically unjustifiable trend is the arbitrary cutoff for no legitimate reasons, of cancer mortality data at the age of 65. Peto (1980) again claims without evidence that mortality figures for persons under 65 are likely to be more accurate. In fact, many cancers have long latency periods and such a cutoff would certainly result in a major underestimate of the effects of occupational exposures to carcinogens.

In fact, a recent study undertaken to determine the accuracy of cancer mortality (Percy et al. 1981) found that the figures on most cancers were accurate and that lung cancer was among the most accurately diagnosed cancers, with a detection rate of 95%. The authors conclude that errors in diagnosis of lung cancer deaths could not possibly affect time trends. Moreover, the authors point out that age, race, and sex had no effect on the accuracy of mortality figures. Hence, there is no scientific justification for the arbitrary elimination of cancer mortality rates for older persons or black persons. The only reason for doing so is to mask rapidly rising cancer death rates, and the occupational component of them.

These various mythologies and methodological limitations in studies on occupational cancer described here tend to trivialize the carcinogenic effect of occupational exposure and thus discourage critically needed research and regulation.

ACKNOWLEDGMENTS

We would like to thank Ms. Christine Riddiough for scientific assistance, Ms. Deborah Schechter for programming assistance, Ms. Kathy Jackson for typing the manuscript, and Mr. Michael Botkin for editorial assistance.

REFERENCES

BEIR (Biological Effects of Ionizing Radiation) Report. 1972. The effects on populations of exposure to low levels of ionizing radiation. Science National Research Council, Washington, D.C.

Carnow, B.W. 1978. The urban factor and lung cancer: Cigarette smoking or air pollution? *Environ. Health Perspect.* **22**:17.

Day, N.E. and C.C. Brown. 1980. Multistage models and primary prevention of cancer. *J. Natl. Cancer Inst.* **64**:977.

Devesa, S.S. and D.T. Silverman. 1978. Cancer incidence and mortality trends in the U.S. 1937-1974. *J. Natl. Cancer Inst.* **60**:545.

Doll, R. 1977. Strategy for the detection of cancer hazards to man. *Nature* **265**:589.

______. 1978. Atmospheric pollution and lung cancer. *Environ. Health Perspect.* **22**:23.

Doll, R. and R. Peto. 1976. Mortality in relation to smoking: 20 years observations on male British doctors. *Br. Med. J.* **2**:105.

Druckrey, H. 1967. Quantitative aspects in chemical carcinogenesis. In *Potential carcinogenic hazards from drugs* (ed. R. Truhaut). p. 707. Springer, Berlin.

Enstrom, J.E. 1979. Rising lung cancer mortality among non-smokers. *J. Natl. Cancer Inst.* **62**:755.

Epstein, S.S. and J.B. Swartz. 1981. Fallacies in the lifestyle theory of cancer. *Nature* **289**:127.

Goffman, J.W., J. Goffman, A. Tamplin, and E. Kovich. 1972. Radiation as an environmental hazard. In *Environment and Cancer,* p. 157. Williams & Wilkins, Baltimore.

Kneale, G.W., T.F. Mancuso, and A.M. Stewart. 1978. Reanalysis of data relating to the Hanford Study of the cancer risks of radiation workers. In *Late biological effects of ionizing radiation*, p. 387. International Atomic Energy Agency, Vienna.

Littlefield, N.A., J. Farmer, D. Gaylor, and W. Sheldon. 1979. Effects of dose and time in a long-term, low-dose carcinogenic study. In *Innovations in cancer risk assessment* (ed. J.A. Staffer and M.A. Mehlman), p. 17. Pathotox, Park Forest South, Illinois.

MacMahon, B., S. Yen, D. Trichopoulos, K. Warren, and G. Nardi. 1981. Coffee and cancer of the pancreas. *New Engl. J. Med.* **304**:630.

Maltoni, C. 1975. The value of predictive experimental bioassays in occupational and environmental carcinogenesis. *Ambio* **4**:10.

Mancusco, T.F. 1979. "Cancer in the workplace." Paper presented at OSHA conference Lost in the Workplace, Chicago, September 14.

Mancuso, T.F. and T.D. Sterling. 1975. Lung cancer among black and white migrants in the U.S. *J. Natl. Med. Assoc.* **67**:107.

Mancuso, T.F., A. Stewart, and G. Kneale. 1977. Radiation exposure of Hanford workers dying of cancer and other causes. *Health Phys.* **33**:369.

Morgan, K.Z. 1980. Appreciation of risks of low-level radiation vs. nuclear energy. *Comments Molec. Cell. Biophys.* **1**:41.

Moss, A.J. 1979. Changes in cigarette smoking and current smoking practices among adults: U.S., 1978. In *Advance data.* National Center for Health Statistics, number 52, September 19.

Pasternack, B.S. and R.E. Shore. 1977. Statistical methods for assessing risk following exposure to environmental carcinogens. In *Environmental health: Quantitative methods* (ed. A. Whittemore), p. 49. SIAM, Philadelphia.

Percy, C., E. Stanek, and L. Gloeckler. 1981. Accuracy of cancer death statistics and its effect on cancer mortality statistics. *Am. J. Public Health* **71**:242.

Peto, R. 1980. Distorting the epidemiology of cancer: The need for a more balanced overview. *Nature* **284**:297.

Pike, M.C., R.J. Gordon, B.E. Henderson, H.R. Menck, and J. SooHoo. 1975. Air pollution. In *Persons at high risk of cancer* (ed. J.F. Fraumeni, Jr.), p. 225. Academic Press, New York.

Saffioffi, U. and P. Shubik. 1956. The effects of concentrations of carcinogens in epidermal carcinogenesis. *J. Natl. Cancer Inst.* **16**:961.

Schneiderman, M. 1978. Trends in incidence and mortality in the U.S. OSHA docket number 090, April 4.

Selikoff, I.J., E. Hammond, and H. Seidman. 1978. Cancer risks of insulation workers in the U.S. In *Biological effects of asbestos* Vol. 64, p. 209. IARC, Lyon.

Shimkin, M., R. Wieder, D. Marzi, N. Gubareff, and V. Suntzeff. 1967. Lung tumors in mice receiving different schedules of urethane. In *Proceedings of the 5th Berkeley symposium on mathematical statistics and probability* (ed. L. LeCam and J. Neyman). University of California Press, Berkeley.

Sterling, T.D. 1978. Does smoking kill workers, or working kill smokers? *Int. J. Health Services* 8:437.

Sterling, T.D. 1980. "Smoking, occupation, and respiratory disease." Paper prepared for the American Lung Association Occupational Task Force meeting, April 9.

Swartz, J.B., C. Ridiough, and S.S. Epstein. 1981. Analysis of dose response relations using dichotomous data: Implications for carcinogenic risk assessment. *Teratogen. Mutagenesis and Carcinogensis* (in press).

Tabershaw, I.R. and W.R. Gaffey. 1974. Mortality study of workers in the manufacturing of vinyl chloride and its polymers. *J. Occup. Med.* **16**:509.

Waxweiler, R.J., W. Stringer, J. Wagoner, J. Jones, H. Falk, and C. Carter. 1976. Neoplastic risk among workers exposed to vinyl chloride. In *Occupational carcinogenesis* (ed. U. Saffiotti and J.K. Wagoner), p. 40. New York Academy of Sciences, New York.

Whittemore, A. 1977. The age distribution of human cancer for carcinogenic exposure of varying intensity. *Am. J. Epidemiol.* **106**:418.

COMMENTS

CAIRNS: I would like to start the discussion with a statement. I think Dr. Swartz, you missed a rather interesting point this morning about Iceland, where the air is virtually free of pollution. Their lung cancer rate is only slightly lower than that of the U.S. and this difference is attributed to the fact that they smoke rather less. I wonder whether you would like to comment about this.

SWARTZ: The statement we have made concerning the importance of air pollution in causing lung cancers is based on a large number of epidemiological studies from many parts of the world—the United States, Great Britain, Ireland, Japan, and South Africa (Carnow 1978). In some instances, the studies were urban-rural studies; in some cases, they compared lung cancer rates between cities with low and high air pollution; in others, they compared rates between more and less polluted areas of the same city. In many cases, the confounding effect of smoking was removed by controlling for this variable, by satisfying for smoking class, or by the use of sampling studies to eliminate the possibility of significant differences in smoking habits between the two areas.

In all cases, there were strong, positive associations between pollutant levels and lung cancer mortality rates. Generally, these were found in both men and women. Although the exact magnitude of the effect varied, estimates from all the studies put the lung cancer risk from exposure to ambient air pollution at at least an order of magnitude greater than what has been calculated by linear extrapolation through the origin. The preponderance of estimates indicates that persons living close to the workplace have at least a 50% increased lung cancer risk from exposure to coke oven emissions.

RADFORD: I wish the BEIR Report were, in fact, looked at more critically. I think that if one does, the fact is that radiation-induced cancers are now quite well understood—although not perfectly at the low-dose rates, admittedly—and we can make reasonably precise risk estimates in terms of the occupationally-induced cancers. Even 0.25% of cancers due to occupational radiation exposure is a major problem. Whether the proportion of occupationally induced cancers is 5%, 10%, or whatever, these cancers are preventable and we should be doing something about it. I don't think much of this argument is really terribly relevant.

SWARTZ: I have found many reports in which the BEIR report is quoted as dogma. I realize there have been revisions to the original BEIR report, but these estimates of the effect of radiation from the original are still quoted, and all the versions give far lower risk estimates than those from the Hanford study (Mancuso et al. 1977; Kneale et al. 1978). Some of the underpinnings of the BEIR estimates, such as the use of data on spondylitis patients, clearly have been shown to be invalid (Morgan 1980).

DAVIS: Getting back to the smoking question, are some of these supposedly smoking-related cancers decreasing, why are others apparently increasing at different rates and why are they different for men and women? These trends suggest to me an occupational etiology, especially when you look at some of the male-female differences for the nonhormone-related cancers.

SWARTZ: We think that the effect of smoking in causing cancer among men, especially lung cancer, is declining because male smoking rates have been declining for at least 25 years and have not increased for over 35 years (Moss 1979). This decline in smoking is not just among young people but appears across the board in men of all ages. Because the excess risk of lung cancer goes down sharply and quickly for persons who have stopped smoking (Doll and Peto 1976; Schneiderman 1978; Day and Brown 1980), we should have already seen a decline in male lung cancer rates if lung cancer were due almost entirely to smoking.

The importance of smoking in causing other "smoking-related" cancers is much more in doubt than lung cancer, although it is certainly a smaller factor. RRs are lower, and there are large discrepancies in the estimates of the RRs (Doll 1977; MacMahon et al. 1981). Also, the trend of pancreatic cancer, one that is labeled a "smoking-related" cancer, does not follow smoking trends the way lung cancer does.

DAVIS: Let me just follow up with the observation that some nonsmoking-related cancers, such as myelomas, are increasing. These have been linked in some fairly careful case-control studies of counties having plastics industry, so that there is some concern that there may be an occupational etiology for some of those.

R. PETO: First, it simply isn't true that lung cancer should be going down now, because there were very large increases in tobacco usage in the first half of this century, and it is tobacco usage in early adult life that imprints a risk of lung cancer on later adult life. In addition to that, smoking affects the second stage of the process of carcinogenesis, and it is the effect on the second stage that produces the rapid decrease when you stop smoking. What is being seen now among the 60-year-olds in this country are the delayed effects of adoption of cigarette smoking by young people about 40 years earlier; these very large increases are larger than the decreases due to decreases in tobacco usage.

Second, it is not true that at least 20% of the lung cancers in this country occur among nonsmokers, if by "nonsmokers" you mean lifelong nonsmokers. That just isn't true.

Third, it is not true that occupation was not considered in the case-control studies of lung cancer. In fact, when those studies were undertaken, occupational factors were thought to be, if anything, more plausible than tobacco as explanations for the increase in lung cancer and it was only the data that drew attention to smoking, and not to occupation. It is not something that was ignored.

WATSON: What is the difference in value between what you say the proportion of lung cancer patients is that have never smoked, and what Joel Swartz says? Would you say 2%, 5%?

R. PETO: I would say probably about 2-4%. But what is the evidence for this 20%, Dr. Swartz, or would you like to withdraw that statement?

SWARTZ: I have no intention of withdrawing my statement. The evidence comes from calculations by Schneiderman (1978). Data from Enstrom (1979) support our contention concerning the high and increasing lung cancer mortality rate among nonsmokers.

EPSTEIN: Let me just comment on these figures.

Point 1: There are some 100,000 lung cancer deaths every year in this country, and it has been estimated that about 80,000 of these occur in smokers, according to figures coming from a wide range of sources, including the American Cancer Society (ACS); and, 20,000 occur in nonsmokers (Schneiderman 1978; Enstrom 1979). That doesn't mean to say that one can definitely exclude the possibility that some of these could have gotten their lung cancers from exposure to sidestream smoke.

Point 2: There are data by Enstrom and others showing a substantial increase in rates of lung cancer in nonsmokers in recent decades.

Point 3: We are seeing an increased number of pulmonary adenocarcinomas in workers who smoke, but who are also exposed to a wide range of occupational carcinogens.

Point 4: We are seeing an increase in incidence of lung cancer cases in working nonsmokers in occupations where you follow them up for lifetime periods.

I don't think there was any question about the fact that the role of smoking in occupation has been overemphasized in the past. There is also no question about the fact that in the majority of studies, that is, retrospective epidemiological studies on smoking and lung cancer, the role of occupation has not been fully documented and has not been fully taken into account. Now, this does not mean to say that smoking isn't a major cause of lung cancer. Nobody in his right mind would deny that. But this doesn't also mean to say, as the life-style advocates seem to think, that occupation is not an important cause of lung cancer.

Essentially, what we are saying very clearly is (1) there is an important role of smoking in lung cancer; and (2) there is an important role of occupation in lung cancer. There is a growing body of scientific data to support that, and it is time that the literature of the life-stylists adequately reflected this. As a nonepidemiologist, I wonder if I could make the following comment: When you examine national figures—rates, trends, mortality, or incidence rates—they express the proper impression of what is happening on an overall basis in the nation. Such overall figures can reflect very major variations, either upwards or downwards, in both high-risk and low-risk populations. So, I think there are certain dangers in looking at overall rate trends, national rate trends, and trying to develop inferences, particularly in relation to high-risk occupations or other such subgroups.

R. PETO: In quoting the 80,000 figure, you are confusing the statement that 80,000 are *occurring* among smokers with the statement that 80,000 are *due to* smoking. If we go back to 1976, which is the year to which these figures relate, then 80,000 were due to smoking out of a total of about 92,000, leaving about 12,000 not due to smoking. But not all of the lung cancers not due to smoking are occurring among nonsmokers; only a fraction of them are. So the discrepancy between my estimate of about 4% and your estimate of 20% is, first, this confusion between occurring among smokers and due to smoking; and, second, the difference between 1976 and the more recent figures, where you have the extra 2 years of increase in lung cancer that is due to smoking. Perhaps that is the discrepancy.

Enstrom compared self-described, lifelong nonsmokers, almost all of whom would have been genuine lifelong nonsmokers, with groups such as active Mormons, one-third of whom are ex-smokers, or people in whom the smoking habits were ascertained from whomever informed the U.S. government of the fact of their deaths. We might well not have known whether these people were smokers, if they had been smokers sometime previously. In both cases, Enstrom is comparing genuine, lifelong non-smokers with people, a proportion of whom are ex-smokers. This produces an impression of trends, because the other studies were later.

If you look among self-described, lifelong nonsmokers, as in the ACS study, or among the study of U.S. veterans, you find no trend within those data.

EPSTEIN: I think it's a good point, when you talk about the 80,000 lung cancer deaths in smokers, to make distinctions between these 80,000 deaths occurring, either on the one hand due to smoking or on the other hand being the 80,000 lung cancer deaths associated with smoking. In the life-style literature, there is an implicit and repeated assumption that these 80,000 deaths in smokers are due to smoking. We challenge that very explicitly.

I say that in these 80,000 lung cancers in smokers we don't know what percentage of these deaths is due to smoking alone, to smoking plus occupation, or to occupation alone. I believe that smoking is an important factor. But we don't know any way of segregating these three elements.

R. PETO: The source that you are quoting says 80,000 due to smoking, not among smokers.

DAVIS: Let me suggest that we're not all that far apart here. You are both saying that aggregate data such as these are a bit of a fishing expedition, that they suggest something. And I think that what we want to end up doing here at the conference is try to propose some more carefully done studies that will answer some of these questions.

What we need to talk about, I think, is how could one go about setting up a study of the case-control type that would address some of these questions, so that we would no longer have to be throwing about county data and historically reconstructed data, and trying to make definitive interpretations of these data. Because there are limits of the aggregate data that we're dealing with right now, we should try to advance epidemiology further by suggesting more appropriate studies be done.

SAMUELS: This morning a colleague said that I have been very silent in this meeting and that I had an obligation, as the health officer for 6 million American workers, to say something.

Let me tell you precisely what is on my mind. This dialogue is extremely boring. It has really very little relevance to what is necessary to be done, and very little relevance scientifically. Let me tell you why.

You have, in effect, two—perhaps more—models. I think you could classify them as a multivariate factor analysis, of the kind done by Bridbord and done by Dr. Swartz and by Sam [Epstein] and by others and a single-cause-single-effect model. Now, as in all models, there really isn't any right or wrong. A model is heuristic based on its predictive value.

What I would suggest is that we spend our time and money doing something constructive, and then wait 10 or 15 years and find out who is right or who is wrong. The reality is that no decisions are going to be made on the basis of what this conference concludes or doesn't conclude. There are some very interesting scientific questions that should be answered, but the important thing is to realize that we are not going to permit decisions to be made simply on the basis of the greatest good for the greatest number, namely, the incidence, or rather the fraction of occupational cancer, or cancer attributed to cancer in the total population. Decisions must be made on what is going on in worker populations. If there is an incidence of bladder cancer of 85% among the working population of dye workers, that is something you act upon.

SWARTZ: I think this discussion has been very interesting, but basically, we stick by our point of view. We think that occupationally caused cancers are important, that they should be studied, and, more importantly, that there should be regulations and protections. We oppose attempts to trivialize them or to confuse people as to their exact importance.

EPSTEIN: I would like to suggest that two major topics need to be considered. First, if you are interested in quantitation of occupational cancer, there cannot be any serious consideration of this topic in the absence of information on exposure. Parenthetically, the life-style advocates and the life-style literature fail to take into account the inescapable fact that there are virtually no data based on exposure. In fact, in this country, the chemical industry still takes the intransigent position that the worker doesn't have the right to know the nature and identity of the chemicals to which he or she is exposed—a position which would appear to be both scientifically and morally intolerable.

The second relates to statements that "occupational cancer can be concentrated among relatively small groups of people," and that "Such risks usually can be reduced, or even eliminated, once they have been identified." This represents a total misconception of the realities. In this country and in England, there are a very wide range of occupational carcinogens that have been identified, and for which little or no regulatory action has been taken to reduce or eliminate exposure.

References

Carnow, B.W. 1978. The urban factor and lung cancer: Cigarette smoking or air pollution? *Environ. Health Perspect.* **22**:17.

Day, N.E. and C.C. Brown. 1980. Multistage models and primary prevention of cancer. *J. Natl. Cancer Inst.* **64**:977.

Doll, R. 1977. Strategy for the detection of cancer hazards to man. *Nature* **265**:589.

Doll, R. and R. Peto. 1976. Mortality in relation to smoking: 20 years observations on male British doctors. *Br. Med. J.* **2**:105.

Enstrom, J.E. 1979. Rising lung cancer mortality among nonsmokers. *J. Natl. Cancer Inst.* **62**:755.

Kneale, G.W., T.F. Mancuso, and A.M. Stewart. 1978. Reanalysis of data relating to the Hanford Study of the cancer risks of radiation workers. In *Late biological effects of ionizing radiation,* p. 387. International Atomic Energy Agency, Vienna.

Mancuso, T.F., A.M. Stewart, and G.W. Kneale. 1977. Radiation exposure of Hanford works dying of cancer and other causes. *Health Phys.* **33**:304.

Morgan, K.Z. 1980. Appreciation of risks of low-level radiation vs. nuclear energy. *Comments Molec. Cell Biophys.* **1**:41.

Moss, A.J. 1979. Changes in cigarette smoking and current smoking practices among adults: U.S., 1978. In *Advance data.* National Center for Health Statistics, #52, September 19.

Schneiderman, M. 1978. Trends in incidence and mortality in the U.S. OSHA docket #090, April 4.

NOTE ADDED IN PROOF (SWARTZ):

The trend of increase in lung cancer mortality rates is demonstrated in the Enstrom paper by comparing two groups of lifelong nonsmokers (1958 and 1966-1968). The data on Mormons are not even needed to demonstrate this increasing trend. Furthermore, Enstrom declares that the Mormon population studied are church leaders who can be considered lifelong nonsmokers, a fact confirmed by actual survey data. The data on Mormon church leaders for the period 1968-1975 indicate that lung cancer mortality has continued to rise sharply among persons who never smoked.

Differentiating Work from Life-style in Cancer Causation

ANTHONY JOHN McMICHAEL
Division of Human Nutrition
Commonwealth Scientific & Industrial Research Organization
Adelaide, South Australia 5000

The famous nineteenth-century demographer-statistician, William Farr, foreshadowed a broad perspective within which to consider occupational cancers:

> Different classes of the population experience very different rates of mortality, and suffer different kinds of diseases. The principal causes of these differences, besides the sex, age, and hereditary organization, must be sought in three sources: ordinary occupations of life, the adequate or inadequate supply of warmth and of food, and the differential degree of exposure to poisonous effluvia and to destructive agents (Farr 1885).

At the least, this view emphasizes the coexistent effects upon health of job, life-style, and the general physical environment. This configuration is an inevitable source of confounding in the epidemiologist's attempt to quantify the occupational contribution to human cancer. Further, it affords many biological interactive possibilities between occupational and nonoccupational factors in the complex and sequential processes of human carcinogenesis. (The above implies a simplistic distinction between job and life-style. In reality, there is an intimate relationship between these two facets of an individual's social existence; but that ideologically loaded question is not directly at issue here. However, "occupational" exposure will refer here to those factors intrinsic to the work environment—and exposure to which is therefore essentially involuntary on the part of the worker.)

In Figure 1 it is assumed that we want to determine the relationship between exposure to job A and cancer X. Notionally, the epidemiologist compares, by nonexperimental observation, the frequency of cancer in job A workers with the frequency in nonjob A workers who are otherwise similar (or who are measurably dissimilar) to the job A workers. Almost inevitably, there will be some off-the-job life-style differences (A′ versus non-A′) between these two occupationally defined groups.

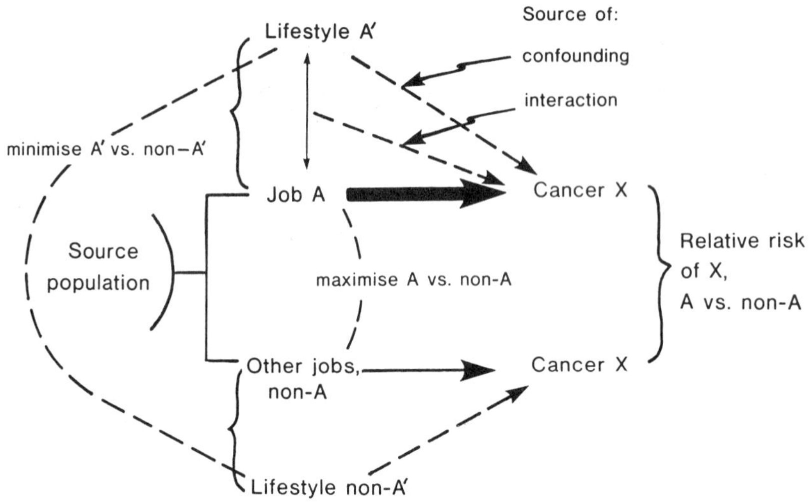

Figure 1
Schematic representation of the interrelated effects of occupational environment and lifestyle upon risk of cancer.

The two consequent problems are, first, confounding, and, second, interaction. Confounding, due to the unequal distribution between the two compared groups of other separately acting, nonoccupational causes of cancer X, will tend to obscure the strength of the true job A-cancer X relationship.

Interaction, whereby the magnitude of the effect of job A upon risk of cancer X is dependent upon the level of other coexistent factors ("effect modifiers"), will tend to produce inconsistency of findings between different study populations, reflecting variation in the prevalence of those interacting factors. Within a study population, it will cause variation in the job A-associated cancer risk between the relevant subgroups of workers.

Unresolved debate about the mathematical formulation of interactive effects, and about the distinction between "interaction" and "synergy" (Rothman et al. 1980), is not crucial here. The term "interaction" is used in reference to those biological processes within carcinogenesis in which the influence of one factor depends wholly or largely upon its potentiation (or suppression) of the effect of another factor. The phenomenon may entail simultaneous effects, as with alcohol perhaps acting as a solvent for chemical carcinogens–tobacco-derived, occupational, or other–in the upper alimentary tract (Tuyns 1979). Or it may entail sequential effects, as with vitamin A deficiency enhancing the posttransformation dedifferentiation of epithelial cells towards frank neoplasia (Schroder and Black 1980).

This presentation briefly considers the rather self-apparent problem of confounding due to life-style, and then examines in more detail ways in which such off-the-job factors, including dietary factors, alter the individual's likelihood of clinical cancer resulting from potentially carcinogenic occupational exposures. Clearly, these latter, interactive phenomena must be considered in any quantitative accounting of the contributory sources of human cancer.

The intention here is not to exonerate occupational exposures; rather, it is to emphasize two other important issues. First, obviously, neglect of confounding effects will lead to an incorrect estimate of the risk attributable to occupational factors. Indeed, the potential for such errors is underscored by various recent estimates that dietary factors account for about half the cancer "excess" in Western populations, and alcohol and cigarettes (separately and together) account for another quarter (Wynder 1977; Higginson and Muir 1979). These life-style factors are thus seen as the major source of environmental cancer etiology.

Second, neglect of interactive effects will lead to a misunderstanding of both the biological role, and, perhaps, the relative importance of the occupational factor within the complex process of carcinogenesis. If the factor is a necessary, but not sufficient, causal factor–such as asbestos in some occupationally related lung cancers–its elimination undoubtedly will reduce the cancer incidence; but the extent of the reduction in that particular example will depend on the smoking profile of the work force. If the occupational factor is one of several cancer-initiating factors for, say, lung cancer, whose several effects each depend (perhaps variably) upon other cocarcinogenic or promotional factors, such as vitamin A status, the quantitative picture then becomes less clear.

In support of that particular hypothetical example, the recent work of Hirayama (1979) in Japan has shown how the cigarette-associated risk of lung cancer is dependent on the individual's intake of dietary micronutrients (especially vitamin A, or, more correctly, dietary retinoids and carotenoids). Equivalent data have not yet been sought in relation to occupational respiratory carcinogenesis.

CONFOUNDING

Social class differences for three major causes of death in males, in contemporary Britain, are shown in Table 1 (Registrar-General 1978). There is a clear-cut gradient for each cause, albeit stronger for cancer.

Because social class is defined by job in these official British statistics, there is presumptive evidence here of a job-related risk gradient for cancer, ischemic heart disease, and diabetes mellitus. However, to the extent that these social class gradients have also been found for married women, classified by husband's job, they may rather more reflect class-related life-style factors than

Table 1
Age-standardized Mortality Ratios for Selected Major Causes of Death, by Social Class, Males Aged 15-64: England and Wales, 1970-1972

	Social class					
Cause of death (ICD code)	I	II	IIIN	IIIM	IV	V
Cancer (140-209)	75	80	91	113	116	131
Ischemic heart disease (410-414)	88	91	114	107	108	111
Diabetes mellitus (250)	84	93	111	98	111	128

SMR for total male population = 100.

job exposures. Thus, any comparison of cancer risks between jobs in different social classes (e.g., foundry workers versus clerical staff in the steel industry) will entail some degree of life-style-related confounding.

Recently, social class adjustment has been incorporated in such comparisons (Fox and Adelstein 1978). Using this social class adjustment, nearly 90% of the variation in cancer rates between Her Majesty's 25 official occupational orders can be eliminated.

However, this approach may well overcorrect. If, by way of extreme example, all blue-collar workers were at approximately equally increased risk of lung cancer because of real, yet distinctive, occupational exposures within specific jobs, then comparisons of blue-collar subgroups would indicate little difference in risk. That is, what might be regarded as shared risk due to similar life-style might actually be, at least partially, a shared risk due to similar levels of occupational carcinogen exposure. In terms of Figure 1, the distance between job A (with a putative lung cancer hazard) and the comparison job has been allowed to contract excessively.

A recent example from a study of large-bowel cancer in Dublin brewery workers, illustrates another facet of Figure 1—the importance of choice of a comparison population in terms of its life-style-derived risk of cancer X relative to that of the job A population.

There is evidence that high consumption of alcoholic drinks may increase the risk of rectal, and perhaps colon, cancer. Beer, in particular, has been implicated (Lancet 1980); a generous free daily ration of beer was available to these brewery workers, which accounted for their demonstrably high intake.

In a 20-year follow-up study (Dean et al. 1979), 32 deaths were observed from colon cancer and 32 from rectal cancer (Table 2). The latter number was clearly higher than the number expected, no matter what comparison population rectal cancer rates were used. However, for colon cancer, the choice of the comparison population was more critical.

Comparing a group of urban blue-collar brewery workers with a largely rural national population introduces substantial confounding due to life-style

Table 2
The Importance of Choosing an Appropriate Comparison Population: Observed and Expected Colorectal Cancer Deaths in a Cohort of Dublin Brewery Workers, 1954-1973

		Deaths expected, based on death rates in:		
Cancer	Deaths observed	Ireland	Dublin County	Dublin blue-collar workers
Colon	32	21.8	27.3	24.1
Rectum	32	13.6	18.2	19.7

differences. Colon cancer rates are generally higher in urban populations, reflecting higher living standards and the associated dietary profile. However, to compare these workers with the entire urban population of Dublin probably reverses the direction of the confounding effect. White collar Dubliners, with their upper- and middle-class diets of 20-30 years' standing, would tend to have higher rates than the lower-class brewery workers.

In this instance, therefore, because occupational carcinogens per se generally are not implicated in colon cancer, the best comparison is with other Dublin blue-collar workers. The ratio of observed to expected deaths (32:24.1 = 1.33) indicates a 33% increase in colon cancer risk in the brewery workers, as compared with the initial overestimate of 47% and the subsequent underestimate of 17%.

INTERACTIVE POSSIBILITIES

Increasingly, carcinogenesis is viewed as a complex multistage process. While, for some cancers (e.g., radiation-induced leukemia), the difference in cancer risks between populations may primarily reflect a difference in exposure to initiating (i.e., cell-transforming) exposures, for many cancers such interpopulation differences probably reflect variation in the rate of growth of subclinical cancers.

In seeking to apportion cancer causality, it is important for epidemiologists to supplement—perhaps replace, even—the conventional empirical approach with one informed by some biological insight. In a recent review of environmental carcinogenesis from an epidemiologic perspective, MacLure and MacMahon (1980) wrote that:

> while others draw subtle distinctions between carcinogens and co-carcinogens, epidemiologists are hardly yet in a position to make operational distinctions between initiators and promoters. These limitations in theory may not be limitations in practice. Knowledge that

an agent increases the risk of cancer is of primary importance; how it does so is usually a secondary question.

Now, that is a seductive, no-nonsense approach, obviously useful to empiricists responsible for primary prevention. However, it invites either imprecision or misinterpretation in the contributory quantification of cancer causation. Indeed, a different approach has been advocated by Higginson and Muir (1979), who conclude, in a review of environmental carcinogenesis, that most cancers of presumed environmental etiology cannot readily be ascribed to industrial exposures, either point source or general, or even to identified cultural habits such as smoking or drinking. They suggest that experimental work with the recently emergent life-style factors that characterize contemporary Western society, such as with dietary fiber deficiency, excess fat and caloric intake, and reproductive and sex hormonal perturbations, imply a multistage carcinogenesis in humans in which the impact of physicochemical initiators is subordinate to cocarcinogenic and promotional factors.

If dietary factors and sex hormones affected predominantly those cancer sites most often implicated in occupational cancer—lung, upper aerodigestive tract, bladder, and hematopoietic tissues—then apportioning causality would become formidable. The fact that they predominantly influence cancers of the gastrointestinal and endocrine-dependent systems makes the task a little simpler.

However, consider again a currently topical example relating to cancer of the lung. (This is one, relatively straightforward, example among many that might have been chosen.) Both animal and human evidence indicate a cancer-protective effect of "vitamin A" precursors or analogs under most circumstances, although tumor enhancement also has been observed (Schroder and Black 1980). For example, Saffiotti et al. (1967) found that oral vitamin A administered to Syrian golden hamsters after intratracheal installation of benzo[*a*]pyrene markedly inhibited not only mucous-to-squamous differentiation, but also the ensuing carcinogenesis. In humans, a protective effect has been reported in both follow-up and case-control epidemiological studies (Bjelke 1975; Basu et al. 1976; Hirayama 1979; Wald et al. 1980), indicating approximately a twofold difference in risk across the range of vitamin A status. Similarly, a twofold risk gradient for human bladder cancer in relation to variation in dietary vitamin A intake has been reported in a large case-control study in the United States (Mettlin and Graham 1979).

Population subgroups eating diets high in meat, dairy foods, and fresh fruit and vegetables have a high intake of vitamin A or its carotenoid precursors. Indeed, not only might such persons be relatively protected by vitamin A against respiratory carcinogens, but the high vegetable intake may well afford other protective effects via the stimulation by other micronutrients (e.g., indoles) of microsomal enzymatic detoxification of carcinogens (Wattenberg 1971, 1978).

There is abundant evidence of intrapopulation variation in vitamin A status. In the United Kingdom earlier this century, a threefold difference in intake of vitamin A was reported across six socioeconomic classes (Orr 1936). The highest class, compared to the lowest class, also had a five times higher intake of fruit and vegetables. More recently, similar, although less striking, dietary gradients were reported across four income-defined strata (National Food Survey Committee 1976).

Likewise, within the United States recently, marked variations in human liver concentrations of vitamin A have been reported between geographic regions and between races. Mean concentrations decreased geographically from 223 μg/g in Missouri, through Ohio, Iowa, and California, to 92 μg/g in Texas (Raica et al. 1972). In males, in each of four age groups, whites had concentrations twice those of blacks (Mitchell et al. 1973).

The U.S. national health and nutrition survey (DHEW 1979) recently demonstrated socioeconomic class and race gradients in dietary vitamin A intake. Whites consume more than blacks; persons above the poverty line consume more than persons below.

Clearly, there is likely to be considerable vitamin A-related variation, between individuals and between subgroups, in susceptibility to occupational respiratory carcinogens. This, if not perceived, could produce a simplistic attribution of sole cancer causality to the occupational factor; and the size of this misestimated attribution would depend on the relative vitamin A status of the compared groups.

Further, if two compared populations differ in both smoking profile and in vitamin A status, "standardization" via the conventional arithmetic for the confounding effects of smoking would be inappropriate. Because the lung cancer-producing effect of the smoking would depend in turn upon the vitamin A status of the smokers, standardization for smoking would merely render the compared groups equal in their "on-paper" exposure to cigarettes, but would not render them equal in their cigarette-related risk of lung cancer. After all, the purpose of such adjustment procedures is to standardize for extraneous risk, not for extraneous risk factors. Specifically, in this example, the adjustment should be for the smoking-related effect, not for the smoking behavior.

This proposition is illustrated in simplified fashion in Figure 2. On the left, the two compared populations (occupationally exposed and nonexposed), with different proportions of smokers (30% and 50%, respectively), have a relative risk (RR) of lung cancer of 1.5. Unknown to the observer, however, their actual smoking-related lung cancer rates are identical, because the population that smokes less is also less vitamin A sufficient, and therefore more susceptible to the carcinogenic effect of smoking. In terms of this biological reality, there is no need to standardize for smoking; indeed, the conventional attempt to do this (Fig. 2, right) actually introduces smoking-related confounding and increases the RR to 2.0.

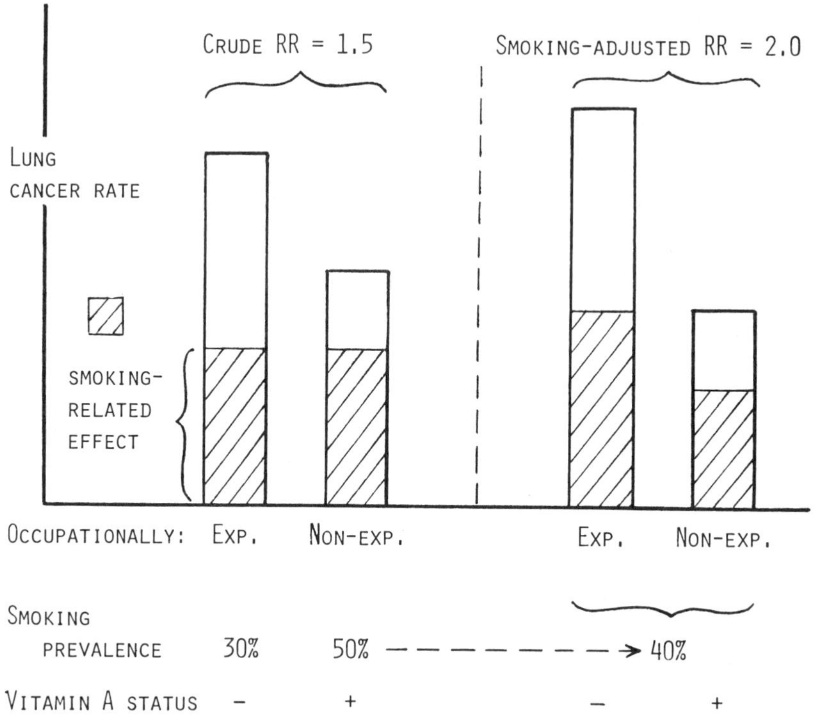

Figure 2
Schematic representation of the effect of inappropriate "standardization" for smoking by ignoring the dependence of its effect upon a second factor (vitamin A status).

Rather, one should make no adjustment for smoking, but instead make an adjustment for the modifying effect of vitamin A upon the extent of the occupation-related cancer risk. If that were done, then the relative difference in the heights of the bars on the left of Figure 2 would actually decrease. That is, the RR would become, say, 1.3.

One can perhaps argue about what this example signifies in terms of conventionally defined confounding effects. However, vitamin A status, not in itself an independent risk factor, is clearly muddying the waters of comparison, and must therefore be taken into account in estimating the occupation-related cancer risk. In more sophisticated data analyses, such effects could be incorporated in multivariate models. The basic point, however, is not to overlook them because of one's preoccupation with the more accessible and conventional, empirical, risk factors.

This one example, vitamin A status in relation to respiratory carcinogenesis, has been chosen because of both the central importance of this malignancy to occupational cancer and the current interest in vitamin A in human carcinogenesis. However, the more general point is that variations in life-style—particularly eating, drinking, and physical activity—directly influence the body's metabolic and hormonal phenomena. On the finely balanced scales of stable cellular biology, the likelihood of malignant transformation or neoplastic progression is very much influenced by these coexistent but often less tangible phenomena.

CONCLUSION

The distinction between "occupation" and "life-style" may be a tenuous one for a sociologist. For an epidemiologist, this distinction must nevertheless be borne in mind when attempting to understand and quantify occupation-related cancers. Interactive effects, or, speaking more broadly, potentiating or suppressing influences, are especially important considerations.

Finally, although many workplace carcinogens clearly derive from the work environment per se, and are therefore experienced involuntarily, where does one draw the occupation-life-style line in some other circumstances?

Table 3 data from Australian male mortality at ages 30-64 during 1968-1976 (McMichael and Hartshorne 1980), that hotel workers and entertainers have elevated risks of cancer of the upper alimentary tract. They also have high mortality from those sentinel diseases of alcohol and tobacco exposure, liver cirrhosis, and lung cancer. The same is true for storemen, freight, and waterside workers. Medical practitioners, administrators and executives, by comparison, appear to have drunk less alcohol and smoked fewer cigarettes and to have had below-average mortality from those cancers. However, their relative abstinence over earlier decades had apparently not encroached upon their upper-

Table 3

Age-standardized RR of Death from Selected Cancers, by Occupation, in Australian Males Aged 30-64, 1968-1976.

	Cause of death			
Occupation	liver cirrhosis	lung cancer	Cancer of mouth, pharynx, and esophagus	colon cancer
Medical practitioners	0.70	0.59	0.71	1.19
Administrators, executives	0.78	0.93	0.77	1.51
Entertainers	1.91	1.32	1.61	0.91
Hotel workers	3.50	1.66	2.28	0.83
Storemen, freight and waterside workers	1.70	1.34	1.54	0.98

Australian male population = 1.00.

class diets high in fat, meat, and fiber-depleted foods, and their colon cancer mortality was noticeably higher than in the three other occupational groups.

Where does occupation end and life-style begin? Consider a barman having a hurried couple of off-duty drinks with his best customers; a nervous entertainer having an offstage smoke; or a businessman clinching a deal over a public relations-inspired steak-and-egg dinner.

In summary, therefore, whether or not we are always able to differentiate life-style from occupation, we must certainly not neglect the confounding and interactive effects of off-the-job factors in our quantification of occupational cancer.

REFERENCES

Basu, T.K., D. Donaldson, H. Jenner, D.C. Williams, and A. Sakula. 1976. Plasma vitamin A in patients with bronchial carcinoma. *Br. J. Cancer* **33**: 119.

Bjelke, E. 1975. Dietary vitamin A and human lung cancer. *Int. J. Cancer* **15**:561.

Dean, G., R. MacLennan, H. McLoughlin, and E. Shelley. 1979. Causes of death of blue-collar workers at a Dublin brewery. *Br. J. Cancer* **40**:581.

DHEW (Department of Health, Education, and Welfare). 1979. *Dietary intake source data. United States, 1971-74,* 1-26. Publication No. (PHS) 79-1221, Hyattsville, Maryland.

Farr, W. 1885. *Vital Statistics,* (ed. N. Humphreys.), p. 150. Edward Stanford, London.

Fox, A.J. and A.M. Adelstein. 1978. Occupational mortality: Work or way of life. *J. Epidemiol. Community Health* **32**:73.

Higginson, J. and C.S. Muir. 1979. Environmental carcinogenesis: Misconceptions and limitations to cancer control. *J. Natl. Cancer Inst.* **63**:1291.

Hirayama, T. 1979. Diet and Cancer. *Nutrition and Cancer* **1**:67.

Lancet. 1980. Beer and bowel cancer. *Lancet* **ii**:1396.

MacLure, K.M. and B. MacMahon. 1980. An epidemiologic perspective of environmental carcinogenesis. *Am. J. Epidemiol.* **2**:19.

McMichael, A.J. and J.M. Hartshorne. 1980. Cardiovascular disease and cancer mortality in Australia, by occupation, in relation to drinking, smoking and eating. *Community Health Studies* **4**:76.

Mettlin, C. and S. Graham. 1979. Dietary risk factors in human bladder cancer. *Am. J. Epidemiol.* **110**:255.

Mitchell, G.V., M. Young, and C.R. Seward. 1973. Vitamin A and carotene levels of a selected population in metropolitan Washington, DC. *Am. J. Clin. Nutr.* **26**:992.

National Food Survey Committee. 1976. *Household food, consumption and expenditure: 1974,* p. 33. Her Majesty's Stationery Office, London.

Orr, J.B. 1936. *Food health and income.* MacMillan and Co., London.

Raica, N., J. Scott, L. Lowry, and H. E. Sauberlich. 1972. Vitamin A concentration in human tissues collected from five areas in the United States. *Am. J. Clin. Nutr.* **25**:291.

Registrar-General. 1978. *Decennial supplement for England and Wales, 1970-72: Occupational mortality,* p. 60. Office of Population Censuses and Surveys, Her Majesty's Stationery Office, London.

Rothman, K.J., S. Greenland, and A.M. Walker. 1980. Concepts of interaction. *Am. J. Epidemiol.* **112**:467.

Saffiotti, U., R. Montesano, A.R. Sellakumar, and S.A. Borg. 1967. Studies on experimental lung cancer: Inhibition by vitamin A of the induction of tracheobronchial squamous metaplasia and squamous cell tumours. *Cancer* **20**:857.

Schroder, E.W. and P.H. Black. 1980. Retinoids: Tumour preventers or tumour enhancers? *J. Natl. Cancer Inst.* **65**:671.

Tuyns, A.J. 1979. Epidemiology of alcohol and cancer. *Cancer Res.* **39**:2840.

Wald, N., M. Idle, J. Boreham, and A. Bailey. 1980. Low serum-vitamin-A and subsequent risk of cancer. *Lancet* **ii**:813.

Wattenberg, L.W. 1971. Studies of polycyclic hydrocarbon hydroxylases of the intestine possibly related to cancer. Effect of diet. *Cancer* **28**:99.

———. 1978. Inhibition of chemical carcinogenesis. *J. Natl. Cancer Inst.* **60**:11.

Wynder, E.L. 1977. Cancer prevention: A question of priorities. *Nature* **268**: 284.

COMMENTS

RADFORD: I think it might be useful for this meeting to focus on a point that Dr. McMichael has stressed here, and that is the extent to which we think environmental factors, to which everybody conventionally associates 80-90% of cancer, are in fact initiators or promoters. It is my perception that, generally speaking, we are talking about initiators. In other words, asbestos may be an exception, but, by and large, most of the carcinogens are perceived as DNA reactors, and this is thought to be related to the initiating step.

Now to give a very specific example, one of the most remarkable facts in carcinogenesis in man occurs in the case of ionizing radiation, for which we have at least some idea of the biochemical steps by which the DNA reaction occurs. When you look at human studies over the globe (and we have enough epidemiology that covers the globe so that we can make this kind of statement), the quantitative risk of induction of cancer in man by radiation is very similar when you compare Swedes to British to Japanese to Americans. This is so against the background of natural cancer rates that are very different in these countries. So it appears that in this case the critical step is the induction of a change at some point, though perhaps not manifested for 40 years afterwards. This change, presumably an initiated cell or cells, controls the subsequent probability of developing a cancer.

McMICHAEL: That seems to be a fair reading of the data; radiation carcinogenesis does seem to be a more clear-cut situation. If there are cocarcinogenic or promotional influences, I don't think we understand them very well. For leukemia, in particular, there are no major social class gradients that would imply "life-style" modulation of radiation effects. However, unlike most of the occupational carcinogens with which we're concerned, radiation is not a chemical carcinogen.

RADFORD: Leukemia is only a minor radiation-induced cancer. There are a lot of other more important cancers induced.

McMICHAEL: Yes. With respect to lung cancer, epidemiologists thought the early data indicated promotional relationships between ionizing radiation and cigarette smoking. This, however, may be a misreading of time-censored data.

CAIRNS: My understanding is that cigarettes have a promoting action and that this helps to explain the curve of incidence against time when people stop smoking.

RADFORD: In addition, the data for radiation tell me that the promoter stages, or the vitamin A influencing viral infections, or whatever, are so widespread in human populations that they no longer become a critical issue in human cancer induction. In other words, the promoters are so widely distributed that it is the initiating step that triggers the whole process and that is required to cause an increased risk of cancer.

SARACCI: There is one point that I want to make about the quantification of cancer and what you are saying about the possible complex interaction or confounding, as in the case of occupation, smoking, and vitamin A. However, we should not lose sight of the situation in which you have a series of interacting factors, and the possibility that a certain amount of cancer could be avoidable by suppressing one or two of the other factors. This was brought home to me very clearly by the classic example of asbestos and smoking. If you look at it in different ways, you can reach very different conclusions. My own conclusion is that, basically, the two have almost the same importance in most situations, but this equal importance doesn't appear if you express it in terms of the relative risk.

McMICHAEL: I can't disagree with you in principle. The problem is that the more we take account of the many etiological components of carcinogenesis, the more we find that we haven't made the measurements necessary to make the refined estimates. Maybe we don't have to worry ourselves about this sort of ultrarefinement. But if we are being too unrefined, as I think we've been in the last 48 hours, in trying to distinguish between just two candidate carcinogens—workplace or cigarettes—then we certainly are going to make mistakes.

SIEMIATYCKI: Quantification of the amount of cancer due to the occupational environment is a somewhat academic issue which is quite subtle. For instance, it is likely that nearly 100% of human cancer is due to genetics and nearly 100% is due to environment. This is because the web of causation of each case probably includes some genetic and some environmental components. Thus, we find that genetics and environment account for 200% of cases. When we start subdividing the environment into occupational, dietary, social and so on, we end up with many hundreds of percent of the cases attributable to various causes. We can get into all kinds of inferrential traps by ignoring the somewhat arbitrary nature of any estimates of proportion of cancer due to occupation. The important issue is: where can you break the chain of events which lead to cancer? This is where the occupational environment may be a particularly important one to study.

McMICHAEL: I must emphasize that we are not just adding simple, independent effects. We also are talking about conditional, or interactive, effects.

Also, we can't be sure of the relative length of the causal chain at the initiational or early stages, and at the later, promotional stages. Incidentally, I wonder if the human body may have, through evolution, become more efficient in its defenses against initiating-type events than against promotional influences. Factors causing chromosomal damage, whether preneoplastic or otherwise, have threatened cellular functioning throughout human evolution; however, the sorts of promotional effects that we have discussed, relating to diet, the hormonal consequences of altered reproductive practices, or massive consumption of cigarettes or alcohol, are relatively recent in human biological experiences—and would have exerted their adverse biological effect mostly after an individual's reproductive life was completed anyway. That is why I take seriously the prospect that promotional effects may make major contributions to variations in the rates of clinically manifest cancers in human populations.

Towards Strategy for the Identification of Occupational Carcinogens in England and Wales — A Preliminary Report

E. DONALD ACHESON, MARTIN J. GARDNER, and PAUL D. WINTER
MRC Environmental Epidemiology Unit
University of Southampton
Southampton, SO9 4XY, England

This paper gives a brief preliminary account of work recently commenced at the Medical Research Council's Environmental Epidemiology Unit at Southampton with special reference to studies on the geography of cancer mortality and its relationship to the distribution of industry and other factors. The design of the studies has been influenced by the work of Dr. Robert Hoover and his colleagues at the National Cancer Institute (Mason and McKay 1973; Hoover et al. 1975). The aim of our work is to seek new clues in the causation of cancer.

MATERIALS AND METHODS

The Unit has obtained from the Office of Population Censuses and Surveys (OPCS) computer tapes of data relating to all deaths that occurred in England and Wales during the 21-year period 1959-1979. Five items of information are available about each death—namely, year, age, sex, place of residence, and underlying cause coded according to the International Classification of Diseases (ICD, 7th, 8th, and 9th revisions). The data relate to almost 12 million deaths. It is planned to prepare maps of the distribution of mortality from cancer by site of tumor and sex for the 1366 Local Authority areas in England and Wales as designated in 1971.

In the analysis of the geographical patterns, correlations will be made with indicators of environmental and social factors such as the distribution of industry, and population density, and data about home amenities and personal possessions derived from the censuses of England and Wales (OPCS 1972). Additional information, for example about smoking and diet, will be obtained from the General Household Survey and other sources, but it is likely that for this part of the analysis it will be necessary to aggregate Local Authority areas (OPCS 1973).

The results described in this paper relate to preparatory work for this analysis. The mortality data used are derived from the Area Mortality analysis for England and Wales for 1969-1973, which gives information about selected causes of death for the principal towns and all the counties (OPCS 1979). Information about the distribution of industry has been derived from data about economic activity collected from a 10% sample of the population of England and Wales at the 1971 Census and supplied by OPCS. The data so far available to us on industry are classified by the geographical location of the place of work, not by place of residence as for deaths. Data relating to smoking and other social factors are not yet available.

The Unit is also engaged in studies designed to identify risk factors for cancer in young men and women. As a first step we have selected men aged 18-54 with cancers of all anatomical sites and resident in areas of England and Wales where 10% or more of the male population is employed in the chemical industry. We are collecting occupational and smoking histories on a sample that we estimate will amount to about 3000 men. At a later stage, the job titles given by the men will be analyzed in terms of the specific chemicals to which they are likely to have been exposed during the relevant periods. For each site of cancer, the combined experience of men with all other types of cancer will be used as controls.

Starting from the lists of substances classified by IARC, we are attempting to produce a short list of those substances for which in terms of size of exposed population, date of introduction, presence of otherwise confounding substances, and other practical considerations, there seems to be a reasonable case for a cohort study. We are studying amosite asbestos, glass fiber, formaldehyde, styrene, and cadmium and have others under consideration.

RESULTS

Geographical Distribution of Cancer Mortality

Standard mortality ratios (SMRs) are available for each of the 83 County Boroughs and 58 Administrative Counties of England and Wales by sex for all cancers and for cancers of 19 individual sites, including bronchus, stomach, bladder, skin, leukemia, etc. Because of the very high frequency with which people travel across area boundaries to work in Greater London, the individual London boroughs have been excluded from this preliminary study.

A study of the geography of the mortality from all cancers combined and from lung cancer reveals some similarities with the geographical pattern of mortality as a whole in England and Wales, with higher rates in the north and west than the south and east. The pattern of mortality from stomach cancer also is similar except that the well-known increased mortality in Wales is clearly seen. These patterns are historically of long standing and have been noted by Stocks, Howe, and others (Stocks 1947; Howe 1970). They are due to a complex of risk factors, many of which are unknown. The pattern of mortality from bladder cancer differs from those already mentioned in that the regions

Table 1
County Boroughs and Administrative Counties with Significantly High SMRs from Bladder Cancer ($p<0.01$) from 141 Areas in England and Wales (1969-1973) by Sex

Men only	Women only	Both sexes
Barrow	Blackburn	Brighton
Huddersfield	Gloucester	
Leeds	Hull	
Liverpool	Oldham	
St. Helens	West Riding	

with high mortality in men are limited to Yorkshire, the northwest, and the southeast.

Although more occupational carcinogens have been identified in the causation of cancer of the bronchus than for any other site, it is fruitless to consider the industrial geography of lung cancer without data about smoking. These are not yet available. Therefore, we have decided to use as an example the mortality from bladder cancer where occupational carcinogens are also important and smoking less so.

Table 1 shows County Boroughs and Administrative Counties in England and Wales with a significantly high ($p < 0.01$) SMR from bladder cancer for the years 1969-1973 by sex. The highest SMRs were 160 for men (Barrow and Huddersfield) and 159 for women (Brighton). As far as the Boroughs where there is a high risk of bladder cancer in men are concerned, Huddersfield and Leeds are two of the principal centers of the British dyestuffs manufacturing industry, St. Helens is a center of the plastics and synthetics industry, and Liverpool has several rubber factories. The reason for the high SMR in Barrow is less obvious as this is virtually a one-industry town where in 1971 40% of the male work force was employed in shipbuilding. However, some dyestuffs were manufactured in the vicinity there at least until 1954. This town also has in common with Huddersfield a concentration of precision engineering manufacturers.

As far as the high SMRs for women are concerned, Oldham and Blackburn are centers of the dyeing and finishing industry for textiles in which women are traditionally employed and Oldham is also a center of the rubber industry. The reasons for the excesses of bladder cancer in Gloucester and in Hull are less obvious although there is small rubber factory in Gloucester and paints, dyes and inks, and rubber are manufactured in Hull. West Riding is the area of Yorkshire where the manufacture of woolen textiles is concentrated and it is possible that the use of dyestuffs in these factories may have increased the SMR from bladder cancer in women in this area.

Table 2
Numbers of Areas with Significantly High SMR for Bladder Cancer (1969-1973) in Which Various Industries Were Located

Industry	SMRs for bladder cancer	
	high areas	low areas
Rubber	6	3
Tires	1	1
Dyestuffs	5	0
Wires and cables	3	8
Paints	3	0
Numbers of areas	11	11

The distribution of the same industries in 11 areas with the lowest SMRs for bladder cancer are also shown.

Data from Blackman (1963).

The substantial excesses of mortality from bladder cancer in both sexes in the seaside town of Brighton on the south coast of England was a surprise. It is being investigated further.

Correlations with the Distribution of Industry

Using an atlas showing the distribution of industry in England and Wales in 1954, we have compared the eleven County Boroughs with significantly high SMRs (1967-1973) in men with the eleven County Boroughs with the lowest SMRs in respect to mentions of dyestuffs, rubber, tire-making, paints, plastics, and cable industries. The results (Table 2) show that more of the towns with low SMRs had firms in the cable and wire industry. One each of the towns with high and low SMRs had a tire factory.

Correlations have been studied for all causes of death, all cancers combined, and for some specific sites of cancer separately with the proportions of men employed in the various orders of industry in 1971. A number of the significant correlations found reflect unfavorable social factors that operate in those parts of the country in which certain industries are concentrated. The interpretation of these must await correction for social factors, smoking, degree of urbanization, etc.

Table 3 shows the significant correlations ($p < 0.05$) between bladder cancer SMRs for 141 County Boroughs and Administrative Counties and the percentage of men employed in various industrial orders in 1971. The correlation coefficients for all malignant neoplasms are also shown. They are all small. All but one of the classes of industry that have a distribution correlated significantly with bladder cancer are also correlated significantly with all malignant neoplasms combined. This fact together with the fact that no significant correlation was found between mortality from bladder cancer and IX Electrical Engineering (which includes the cable industry) or XIX Other Manufacturing (which includes the rubber industry) suggests that the study of correlations between cancer mortality and aggregations of industry classified in this way is too insensitive a method to be of much practical value. Our future studies will, however, disaggregate the 29 industrial orders into some 200 smaller components. At present, there is no obvious explanation for the correlation (for which there is no parallel with all malignant neoplasms) between bladder cancer and the distributive trades.

Bladder Cancer and the Chemical Industry

Hoover and Fraumeni have studied cancer mortality in U.S. counties with chemical industries (Hoover and Fraumeni 1975). We are carrying out similar studies in England. In the British Classification of Industry, the manufacture of chemicals and allied products is divided into nine subgroups–general chemicals, pharmaceuticals, toilet preparations, paint, synthetic resins, dyestuffs and pigments, fertilizers, and other chemicals. Table 4 shows the significant relationships between SMRs (men, all ages) from bladder cancer and the percentages of men employed in the subgroups of the chemical industry in 141 county boroughs and administrative counties. The strongest correlation (r = 0.30, $p < 0.01$) was with employment in the dyestuffs and pigments industry. Taking this figure at its face value, it suggests that not more than about 10% of the variation between the areas is associated with the dyestuffs industry. A significant correlation was also found with the manufacture of soaps and

Table 3
Significant Correlations ($p < 0.05$) between SMRs for Bladder Cancer in Men (1969-1973) and Percentage of Men Employed in 141 Areas in England and Wales by Industrial Order

	Category of industry	Bladder cancer	All malignant neoplasms
V	Chemicals	0.16	0.18
VII	Mechanical engineering	0.18	0.18
X	Shipbuilding	0.22	0.22
XVIII	Paper, printing	0.26	0.15
XXII	Transport	0.38	0.52
XXIII	Distributive	0.26	0.05
XXIV	Insurance, banking	0.20	0.22

Correlation coefficients for all malignant neoplasms are also shown.

Table 4
Relationship between SMRs (males, all ages) from Bladder Cancer (1969-1973) and Percentages of Men Employed in Chemical Industry (1971) in 141 County Boroughs and Administrative Counties in England and Wales

Category within chemical industry	SMR from bladder cancer				Correlation coefficient
	< 80	80-99	100-119	120+	
General chemicals	0.7	0.9	1.2	0.5	0.04
Pharmaceuticals	0.2	0.3	0.3	0.3	0.09
Toilet preparations	0.05	0.07	0.04	0.1	-0.03
Paint	0.2	0.1	0.09	0.2	0.04
Soap and detergents	0.01	0.1	0.07	0.2	0.19[a]
Synthetic resins	0.2	0.4	0.4	0.1	0.03
Dyestuffs and pigments	0.03	0.05	0.2	0.4	0.30[b]
Fertilizers	0.03	0.06	0.2	0.1	0.06
Other chemicals	0.2	0.3	0.1	0.2	-0.09
All categories	1.7	2.3	2.7	2.0	0.16[a]
Number of areas	21	59	44	17	

[a] $p < 0.05$
[b] $p < 0.01$

detergents ($r = 0.19, p = < 0.05$). The latter relationship may be nonspecific as there is also a significant correlation ($r = 0.28, p < 0.01$) with mortality from all malignant neoplasms combined, unlike the dyestuffs and pigments industry where the correlation coefficient with all malignant neoplasms is small ($r = 0.05$, $p > 0.05$). No significant correlations were found between SMRs for bladder cancer in women and the proportions of men employed in the various divisions of the chemical industry in the 141 areas. Unlike the U. S. material, the British analysis has not shown a relationship between bladder cancer mortality and the manufacture of toilet preparations or pharmaceuticals.

DISCUSSION

The geographical pattern of bladder cancer in England and Wales during the years 1969-1973 demonstrated in this paper shows signs of the influence of exposure of men and women in the workplace to carcinogenic aromatic amines manufactured in the dyestuffs industry and used in the textile and rubber industries. Correlation of bladder cancer mortality with the proportions of men employed in the 29 orders of industry did not yield a pattern that pointed clearly to the influence of the aromatic amines. However, when the relationship of the employment of men in the component divisions of the chemical industry to the mortality from bladder cancer was studied, a highly significant correlation was found. More detailed studies of other sections of industry may reveal correlations with work in the rubber and cable industries.

The industrial data currently available to us are unsatisfactory because they are classified according to place of work, whereas the mortality data are classified according to place of residence at death. The effect of cross-boundary movement from home to work reduces the sensitivity of the method.

In view of the period of years that usually elapses between exposure to a carcinogen and the appearance of a related tumor, it is unfortunate that the industrial and mortality data are derived from the same period. Industrial data from the censuses of 1951 or 1961 would have been more appropriate but the information is not easily accessible to computers. As 2-naphthylamine and benzidine were not withdrawn from use until 1954 and 1968, respectively, it is possible that the excess mortality noted in 1969-1973 was related to the manufacture and use of these substances.

Another reason for lack of sensitivity when dealing with only 5 years mortality experience (1969-1973) is that the number of deaths on which the SMRs are based are quite small for many cancers with lower mortality rates. Thus, for bladder cancer, typically 30 deaths would occur in an average county borough over 5 years. Determining high areas on the basis solely of the statistical significance of the SMR, as we have done in this paper, will necessarily exclude some areas with a real excess but which do not, because of small numbers, reach significance. Extra years data, together with taking account of an area's ranking in the SMRs, will improve the situation.

It is also possible that an improvement in sensitivity of the method may be obtained by extending the analysis from 141 large areas to 1366 much smaller areas by splitting down the Administrative Counties into their component parts (Urban Districts, Municipal Boroughs, and Rural Districts). This will produce greater homogeneity in that other major industrial centers will be identified individually and separated from more rural areas. Also, the effects of exposure to multiple carcinogens in the same small area will be less–whether they be other industrial or occupational exposures or personal, social, or general environmental factors–and relationships between mortality and industry should become clearer. The most that can be expected from this approach, however, is the identification of clues that can form the basis of hypotheses to be tested by other more rigorous methods, e.g., case-control and cohort studies (Blot et al. 1979).

ACKNOWLEDGMENTS

We would like to thank Miss R. Kirby for compiling the data and assistance with computer programming.

REFERENCES

Blackman, G.E. (ed.) 1963. *Atlas of Britain and Northern Ireland*, p. 193. University Press, Oxford.

Blot, W.J., J. F. Fraumeni, Jr., T.J. Mason, and R.N. Hoover. 1979. Developing clues to environmental cancer: A stepwise approach with the use of cancer mortality data. *Environ. Health Perspect.* **32**:53.

Hoover, R. and J.F. Fraumeni. 1975. Cancer mortality in U.S. counties with chemical industries. *Environ. Res.* **9**:196.

Hoover, R., T.J. Mason, F.W. McKay, and J.F. Fraumeni. 1975. Geographic patterns of cancer mortality in the United States. In *Persons at high risk of cancer: An approach to cancer aetiology and control* (ed. J.F. Fraumeni), p. 343. Academic Press, London.

Howe, G.M. 1970. *National atlas of disease mortality in the United Kingdom*. Nelson, London.

Mason, T.J. and F.W. McKay. 1973. *U.S. cancer mortality by county: 1950-69.* U.S. Government Printing Office, Washington, D.C.

Office of Population Censuses and Surveys (OPCS). 1972. *Census 1971, England and Wales, County Reports.* HMSO, London.

———. 1973. *The general household survey*. HMSO, London.

———. 1979. *Area mortality tables: The Registrar-General's decennial supplement for England and Wales 1969-73.* Series DS No. 3. HMSO, London.

Stocks, P. 1947. *Regional and local differences in cancer death rates: General Register Office studies on medical and population subjects No. 1.* HMSO, London.

Occupational Studies — The Use of National and Industrial Comparisons or an Internal Analysis

MICHAEL ALDERSON
Division of Epidemiology
Institute of Cancer Research: Royal Cancer Hospital
Sutton, Surrey SM2 5PX England

HISTORICAL ASPECTS

For over 100 years, there has been gradual progress in the way studies may be done to compare the mortality of different populations. The Registrar General (1855) wrote, "The professions and occupations of men open a new field of enquiry, on which we are now prepared to enter, not unconscious, however, of peculiar difficulties that beset all enquiries into the mortality of limited, fluctuating, and sometimes ill-defined sections of the population." Attention was drawn to the inaccuracy of the Classification of Occupations and the need to study age-specific mortality rates rather than crude rates when comparing different occupations. Neison (1844) advocated a method whereby the difference in the age distribution of the population at risk could be taken into account by a method of standardization. This was the technique subsequently used for the Registrar General's Decennial Supplements from 1851 onwards when comparing either occupation or location (Farr 1859).

Limited attention was paid to subsequent statistics by Farr (1864, 1875). The first detailed analysis of the problems involved in the interpretation of occupational mortality data was by Ogle (1885); he gave a clear description of the selection processes into and out of occupations. Further attention was paid to this problem of selection into and out of occupation by Tatham (1902, 1908) and Collis and Greenwood (1921).

Stocks (1938) presented evidence suggesting that variation in male mortality in England and Wales was influenced by housing, and to a lesser extent by social class and latitude. Attempts were made to distinguish the influence of a man's work, the industry in which he worked, and his general environment. Separate analyses of mortality by occupation and industry were carried out. The 1930-1932 Decennial Supplement attempted to permit examination of the influence of job, independent of industry and locality, by presenting cause-specific mortality for wives. Comparison of the direct influence of occupation was possible from the standardized mortality ratios (SMR) of men and their wives. It was accepted that the influence of selection might be responsible for farmers having a lower SMR than their wives, rather than from benefit of their actual work. (See Alderson [1972] for further discussion of the problems of such statistics.)

DEVELOPMENT OF CONVENTIONAL METHOD

The general method of using national mortality to generate an expected number of deaths in a particular occupation and thus derive an SMR was known long before there was an expansion in interest in carrying out specific studies on the health of groups of workers. For someone familiar with the application of the technique of standardization, it required only a little ingenuity to see that for groups followed over time (with the addition of recruits and deletion of leavers) the national mortality rates over the calendar period of follow-up could be applied to an estimate of the "population-at-risk" classified by age and calendar period. Case and Lea (1955) set out the technique for such studies. They acknowledged that an external standard may not be applicable to men in a particular study, and demonstrate how "industrial comparisons" could be made.

Many authors began to use this approach; the use of national mortality rates for succeeding specific time periods introduces a subtle but distinct change from the classic method of indirect standardization. Many authors still incorrectly refer to the results of $\frac{O}{E} \times 100$ as an SMR. Liddell (1960) reviewed the application of four methods of age-standardization and commented that no mortality index should be used without a knowledge of the inherent inadequacy due to variation in the relative death rates. Chiazze (1976) noted that an "SMR" is a statistic frequently used in evaluating industrial mortality, but interpretation only relates to the comparison population. Gaffey (1976) pointed out the difference between relative risk (RR), SMR, and life expectancy statistics and emphasized the care required in interpreting an SMR.

In the early 1950s there was considerable development in occupational mortality studies. In a note on statistical considerations, Cutler et al. (1954) discussed (1) calculation of the size of the study required, (2) sources of data, (3) comparison of the observed number of the deaths in a study with confidence limits and the overlap of the "expected" data. In a series of papers by Mancuso and his colleagues (1959, 1963, 1966, 1968), a number of topics were raised: dilution due to imprecise job descriptions; bias in follow-up with loss of death of some categories of individuals; the advantages of cross-checking death details, or multiple cause coding; the use of morbidity as an alternative end point; the healthy-worker effect and use of "worker's" rates; and the influence of age at entry, length of follow-up, age at death, and latent interval on the results. No solution to the latter problem was provided. Redmond and Breslin (1975) presented data indicating that an internally based "SMR" or RR was preferable to an internally based proportionate mortality ratio (PMR). Enterline (1976) also suggested that an internal comparison was ideal, but in its absence national rates may be adequate (depending on the selection into the study population, and whether the agent being studied had a constant effect on the absolute or relative risk of disease). Wong et al. (1978) had concluded that multiple-cause coding may not lead to a justifiable gain in information, in relation to cost.

Ott et al. (1976) used an external comparison as a preliminary to more detailed cohort analysis of Dow chemical workers. They acknowledged the influence of a range of factors contributing to differences in mortality between an industrial and general population.

In the period 1950-1975, there was only limited innovation in techniques for statistical analysis. For example, Knox et al. (1968) separated the subjects in their study into three categories of exposure. Expected values were obtained and a test for trend was applied to the observed and expected deaths across the categories of exposure. Unfortunately, no discussion is provided in their paper about the power of such analysis, nor alternative ways of analyzing such material.

In recent years there has been increasing disquiet about the suitability of the national rates to generate a valid expected number of deaths. In many studies this has resulted in a ratio of O/E considerably less than 1; often the all-cause figure is about 0.75 and some recent studies have reported even lower figures. This creates confusion in the interpretation of the data, because the lower figure should not be interpreted automatically as indicating absence of a health hazard. Also, when specific causes of death are examined, it has been suggested that the all-cause ratio may be used as a yardstick against which to measure results from specific causes. Thus, with an all-cause figure of 0.75, it has been claimed that a ratio of 1.00 for cancers is raised (i.e., represents an increment of one-third over the expected figure of 0.75). This will produce considerable argument over the interpretation of the data, especially where the results are based upon large numbers of deaths and such differences are statistically significant.

THE HEALTHY-WORKER EFFECT

Goldsmith (1975) criticized a number of authors for their use of expected deaths calculated from external rates and advocated (1) proportional mortality, (2) scaling of the ratio O/E down to 90%, and (3) use of pooled worker mortality rates. Enterline (1975) responded that worker populations did not usually have uniformly lowered rates for each cause of death, and that lack of "internal control rates" did not introduce a serious bias. Gaffey (1975) believed that worker rates would be of great benefit, but he also hinted at problems with the "SMR." He did not advocate use of proportional mortality. McMichael et al. (1975) indicated that the healthy-worker effect is linked to age of the cohort, bias may be greater for certain chronic disabling diseases rather than cancer, and adjustment for education, socioeconomic status, and region of residence may be required.

Fox and Collier (1976) used data from a vinyl chloride monomer study to quantify the relative influences of selection of people fit for work into industry, their continuing employment in industry, and the length of time over which the men had been followed. They suggested that mathematical models were an alternative method for analyzing mortality studies to assess the influence of these factors. Despite the use of the expression "healthy worker," it must be emphasized that some industries may recruit individuals of poor physique at risk of particular diseases; an example with risk of tuberculosis in shoemakers was described by Cairns and Stewart (1951). McMichael (1976) showed that the healthy-worker effect is marked in those recently recruited to an industry; if premature retirees are excluded, the "SMR" of those remaining at work is lower at age 64 than 58. He also emphasized the confounding between race and social class in the expected figures. Vinni and Hakama (1980) examined the influence of (1) the healthy population selection effect, and (2) the survivor population effect. They suggest that the combined effect can be quantified by examining the ratio of the SMR for all entrants to the SMR of those changing occupation or retiring prior to the age of 65.

Analyses may be done on a fictitious plant, with equal numbers of workers in four 10-year age groups, 20-29, 30-39, 40-49, 50-60, in the initial quinquennium. A turnover rate of 1.7% per annum in each age group occurs, with replacement of men of the same age. The national rates for a particular cancer are known, which double from one 10-year age group to the next; the plant hazard adds a risk of cancer equal to the initial population rate and remains constant throughout a 25-year period. The national rate is increasing at 1.7% per annum over the 25 years. The conventionally calculated ratios of O/E for the initial and four "replacement" cohorts are 1.68, 1.66, 1.63, 1.60, 1.59. Using the first quinquennia rates as standard, the ratios of O/E are 2.47, 2.52, 2.58, 2.66, 2.75.

These different trends are a reflection of the cohorts' aging across different quinquennia and the difference in the slight increase in population trend and the constant plant hazard over a 25-year period. It is suggested that neither the "conventional" O/E, nor an SMR should be used, but the difference in O - E after a second standardization for the cohort mortality trend. Work on this issue is being done in the Division of Epidemiology.

SOME INTERNAL ANALYSES

Oldham and Rossiter (1965) used a discriminant function (canonical variates of Rao) to give a linear combination of 18 measurements made on a sample of men, to distinguish those who died at various periods of follow-up. They obtained results that facilitated interpretation of the data and did not appear to be very dependent upon the distributional assumptions involved.

Liddell (1975) reported on a discussion held with a number of statisticians about the appropriate analysis of occupational cohort studies. This suggested (1) an a posteriori analysis (from effects to causal variates) to determine the best hypothesis, with probability statements adjusted for simultaneous inference; (2) a priori analysis (from hypothesized causes to effects) to obtain mortality rates for defined subcohorts; (3) summarization of the calculated rates in life-table form to compare subcohorts. Steps (2) and (3) were advocated without statistical testing. Application of such a strategy was reported by Liddell et al. (1977), who used a case-control method and the regression models of Cox (1972) for step (1). For the conventional a priori analysis, they used both province and industrial rates to calculate expected deaths. They suggested that it was useful to place the cohort in demographic context using the conventional analysis; the regression analysis was more complex than that of the case-control study, but could provide absolute risks if the complete data set were used. Cox (1972), in a mathematical paper on the use of regression models and life-tables, had pointed out that larger sample sizes and increase in the number of explanatory variables would make application more complicated.

McDonald et al. (1980) reported a further study where they contrasted the external and internal analyses. They suggested that the a posteriori analyses had the advantages that interaction between several variables could be examined and they avoided the requirement of external rates. The healthy-worker effect was commented upon, and it was stated that no observational study in epidemiology could correct for the influence of this.

Darby and Reissland (1981) studied men exposed to low-level irradiation at work; they developed a test for trend that examined the distribution of observed and expected deaths in dose categories across age (calendar period) and time since first employment strata. The expected values were calculated assuming no-dose effect. Strata with no deaths, or all-person years in one-dose category were excluded. It was not clear to what extent this restricted the use of the complete data set, but it was obviously part way between the case-control and regression approaches discussed above. These authors also carried out a conventional analysis with U.S. national rates; comparable results were obtained from both approaches. The authors drew attention to the tendency for healthier men to remain in the industry, and yet such men accumulated higher exposure to the hazard.

Alderson et al. (1981) were asked by the U.K. bichromate industry to check if control of environmental exposure had reduced the risk of lung cancer to an acceptable level. There was confounding between the duration of employment, length of follow-up, calendar period of employment, age at entry to work, and degree of chromate exposure. In addition, three locations were involved with a difference in the risk of lung cancer at each factory. In an attempt to quantify the relative importance of these different factors, a multiple regression analysis was performed. This used the scores for each individual on the various independent variates, and the dependent variate was recorded as "yes" or "no" to the question: Died from lung cancer? This permitted estimates to be made of the relative importance of the factors, but raised considerable problems in discussing the results with the industry concerned. The results were very different from the conventional ratios of O/E; this ratio was a biased estimate of risk for men who had only worked after the plant had been modified (though it was clear from the regression analysis that plant modification had made an appreciable impact upon the risk of lung cancer). The results of the usual analysis were used to present some answers to the industry concerned, but the internal analysis helped interpret the results and formulate sounder conclusions.

A very different approach to the above, which uses all the data available, is a case-control study within a major historical prospective study. Rushton and Alderson (1981) had carried out a follow-up of over 35,000 workers in U.K. oil refineries from 1950-1975; only limited details were available on the last job of each individual. For 36 men whose death certificates mentioned leukemia and two sets of matched controls, detailed job histories were obtained by special enquiry in each refinery; this permitted a working party to classify the potential benzene exposure of cases and controls. A logistic regression model was fitted to test the RR associated with benzene exposure and the influence of year of entry and length of service. Such an approach has two quite separate advantages over the conventional comparison of O and E for the complete set of workers: (1) detailed job history was only required for 252 individuals out of the 35,000 workers, (2) a much more flexible analysis is permitted by fitting the logistic regression model.

DISCUSSION

It is important to clarify what is the actual aim of the analysis; the technique used will be determined to some extent by the precise needs of the study. In general, the comparison of observed and expected deaths will be carried out in an occupational study in order to clarify one of the following:

1. Is there an etiological relationship? What is the influence of the selected independent variates upon the dependent variate? There will be need to quantify the influence of various confounding, intervening, and moderating factors.
2. Who is at risk? Are there specific categories of worker who are at risk? This may be influenced by the jobs they do, a particular age or sex susceptibility, pregnancy, other characteristics of the worker, and the distribution of the latent period.
3. How large is the risk? Though not necessarily explicitly requested, this will

require some indication of either the absolute or relative risk of the disease being studied.

4. What is happening to the risk? This may be the most important question for both management and unions; they will wish to know if the steps taken to control the environmental hazard are having a major or minor impact on the problem.

Use of National Comparison

It is accepted that use of national rates will generate an expected number of deaths on the low side for many industries. The reasons for this have already been described. In addition to age, there are a number of other demographic factors that are directly or indirectly linked to variation in mortality (e.g., social class and region of the country). The technique for adjustment for such factors exists, though the lack of relevant rates can pose a problem. For example, in England and Wales the mortality rates by region or social class have not been tabulated by as fine a classification of cause of death as for the country. Thus, it may be possible to adjust for the regional (or social class) variation in mortality for lung cancer, but not for cancer of the larynx. A rather different consideration is whether the statistics on social class variation in mortality are sufficiently valid to use for such an adjustment procedure. Comparison of patterns of mortality may be made with those individuals who only stay in industry a short period of time, the argument being that such individuals are more like those who remain in the industry than males from the country as a whole. However, there is the difficulty that those who stay in any industry only a short while are likely to be a very biased subgroup of the work force. They may differ in many characteristics themselves, they may have some specific allergy to the work conditions of the industry, or they may move to or from a job with other health hazards.

An Industry Comparison

One approach to overcome the defects of the use of national data has been to use industry-wide mortality rates to generate the expected number of deaths for particular groups of workers. The chief disadvantages are, presently, lack of available industry mortality rates and the fact that when calculated they may be based on relatively few deaths for many causes.

Use of an Internal Analysis

Conceptually quite different is the use of an internal comparison to analyze the influence of the occupational hazard. The general principle is that only the data collected in the specific study is used in an analysis of the relation of exposure to outcome. This is a relatively simple issue to explore where there is a single known or suspected industrial hazard affecting a specific cause of death. This approach provides the opportunity to collect detailed information about a subset of the study population—cases and controls; there also is a range of statistical analysis that may be explored that probes the data much more thoroughly than the descriptive presentation of ratios of O/E.

ACKNOWLEDGMENTS

I thank my colleagues in the Division of Epidemiology and in industry for discussion of points raised in this brief paper. My secretary, Mrs. D. Folkes, typed the material. It is a pleasure to record financial support from the Cancer Research Campaign.

REFERENCES

Alderson, M.R. 1972. Some sources of error in British occupational mortality data. *Br. J. Ind. Med.* **29**:245.

Alderson, M.R., N.S. Rattan, and L. Bidstrup. 1981. Health of workmen in the chromate-producing industry in Britain. *Br. J. Ind. Med.* (in press).

Cairns, M. and A. Stewart. 1951. Pulmonary tuberculosis mortality in the printing and shoemaking trades: Historical survey, 1881-1931. *Br. J. Soc. Med.* **5**:73.

Case, R.A.M. and A.J. Lea. 1955. Mustard gas poisoning, chronic bronchitis, and lung cancer. *Br. J. Prev. Soc. Med.* **9**:62.

Chiazze, L. 1976. Problems of study design and interpretation of industrial mortality experience. *J. Occup. Med.* **18**:169.

Collis, E.L. and M. Greenwood. 1921. *The health of the industrial worker,* p. 72. Churchill, London.

Cox, D.R. 1972. Regression models and life-tables. *J. R. Statis. Soc.* **34**:187.

Cutler, S.J., M.A. Schneiderman, and S.W. Greenhouse. 1954. Some statistical considerations in the study of cancer in industry. *Am. J. Public Health* **44**:1159.

Darby, S.C. and J.A. Reissland. 1981. Low levels of ionising radiation and cancer—are we underestimating the risk. *J. R. Stat. Soc. Series A.* (in press).

Enterline, P.E. 1975. Not uniformly true for each cause of death. *J. Occup. Med.* **17**:127.

———. 1976. What do we expect from an industrial cohort? Pitfalls in epidemiological research—an examination of the asbestos literature. *J. Occup. Med.* **18**:150.

Farr, W. 1859. Method of comparing the local rates of mortality with the standard rate. In *Annual report of the Registrar General of births, deaths, and marriages in England,* p. 174. Her Majesty's Stationery Office, London.

_____. 1864. *Supplement to the 25th Annual Report of the Registrar General*, p. 440. Her Majesty's Stationery Office, London.

_____. 1875. *Supplement to the 35th Annual Report of the Registrar General*, p. lii. Her Majesty's Stationery Office, London.

Fox, A.J. and P.F. Collier. 1976. Low mortality rates in industrial cohort studies due to selection for work and survival in the industry. *Br. J. Prev. Soc. Med.* **30**:225.

Gaffey, W.R. 1975. What do we expect from an occupational cohort? Cause specific mortality. *J. Occup. Med.* **17**:128.

_____. 1976. A critique of the standardised mortality rate. *J. Occup. Med.* **18**:157.

Goldsmith, J.R. 1975. What do we expect from an occupational cohort? *J. Occup. Med.* **17**:126.

Knox, J.F., S. Holmes, R. Doll, and I.D. Hill. 1968. Mortality from lung cancer and other causes among workers in an asbestos textile factory. *Br. J. Ind. Med.* **25**:293.

Liddell, F.D.K. 1960. The measurement of occupational mortality. *Br. J. Ind. Med.* **17**:228.

_____. 1975. Occupational mortality in relation to exposure. *Arch. Environ. Health* **30**:266.

Liddell, F.D.K., J.C. McDonald, and D.S. Thomas. 1977. Methods of cohort analysis: Appraised by application to asbestos mining. *J. R. Stat Soc. Series A.* **140**:469.

McDonald, J.C., F.D.K. Liddell, G.W. Gibbs, G.E. Eyssen, and A.D. McDonald. Dust exposure and mortality in chrysotile mining. *Br. J. Ind. Med.* **37**:11.

McMichael, A.J. 1976. Standardised mortality rates and the 'healthy worker effect'; scratching beneath the surface. *J. Occup. Med.* **18**:165.

McMichael, A.J., S.G. Haynes, and H.A. Tyroler. 1975. What do we expect from an occupational cohort? Observations on the evaluation of occupational mortality data. *J. Occup. Med.* **17**:128.

Mancuso, T.F. and E.J. Coulter. 1959. Methods of studying the relation of employment and long-term illness—cohort analysis. *Am. J. Public Health* **49**:1525.

_____. 1963. Methodology in industrial health: The cohort approach with special reference to an asbestos company. *Arch. Environ. Health* **6**:210.

Mancuso, T.F. and A.A. El Attar. 1966. Dynamic changes in industrial cohort. *Indust. Med. Surg.* **35**:1059.

Mancuso, T.F., A. Ciocco, and A.A. El Attar. 1968. An epidemiologic approach to the rubber industry: A study based on departmental experience. *J. Occup. Med.* **10**:213.

Neison, F.G.P. 1844. On a method for conducting enquiries into the comparative sanitary condition of various districts, with illustrations, derived from numerous places in Great Britain at the period of the last census. *J. Stat. Soc.* **7**:40.

Ogle, W. 1885. Supplement to the 45th Annual Report of the Registrar General, p. xxiv. Her Majesty's Stationery Office, London.

Oldham, P.D. and C.E. Rossiter. 1965. Mortality in coalworkers' pneumoconiosis related to lung function: A prospective study. *Br. J. Ind. Med.* 22:92.

Ott, M.G., B.B. Holder, and R.R. Langner. 1976. Determinants of mortality in an industrial population. *J. Occup. Med.* **18**:171.

Redmond, C.K. and P.P. Breslin. 1975. Comparison of methods for assessing occupational hazards. *J. Occup. Med.* **17**:313.

Registrar General. 1855. 14th Annual Report of the Registrar General of births, deaths, and marriages in England. Her Majesty's Stationery Office, London.

Rushton, L. and M.R. Alderson. 1981. A case-control study to investigate the association between exposure to benzene and deaths from leukaemia in oil refinery workers. *Br. J. Cancer* **43**:77.

Stocks, P. 1938. The effects of occupation and of its accompanying environment on mortality. *J. Roy. Stat. Soc.* **101**:669.

Tatham, J. 1902. Mortality of occupations. In *Dangerous trades* (ed. T. Oliver), p. 121. Murray, London.

———. 1908. Supplement to the 65th Annual Report of the Registrar General of births, deaths, and marriages in England and Wales, p. xiii. Her Majesty's Stationery Office, London.

Vinni, K. and M. Hakama. 1980. Healthy worker effect in the total Finnish population. *Br. J. Ind. Med.* **37**:180.

Wong, O., H.E. Rockette, C.K. Redmond, and M. Heid. 1978. Evaluation of multiple causes of death in occupational mortality studies. *J. Chronic Dis.* **31**:183.

COMMENTS

WAXWEILER: I am curious as to how you would interpret your findings.

ALDERSON: It is compatible with a subset within that work force having a modest increment in risk. There is a major degree of dilution, perhaps, and there may have been a small group exposed to 10-100 ppm benzene at least at peak levels in their working time. It may also be compatible with the changing environmental control, but it is compatible with that small risk lost within the total workforce.

WAXWEILER: To what would you attribute, then, the deficit in the rest of the oil refining population?

ALDERSON: Well, I am not happy that the national figure gives an absolutely precise O/E, but it shows that it is around no obvious overall work-force risk.

EPSTEIN: Do you have any data on the benzene levels for the median and the peak values? Also do you have any information on incidence of aplastic anemia in this particular population?

ALDERSON: Yes, cytology of the leukemia as well. It isn't the leukemia predominantly associated in the past with benzene exposure. There is no evidence of an increased rate of aplastic anemia. This study was from 1950 to 1975, but 1950 involved a cross-sectional in-post cohort, and some of these men had been working for 20 and 30 years. So it does go back. They have had long-term exposure.

Measurement in the industry, we just have to confess, hasn't been done adequately. There has been much more measurement in the industry—and this is where we are following it through—on the tanker loaders in the distribution side. But it is felt that the levels that existed in the past certainly may have been more harmful than present ones.

EPSTEIN: You did make reference to peak levels. I wonder what kind of estimates you are talking about.

ALDERSON: I think you are pushing the data beyond its limits. I said that the case-control study might be compatible with a very small group that has peak levels that are associated with a hazard by other people.

J. PETO: How many of them were myeloid leukemias? Were these all forms of leukemia?

ALDERSON: It was all forms of leukemia mentioned on the death certificate. I think there were three or four that hadn't been given as the underlying cause of death. There was no overt relationship with cytological type normally associated with the hazard.

R. PETO: There is a reason why observed and expected numbers, I think, are generally preferable. It is because you quite often get a sort of proportional hazard relationship, for example, among the A-bomb survivors and so on, and the comparison of observed with expected numbers is of maximum statistical sensitivity at detecting any such effects. So that is one strong reason for sticking with them.

The second thing is, on your Cox regression, I agree that you cannot explain the results of the Cox regression on maximizing log likelihood to anybody who isn't especially a statistician, nor even to quite a lot of people who are.

ALDERSON: They can't explain it to me, I am sure, Richard [Peto].

R. PETO: The point is that you can actually present the results of what is essentially a Cox analysis in terms of observed and expected numbers. In his paper Cox says that if you look at the first derivative with respect to whatever is the final thing of interest to you, this gives you as efficient a test as fitting the first derivative; giving an algebraic identity to the first derivative with respect to the thing that is of interest to you is equal to an O - E number. So you can do a Cox thing on the quiet and present the results in terms of O - E.

ALDERSON: Yes. If someone cross-questions you and thought you had done that, you are immediately getting accused of laundering the data. This is one of the difficulties. I accept that general point. What I didn't bring out, though, is the Liddell symposium agreed that you shouldn't use that approach to provide tests of significance.

There is another point, of course. I think this comes to your maximizing its efficiency. It depends whether the total risk you are looking at is the population mortality times the hazard or plus the hazard. Is the hazard additive, multiplicative, or interactive?

I was suggesting this: Use it where people are not saying, "Is there an increased risk?" but, "Is there a risk that is linked to duration of exposure, frequency of exposure, degree of exposure, latent interval, et cetera?" I am not sure that that is the same as the issue that you are talking about. Once you have clarified what you are trying to find out, you may then decide what is the most appropriate way to go about it.

The Value of Contemporary Demographic Controls in Evaluating Cancer Incidence and Mortality Rates in Heavily Industrialized Urban Areas in the United States

HARRY B. DEMOPOULOS* AND EVELYN G. GUTMAN†
Department of Pathology* and Coordinated Tumor Registry†
New York University Medical Center
New York, New York 10016

Our presentation is related only indirectly to the primary question of this conference–What is the proportion of cancers that are due to occupational exposures? However, it is related directly to the secondary question–What is the risk to communities that are situated near or are in juxtaposition to heavy industrial facilities where carcinogens and possible occupational exposures might raise the cancer risk?

Our exposure to this question arose in 1976, when Demopoulos was invited by the medical schools in New Jersey and other interested parties to attempt to develop a comprehensive cancer center, statewide, in New Jersey. The main impetus for this was the fact that the National Cancer Institute (NCI) cancer mortality study by county from 1950 to 1969 (Mason and McKay 1974) had been released and analyzed; a number of individuals had quickly done some simple arithmetic and labeled New Jersey . . ."the Number 1 cancer state."

Because there is an extensive petrochemical industry, particularly chemicals, in New Jersey, a link was made between this and New Jersey's high cancer rates. Various officials in New Jersey's Departments of Health and of Environmental Protection were quoted several times as ascribing New Jersey's cancer rates to carcinogens in the air and water. Headlines appeared several times proclaiming, "It's In The Air," "It's In The Water."

Another reference to this idea was found in an article in *The New York Times* (Sullivan 1979), which included the map shown in Figure 1. This map was the result of a study conducted by the New York City Department of Health and purported to show that polluted air wafting over from New Jersey (prevailing winds blow from west to east) was responsible for the "extraordinarily high lung cancer mortality rates in the areas denoted in black." The fact that skip areas were represented on this map did not bother them. Furthermore, it was stated that the high lung cancer rates in central Harlem were due to cigarette

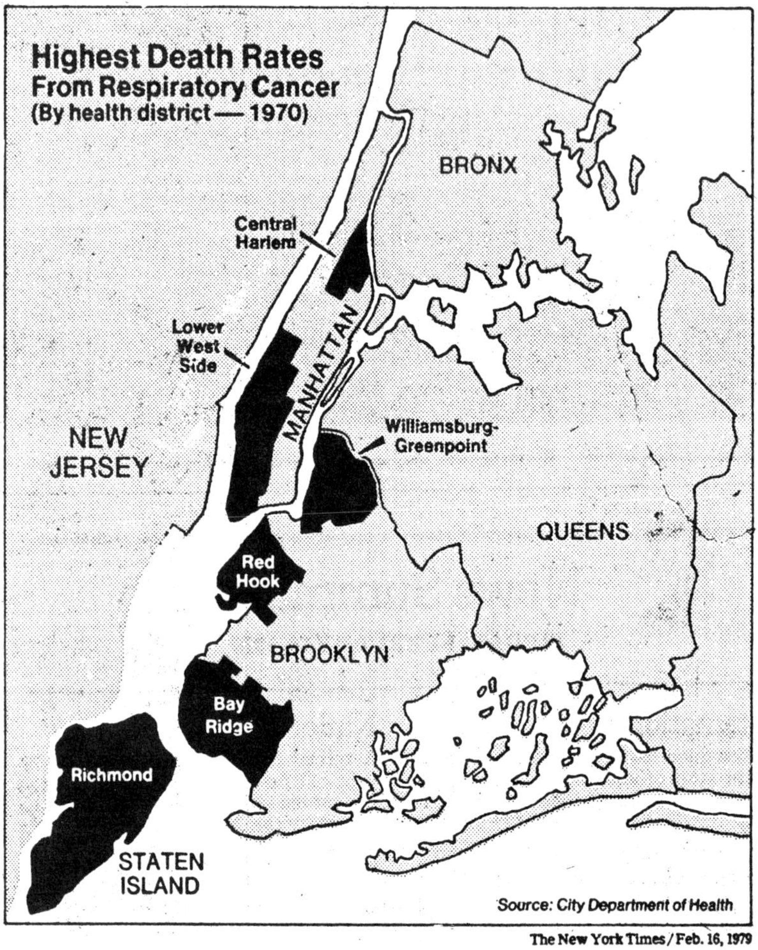

Figure 1
Map of New York City indicating regions that have highest lung cancer rates (■). These are in proximity to New Jersey and are said to receive polluted industrial air. Central Harlem is not within such an air flow pattern and cigarette smoking is given the predominant blame in that area. This particular study did not separate the data according to race, nor does it explain apparent skip areas, for example, the Lower East Side of Manhattan (□) which is between two "high cancer" areas, the Lower West Side of Manhattan and the Williamsburg-Greenpoint section of Brooklyn, on a direct west-to-east line. (Figure reprinted, with permission, from *The New York Times* (Sullivan 1979); Legend reprinted, with permission, from Demopoulos and Gutman (1980).

smoking, whereas the high rates in Staten Island were due to New Jersey's air (Israel et al. 1979).

The study was not race-corrected, and it obviously was not interested in consistency, because different causes were ascribed to different areas. It is an example of the kinds of anxieties that have been raised by the question of air pollution and industrial causes of cancer as they may affect communities.

The agencies in New Jersey and New York City, however, have not been the only ones to seize upon the notion that general environmental pollution causes many human cancer deaths and afflicts industrial communities more heavily. The *Federal Register* that dealt with the Occupational Safety and Health Agency's (OSHAs) proposed occupational carcinogen policy stated, "In general, however, states with high (cancer) rates are the more industrialized states, . . . and the excess disease risk in such states is attributable . . . to occupation, to the environment of cities . . ."[1] Similar statements can be found in the *Federal Register* dealing with the Environmental Protection Agency's (EPAs) proposed regulations for airborne carcinogenic substances.[2]

REVIEW OF THE DATA

Virtually all of the figures in the present work are white male cancer mortality rates or white male cancer incidence rates, expressed per 100,000 and derived from tabular data from the NCI studies on mortality (Mason and McKay 1974) and incidence (Cutler and Young 1975). The first region we studied was New Jersey because the NCI mortality study demonstrated that the annual nationwide rate for overall cancer rates for white males from 1950-1969 was 174/100,000, whereas in New Jersey it was 17% higher, or 205/100,000. This 17% increase was blamed on industry.

Although at first we thought that industry was probably responsible, we started to look at some other factors and to consider using contemporary demographic controls to evaluate whether N.J. communities really faced an increased risk for cancers as a result of general, industrial air pollution.

For example, we asked the question: What is the Number 2 cancer state? The Number 2 state turned out to be Rhode Island, with the rate of 203 white male cancer deaths (see Table 1) per 100,000. Of further curiosity was the fact that Pennsylvania and Ohio shared certain features with New Jersey, according to the U.S. Census (Department of Commerce 1951), particularly in terms of the proportion of workers in the work force who were engaged in heavy industry that involved manufacture of durable and nondurable goods, mining, chemicals, petroleum, and rubber industries. These three states, New Jersey, Pennsylvania, and Ohio, also shared the same proportion of residents in communities juxtaposed to heavy, industrialized facilities (see Tables 2-5).

[1] 42 *Fed. Reg.* 54148 (October 4, 1977)
[2] 44 *Fed. Reg.* 58642 (October 10, 1979)

Table 1
States with the Highest Cancer Mortality Rates—1950-1969

	White males		White females	
	number[a]	annual rate (per 100,000)	number	annual rate (per 100,000)
1. New Jersey	106,900	205.01	93,379	147.92
2. Rhode Island	16,434	203.17	14,770	143.37
3. New York	307,997	199.24	273,316	148.01
4. Connecticut	44,501	195.68	38,333	138.64
5. Maryland	39,157	192.43	35,366	138.66
6. Massachusetts	95,772	192.23	90,506	139.47
7. Louisiana	32,662	190.39	24,611	118.98
8. New Hampshire	11,944	189.19	10,655	140.20

Reprinted, with permission, from Demopoulos and Gutman (1980).
[a]This number is the total deaths, from 1950-1969.

Table 2
Lack of Correlation Between High Cancer Rates and Industrialized States

State	Rate[a]	Relation to national average[a]	Predominant business
New Jersey	205	17% higher	chemical/pharmaceutical/petroleum
Rhode Island	203	16% higher	light industry and light manufacturing
New York	199	13% higher	light industry and light manufacturing
Pennsylvania	183	4% higher	heavy industry[b], including iron and steel
Ohio	178	1% higher	heavy industry[b], including steel, chemicals, rubber

[a]The U.S. average cancer mortality rate for white males is 174/100,000 (Mason and McKay 1974).
[b]Heavy industry includes mining, construction, and manufacturing of durable and nondurable goods when more than 30% of work force is in this category, or when more than 20% of the male workers in the nondurable manufacturing work force are engaged in chemical, petroleum, and rubber industries (N.J. 37.4%; R.I. 12.1; N.Y. 13.2%; Penn. 20.4%; Ohio 42.0%; from Table 79 (Department of Commerce 1951).
Reprinted, with permission, from Demopoulos and Gutman (1980).

Table 3
Total Males Employed in Heavy Industry as a Percent of Total Number of People Employed in the Work Force 1950

New Jersey	32.63%
New York	25.56%
Ohio	35.31%
Pennsylvania	36.13%

Heavy industry includes mining, construction, and manufacturing of durable and nondurable goods.
Data from Department of Commerce (1951).

Table 4
Percent of Population of Pennsylvania, Living in Heavy Industry Areas

City	Population
Philadelphia	2,000,000
Pittsburgh	600,000
Erie	140,000
Scranton	110,000
Reading	100,000
Allentown	110,000
Bethlehem	75,000
Chester	64,000
Wilkes-Barre	64,000
New Castle	45,000
Lanchester	60,000
Harrisburg	80,000
York	55,000
Altona	70,000
Williamsport	42,000
Total	3,615,000

Table reprinted, with permission, from Demopoulos and Gutman (1980).
Population, 11,000,000; 33% of population lives in heavy industry areas.

Table 5
Percent of Population of Ohio, Living in Heavy Industry Areas

City	Population
Cleveland	900,000
Akron	300,000
Youngstown	170,000
Cincinnati	500,000
Columbus	500,000
Toledo	300,000
Lorain	70,000
Dayton	260,000
Canton	115,000
East Liverpool	20,000
Marietta	16,000
Steubenville	32,000
Bellaire	10,000
Ironton	15,000
Total	3,208,000

Table reprinted, with permission, from Demopoulos and Gutman (1980).
Population 9,700,000; 33% of population lives in heavy industry area.

New Jersey, Pennsylvania, and Ohio have approximately one-third of their work force engaged in such industry; furthermore, about 33% of the population of New Jersey, Pennsylvania, and Ohio lived in proximity to industrial facilities, thus raising a question of whether the community might be a risk. Yet, when the NCI's cancer mortality data are examined, Pennsylvania and Ohio are 4% and 1%, respectively, higher than the national cancer rate for white males, whereas New Jersey is the only one that has a 17% higher rate.

We wondered about the difference and looked again at the U.S. Census, and found that 90% of the New Jersey population is urbanized, making it the most urbanized state in the country. (It is also the most densely urbanized.) Pennsylvania and Ohio are about 60-70% urbanized.

When you look further at New Jersey, the majority of the state's population (about 7 million people), or about 5.6 million, live in the northeast portion of New Jersey. Demographically, such a land mass with such a density of people in it really corresponds much more to a metropolitan area, and comparisons among states is ludicrous.

If one examines the NCI mortality studies and other dense metropolitan areas that might serve as approximate demographic controls for New Jersey's 5.6 million people, one finds that areas like Nassau County have white male cancer mortality rates that exceed those in New Jersey, but areas like the District of Columbia and Westchester County do not have rates that are significantly different from those in New Jersey. Thus, places that approximate New Jersey demographically but lack industry have cancer rates that are approximately the same are not significantly different, or in fact, in the case of San Francisco and Nassau County, have rates that are equal or higher (see Table 6).

Table 6

A Comparison of Cancer Mortality Rates, 1950-1969, Among Urban Areas That Are Similar to New Jersey's Density

Philadelphia	221/100,000
St. Louis, Missouri	220/100,000
New York City	215/100,000
Nassau County (an eastern suburb of New York City)[a]	212/100,000
San Francisco[a]	206/100,000
Chicago	206/100,000
New Jersey[a]	205/100,000
District of Columbia	203/100,000
Westchester County (a northern suburb of New York City)[a]	200/100,000
U.S. nationwide	174/100,000

Table reprinted, with permission, from Demopoulos and Gutman (1980).

[a]Areas such as Nassau County, San Francisco, and Westchester County are predominantly residential with business trades, yet their cancer rates exceed, or closely match, New Jersey's.

In studying New Jersey's cancer mortality rates, it became apparent to us that there was no pattern of excess cancer rates that could be ascribed to industrial exposures (Louria 1976). Curiously, the only cancer category, aside from uterine cervical carcinoma, that was not elevated in New Jersey compared to the national average was that of lymphomas and leukemias (see Table 7). Benzene, as part of polluted industrial air, is alleged to pose a community risk because it supposedly creates an occupational leukemia risk. New Jersey has significant benzene air pollution, and despite several decades of such pollution, the leukemia and lymphoma rates were not elevated above the national average.

We wondered about the origin of the notion, expressed in the *Federal Register* cited previously, that there is more cancer where there is more industry, and thus we decided to look at incidence data and not just at mortality.

Fortunately, the Third National Cancer Survey (TNCS), although it was not originally planned that way, provided some interesting comparisons between cities with heavy polluting industries and cities with far less pollution (see Tables 8 and 9). Out of the 20 million people that formed the basis for the TNCS, 16 million of those people were in seven cities in the TNCS that was conducted in 1969, 1970, and 1971.

Three of those cities—Detroit, Pittsburgh, and Birmingham—were interesting, because about 44% of the work force in Detroit, Pittsburgh, and Birmingham are engaged in possible high-risk industries. Approximately 22% of the work force in Atlanta, San Francisco, Dallas, and Minneapolis, cities that are not noted for their heavy industry, were engaged in work that might be worrisome (see Table 10).

It is also interesting to point out that the TNCS, falling as it did in 1969, 1970, and 1971, really represented cancers that started to develop in the late 1940s, 1950s, and even the early 1960s. That period of time in Detroit, Pittsburgh, and Birmingham was marked by very few, if any, controls over

Table 7
Lymphoma and Leukemia Mortality Rates in New Jersey

	New Jersey	U.S. average
Lymphomas (white males)	4.93	4.89
Leukemias (white males)	8.74	8.81

Table reprinted, with permission, from Demopoulos and Gutman (1980).

Benzene is supposed to be a common air pollutant where there is extensive petroleum refining; this chemical is also thought by some to be leukemogenic in chronic, low-dose exposures. Examination of heavy petroleum counties within New Jersey also fails to reveal any "excess" above the U.S. average. These neoplasms and a few other types were not in "excess" in New Jersey, compared with national averages.

Table 8
Average Annual Cancer Incidence in Urban Areas, with and without Heavy Industry

	All cancers	Lung	Naso-pharynx	Stomach
Urban Areas with heavy industry[a]				
Detroit	303	67	0.3	13.5
Pittsburgh	299	67	0.8	14.5
Birmingham	294	83	0.4	7.6
Average	299	72	0.7	11.9
Urban Areas without heavy industry				
Atlanta	304	72	1.1	7.4
San Francisco[b]	330	68	0.8	14.2
Dallas	321	78	1.0	9.2
Minneapolis	311	57	0.3	13.3
Average	314	69	0.8	11.0

Table reprinted, with permission, from Demopoulos and Gutman (1980).

[a]Data for white males, age-adjusted, per 100,000. Data from Cutler and Young (1975).

[b]San Francisco-Oakland standard metropolitan statistical area includes the counties of Alameda, Contra Costa, Marin and San Mateo, which is the data base used in the TNCS, 1969-1971; San Francisco's death rates, from Mason and McKay (1974) for 20 years, were 212/100,000, compared with 174-179/100,000 for the other four counties (Alameda, Contra Costa, Marin, and San Mateo). Therefore, the incidence data in this SMSA dilutes the San Francisco city data which is not published alone, as it was in the mortality study.

industry, in terms of pollution, and very little regard, if any, for worker protection against point sources of exposure.

We have, therefore, the possibility that the TNCS might represent a worst-case scenario for the cancers that might develop in places like Detroit, Pittsburgh, and Birmingham when there were no controls. The other attribute of these three so-called "dirty" cities is that they have been in the business of heavy industry for a long time, so that there was sufficient time to take up the lag phase for human carcinogenesis, of somewhere between 15 and 30 years.

The data is interesting, in that if one examines cancer incidence in Detroit, Pittsburgh, and Birmingham, the overall number of cancers on the average is 299/100,000. The four so-called "clean" cities that had fewer exposed workers and less industry, had cancer rates that were, overall, 8% higher, or 314/100,000, than the three dirty cities. Although the 8% difference is not significant, the point is that the three dirty cities did not show us any kind of outstanding high cancer rates compared with the four clean cities.

Because we are dealing with 16 million people in seven cities and a situation in these three dirty cities where we probably had worst-case scenarios,

Table 9
Average Annual Age-Specific Incidence Rates per 100,000 Population, Males, Whites, 1969-1971

	Age groups									
	40-44	45-49	50-54	55-59	60-64	65-69	70-74	75-79	80-84	85+
Urban with heavy industry										
Detroit	119	226	404	701	993	1573	2073	2578	2984	2407
Pittsburgh	116	256	408	666	1070	1490	1951	2063	2706	2571
Birmingham	158	228	430	632	1031	1579	1878	2343	2350	2621
Urban without heavy industry										
Atlanta	126	247	456	677	1068	1589	1912	2334	3024	2323
San Francisco	130	233	433	697	1140	1653	2204	2858	3165	3027
Dallas	142	301	446	748	1113	1643	2069	2567	2674	2500
Minneapolis-St. Paul	111	219	371	654	1102	1534	2044	2848	3207	3684

Table reprinted, with permission, from Demopoulos and Gutman (1980).

Table 10
Total Males Employed in Heavy Industry as a Percent of Total Number of People Employed in the Work Force for Urban Areas, with and without Heavy Industry, 1950

With	Without	1950
Detroit		44.76%
Pittsburgh		42.06%
Birmingham		37.11%
	Atlanta	21.78%
	San Francisco-Oakland	22.58%
	Dallas-Ft. Worth	25.61%
	Minneapolis-St. Paul	24.14%

Data from Department of Commerce (1951).
Heavy industry includes mining, construction, and manufacturing durable and nondurable goods.

we calculated that if, in fact, the hypothesis that the kinds of industries and the lack of controls that were rife in these three cities really posed a carcinogenic risk of increasing the cancer rate by even 50% were correct, then we should have seen somewhere around 7% higher cancer rates here as compared with the four clean cities (Demopoulos and Gutman 1980).

We found, however, no significant difference for lung, nasopharynx, stomach, or overall cancer rates (see Tables 8 and 9).

If the rates are examined by 5-year groupings, again there were no significant differences between the three dirty cities and the four clean cities (see Table 9). This point about age-distribution is critical not only because there is no skewing in the data, but also because the older age groups in the three so-called dirty cities show the same consistently lower incidence rates compared with the four clean cities. The importance of this is in the question of whether the cancer rates might be lower in the three dirty cities because of out-migration of white workers, and higher in the clean cities because of in-migration by workers seeking better living conditions. Although there have been considerable movements among urban dwellers, it is not likely that only those who worked in the heavy polluting industries migrated out. The data presented is per 100,000, and it is similar for whites (see Tables 8 and 9) and for blacks (see Table 11), i.e., consistently lower in the three so-called dirty cities.

We also turned our attention to the question of Los Angeles and San Francisco. San Francisco and its surrounding counties pose informative comparisons of cancer mortalities, particularly as some of the surrounding counties are industrialized heavily (see Table 12). Despite the comparative lack of extensive polluting industries, San Francisco had higher rates than Alameda County, which is industrialized.

Table 11
Black Males—TNCS Incidence Data, 1969-1971

	All cancers	Prostate	Lung	Nasopharynx	Larynx	Esophagus	Stomach
Urban areas with heavy industry							
Detroit	360	77	87	0.2	8.6	15.8	18.1
Pittsburgh	378	69	99	0.2	5.9	20.8	20.6
Birmingham	296	71	70	0.4	5.1	7.4	21.4
Averages	345	72	85	0.3	6.5	14.6	20
Urban areas without heavy industry							
Atlanta	333	80	75	0.9	6	20.1	19.2
San Francisco	365	82	79	1.3	11.8	15.4	22
Dallas	377	87	87	0.6	7.4	15	19.1
Minneapolis	355	63	88	—	6.6	12.8	13.1
Averages	360	75	80	0.9	8	15.8	18.3

Table 12
Comparative Rates in Northern California

Area	Rate
All types of cancers	
San Francisco	212/100,000
Alameda	179/100,000
Contra Costa	174/100,000
Marin	174/100,000
San Mateo	176/100,000
U.S. nationwide	174/100,000
Nose, nasal cavity, middle ear, and sinuses	
San Francisco	0.6/100,000
Alameda	0.4/100,000
Contra Costa	0.4/100,000
Marin	0.5/100,000
San Mateo	0.2/100,000
U.S. nationwide	0.43/100,000
Larynx	
San Francisco	3.8/100,000
Alameda	2.5/100,000
Contra Costa	2.3/100,000
Marin	2.6/100,000
San Mateo	1.9/100,000
U.S. nationwide	2.59/100,000

Data from Mason and McKay (1974).

Despite the substantive petroleum, chemical industry of Alameda County, its over-all cancer death rates, as well as the sites that Blot suggests are related to petroleum and chemical industry, are at or below the nationwide rates. San Francisco, with retailing, commerce, trades, minimal chemical industry and Pacific Ocean air, has significantly higher rates. It is noteworthy, perhaps that San Francisco crowds 715,674 people into a relatively small area, whereas the surrounding counties have low-density populations.

The National Wildlife Federation records the number of unhealthy days of polluted air, particularly in Los Angeles, and they have cataloged approximately 320 days a year of unhealthy days for Los Angeles. San Francisco is relatively more blessed, because it is bathed by Pacific Ocean air flowing in from west to east; it has only about 125 such days a year. Furthermore, Los Angeles is interesting, not only because of its smog, but also because the oil refineries in this major petroleum county are located along the seacoast and the prevailing winds carry whatever pollutants come out of the petroleum plants into the Pacific Basin and mix it with automotive smog. The net result is pretty astounding levels of irritants.

Yet, despite the fact that smog has been a problem in Los Angeles since the late 1940s and we have had sufficient time for cancers to develop, the fact of the matter is that overall Los Angeles white male cancer deaths are 175/100,000. San Francisco, with its much cleaner air and being virtually devoid of any contaminating or polluting industries, has cancer rates that are 212/100,000 (see Table 13).

Similarly, when the lung, nasopharynx, and stomach cancer rates in Los Angeles are examined, they are not different from the nationwide cancer rate, whereas, San Francisco's are elevated.

The absence of any correlation between general industrial air pollution and cancer risks has been substantiated by other independent investigators. Aoki and Shimizu (1977) showed that lung cancer rates in Japan did not correlate with industrialized areas and rather showed a gradation in incidence that paralleled the density of population. Similarly, Hammond and Garfinkel (1980) found no relationship between general air pollution and cancer.

Table 13
Comparison of San Francisco and Los Angeles

Area	Rate
All types of cancers	
Los Angeles	175/100,000
San Francisco (alone)	212/100,000
U.S. nationwide	174/100,000
Lung	
Los Angeles	41/100,000
San Francisco (alone)	47/100,000
U.S. nationwide	38/100,000
Nasopharynx	
Los Angeles	0.4/100,000
San Francisco (alone)	0.6/100,000
U.S. nationwide	0.38/100,000
Stomach	
Los Angeles	15/100,000
San Francisco (alone)	20/100,000
U.S. nationwide	15/100,000

Data from Mason and McKay (1974).

As in other comparisons, there is no consistent correlation between petroleum, chemical industries, and cancer death rates. The most consistent correlation appears to be with population density. Los Angeles, for example, has a low density, whereas San Francisco's is high. The serious air pollution and extensive petroleum industry in Los Angeles do not appear to have had an effect as far as raising the cancer rates above the national average.

Of considerable interest with regard to the heavily industrialized area of New Jersey, New York City, and Philadelphia, is a recently completed report demonstrating that this region's overall cancer mortality rates for white males were unchanged for the period 1950-1975, studied at 5-year intervals (Greenberg and Caruana 1981). This included lung cancers.

CONCLUSION

The question of the role of general industrial pollution in cancer causation is far from proven, and if one makes an attempt by using NCI mortality and incidence studies, the latter probably representing worst-case environmental circumstances, one is hard put to find any justification for the comments that have often appeared in the *Federal Register* cited previously by various Federal regulatory agencies, that where there is more industry there is more cancer. That does not appear to be accurate. As a matter of fact, the statistics indicate that the opposite seems to be the case.

We have not been able to find any correlation between the extent of industry in this country and elevated cancer rates. We think that there is a level of mythology in this business of cancer and the environment, and it deserves close examination because it does confuse people, it does detract from cancer prevention efforts, and if we are going to prevent cancer we really need to know what tactics to use. Higginson (1979) has clearly enunciated what he and the World Health Organization meant by the term, "Environmental Cancer." He meant the individual's total environment, in particular that which is constructed by the choices of life-style, habits, and diet. Two recent symposia (Journal of Environmental Pathology and Toxicology 1980; Preventive Medicine 1980) also have delineated major avenues of approach for the prevention of cancer, and much emphasis has been placed on the factors described by Higginson.

ACKNOWLEDGMENTS

The majority of this work was performed while Dr. Demopoulos was director of the Cancer Institute of New Jersey, supported by a Cancer Center Development Grant from the National Cancer Institute, Cancer Centers Program, Bethesda, Maryland.

REFERENCES

Aoki, K. and H. Shimizu. 1977. Lung cancer and air pollution. *Natl. Cancer Inst. Monogr.* **47**:17.

Cutler, S.J. and J.L. Young (ed.). 1975. Third National Cancer Survey: Incidence data. *Natl. Cancer Inst. Monogr.* **41**.

Demopoulos, H.B. and E.G. Gutman. 1980. Cancer in New Jersey and other complex urban/industrial areas. *J. Environ. Pathol. Toxicol.* **3**:219.

Department of Commerce. 1951. *1950 census of population.* Government Printing Office, Washington, D.C.

Greenberg, M. and J. Caruana. 1981. *Trends in cancer mortality in the New Jersey-New York-Philadelphia regions 1950-1975.* New Jersey Department of Environmental Protection, Office of Cancer and Toxic Substances Research, March.

Hammond, E.C. and L. Garfinkel. 1980. General air pollution and cancer in the United States. *Prev. Med.* **9**:206.

Higginson, J. 1979. Cancer and the environment. *Science* **205**:1363.

Israel, M., J. Gibbons, and T. Chen. 1979. *Trends in respiratory cancer deaths: New York City, 1960-1977.* New York City Department of Health, Office of Biostatistics.

Journal of Environmental Pathology and Toxicology. 1980. *J. Environ. Pathol. Toxicol.* **3**.

Louria, D.B. 1976. "Cancer in New Jersey: An overview." Paper presented at the Seminar for Physicians: Cancer risk identification within New Jersey, and methods of cancer control, May 1-2. Cherry Hill, New Jersey.

Mason, T.J. and F.W. McKay. 1974. *U.S. cancer mortality by county: 1950-1969.* DHEW Publication No. (NIH) 74-615, Washington, D.C.

Preventive Medicine. 1980. *Prev. Med.* **9**.

Sullivan, R. 1979. New York areas cited in a study on fatal cancer. *The New York Times,* p. B1-B2, February 16.

42 *Fed. Reg.* 54148 (October 4, 1977)

44 *Fed. Reg.* 58642 (October 10, 1979)

COMMENTS

DAVIS: I would like to point out that the aggregate measures of the dirty and clean cities that you looked at are too large to allow definitive resolution of any hypotheses. Moreover, these cities have some other characteristics besides being dirty and heavy which might partly account for their lower mortality rates than clean cities. One of these is that the out-migration pattern in Detroit, Pittsburgh, and Birmingham in the period that you looked at them was enormous; they all lost substantial portions of their populations. That is evident in the latest census. Further, your clean cities of Atlanta, San Francisco, and Dallas all gained substantially in population during this same period of time. Their increased mortality might reflect exposures of these immigrants.

Now, again, I cannot take away from you with one hand what I want to give to myself and say, therefore it proves that migration patterns are the explanation for the differences you present, but I simply want to suggest that by not taking these migration factors into account, your analysis does not take into account all factors. With respect to Los Angeles and San Francisco, we should note that there is a tremendous in-migration to San Francisco so that you get people in San Francisco who have been in lots of other places. Let me suggest that we have to look at the migration patterns and the counting problems with younger aliens in Los Angeles, as well. Some of these things might be explaining it.

With respect to industry, there have been some case-control studies that compared counties, but were more closely controlled for variation between them—for example, the work of Blot with case-control studies on effects of asbestos, and the work of others at NCI on the effects of the plastics industry. Because these studies have controlled more closely and have looked at white males, they give some indication of some effect. Although you suggest some interesting hypotheses, I would just say that we need to do further work before we can confirm it.

DEMOPOULOS: To answer your points, the data I showed was white male mortality or incidence data per 100,000. No matter how you stretch the out-migration that may have occurred before the TNCS, you couldn't have produced a reversal of expected rates.

Furthermore, in comparing Los Angeles with San Francisco and in comparing New Jersey with other demographic areas, we used the NCI mortality study from 1950-1969 (Mason and McKay 1974). The rates were not different during the cancer mortality study from 1950-1960 if lung cancer, which is due to increased cigarette smoking, is excluded.

So that this question of migration, when you look at New Jersey and its demographic controls, or when you look at San Francisco and Los Angeles, is a nonissue because the rates, minus lung cancer, were the same for 20 years (see Devesa and Silverman 1980).

DAVIS: You are saying there was no change in the rates between 1950 and 1969?

DEMOPOULOS: No significant changes. That's what I'm told in the NCI cancer mortality studies, if lung cancers are not included.

CAIRNS: Are you talking about trends for each of these places, or the relative risk?

DEMOPOULOS: I'm saying that if you take one county, or if you take San Francisco, and look at the cancer mortality rates minus lung cancer over a 20-year period of time, the rates did not change substantially.

GOTTLIEB: Can I make just a point of methodology here? You are talking about trends within that 20-year period?

DEMOPOULOS: Yes.

GOTTLIEB: So the reason for taking 20 years was that you needed that period of time to have enough cases or deaths to make the period valid. I fail to see how they can comment accurately about any time point within it because the whole point of taking the whole 20 years was to get validity to your data base.

DEMOPOULOS: Devra [Davis], I don't quite understand your point in terms of explaining the differences between the three dirty cities and the four clean cities based on your hypothesis. Would it be that the people who were at risk of developing high cancer rates in those three dirty cities out-migrated?

DAVIS: Not necessarily.

DEMOPOULOS: But you are raising that as a possibility.

DAVIS: I am simply saying that that is one factor that needs to be looked into.

DEMOPOULOS: John Goldsmith (1980) reported that in the case of this question of lifelong residents in urban centers versus people who moved in, the lifelong urban dwellers had lower lung cancer rates than people who moved in recently. I am not sure that there is anything to support the contention that the explanation that the three dirty cities had an 8% lower cancer rate or didn't have a significantly higher cancer rate is due to out-migration.

You would have to demonstrate to me that the percentage of people that out-migrated was sufficient to negate the increase that you would expect to see, and I don't think that the numbers are there. It would also have to have been a selected out-migration of just the exposed workers.

R. PETO: The point you're making isn't that you are trying to account for the differences between cities, but merely that these differences that have been used as clear evidence of chemical contamination cannot properly be so used. But this is not to guarantee that there is no effect of chemical contamination.

DEMOPOULOS: Yes. As I said, my conclusion was just that we cannot find evidence from the mortality and incidence studies in these areas to support the statement that has appeared repeatedly in regulatory issues and elsewhere as a rationale for the regulation, that is, where there is heavy industry there is a lot more cancer.

We looked at bladder cancers and they were like the lung, the nasopharynx, and stomach. We also looked at leukemias, but we couldn't discern any differences. We didn't feel that we should put all the anatomic sites across, but you can check TNCS for these things. Urinary bladder cancer was not elevated in those three dirty cities, nor were the leukemias and lymphomas.

SAMUELS: I have heard you give this presentation before, and the premises are rather disturbing. First of all, as a fervent reader of the *Federal Register,* I don't know what governmental message is as simplistic as the one which you imply.

Second, the term "due to" seems to be sometimes a synonym for "cause." I think usually the government agencies are smarter than that; they use the term "associate," which has an entirely different meaning.

As for looking at county death rates, at least among the people I represent, people very often don't die where they work. They go to another place when they retire and they die there.

References

Devesa, S. and D.T. Silverman. 1980. Trends in incidence and mortality in the United States. *J. Environ. Pathol. Toxicol.* 3:127.

Goldsmith, J.R. 1980. The "urban factor" in cancer: Smoking, industrial exposures, and air pollution as possible explanations. *J. Environ. Pathol. Toxicol.* **3**:205.

Mason, T.J. and F.W. McKay. 1974. *U.S. cancer mortality by county: 1950-1969.* DHEW Publication No. (NIH) 74-615, Washington, D.C.

Proportion of Cancer Attributable to Occupation Obtained from a Census, Population-based, Large Cohort Study in Japan

TAKESHI HIRAYAMA
Epidemiology Division
National Cancer Center Research Institute
Tokyo, Japan

The proportion of cancer attributable to occupation is undoubtedly an important subject to be studied, particularly from the standpoint of public health and preventive medicine. However, actual determination of such a measurement is not an easy task. In the case of cigarette smoking, population attributable risk (AR) is obtained readily. For instance, in our large-scale cohort study in Japan, the standardized mortality (SM) rate for cancer of all sites in males was 445.9 per 100,000(1_t), while the rate in nonsmokers was 304.3(1_0) (13-year follow-up results). The population AR was calculated as $(1_t - 1_0)/1_t$ or 31.8%. In case of the problem of occupation, similar calculation of AR is not as easily applied because the term "occupation" is quite general, often vague, and difficult to be defined.

In this presentation, the relative risk (RR) and the AR for various categories of occupation were calculated to approach the problem, taking into consideration the effect of cigarette smoking. Materials used were taken from the on-going cohort study in Japan.

METHODS AND MATERIALS

A large-scale population prospective study on the influence of life-styles on major causes of death has been in progress in Japan (Hirayama 1975, 1977a, 1981). In the fall of 1965, right at the time of national census, 265,118 adults aged 40 and above residing in 29 Health Center Districts in Japan were interviewed with standard questionnaires containing such items as smoking, drinking, diet, marital status, reproduction history, and occupation. Response rates were 94.8%. These people have been followed by establishing record linkage among original risk-factor records, results of an annual residence survey, and death certificates. During 13 years of follow-up, 1966-1978, over 10,000 cancer deaths took place out of over 3 million observed person-years (Table 1). The age-standardized mortality rates for cancer of all sites and each site were calculated according to the initial risk-factor categories (Hirayama 1976).

Table 1
Observed Person-years and Number of Deaths during 13-Year Follow-up Period, 1966-78, Japan

	Male	Female	Total
Observed person-years	1,369,937	1,690,562	3,060,499
Number of deaths in 13 years	22,946	16,181	39,127
Apoplexy (stroke)	6455	4730	11,185
Cancer	6175	4156	10,331
Heart disease	3351	2653	6,004
Number of cancer deaths (all sites)	6,175	4,156	10,331
Stomach	2,562	1,351	3,913
Lung	940	304	1,244
Liver	549	316	865
Esophagus	314	104	418
Pancreas	251	166	417
Rectum	218	165	383
Colon	151	192	343
Gallbladder	148	164	312
Urinary bladder	117	55	172
Prostate	112	–	112
Uterus	–	478	478
Breast	–	183	183
Other			1,491

RESULTS

Standardized mortality ratio for Cancer of All Sites and Each Site by Occupation

The observed person-years, number of deaths, and age-standardized mortality rate for cancer of all sites for various categories in males in the present study were shown in Table 2. The standardized mortality ratio (SMR) by each occupation is illustrated in Figure 1. Similar graphs were made for cancer of the lung and stomach (Figs. 2 and 3). Such analysis was done for each cancer site. Selected occupations showing significantly elevated cancer risk were listed by each site in Table 3.

SMR by Occupation in Comparison with SMR by Other Risk Factors

In this cohort study, the SMR for cancer of all sites and for each site was calculated according to various life-style risk factors. Among many factors studied, cigarette smoking was found to be the most important risk factor for increasing the SMR for cancer of all sites (Fig. 4), and other cancers such

Table 2
Standardized Mortality Rate and Ratio for Cancer of All Sites by Occupation

Occupation		Population	Number of deaths	SM rate	SMR
	Total	1,369,928	6175	445.9	
1	Professional and technical workers	53,050	175	358.2*	0.803*
1.1	Technicians and engineers	4,823	16	458.5*	1.028
1.2	Professors and teachers	24,514	53	259.8*	0.582*
1.3	Medical and public health technicians	10,475	50	478.1*	1.072
1.4	Artists and public entertainers	817	8	878.1*	1.969
1.5	Other professional workers	12,415	48	321.2*	0.720*
2	Managers and officials	25,471	117	474.8*	1.064
3	Clerical and related workers	153,289	499	453.7*	1.017
4	Sales workers	112,556	546	491.7*	1.102
5	Farmers, lumbermen, and fishermen	614,456	2980	437.7*	0.981
6	Workers in mining and quarrying occupations	7,735	19	339.8*	0.762
7	Workers in transport and communicating occupations	29,225	74	375.6*	0.842
8	Craftsmen, production process workers, and laborers	259,301	1093	472.4*	1.059
8.1	Metal material workers	8,491	62	750.6*	1.683*
8.2	Metal processing, machine repairing, and assembling workers	42,184	149	449.7	1.008
8.3	Electric and electronic machine repairing and assembling workers	2,442	6	283.8*	0.636
8.4	Transportation equipment repairing and assembling workers	7,070	40	775.9*	1.740*
8.5	Meter and optical instrument repairing and assembling workers	2,117	9	477.6*	1.071
8.6	Silk reel and textile workers	26,251	108	483.6*	1.084
8.7	Garment and related textile fabric workers	12,557	48	429.4*	0.962
8.8	Wood, bamboo, grass, and vine products workers	20,673	100	490.1*	1.099
8.9	Pulp, paper, and paper products workers	2,485	11	482.8*	1.082
8.10	Printing and bookbinding workers	4,374	16	398.0*	0.892
8.11	Rubber and plastic products workers	2,194	7	357.8*	0.802
8.12	Leather and leather products workers	4,608	17	435.0*	0.975
8.13	Ceramic, clay, and stone products workers	7,843	30	417.5*	0.936
8.14	Food and beverage manufacturing workers	14,604	61	425.3*	0.953
8.15	Chemical products workers	2,621	16	675.9*	1.515
8.16	Construction workers	43,560	181	427.7*	0.959
8.17	Stationary engine and construction machinery operators	1,175	5	713.8*	1.600
8.18	Electrical workers	3,691	12	540.8*	1.212
8.19	Miscellaneous craftsmen and production process workers	11,373	50	493.9*	1.107
8.20	Laborers not elsewhere classified	38,946	165	471.4*	1.057
9	Service workers	28,470	101	367.7*	0.824
10	Not classifiable and not reported	86,375	571	474.4*	1.063

Data from Prospective Study, 1966-1978, Japan.

Table 3
Occupational Groups with Significantly Elevated Risk

Site	Occupation	SMR	Number
Cancer of all sites	metal material workers	1.683	62
	transportation equipment repairing and assembling workers	1.740	40
Mouth and pharynx	metal material workers	4.977	2
	food and beverage manufacturing workers	4.533	3
	electric workers	5.600	1
	miscellaneous craftsmen and reproduction process workers	4.022	2
Esophagus	technicians and engineers	4.141	3
Stomach	metal material workers	2.042	31
	transportation equipment repairing and assembling workers	1.733	17
	chemical product workers	2.050	9
Colon-rectum	none		
Bile duct and gall bladder	sales workers	1.700	20
	medical and public health technicians	3.560	4
	garment and related textile fabric workers	3.074	3
Liver	clerical and related workers	1.417	60
Pancreas	artists and public entertainers	6.651	1
	silk reel and textile workers	2.502	10
	electrical workers	7.276	3

Nasal sinus	craftsmen, production process workers	1.710	16
	artists and public entertainers	26.105	1
	metal processing, machine repairing and assembling workers	3.236	5
	transportation equipment repairing and assembling workers	6.657	1
	leather and leather product workers	10.210	1
	(wood, bamboo, grass and vine products workers)[a]	2.815	2
	miscellaneous craftsmen and production process workers	4.894	2
Larynx	transportation equipment repairing and assembling workers	16.022	3
	miscellaneous craftsmen and production process workers	4.822	2
Lung	(leather and leather products workers)[a]	2.324	5
	(stationary engine and construction machinery operators)[a]	3.472	2
Prostate	electric and electronic machine repairing and assembling workers	7.012	1
	pulp, paper, and paper product workers	5.975	1
Kidney	miscellaneous craftsmen and production process workers	8.062	3
Urinary bladder	sales workers	1.642	15
	artists and public entertainers	14.333	1
Skin	wood, bamboo, grass, and vine products workers	4.750	2
	leather and leather products workers	7.916	1
Malignant lymphoma	craftsmen, production process workers	1.435	38
	construction workers	2.324	11
Leukemia	(professors and teachers)[a]	2.836	3

[a]( ) = of borderline significance.

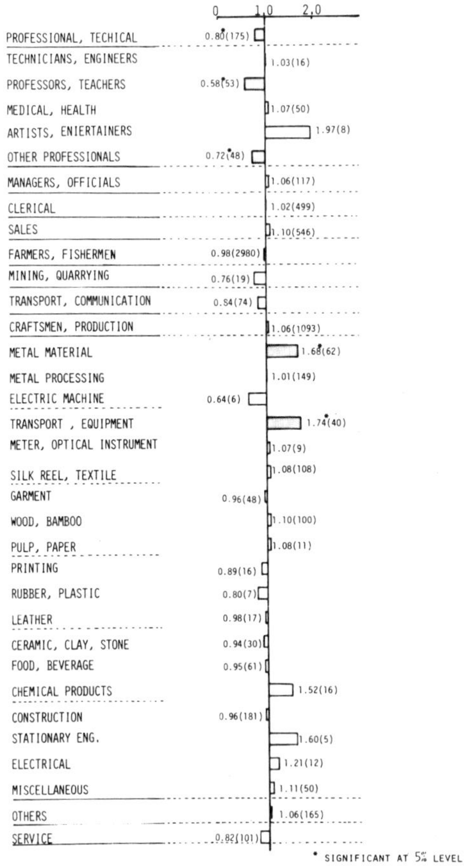

Figure 1
SMR for cancer of all sites by occupation (Prospective Study, 1966-1978, Japan).

as stomach (Fig. 5), liver (Fig. 6), pancreas (Fig. 7), larynx (Fig. 8), and lung (Fig. 9). Craftsmen, production process workers, and laborers, categories that include various types of workers in different industries, were labeled as "Factory Workers" in these figures. The SMR for such factory workers as a whole was not so high as seen in Figures 4-9. The SMR for each cancer site for such factory workers is summarized in Figure 10, including other minor sites.

Population AR Due to Industrial Occupation

Population AR was also calculated and listed in Figure 10. Among cancers of many sites studied, the highest SMR and AR, 1.71 and 11.9% respectively, were

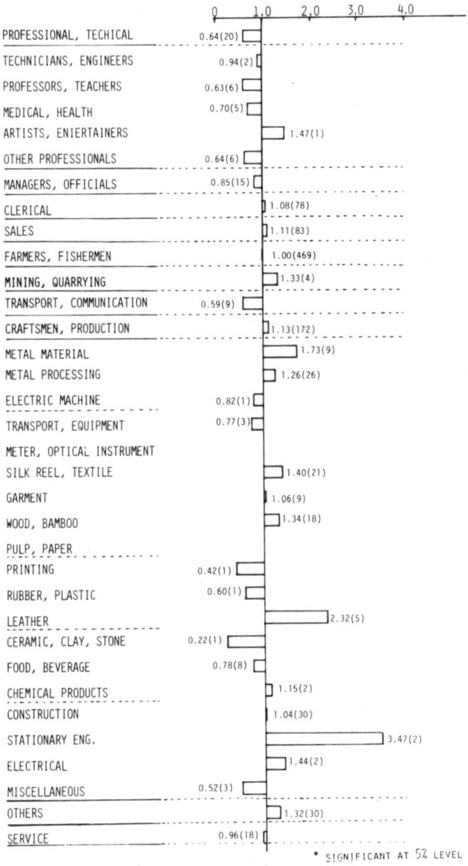

Figure 2
SMR for lung cancer by occupation (Prospective Study, 1966-1978, Japan).

observed for cancer of nasal sinus, followed by malignant lymphoma, (1.44 and 7.6% respectively). The SMR and AR for cancer of all sites were 1.06 and 1.1% respectively. Thus, 1.1% of cancer of all sites was observed to be attributed to total occupational exposure in various industries. As certain occupational factors are known to interact with cigarette smoking, the SMR and AR were calculated for factory workers who smoke cigarettes daily (Fig. 11). Again cancer of the nasal sinus showed the highest SMR and AR, 1.97% and 15.5% respectively. The SMR and AR of cancer of all sites for these factory workers who smoke daily were 1.17 and 3.1% respectively. Thus, 3.1% of cancer of all sites was observed to be attributed to industrial occupation when interaction with cigarette smoking was taken into consideration.

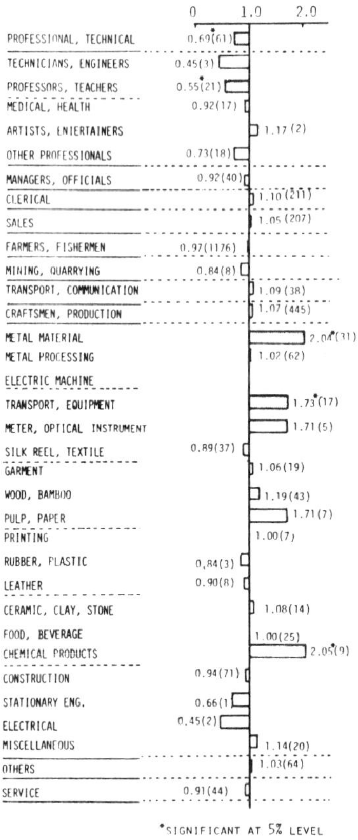

Figure 3
SMR for stomach cancer by occupation (Prospective Study, 1966-1978, Japan).

The SM Rate and 95% Confidence Interval by Occupation

The SM rates and their 95% confidence intervals (CI) were calculated by occupation for cancer of all sites (Fig. 12) and cancer of the lung (Fig. 13). Similar calculation was done for daily smokers (Figs. 14 and 15), and for nonsmokers (Figs. 16 and 17) in each occupation. These analyses demonstrate the extent and pattern of interaction of cigarette smoking and occupational exposure on cancer of all sites and cancer of the lung. The solid vertical line in these figures represents the average rate for total population. For instance in figures for daily smokers (Figs. 14 or 15), the risk for the total population itself goes up when cigarettes are smoked daily, as shown by dotted line.

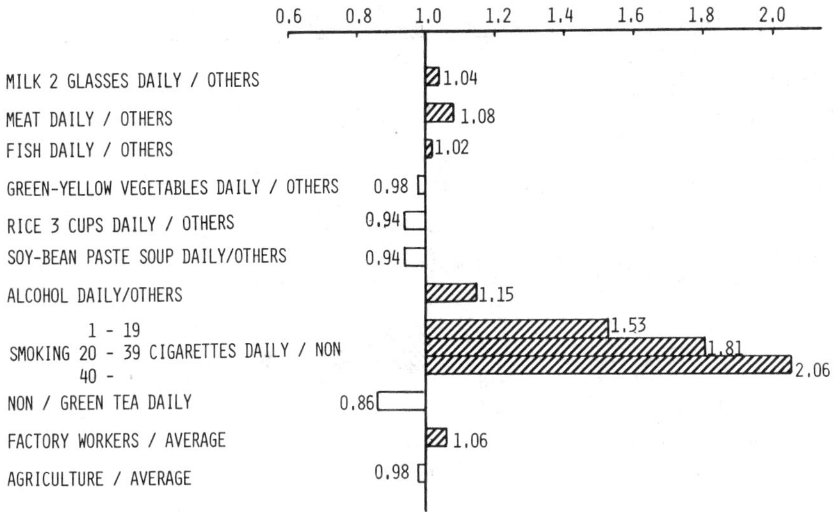

Figure 4
SMR for cancer of all sites by selected risk factors (Prospective Study, 1966-1978, male).

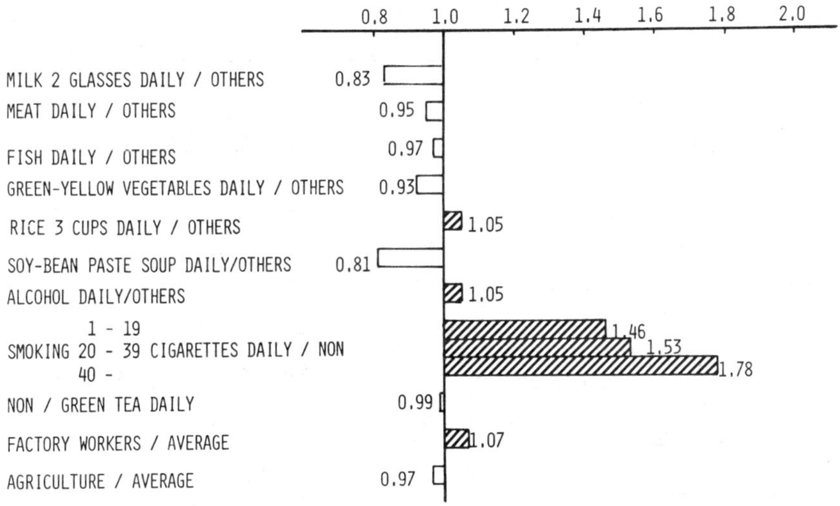

Figure 5
SMR for stomach cancer by selected risk factors (Prospective Study, 1966-1978, male).

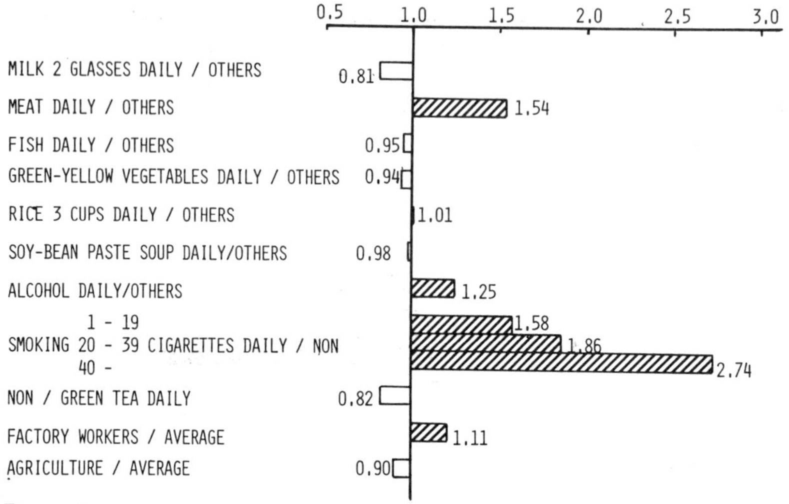

Figure 6
SMR for cancer of liver by selected risk factors (Prospective Study, 1966-1978, male).

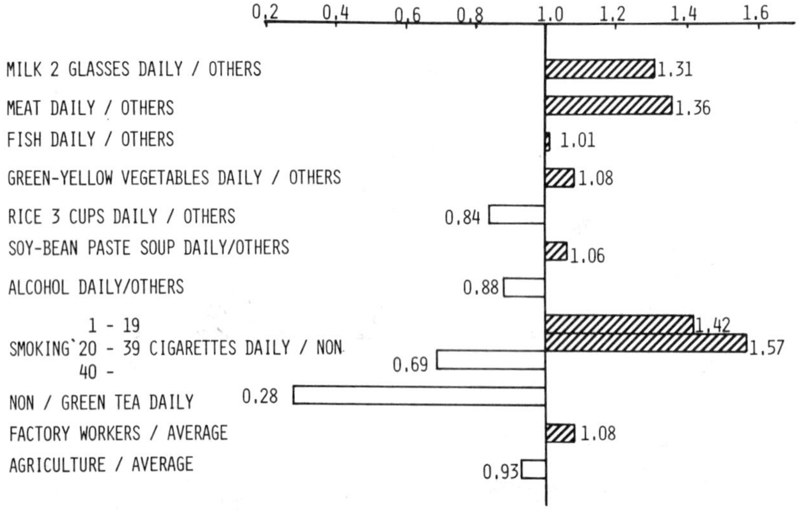

Figure 7
SMR for cancer of pancreas by selected risk factors (Prospective Study, 1966-1978, male).

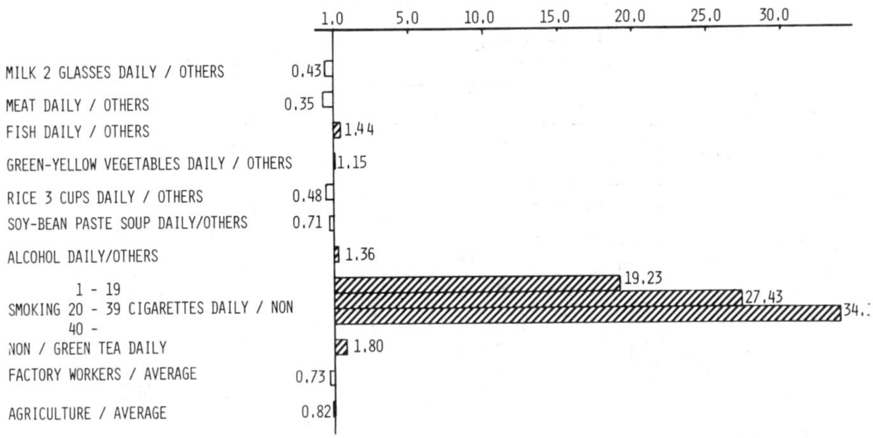

Figure 8
SMR for cancer of larynx by selected risk factors (Prospective Study, 1966-1978, male).

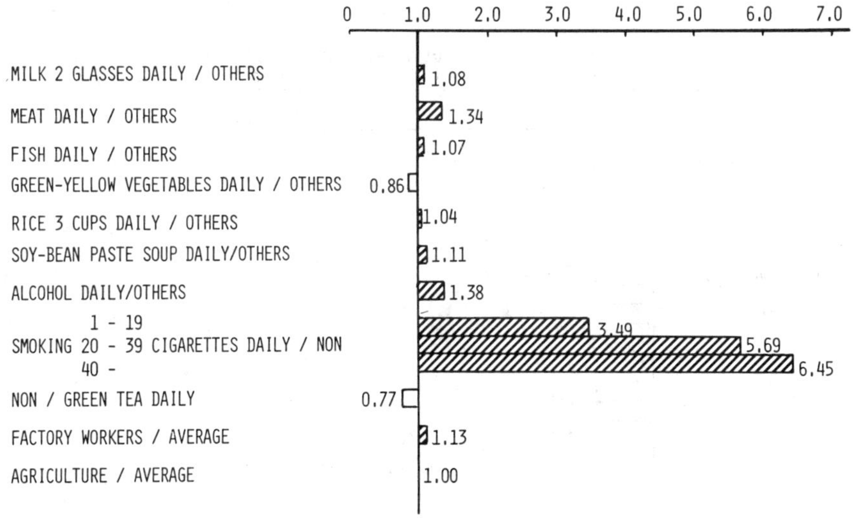

Figure 9
SMR for lung cancer by selected risk factors (Prospective Study, 1966-1978, male).

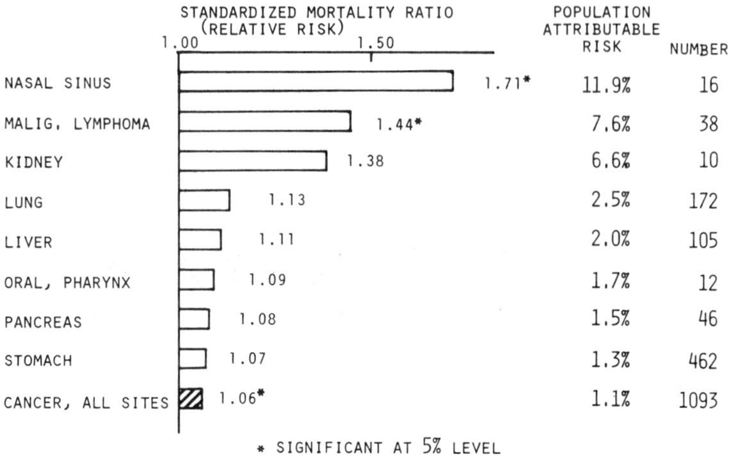

Figure 10
SMR (RR) and population AR of cancer of selected sites for industry workers

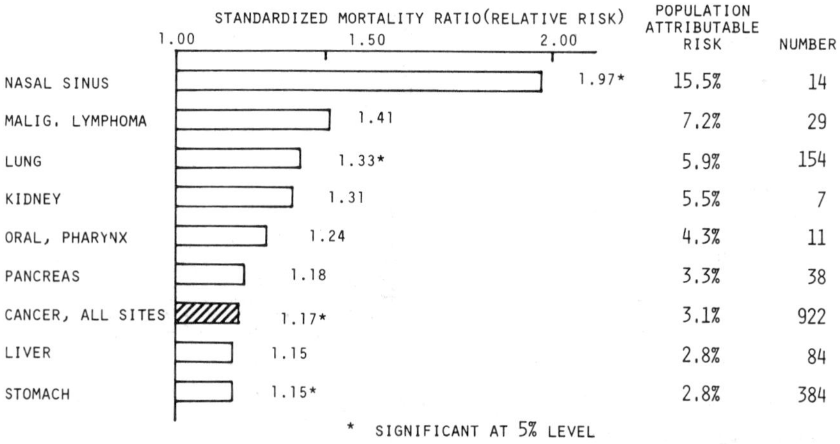

Figure 11
SMR (RR) and population AR of cancer of selected sites for industry workers–daily smokers

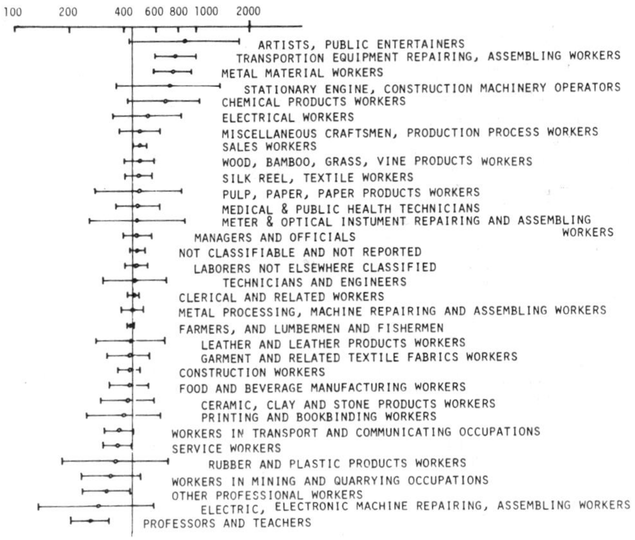

Figure 12

SM rate per 100,000 for cancer of all sites with 95% CI by occupation for males (Prospective Study, 1966-1978, Japan).

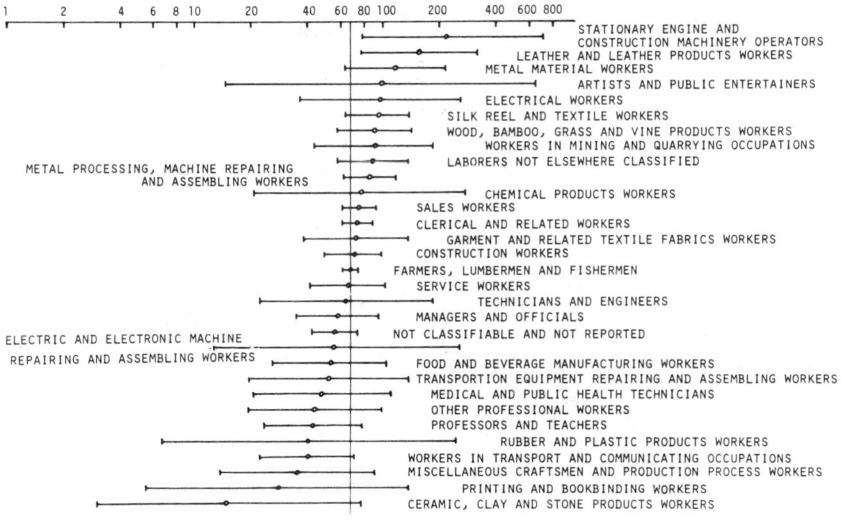

Figure 13

SM rate per 100,000 for cancer of the lung with 95% CI by occupation for males (Prospective Study, 1966-1978, Japan).

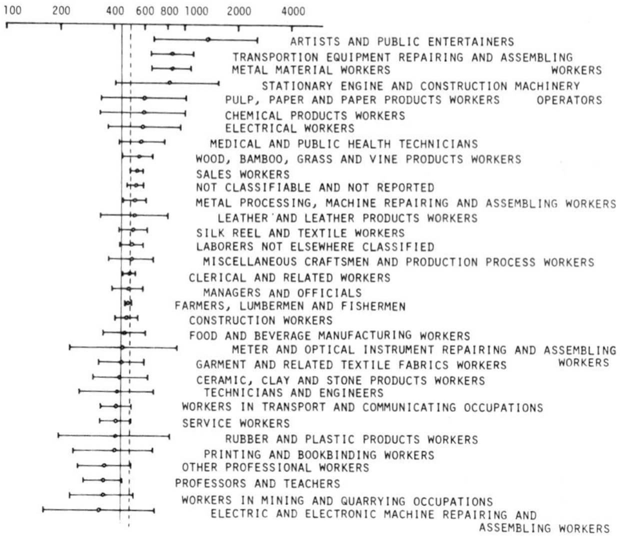

Figure 14

SM rate per 100,000 for cancer of all sites with 95% CI by occupation for daily smokers, males (Prospective Study, 1966-1978, Japan).

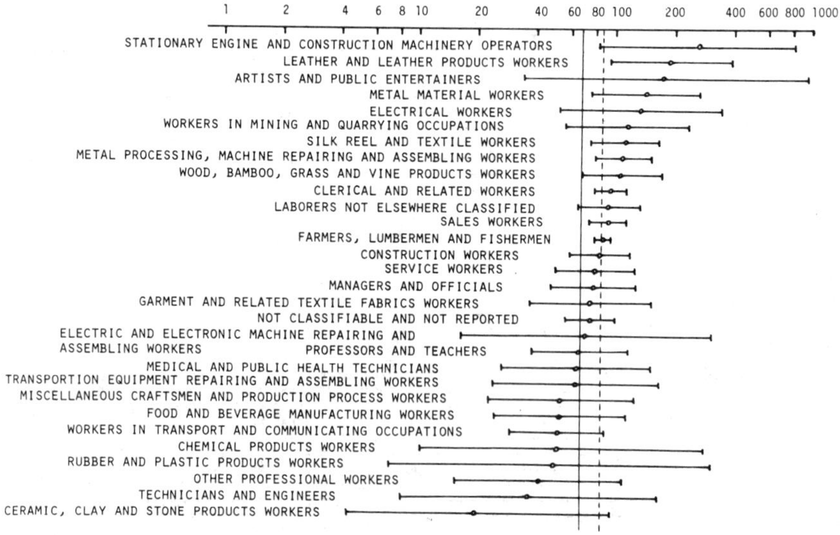

Figure 15

SM rate per 100,000 for cancer of the lung with 95% CI by occupation for daily smokers, males (Prospective Study, 1966-1978, Japan).

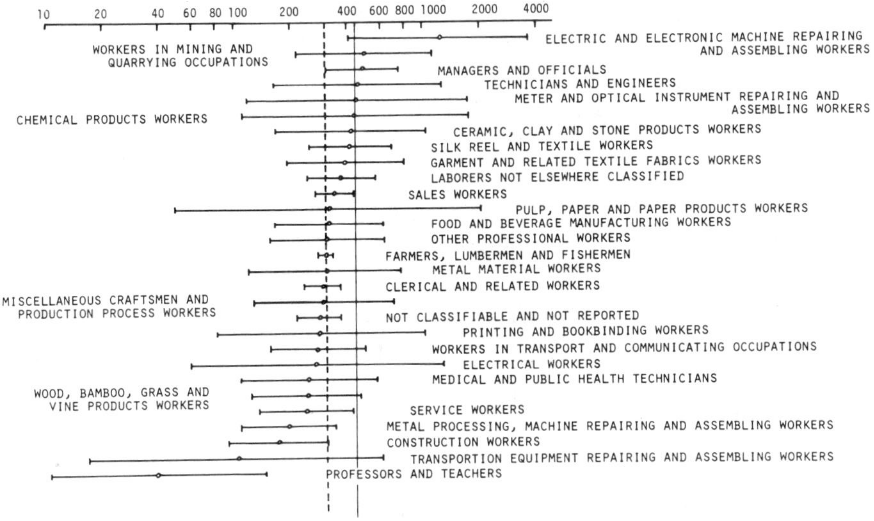

Figure 16

SM rate per 100,000 for cancer of all sites with 95% CI by occupation for nonsmokers, males (Prospective Study, 1966-1978, Japan).

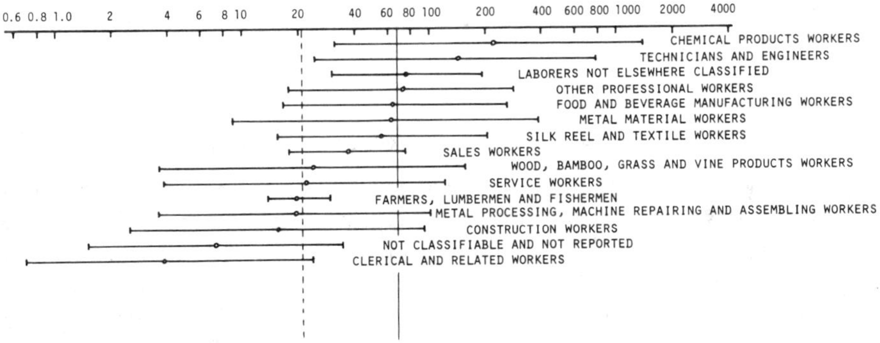

Figure 17

SM rate per 100,000 for cancer of the lung with 95% CI by occupation for nonsmokers, males (Prospective Study, 1966-1978, Japan).

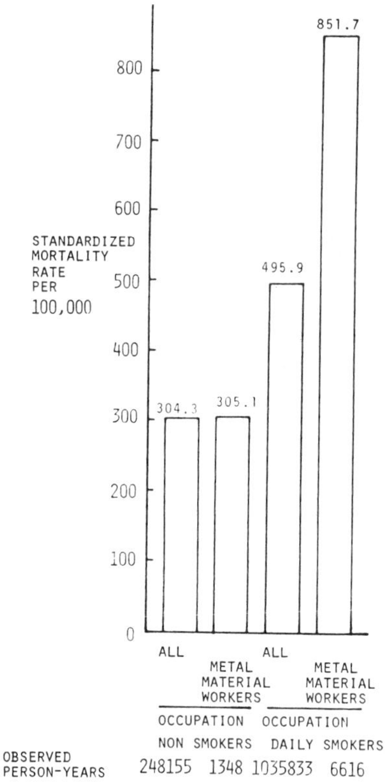

Figure 18
SM rate for cancer of all sites in metal material workers by smoking habit (Prospective Study, 1966-1978).

Interaction of Cigarette Smoking and Occupational Exposure

As metal material workers are found to carry higher risk of cancer of all sites and selected sites, the interaction with cigarette smoking was studied and shown in Figures 18, 19 and 20. For cancer of all sites (Fig. 18), no elevation of risk in metal material workers was observed for nonsmokers, but a rather striking risk elevation was noted in daily smokers. The effect of interaction is apparent in this case, the pattern being far over multiplicative. For cancer of the lung (Fig. 19), the effect of interaction appeared to be additive (expected 127.3, actual 142.1) rather than multiplicative (expected 258.15, actual 142.1). For cancer of the stomach (Fig. 20), the effect of interaction is far over multiplicative. The population AR of cancer of all sites, cancers of lung, and stomach for metal material workers with or without habits of cigarette smoking is calculated and the results are shown in Table 4. Compared to the AR due to cigarette smoking, AR due to this particular occupation is observed to be of quite limited magnitude.

SUMMARY

The proportion of cancer deaths attributed to occupation of various categories was studied using a large-scale, census population-based cohort study on-going in Japan since 1965 as material.

As a result, 1.1% of deaths from cancer of all sites were observed to be attributed to industrial occupation. When interaction with cigarette smoking was considered, the percentage went up to 3.1%. Type of occupation showed

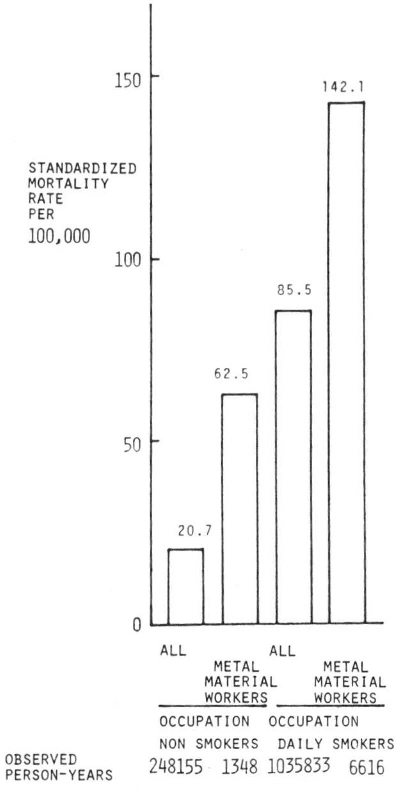

Figure 19
SM rate for lung cancer in metal material workers by smoking habit (Prospective Study, 1966-1978).

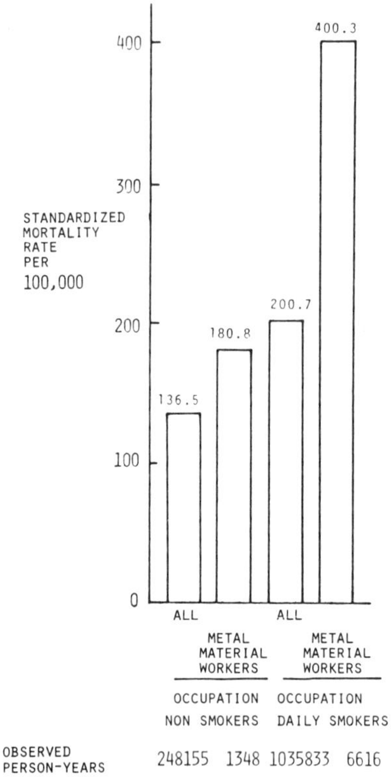

Figure 20
SM rate for stomach cancer in metal material workers by smoking habit (Prospective Study, 1966-1978).

Table 4
RR and Population AR for Metal Material Workers (males)

	Cancer, all sites		Cancer, lung		Cancer, stomach	
	RR	AR %	RR	AR %	RR	AR %
Metal material workers						
Daily smokers	2.87	0.96	6.94	3.00	2.94	1.00
Nonsmokers	1.03	0.003	3.05	0.20	1.33	0.03
Other workers						
Daily smokers	1.66	34.90	4.16	71.82	1.46	27.21
Nonsmokers	1.00		1.00		1.00	
Occupation-smoking combined AR		35.31		72.08		27.76

Data from Prospective Study, 1966-1978, Japan.

significantly elevated risk for cancer of each site listed. An SMR and 95% CI were calculated for cancer of all sites and cancer of the lung. A special analysis was done on the SMR for cancer of all sites, lung, and stomach in metal material workers, taking into consideration interaction with cigarette smoking.

Population AR due to occupational exposure was observed to be of limited magnitude. However, because primary prevention is quite promising in the case of occupational cancer, the detection and control of occupational hazard must have a high priority in any program of cancer prevention. This study is a testament to the precious value of a carefully planned population prospective study or a cohort study for the purpose of detection and monitoring of life-style risk factors, including occupational exposure (Hirayama 1981).

REFERENCES

Hirayama, T. 1975. Prospective studies on cancer epidemiology based on census population in Japan. *Proc. XI Int. Cancer Conf. Florence* **3**:26.

_____. 1976. Metal-material workers and lung cancer in Japan. Occupational carcinogenesis. *Ann. N.Y. Acad. Sci.* **271**:269.

_____. 1977a. Smoking and cancer. A prospective study on cancer epidemiology based on census population in Japan. In *Proc. 3rd World Conf. on Smoking and Health 1975,* 2:65. DHEW Publication No. (NIH) 77-1413.

_____. 1977b. Prospective studies on cancer epidemiology based on census population in Japan. In *Prevention and detection of cancer* (ed. H.E. Nieburg), part 1, vol. 1, p. 1139.

_____. 1981. Operational epidemiology of Japan. *J. Cancer Res. Clin. Oncol.* **99**:15.

Considerations for Designing a Large-scale Case-control Lung Cancer Study to Explore Occupational Cancer Risks

RICHARD PETO
Radcliffe Infirmary
University of Oxford
Oxford OX2 6HE, England

I have been hoping for two things from this meeting. The first may appear more sterile than the second, but both are necessary steps towards our overall aim of the quantification of occupational cancer.

First, where extremely different views continue to be widely propounded I hope we can, after discussion, agree that at least some of the things that are currently being maintained are wholly unjustifiable, and thereby limit the range of *reasonable* uncertainty that remains. For example, at this meeting we have already taken substantial steps towards a consensus about the net effects of asbestos on current U.S. cancer mortality and about the need to analyze the data on the Hanford radiation workers by life-table methods, and I hope we can now add to these a consensus that we do not accept the methodology that underlay the 1978 NCI/NIEHS/NIOSH "Estimates" paper (which is reproduced as an appendix to this volume, since it has been cited widely but never published).

Second, having briefly drawn attention to some of the defects of that 1978 paper (and those who do not want to hear any more about that paper should skip the following section!), I would like to move on to the far more important question of what studies we can recommend that will more accurately quantify the effects of occupational carcinogens, and perhaps to detect some that have thus far been overlooked.

THE 1978 ESTIMATES PAPER

In 1978, at a time when most epidemiologists estimated that occupational factors were causes of "only" a few percent of all cancer deaths, a manuscript appeared (prepared as a contribution to the OSHA hearings on proposals for generic regulation of occupational exposure to animal carcinogens) that suggested that about 23-38% of all U.S. cancers are, or would soon be, due to certain occupational factors. Although (or perhaps, in view of the criticisms that can be made of it, because) it was unpublished it was, and continues to be, cited widely. It considered half a dozen agents, although there are many others it could have studied, and first estimated the numbers of millions of Americans employed in the early 1970s (ignoring, until later, former employees) in industries using these agents. Many of these employees would have had little or no exposure to the agent of interest, but despite this the 1978 paper assumed that all would suffer risks of cancer (e.g. a fivefold excess of lung cancer) as great as those of heavily exposed long-term employees. If true, this would on average over the next few decades imply that each year some tens of thousands of cancers (or cancer deaths: there is some confusion between the two) would be due to these agents alone. What many readers have found unacceptable about the methods used in the 1978 paper is that the number of people exposed in any way to these agents was multiplied by risk ratios carried over from studies of people who had been heavily exposed to those agents for long periods. As Marvin Schneiderman (one of the principal contributors to this paper) and I have agreed in the Afterword of this volume), "the 1978 report took insufficient account of intensity and duration of exposure to the agents that were studied. Any study neglecting this kind of exposure information will be inappropriate." In addition, the 1978 paper included the suggestion that about 13-18% of all U.S. cancer deaths are, or would soon be, due to asbestos alone, an estimate about ten times as large as that which has emerged from this meeting.

More detailed criticism of the 1978 paper may be found in Appendix F of Doll and Peto (1981; in Section 5.6) of which we suggest that the degree of overestimation is probably by a factor of about one order of magnitude. My present purpose, however, is merely to suggest that we agree to dismiss the *arguments* in the 1978 paper, and not to suggest that we agree on the most plausible estimate, for it is clear that we at this meeting cannot yet agree on this among ourselves.

THE VALUE OF A LARGE CASE-CONTROL STUDY OF LUNG CANCER

Wide quantitative disagreement about the likely *future* role of present and past exposure to occupational carcinogens is likely to persist indefinitely, but wide disagreement about their approximate *present* effects could be almost eliminated by the use of standard epidemiological methods. It is not difficult to discover what is really happening to people; the methodology for doing so has been available for more than a quarter of a century, and I suggest that it would really pay, in the context of the amount of money that is being spent on occupational carcinogens, to find out in a systematic way what is currently happening to people. This is not to say that the only way to find out what causes cancer is to follow the workers for decades and count the dead. Obviously, there must be a lot of laboratory testing and some restriction of suspected agents based on laboratory evidence. But we must also look at what happens to humans. The causes of cancer today may differ from the

CASE-CONTROL STUDY—EVERY 10 YEARS

STUDY AT LEAST 10,000 LUNG CANCERS plus a similar number of controls —occupation, tobacco (including type of cigarette), residential history, "usual diet," specific inquiry about certain agents such as asbestos, radiation, etc.

* Quantifies current (but not future) effects of some known occupational exposures
* Picks up some new ones, and quantifies them
* Resolves 1% to 50% controversy
* Quantifies tobacco *and compares different types of cigarettes*

Figure 1
Suggested case-control study

causes of cancer in 10 or 20 years' time; therefore we examine these people on a reasonably regular basis to be aware of what is actually killing people and thus pick it up in time to do something about it. No matter what testing is done, some things are going to fall through the net. For example, there is no animal test at all that would have picked up arsenic, and alcohol is inert in virtually every animal test, although it causes cancer in humans. There is no way to prevent every single occupational carcinogen.

My recommendation is that we should undertake a case-control study about every 10 years that would study at least 10,000 lung cancers (preferably more) plus a similar number of controls. For example, a study of 15,000 subjects and 15,000 controls, that is, 30,000 subjects being interviewed, is about three times as big as the National Bladder Cancer Study that Sheila Hoar (this volume) just described to us. That study cost $1.3 million. A study of the size I am suggesting would cost about $4 million (see Fig. 1). Once you have actually got the people in such a study, it does not cost very much to give them a fairly thorough working over. Information that would be obtained from these people should include: Occupational history in very considerable detail; residential history (which may be significant in relation to air pollution, radioactivity from the rocks, contamination from chemical dumps, etc.); details of smoking, including particularly the type of cigarette (because the cigarette is changing rapidly all the time, and killing about a quarter of a million Americans annually; this would provide a systematic method to find out what these changes in smoking are actually doing to humans); dietary history; and a specific inquiry about certain things that you know are enormous disasters, like asbestos, perhaps radiation exposure, and so on. This reads almost exactly like an independent prescription for the study that the National Cancer Institute is just beginning in New Jersey, but on a tenfold larger scale, so that the New Jersey study would be a perfect pilot for what I have proposed.

Such a study would get rid of the absurd situation where some people are saying that less than 1% of all cancers are due to occupational factors and other people seem to be saying that the majority of all cancers are due to occupational factors.

The National Bladder Cancer Study has given us a pretty good estimate of about what proportion of the bladder cancers are due to occupational factors—about 8 or 9%. If we did the same thing for lung cancer, then we would have a consensus to within a factor of at most 2 on what proportion of current cancers is caused by occupational factors. Such a study would quantify the current, but not future, effects of the known occupational exposures, and it will pick up any new ones that we have missed that are accounting for substantial percentages of lung cancer. But it is not going to solve everything of course, because it would probably not pick up things which affect only a very small number of workers, even if these things were really terrible for the few workers exposed to them. For example, just recently I was down (at the request of a trade union safety officer) at a South Wales plant with a couple of hundred workers, and I wouldn't be surprised if half of those guys died from the past effects of what has happened to them. Some rare causes could be missed in a study such as this. But you will pick up anything that is killing a substantial number of workers, and you will generate a variety of leads, three-quarters of which will turn out to be false, perhaps, and one-quarter of which will turn out to be true. If there are any substantial new things around there waiting to be discovered, the large case/control study I am proposing should point to them and help quantify them although each may then need a special study to point to them and check which ones are real and which ones are bogus. (Robert Hoover said the best way of preventing cancer is to go into one of those places where there is a hot spot on the cancer maps and do a study, because it always disappears when you do.)

In Figure 1, I have listed some of the main advantages of the study I have proposed, and others may be found in Doll and Peto (1981).

REFERENCES

Doll, R. and R. Peto. 1981. The causes of cancer: Quantitative estimates of avoidable risks of cancer in the United States today. *J. Natl. Cancer Inst.* **66**:1191.

COMMENTS

FALK: I think one difference between what you are suggesting, perhaps, and the National Bladder Cancer Study is that, if I understand the bladder cancer study correctly, they chose certain regions.

R. PETO: You would have to do the same here, for practical reasons. For example, you could take something like the SEER areas, where some kind of registration program is established. The study wouldn't be absolutely nationally representative.

FALK: You might miss some very major industrial areas doing this.

R. PETO: Yes, unfortunately.

HIRAYAMA: Could you explain, first, why those large numbers of cases are necessary and, second, what proportion of these numbers would be under age 65.

R. PETO: About half of lung cancer is under age 65. And why so many cases? Well, you had 1,000 lung cancers in your Japanese study (this volume), and there were many things there that might have been real, but you really didn't know whether they were real or not. Sam Milham had 20,000 lung cancers in the study he presented this morning. But he only just about picked out some things that turned out to be quite major occupational hazards.

I think you need these large numbers because, contrary to what many other people suppose, I think that the actual proportion of cancers caused by occupational factors is not likely to be large. I don't really think any of these 20-40% estimates are plausible. But if they are, this study will support them. It should be a study that everybody, from the American Industrial Health Council to the other extreme, could agree on, because everybody is sure that everybody else is talking rubbish.

GOTTLIEB: I agree with you as far as the number of people required for a useful study. Whether case collection is for one period or whether you collect cases from a smaller area for a longer period is open to discussion. I would suspect you probably are better off doing a somewhat longer time period for a selected smaller population base so that you would have a better chance of being sure of your ascertainment. But one of the big problems with the bladder cancer study is that of incomplete ascertainment and associated inherent bias because the subjects were in and they were out. That study was done in that way because there was a mandate to get a fast answer on a particular question. But the way the study was performed leaves doubts that it is adequate to provide answers to all the questions that they tried to include. Therefore, I am concerned about some of these major efforts because they really do have to be done well and at a cost that is a lot more than you are predicting.

For example, there are some other studies being done by the National Heart, Lung, and Blood Institute, large multicenter studies, which have similar problems in coordination and uniformity, that will probably be done a lot more carefully than what appears to have occurred in the case of the National Bladder Cancer Study. If you want to be prudent in your financial predictions, you might get some estimates of what some of these studies are costing. You have got to be careful. If you are going to go into something like this, you have got to really make sure your data are good.

R. PETO: Yes, but, as Jack [Siemiatycki] was saying, the cost of actually being careful about what you record from people is not a very large fraction of the cost of running such a study. Most of the cost is connected with getting the organization and machinery and getting to the people, not with the length of the interview or the coding. That cost could be cut by using the SEER program.

GOTTLIEB: But the SEER program isn't geared up for the type of work that you are talking about, and other areas that have no SEER programs would have to be included.

DAVIS: I think it is also necessary to do a pilot with respect to the history and a pilot with respect to the control. Dr. McMichael, could you tell us to how you would go about choosing control populations, given what you have told us about the importance of nutrition, along with all these other things?

How would you propose on a large scale controlling for something of that sort that would allow us, then, the luxury of doing what I think needs to be done?

McMICHAEL: One either controls in the design or controls in the analysis. As long as we have got our wits about us in measuring our things and believe that we have got valid measurements or measurements that will do, then we at least have a chance to control for them in the multivariate modeling in the analysis.

SIEMIATYCKI: Let me point up one other problem, Richard [Peto], that the bladder cancer study might not have run into—that is the much worse survival of lung cancer patients. Ascertaining them and getting to them quickly will be much more expensive.

R. PETO: Yes, but a lot of case-control studies of lung cancer patients have been done; for example, Doll got 1500 in one of the original studies (Doll and Hill 1952). It wasn't so difficult to interview them, and they picked up the hazard of working in gas works in Britain. They then did a prospective study to confirm it, which it did.

SAMUELS: You are not saying, are you, Dr. Peto, that we should not control known agents to the extent feasible until we have finished such a study?

R. PETO: I am *not* arguing that the method of choice for controlling industrial carcinogens is to wait and see their effects on humans before anything is done. I am not arguing that, I do not think that, and I would recommend specifically not doing it. But I would say, let's also find out what is happening to humans.

SAMUELS: Well, that is what I thought you said. But, you see, the implication of that is, then, that the decision for control will not be based on the study.

R. PETO: It depends what you find. If you find something new, then the decision to control that may be 10 years ahead of what it would have been.

SAMUELS: But, you see, epidemiologically we never find something that is new. We always find the effect of a past exposure.

CAIRNS: I am a little bit confused here about this, because it seems there are some things that are known to be hazards, which presumably one would control. But there are also presumably things that are hazards you don't know about. I can see no way of finding out about these unless you look. So I cannot believe that a program to look for the unknown would ever neutralize your capacity to deal with the knowns. If you believe that, then, in fact, by definition, we will never find out about any more unknowns.

SAMUELS: I agree, but the unfortunate fact is that we will get, in the regulatory process, the argument, "Don't do anything until we have counted the bodies." And I assure you, we are not going to wait if we can.

References

Doll, R. and A.B. Hill. 1952. A study of the aetiology of carcinoma of the lung. *Brit. Med. J.* 2:271.

SESSION 8:
Future Needs

Record Linkage and Needed Improvements in Existing Data Resources

GILBERT W. BEEBE
Clinical Epidemiology Branch
National Cancer Institute-National Institutes of Health
Bethesda, Maryland 20205

Whatever view one takes of the importance of occupational exposures in the total cancer picture at this time, it is hard to escape the conclusion that cancers of occupational origin may well become a more serious problem in the future, if only because of the rapidity with which new chemicals have been introduced into industry and commerce in recent years (Davis and Magee 1979). Hence, I am a strong advocate of systematic monitoring and surveillance systems that would alert us to important occupational exposures as well as enable us to chart the progress of control measures. Epidemiology and industrial hygiene have a major role to play in such surveillance; experimental methods are still too uncertain and ill-suited to the magnitude of the problem.

The epidemiologic approach to determining the influence of occupation on cancer incidence and mortality has two aspects. First, it can create monitoring devices for surveillance, ways of bringing to light large apparent variations in risk that generate hypotheses deserving to be tested. And, second, it provides methods for testing those hypotheses and thus pinpointing specific jobs, identifying suspected carcinogens, occasionally uncovering interactions between a chemical carcinogen and, say, a life-style factor like smoking, and, rarely, providing information on dose-response or host factors in susceptibility.

The long latent period for chemical carcinogenesis certainly impairs the usefulness of epidemiologic methods of monitoring and surveillance. And it has been pointed out (Acheson 1979) that none of the known carcinogens of the workplace was first brought to light by examination of the decennial British Occupational Mortality tables (Registrar General 1978), despite their long history. Although we cannot expect too much from such surveillance methods, and may hope that the alert practitioner (Miller 1977), the laboratory scientist, or the epidemiologist will sound the alarm before any routine monitoring of mortality by occupation can arouse suspicion, we do need an efficient national surveillance system to minimize the risk that exposure hazards will go undetected for a long time.

I would like to examine with you some of the possibilities I see for large-scale monitoring of occupational cancer, primarily by linking existing administrative and statistical records. One of the great advantages of linking such records is that we do not increase the respondent burden of duplicate data collection and the data processing costs. Record linkage can also serve the needs of investigators testing hypotheses concerning occupational cancer, as we are hoping the National Death Index (NDI) (Patterson 1980) will illustrate shortly. But there are barriers to record linkage that impair the efficiency of research, barriers of a technical, administrative, or legal nature that will have to be overcome if we are to have more effective epidemiologic research. The content of routine administrative records also deserves scrutiny if we are to use such records and record systems more effectively.

POSSIBLE SYSTEMS FOR MONITORING OCCUPATIONAL CANCER

The systems with some chance of becoming operational in this decade would involve mortality, not morbidity, would yield information on all the causes of death, not merely cancer, and would rest on existing administrative records, not on records newly created for the purpose. In this discussion, I am putting the emphasis on the records of the individual where I believe the need is most acute. But in doing so, I do not want to overlook the usefulness of other approaches, e.g., the cancer maps that have stimulated National Cancer Institute epidemiologists to undertake studies that have linked specific occupational hazards with cancer in certain high-risk counties (Blot et al. 1977; Blot et al. 1978). Table 1 lists the present possibilities as I see them developing, but I should warn you at the outset that none of them is ideal and that each of them would require considerable technical work, negotiation, and time before it could bear fruit.

Linking the 1980 Census, the NDI, and Death Certificates

In the first option, a sufficiently large segment of the long forms of the 1980 census would be matched with the NDI periodically to identify deaths; the cause of death would be obtained from the states. It would be impractical to use earlier censuses in this way. The long form has good information on industry and occupation, and in addition has demographic and socioeconomic information that would strengthen mortality analyses by occupation and industry. The National Institutes of Health have proposed this plan to the Census Bureau and the National Center for Health Statistics (NCHS) where it is receiving serious consideration. On the technical side, there is uncertainty as to the quality of the match that can be made in the absence of the Social Security number (SSN) (Rosenberg et al. 1980) on both records. The great majority of

Table 1
Linkage Options for Monitoring Mortality by Occupation

	Source of information				
			death		
Option	occupation	industry	fact	cause	Problems
I	census	census	NDI	DC	quality of match
II	IRS[a]	CWHS[c]	CWHS	DC	quality, occ info; size of CWHS
III	DC[b]	DC	DC	DC	quality, occupation/industry; no denominator
IV	state unemployment insurance	state unemployment insurance	DC/NDI[d]	DC	size?
V	census surveys	census surveys	NDI	DC	size

[a]Internal Revenue Service Form 1040.
[b]State death certificates.
[c]Continuous Work History Sample, SSA.
[d]National Death Index.

the death certificates carry the SSN but the census does not. In the Kitagawa-Hauser study (1973), deaths occurring shortly after the 1960 census were used so that matching to the census could take advantage of the likelihood that residence would remain unchanged in that period. Even so, the success rate was only 74%. At present the Census Bureau and NCHS are seeking a solution to the problem posed by the confidential nature of each file. Should the quality of the direct match of the census sample and the NDI fall below an acceptable level, consideration might be given to matching the census sample to the 1980 income tax returns so as to obtain the SSN for the census sample, as both files contain a 1980 address.

Linking the Internal Revenue Service Form 1040, the Continuous Work History Sample, the NDI, and Death Certificates

The second option is more complex. The 1% Continuous Work History Sample (CWHS) brings together more of the requisite information than any other Social Security Administration (SSA) file. It contains the fact of death (Alvey and Aziz 1980), which the SSA records in connection with death claims, and the industries of employment since 1957, derived from the employer's identification on the tax record. But cause of death would have to be obtained from the states directly or through NCHS. And the only ready source of occupation is the Internal Revenue Service (IRS) Form 1040, where the taxpayer is asked to specify his occupation but no instruction is provided. The occupational statement on the 1040 has been shown to be reasonably adequate as an index of socioeconomic status, but that it would suffice at the 3- or 4-digit level of coding may be doubted. To determine its adequacy for this purpose, IRS has planned a coding experiment in which the coder would have not only the 1040 entry on occupation, but also the SSA information on industry of employer. The combined information should extend significantly the codability of the 1040 entry for occupation, but whether even the combination would be sufficient remains to be seen. Fortunately, the IRS is showing interest in occupation in connection with its own economic analyses of income and wealth (Sailer et al. 1981), and it seems conceivable that it might move to improve the entry if the coding experiment were to show the need for it.

State Death Certificates Coded for Industry and Occupation

The utility of the death certificate approach, without a matching denominator, has been demonstrated by Milham in his study of death certificates in Washington state over the period 1950-1971 (Milham 1976). Although this requires that one depend on the proportional mortality ratio (PMR) approach, I see no reason not to rely on PMRs in screening and surveillance work. Moreover, although Guralnick showed in her 1950 study that the "usual" occupation on the death certificate did not fit too well with the present occupation of the census schedule (Guralnick 1962, 1963a,b), in the British decennial tables of mortality by occupation, the deaths are classified by occupation according to the death certificate and the population according to the census.

Fortunately, NCHS is currently looking with favor on a proposal, funded by National Institute for Occupational Safety and Health (NIOSH), to encourage the states to code occupation and mortality under guidelines to be provided by the Census Bureau. A number of states have responded favorably to this initiative, which is consonant with recommendations of the National Committee on Vital and Health Statistics (National Center for Health Statistics 1977) and with recent legislation requiring that NCHS "develop a plan for collection and coordination of statistical and epidemiological data on the effects of the environment on health" (P.L. 95-623, §8). The NCHS response to this mandate (National Center for Health Statistics 1980) suggests a commitment to the extension of the ongoing vital statistics system to include occupational mortality, beginning with perhaps 5-10 states and expanding in time as the individual states develop interest and the capability for occupational coding.

Linkage of State Unemployment Insurance Files, the NDI, and Death Certificates

I can say little about the possible use of state unemployment insurance files, together with the NDI, except that some states have files that in theory could be linked with state death certificate files and the NDI to yield denominator-based mortality estimates by occupation and industry.

Linking the Current Surveys of the Census Bureau, the NDI, and Death Certificates

The Census Bureau performs a number of current surveys for other agencies, e.g., the Current Population Survey (CPS), the Annual Housing Survey, and the Health Interview Survey, all of which could obtain not only good identifying information for linkage purposes but also information on industry and occupation. The best known is the CPS, which has excellent information on occupation and industry but generates less than 100,000 new SSNs annually. But in the aggregate, such surveys, plus special surveys that the Bureau may undertake from time to time, might be organized to provide an attractive cohort for future studies of occupation and mortality.

Overall, then, immediate prospects are poor, but there is increasing recognition among technical people in government that a mortality surveillance system is needed for occupational hazards and that all the necessary data elements exist in administrative and statistical records now available.

Nevertheless, the complexity and fragmentation of federal statistical programs prohibit easy solutions at the federal level. Perhaps the most promising prospect is that the states may be willing to code industry and occupation on the death certificate. In time, such a system could provide essentially complete coverage of the population.

BARRIERS TO RECORD LINKAGE

Although record linkage is by no means a sufficient tool for either surveillance or hypothesis-oriented research in occupational cancer, it is often a necessary one without which the latency gap cannot be bridged. For more than a decade now the feasibility of record linkage has been increasingly limited by the growing social and political pressures to ensure privacy and maintain the confidentiality of the records of individuals. These pressures stem from abuses in areas other than medical research. One looks in vain through the Report of the Privacy Protection Study Commission (1977) for a catalog of abuses traceable to medical research. Although the results of epidemiologic studies now are reported commonly in the public press and on television programs, I doubt that the general public or even the Congress understands that because the health consequences of environmental exposures are often long-delayed, and not uniquely associated with single agents, record linkage is often the only way of establishing relationships. But when these matters do become more generally understood, I believe epidemiologists would be well advised to have in place a professional ethic and guidelines for record handling that would inspire trust.

Legal Barriers

Although there are technical and administrative barriers to effective record linkage, the most difficult ones to overcome are those rooted in law. It is not even the Privacy Act of 1974 (P.L. 93-579) that constitutes the major barrier here, for that legislation contains a "routine use" provision under which the managers of the federal record systems registered under the law have considerable latitude in defining the legitimate uses that may be made of their records. Laws that are even more restrictive are those governing the records of individual agencies, especially the Census Bureau (13 U.S.C. 8, 9), the IRS (26 U.S.C. 6103), the SSA (42 U.S.C. 1306), and the NCHS (42 U.S.C. 242m 1306). For example, because much of the information maintained by SSA is derived from tax records, access to Social Security data has been severely restricted by provisions added to the Internal Revenue Code by the Tax Reform Act of 1976 (P.L. 94-455). Formerly, in collaboration with Mancuso (Mancuso and Coulter 1959) and other investigators, SSA was willing to define cohorts of workers in a specific industry from the quarterly earnings reports submitted by employers, trace these cohorts forward for mortality, and inform the investigator of date and place of death so that cause of death could be obtained. The limiting factor then was the SSA workload, as these studies were external to its mission. Today, with the quarterly earnings reports of even 40 years ago being regarded as tax records, SSA appears to be unable to provide the basis for such cohort studies as Mancuso and others conducted during the 1950s and 1960s.

Critical to our understanding of the present situation is the recognition that it is not just access by the public that is prohibited by the legislation protecting the records of each federal agency, but also access by other federal agencies. The statistical responsibilities of the federal government are scattered among many agencies with little provision for coordination or integration. A single U.S. statistical agency seems out of the question for us, but we should be able to devise an integrating mechanism that would satisfy broader interests than those served by the agencies individually. An effort in this direction was made in 1979 with the drafting of an Administration bill, to be entitled "Confidentiality of Federal Statistical Records Act," that would have established an enclave of the major statistical agencies within which they could have exchanged and linked individually identifiable records for statistical purposes. Unfortunately, the Administration never submitted the bill to the Congress and I know of no similar effort at the present time. One possibility would be a national analog to the Institutional Review Board (P.L. 93-348), something like the proposed British Data Protection Authority (Report of the Committee on Data Protection 1978), with power to control linkage and access in the service of broad societal interests. Meanwhile, as suggested in the report of the Privacy Protection Study Commission (1977) and in the report of the Interagency Task Force on Ionizing Radiation (DHEW 1979), research on occupational health would benefit from changes in particularly restrictive laws, especially the Internal Revenue Code and the Privacy Act of 1974. The latter might profitably be amended to establish a clearer basis for disclosing information for research than the routine uses defined by the holding agency. It will be interesting to see what the Office of Management and Budget does with its mandate under the Paper Work Reduction Act of 1978 (P.L. 96-511) to submit legislative proposals to remove inconsistencies in law and practice regarding privacy, confidentiality, and disclosure of information.

Administrative Barriers

Although on the whole the records of the federal government are rationally retired, arranged, and preserved by the National Archives and Records Service, this cannot be said of other records that may be useful sources of information on exposure in the workplace, on the identity of the exposed, or on the medical care of the exposed. There can be no measure of the impact of record loss on the progress of knowledge in this field, but I believe the preservation of essential records deserves more attention than I have seen it given.

One important administrative barrier to efficient record linkage is an aspect of the fragmented federal responsibility for statistical programs: A narrow mission may not permit the appropriation of the funds that would be necessary to code, organize, and store information in ways that would enhance the possibilities for record linkage. Another is the catalog of missed opportunities to acquire information that would make a record or record system useful in linking records to create new information on occupational hazards. An example is the failure of SSA to require a copy of the death certificate in support of a death claim.

The centerpiece of record linkage (Miller 1971) in the service of medical research is the proposed NDI (Patterson 1980). Although formally proposed by a subcommittee of the National Committee on Vital and Health Statistics in 1968 (NCHS 1968), it was not until 1978 that a decision was made to proceed with its development. The 10-year delay means that the file now begins with deaths in 1979 rather than 1969. And even now it will not be possible to obtain the cause of death from NCHS; it will still be necessary to request the cause of death from the state of registration. Thus, the NDI will be useful for cohort studies but not for defining samples for case-control studies.

Another administrative factor impeding record linkage is the failure to code information available in hard-copy records. There are many examples: Few states code the death certificate information on industry and occupation; neither the Army nor the Veterans Administration (VA) codes the occupation recorded on the standard federal hospital record; the IRS does not code the occupation of the taxpayer given on the Form 1040; etc.

RECORD CONTENT

One way to accelerate the pace of research into the health effects of occupational exposures would be to improve records and record systems with respect to identifiers and occupational exposure.

Records Lacking Adequate Identifiers for Record Linkage

There are several important records or classes of records that lack adequate identifiers or for which the recording of identifiers needs to be improved. The decennial population schedule is one; because it lacks the SSN and the day of birth, matching of high quality tends to be limited to contemporary records for which an address can be used. Union records are, of course, extremely variable. Although excellent epidemiologic studies have been based on union records, e.g., Selikoff's studies of asbestos exposure on the part of the members of the International Association of Heat and Frost Insulators and Asbestos Workers (Selikoff et al. 1979), in many instances membership records lack SSN or date of birth, which would be needed for good results in a long-term cohort study.

Union records are an especially valuable resource because they may provide evidence of continuous occupational exposure despite changes in employment. The standard death certificate has a provision for the SSN, but perhaps only 80% of certificates contain it.

Records Lacking Information on Occupation and (or) Industry

Records or record systems lacking these items are more numerous. The federal clinical record form provides for occupation but not for industry, and with no instruction. The birth certificate contains the education of both parents but not their occupations. The SSA collects information on industry for all those in covered employment but occupation only for those who file for disability awards. It is a remarkable fact that the Medicare record system has no provision for either industry or occupation. The Hospital Discharge Survey of NCHS does not include information on occupation and industry; such information is often not found in the hospital records sampled and has no standard format. All but one of the 10 cancer registries in the Cancer Surveillance, Epidemiology, and End Results (SEER) Program of the National Cancer Institute collect information on occupation from the hospital record, but this has not been a required data element for the SEER system. Currently, however, an investigation of the completeness and usefulness of this information is being made.

Federal systems that may be of more interest in the future are those covering U.S. government civilian employees and U.S. military personnel. For civilian employees, both white- and blue-collar, the Office of Personnel Management maintains a central personnel data file dating back to 1972 that contains occupational specialty. In addition, under the terms of the Federal Employees Compensation Act (P.L. 93-416), the Department of Labor maintains an automated file of disability claims with information coded according to an abbreviated classification. Each of the armed services maintains personnel tapes containing military occupational specialty; these also are available for about a decade or more.

The Nature and Intensity of Occupational Exposure

Even a good occupational history may not provide adequately specific information on the substances or other environmental influences to which many workers are exposed and will have no measure of intensity of exposure except time spent in that kind of work. One must often go to employers or to state or federal inspection programs to learn the specific nature of the exposure and will seldom find measurements of specific exposures to the individual akin to those derived from the badges worn by radiation workers, for whom I would suppose we have the best data on individual occupational exposure. I understand that the best current source of such information is the National Occupational Hazards Survey (NOHS) (NIOSH 1974) conducted by NIOSH in 1972-1974 in which almost 5000 establishments in 67 metropolitan areas were inspected for exposure to chemical and other environmental influences potentially hazardous to human health. Certainly it is too much to expect the record of the individual worker to carry the detail of such exposure. This is another application for record linkage. I assume that under the Toxic Substances Control Act of 1976 (P.L. 94-469) many employers are making measurements of the working environment that can be tied to the individuals working there at the time, so that in the future, if such records are kept, it would be possible to have more quantitative data for dose-response analysis. Meanwhile, progress is being made in the direction of an occupational classification indexed to specific exposures (Hoar et al. 1980). Registries are being suggested (Doll 1977) for workers exposed to chemicals suspected of being carcinogenic. Since Three Mile Island, pressure has been building for a registry of radiation workers in the United States; Canada has such a registry with cumulative dose information dating back to about 1950.

Other Risk Factors

At this meeting especially, where we are trying to quantitate the separate contributions of occupational hazards and life-style factors to the total cancer burden, risk factors other than those implicit in occupational exposure are of particular importance. For the most part, we must look to special situations and to direct inquiry of subjects of investigation if we are to obtain information on such factors. Even so simple a characteristic as smoking status is rarely found in the major record systems.

Acheson (1979) has argued for the registration of women employed in industry during pregnancy so that malformations, stillbirths, and infant deaths could be monitored for the possible effects of occupational exposures. Such a registry might also be useful in the continuing surveillance of the workplace for its carcinogenic effects.

SUMMARY

Whatever our views may be as to the partitioning of cancer incidence attributable to environmental influences into its occupational vs life-style components, the rapid introduction of new chemicals into the workplace in recent decades requires that we be more alert to possibly occupational influences. A useful strategy would include not only the clinical observations of etiologically minded practitioners, continued development of experimental test systems, and careful epidemiologic studies to test specific hypotheses, but also a national monitoring of occupational mortality that might bring into view potential hazards not otherwise identified. A number of contemporary possibilities for monitoring mortality in relation to industry and occupation have been reviewed. None seems both readily attainable and ideal for the purpose, but an NCHS system based on state coding of occupation and industry on the death certificate seems to have the most immediate promise.

Although linking available administrative and statistical records to bring together at least the fact of occupational exposure and subsequent cancer should be technically feasible and inexpensive on a large scale, examination of all major files reveals that many are flawed in one way or another and either permit only partial solutions or require developmental work to determine feasibility of linkage or adequacy of the information produced by linkage. These flaws not only militate against the achievement of an adequate federal system for monitoring occupational mortality but also limit the resources available to the epidemiologist testing specific hypotheses.

There are, in addition, barriers to record linkage that derive from the multiplicity of federal agencies gathering statistics and the limits placed on their individual missions and from legislation designed to protect the privacy of the individual and of the private employer and the confidentiality of their records. Information that would be useful for health programs may not be collected by an agency with no health mission, and a medical care agency may show little interest in the occupational origin of disease. And the integration and standardization of statistical practice and programs takes place at a technical level where larger national interests are difficult to serve.

Research on the connection between occupation and cancer would be enhanced not only by easier and more imaginative linkage of administrative records but also by improvements in records and record systems. A number of key records have inadequate identifiers for record linkage. Others lack information on occupation and industry. And few records index occupational exposure in any terms except the occupational rubric itself: Other records needed for information on specific chemical or other environmental exposure generally are in the workplace, and these have been sparse and generally non-quantitative. Only for exposure to ionizing radiation in some installations are there long-term, cumulative records of individual exposure. The lesson is plain: If we are serious about chronic disease arising from exposure in the workplace, we need to reform our records and record systems, and weaken the barriers to record linkage for research purposes.

REFERENCES

Acheson, E.D. 1979. Record linkage and the identification of long-term environmental hazards. *Proc. R. Soc. Lond. B. Sci.* **205**:165.

Alvey, W. and F. Aziz. 1980. Quality of mortality reporting in SSA linked data: Some preliminary descriptive results. In *American Statistical*

Association 1979 proceedings of the section on survey research methods, p. 275. American Statistical Association, Washington, D.C.

Blot, W.J., L.A. Brinton, J.F. Fraumeni, Jr, and B.J. Stone. 1977. Cancer mortality in U.S. counties with petroleum industries. *Science* **198**:51.

Blot, W.J., J.M. Harrington, A. Toledo, R. Hoover, C.W. Heath, Jr, and J.F. Fraumeni, Jr. 1978. Lung cancer after employment in shipyards during World War II. *N. Engl. J. Med.* **299**:620.

Davis, D.L. and B.H. Magee. 1979. Cancer and industrial chemical production. *Science* **206**:1356.

Department of Health, Education and Welfare (DHEW). 1979. *Report of the interagency task force on the health effects of ionizing radiation.* Office of the Secretary, H.E.W., Washington, D.C.

Doll, R. 1977. Strategy for detection of cancer hazards to man. *Nature* **265**: 589.

Guralnick, L. 1962. *Mortality by occupation and industry among men 20 to 64 years of age: United States, 1950.* Vital statistics–special reports, vol. 53, no. 2. Government Printing Office, Washington, D.C.

______. 1963a. *Mortality by occupation level and cause of death among men 20 to 64 years of age: United States, 1950.* Vital statistics–special reports, vol. 53, no. 3. Government Printing Office, Washington, D.C.

______. 1963b. *Mortality by industry and cause of death among men 20 to 64 years of age: United States, 1950.* Vital statistics–special reports, vol. 53, no. 4. Government Printing Office, Washington, D.C.

Hoar, S.K., A.S. Morrison, P. Cole, and D.T. Silverman. 1980. An occupation and exposure linkage system for the study of occupational carcinogenesis. *J. Occup. Med.* **22**:722.

Kitagawa, E.M. and P.M. Hauser. 1973. *Differential mortality in the United States: A study in socioeconomic epidemiology.* Harvard University Press, Cambridge, Massachusetts.

Mancuso, T.F. and E.J. Coulter. 1959. Methods of studying the relation of employment and long-term illness–Cohort analysis. *Am. J. Public Health* **49**:1525.

Milham, S., Jr. 1976. *Occupational mortality in Washington state, 1950-1971.* DHEW Publication No. (NIOSH) 76-175-A-C, 3 vols. Government Printing Office, Washington, D.C.

Miller, R.W. 1971. Occupational cancer epidemiology: Its potential and problems. In *XVI international congress on occupational health,* p. 243. Japan Industrial Safety Association, Tokyo.

______. 1977. The alert practitioner as a cancer etiologist. *Cancer Bull.* **29**:183.

National Center for Health Statistics (NCHS). 1968. *Use of vital and health records in epidemiologic research.* NCHS series 4, no. 7. Public Health Service Publication No. 1000. Government Printing Office, Washington, D.C.

______. 1977. *Statistics needed for determining the effects of the environment on health: Report of the Technical Consultant Panel to the U.S. National Committee on Vital and Health Statistics.* Vital and Health Statistics

Documents and Committee Reports, series 4, no. 20. Government Printing Office, Washington, D.C.

———. 1980. *Environmental health–a plan for collecting and coordinating statistical and epidemiological data.* DHHS Publication No. (PHS) 80-1248. Government Printing Office, Washington, D.C.

National Institute of Occupational Safety and Health (NIOSH). 1974. *National occupational hazard survey.* DHEW Publication No. (NIOSH) 74-127. Government Printing Office, Washington, D.C.

Patterson, J.E. 1980. The establishment of a National Death Index in the United States. *Banbury Rep.* **4**:443.

Privacy Protection Study Commission. 1977. *Personal privacy in an information society.* Government Printing Office, Washington, D.C.

Registrar General. 1978. *Occupational mortality, the Registrar General's decennial supplement for England and Wales, 1970-72.* Series DS No. 1. Her Majesty's Stationery Office, London.

Report of the Committee on Data Protection. 1978. Her Majesty's Stationery Office, London.

Rosenberg, H.M., D. Burnham, R. Spirtas and V. Valdisera. 1980. Occupation and industry information from the death certificate: Assessment of the completeness of reporting. In *American Statistical Association 1979 proceedings of the section on survey research methods,* p. 286. American Statistical Association, Washington, D.C.

Sailer, P., H. Orcutt, and P. Clark. 1981. Coming soon: Taxpayer data classified by occupation. In *American Statistical Association 1980 proceedings of the section on survey research methods.* American Statistical Association, Washington, D.C.

Selikoff, I.J., E.C. Hammond, and H. Seidman. 1979. Mortality experience of insulation workers in the U.S. and Canada, 1943-1976. *Ann. N.Y. Acad. Sci.* **330**:91.

P.L. 93-348

P.L. 93-416

P.L. 93-579

P.L. 94-455

P.L. 94-469

P.L. 95-623 §8

P.L. 96-511

13 U.S.C. 8, 9

26 U.S.C. 6103

42 U.S.C. 242m, 1306

Long-term Medical Follow-up in Canada

MARTHA E. SMITH
Vital Statistics and Disease Registries Section
Health Division
Statistics Canada
Ottawa, Ontario K1A 0Z5

There is increasing demand for human epidemiology studies for better detection and estimation of possible risks to individuals exposed to potentially harmful agents and to occupational, environmental, and social influences upon health. The difficulty in studying these effects is greatest where the harm does not become apparent until some years or decades after the initiating exposures, as is the case with many cancers and genetic defects. Detection and measurements of the effects of potentially harmful agents are dependent in such situations on the ability to follow large numbers of exposed and unexposed people to find out what happens to them. Such investigations require some knowledge of work histories, dose histories, and the personal identification of the individual concerned.

The present account describes three interrelated computer systems developed at Statistics Canada that have been designed to permit optimal use of a number of different files of routine records for an entire country for health-related research. The development of a Canadian Mortality Data Base file, a National Cancer Incidence Reporting System, and a unique Generalized Iterative Record Linkage System have helped to reduce the cost and increase the scale and efficiency of automated follow-up in Canada. These computer systems have already been implemented, and references are made to studies currently being conducted using these data resources, e.g., a study of all Ontario miners and a large study to monitor the whole of Canadian industry for possible delayed effects on health and well-being. By sharing our experience, we hope it may be beneficial to those who are setting up new files in other countries and to those who are interested in the probabilistic matching approach, which we are adapting to the various sorts of follow-up.

We are rather excited about the potential these kinds of studies have in their humanitarian objectives (e.g., identifying diseases that may be preventable), their potential scientific output (e.g., in obtaining human data for estimating dose-response relationships), and in the development of new computer files and facilities for carrying out epidemiological research. Research in occupational health not only is important to protect the worker, but also has wider implications for protecting the general public. It is relevant to ask whether current safety standards are appropriate and to estimate any health risks involved. Quantitative estimates are required to assess whether the problems of certain agents or conditions in the workplace are important or trivial. Critical to answering these kinds of problems are the quality and extent of statistical and personal records based on monitoring of environmental contaminants and on the biological surveillance of the individual worker.

THE UNIQUE OPPORTUNITY IN CANADA

Statistics Canada is a centralized federal statistical agency whose mandate (Statistics Act 1970-71-72, c.15) includes collecting, compiling, analyzing, abstracting and publishing social, economic, and health statistics at the national level for all Canadians, in addition to conducting regularly a census of population and agriculture of Canada. Also, the agency has a mandate to promote the avoidance of duplication in the information collected by departments of government, and generally to promote and develop integrated social and economic statistics pertaining to the whole of Canada and to each of the provinces thereof and to coordinate plans for the integration of such statistics.

Nowhere is the cooperation more evident and more critical than in the area of vital and health statistics. Many countries produce similar health statistics, but in Canada in recent years the machine-readable vital records in particular have been planned to carry enough information to identify the individual and family to whom they refer.

Computer storage techniques and the speed of computers have advanced markedly in the last few years, and this makes it easier to store and retrieve large volumes of data over long periods of time. It is now technically feasible to implement some of the studies being talked about several years ago (Medical Research Council of Canada 1968).

It is important to note that Canadians do not have lifetime unique identifiers. All Canadian death records, for example, do not have the social insurance number recorded on them. Therefore, it has been necessary to develop computer-matching techniques. Again Canada is fortunate in that much of the pioneering work in record linkage was developed and tested using Canadian vital records. One of the first detailed proposals for doing this kind of thing by computer using the vital statistics registration records was by Dr. H. B. Newcombe in the late 1950s (Newcombe et al. 1959). The proposal at that time was to get family data relevant to the genetic risks of irradiation based on a whole population or a particular province. In the family studies, birth records were linked into sibship groups, along with parental records and various other health records.

Individual follow-up, however, is in much greater demand now at the national level. The following sections summarize recent developmental work within Statistics Canada that has been described in detail elsewhere (Smith 1979, 1980a,b; Smith and Newcombe 1980; Smith et al. 1980; Howe and Lindsay 1981; M. E. Smith and H. B. Newcombe, unpubl.).

THE RECORDS USED

The records typically used in occupational and environmental health studies may be divided into two classes: (1) Those containing outcome information about sickness and death and (2) those from which inferences may be made about exposure to a particular substance (e.g., pertaining to certain medical treatment, nickel miners, uranium miners, workers in particular geographic areas).

At Statistics Canada, our emphasis to date has been in the organization of the outcome files on a national scale, because this is a function that other institutions are unable to perform due to the confidentiality laws governing the use of such information. Other outside organizations generally come to us with detailed exposure records which relate to some specific group under study. We carry out these epidemiological studies on a cost-recovery basis. In these studies we are looking for statistical associations between agents and particular causes of cancer or death that may confirm or indicate a need for further experimental or clinical study, or for preventive measures.

THE MORTALITY DATA BASE AND THE NATIONAL CANCER INCIDENCE REPORTING SYSTEM

Both death and cancer incidence records form fundamental ingredients in the design of any systematic investigation of the risk of cancer in large groups of people. The design and function of the Canadian Mortality Data Base file containing information from all Canadian death registrations and of the National Cancer Incidence Reporting System have been described in Smith and Newcombe (1980).

Consolidation of a historical mortality file on a national level is highly desirable in view of the potential multiple uses it could serve for epidemiological studies. Canadians are very mobile, and as a result death often occurs far from the place of exposure to the hazardous substance that may have caused the death; the same is true of diagnoses of environmentally induced diseases. For example, in the Royal Commission Study on the Health and Safety of Workers in Mines in Ontario (Ham 1976), only 72% of deaths to Ontario uranium miners occurred in Ontario.

It may be helpful to review the overall flow of death information in Canada. Registration of vital events is a provincial responsibility, but under Orders-in-Council dating back to 1919 a viable mechanism was set into place resulting in the uniform registration of vital events, the transmission of copies of vital records to Statistics Canada, and the publication of vital statistics starting with 1921 (Rowebottom 1979).

At the present time, the original source documents are collected in provinces and transmitted to Statistics Canada using magnetic tape, microfilm, and (or) copies of the original forms. In anticipation of new federal social legislation, provision was made in 1945 to transmit actual micrographic copies of all vital registrations together with appropriate amendments to the central statistical agency. Administrative needs of the day dictated that respondent agencies had to microfilm all registrations filed since 1926. It is from these records that nominal machine-readable abstracts were prepared for the period 1926-1949. From 1950 to the present, the machine-readable abstracts also incorporate statistical data for each event. These data are used to produce the routine annual national statistical tabulations.

Work in organizing a historical Mortality Data Base file in a standard format began in 1975. The objective of the current project is to create and maintain a death file that will facilitate computer and manual follow-up studies, as well as generation of special historical tabulations.

The file is in two forms: (1) Compact microfiche, alphabetic listings dating back to 1926 that are used for small research studies (coded cause of death is missing prior to 1950) and (2) the machine-readable file of over 4 million records in the period 1950-1977 with coded cause of death. This latter file is basically in a standard format, is consolidated over all Canadian provinces and over a span of years to facilitate searching by computer, and is increasing at a rate of about 170,000 events per year. An historical summary file is being planned to serve special requests for historical tabulations. A typical product of the use of such a file is in the production of mortality atlas data to illustrate the spatial variation of mortality rates in Canada and facilitate the detection of high-risk regions and any general pattern of disease distribution (Minister of Supply and Services Canada 1980a, b).

The National Cancer Incidence Reporting System, which has been in operation since 1969, is based on reports from provincial cancer registries and covers all of Canada except Ontario. Each province in Canada has a central cancer registry that tries to record each newly diagnosed primary cancer. Most provincial registries also are responsible for recording treatment and other follow-up information. There are about 43,000 notifications each year, and the file for 1969-1977 contains a total of about 400,000 cancer registrations. Less experience has been gained in utilizing the cancer incidence files, but several are in the planning stage. This file will be particularly valuable where the survival rate is high or where the cancer is rare.

THE GENERALIZED ITERATIVE RECORD LINKAGE SYSTEM

The development of a generalized iterative record linkage system (GIRLS) for use in follow-up of cohorts in epidemiological studies and the statistical theory behind the methods used for linkage have been described earlier (Newcombe et al. 1959; Kennedy et al. 1965; Newcombe 1967; Fellegi and Sunter 1969; Smith 1980a; Howe and Lindsay 1981). Previous linkage systems have been restrictive in that they have been tied to specific algorithms and application requirements. The GIRLS system uses new data base technology, operates in either batch or on-line mode, is modular in development, has been designed to be simple to use, and utilizes weights to produce a quantitative measure of the total probability that two records being compared do or do not relate to the same entity. These weights are modified easily. The particular rules used in the linkage are tailored to the files coming to us from a wide variety of research areas. The system has been designed and tested using real data from a fluroscopy study, with Dr. G. Howe from the National Cancer Institute of Canada collaborating with Statistics Canada in its development. Since 1979, production runs for several large projects have been successfully completed using this system.

In developing a computer strategy for linking records, it was found that the rules of subjective judgment that a human clerk uses when matching records fortunately are simpler to simulate by computer than one might originally have supposed.

To get around spelling variations in surnames, a phonetic New York State Identification and Intelligence System (NYSIIS) code is used (Lynch and Arends 1977). To aid in deciding whether pairs of records do or do not relate to the same individual, we use the fact that rare names and rare birthplaces carry more discriminating power when they agree than do their commoner counterparts. We have calculated weights for surname and forename spellings based on frequencies from the death files. The weights for forenames are calculated separately for females. For example, if we have two records with "J. Smith" on them, subjectively, we would not be sure that they relate to the same individual, but if the name were rare, such as "Zacharias Orvil Krawczyk," we would have greater assurance the pair belongs to the same individual. Logarithms to the base two are used as in information theory, the weights are additive, and a total weight is achieved at the end indicating whether the pairs are linked, possibly linked, or nonlinked.

The user defines the comparison space of those records that will be physically compared to each other, e.g., all records with the same phonetic NYSIIS surname code. But there are certain instances where this code may differ due to major surname spelling changes. In these cases, one may have an option, at more cost, of using alternate sort sequences to define the pockets within which records are compared, e.g., birth date and first forename spelling.

Rejection rules can be used to reduce the number of comparisons. For example, if you have an occupational file where a worker was known to be alive in 1975, then there is no use searching the 1950-1974 death records. Thus "last known alive date" is a valuable item that is often overlooked when creating occupational nominal roll files. This variable can help reduce the cost of the mortality search.

The system is modular in development and allows the user to adjust parameters and weights easily until optimum linkage results are achieved for a particular application. The system is also designed such that unwanted repetition of successfully completed steps is unnecessary.

DESIGN OF EMPLOYEE NOMINAL ROLLS

When a study of the delayed effects of a working environment is initiated, there are often major problems in establishing who had worked in the past in the industry involved and in gathering identifying information with sufficient specificity to reduce the low level and the likelihood of mistaken identity when searching large files. This lack of adequate recorded information is a major stumbling block in epidemiology (Science Council of Canada 1977). Even today, the information being collected regarding many employees in the workplace is often inadequate (particularly for women employees who may change their surnames), or it is stored in a fragmented fashion, which substantially reduces its utility.

Such difficulties could be greatly reduced in the future if adequate personal identifying information were obtained routinely in compact form from each employee at the time of hiring. A list of items to be included in such a questionnaire is shown in Table 1. Other information relating to work histories, exposure histories, and updates to the items (e.g., place of residence) should be added later. Termination dates should be recorded, and if the employee dies, the complete date and place of death recorded. Although some items such as the Social Insurance Number and Health Insurance Number are not used in the mortality search, these items are of value because they simplify the removal of duplicate entries in such a nominal roll and facilitate the compilation of work histories involving more than one employer.

The availability of identifying and statistical items is not consistent over time. It is highly desirable to monitor the reporting of all items on the Mortality Data Base file and the cancer file by year and province. We also recommend preparation of this kind of report for the exposure file, as it will give one an indication of the likelihood of linkage success for these files. The availability of identifying items on the linked output file can be used to facilitate the analysis of comparable subgroups of the file.

It is very important to edit the fields on the nominal roll files (e.g., month of birth should have numeric values in the range 01-12). Standard rules are needed for keypunching this information (e.g., indicating how to handle double-barreled surnames, prefixes, titles such as junior, etc.). In addition, abbreviations for forenames should be avoided (e.g., Wm. for William).

Table 1

A List of Items to be Included in an Employee Health-identifying questionnaire

1. Surname
2. Previous surname (if any)
3. First given name
4. Second and other given names
5. Usual name (or nickname)

6. Sex
7. Birth date (year, month, day)
8. Birth province or country
9. Birth city or place

10. Father's surname
11. Father's first given name
12. Father's second given name
13. Father's birth province or country

14. Mother's maiden surname
15. Mother's first given name
16. Mother's second given name
17. Mother's birth province or country

18. Marital status
19. Spouse's birth surname
20. Spouse's first given name
21. Spouse's second given name
22. Spouse's birth province or country

23. Social Insurance Number
24. Health Insurance Number
25. Pension plan number

26. Current complete address including postal code

Signature: ______________________________

Date: ______________________________
Year Month Day

This form is designed to be filled out when the employee is hired. Other information relating to work histories, exposure histories, and updates should be added later. A control code to indicate the work site, a control code digit to indicate alternative entries for the same event (e.g., cases where an individual may have an alternate spelling for surname), and a unique employee number are optional additional items. Termination dates and address changes should be added. A "last known alive date" is of value to reduce the amount of searching required in the death file. If the employee dies, the date of death and province or country of death should be added to the nominal roll file.

THE PRODUCTS

Most of the studies undertaken to date relate to groups of people numbering in the tens of thousands to hundreds of thousands. The studies are concerned with the long-term consequences of various occupations, medical treatments and diagnostic procedures, and circumstances of other kinds that may contribute to death from cancer, cardiovascular disease and other causes. Table 2 indicates the wide range of topics of interest and also the size of the studies being carried out. The industrial groups include uranium miners, nickel workers, hard-rock miners, and radiation workers, plus some who are exposed to asbestos, fiberglass, vinyl chloride, and formaldehyde vapor. The medical patients include persons exposed repeatedly to fluoroscopic X-rays and others treated with a potentially carcinogenic drug, isoniazid. Similar follow-up is planned for participants in a large nutritional survey, as well as other studies using various provincial cancer registries. An expanded list of reference for these studies is given in (Smith 1979; Smith et al. 1980; M.E. Smith and H.B. Newcombe, unpubl.).

In Ontario, the recent report of the Royal Commission on the Health and Safety of Workers in Mines (Ham 1976) indicated an excess of lung cancer among uranium miners. The study currently in progress is more comprehensive and will attempt to calculate the relationship between the time course of exposure to short-lived radon daughters and the time course of excess lung cancer risk. Several control populations will be used: Ontario males, northern

Table 2
Long-term Medical Follow-up Studies

Study	Number of individuals
1. Infant death-birth linkage (1971 births)	6,000
2. Ontario uranium miners	16,000
3. Isoniazid and cancer in tuberculosis patients	64,000
4. Canadian labor force—10% sample	700,000
5. Fluoroscopy and cancer in tuberculosis patients	100,000
6. INCO nickel workers	62,000
7. Falconbridge nickel workers	12,000
8. Eldorado uranium workers	16,000
9. Ontario miners nominal roll	57,000
10. Newfoundland fluorspar miners	2,000
11. Railway workers	18,000
12. Ontario morticians	1,500
13. Nutrition Canada Survey participants	20,000
14. Breast cancer and age at first birth	300,000
15. Alberta Cancer Registry Death Clearance	175,000
16. Ontario Cancer Registry Reporting System	125,000

Ontario males, and Ontario miners who have not worked in a uranium mine. Information concerning death in the study population of about 57,000 miners is being obtained by matching the personal identifying information of each miner with that contained on the Mortality Data Base file. The study is ongoing and the data are to be reviewed regularly.

There is existing scientific evidence, although by no means conclusive, suggesting that the various sulfide forms of nickel are carcinogenic. The initiative for an INCO study of nickel workers came from a joint union-management committee on occupational health set up by INCO Metals Limited and the United Steelworkers of America, and was funded as a result of the 1975 negotiation over renewal of their 3-year agreement. McMaster University was chosen to conduct the work. Falconbridge Nickel Limited made a similar request to the university. The employment records for the cohort populations of about 62,000 and 12,000 individuals respectively are currently being matched against the Mortality Data Base file. Because INCO has produced in earlier years up to 75% of the western world's nickel and still accounts for 40%, its potential contribution to the study of the effect of nickel on humans should be great.

The Eldorado Nuclear uranium workers, who are being followed in a similar fashion, include those employed in mining, milling, the extraction of radium for medical purposes, and the refining of uranium as a nuclear fuel. A nominal roll has been prepared of past and present employees from personnel records, pay records, and all other available sources (Abbatt et al. 1980) representing the Port Radium mine in the Northwest Territories which operated from 1932-1960, the Beaverlodge mine in northen Saskatchewan, and the Port Hope refinery, which have been operating since 1953 and 1933 respectively. As the operator of Canada's first uranium mine, in Port Radium, and the country's only refinery over a 50-year period at Port Hope, they are in a good position to make an important contribution to the scientific knowledge of the health effects of the uranium industry on its workforce.

This study, like many others, serves to stress the need for industry to retain adequate name rosters of past employees in compact, easily retrievable form. Extensive work has been involved in compiling the nominal roll file. Many institutions now routinely destroy old personnel files a few years after employees have terminated. In an ongoing study of the employees of a company, a cumulative name roster should be maintained and updated routinely.

Ontario morticians are of special interest as a study group because of their exposure to formaldehyde vapor. Use is being made of records for 1500 licenses issued to embalmers and funeral directors in Ontario from the period 1928-1957. We are doing a manual research using the early microfiche file, as well as a computer search for deaths after 1950.

In addition to the suspected high-risk occupational groups, there is a need for a systematic investigation of substantial numbers of persons in the working environment to determine whether new risks might be identified. Survey records based on a 5-10% sample of the Canadian labor force were keypunched, including codes for occupation and industry for the period 1965-1971. These records have been used to form composite work histories for each individual. The volume of records at the start was about 3 million, which was reduced to form 700,000 individual work histories. These histories were then linked to a file of about 2 million death records.

A detailed plan for this study was prepared initially by Dr. Newcombe (1974) and the actual study has been undertaken by Dr. G. Howe of the National Cancer Institute of Canada (Howe et al. 1980). Analysis of the results of this study is currently in progress, and it is anticipated that further updates to the follow-up of the survey group will be of particular interest.

Added to the demands for occupational studies, there is a growing interest in the extents to which other circumstances including diet, food additives, life-styles, and other variables may contribute to killing conditions such as cancer and cardiovascular disease. About 20,000 Canadians participated in a Nutrition Canada Survey conducted in 1970-1972, and the subsequent mortality experience of these persons is being investigated. A breast cancer study will compare the ages of women bearing their first child, as indicated on British Columbia birth registration tape, with the causes of their eventual death.

The efficiency and cost of any follow-up study depends on the availability and quality of identifying information that is common to the two files being brought together. In certain mortality studies, cases known to be alive are included in the death search to assist estimation of possible linkage errors.

In general, the larger the number of records in a cohort file, the lower the cost per search. Unit costs in the vicinity of a dollar or two per search may be encountered. This includes the overall steps of preprocessing the files, encoding surnames, sorting, and preparing a file in a format suitable for analysis, in addition to the linkage steps. There are fixed costs for the personnel time required to do the computer programming and tailoring of the linkage techniques to make maximum use of the items available.

THE LAW

Statistics Canada does carry responsibility for the confidentiality of the vital and health records that are entrusted to it, and there are several pieces of legislation that define what we may or may not do. Most important are the Statistics Act, the recent federal Human Rights Act, Orders-in-Council pertaining to vital statistics, and the various provincial statistics acts or their equivalents.

CONCLUSION

If one wants to know whether various agents to which people are exposed are good or bad for them, there is only one way to be certain, and that is to follow them up. This is particularly true for any agent with delayed effects and where numbers of individuals must be observed to detect small excess risks. Long-term medical follow-up implies the organization of certain outcome files at a national level that are centralized, searchable, and contain adequate identifying information.

Collaboration and cooperation among a number of different agencies often are necessary. Various federal and provincial departments and agencies such as the National Cancer Institute of Canada, the Department of Health and Welfare, the various provincial vital statistics departments, and cancer agencies have all contributed in the development of the files and facilities at Statistics Canada.

REFERENCES

Abbatt, J.D. and ENL Project Team. 1980. *The Eldorado epidemiology project: Health follow-up of Eldorado uranium workers.* Eldorado Nuclear Ltd., Ottawa.

Fellegi, I.P. and A.B. Sunter. 1969. A theory of record linkage. *J. Am. Stat. Assoc.* **64**:1183.

Ham, J.M. 1976. *Report of the Royal Commission on the Health and Safety in Miners.* The Attorney-General, Province of Ontario, Toronto.

Howe, G.R. and J. Lindsay. 1981. A generalized iterative record linkage system for use in medical follow-up studies. *Comput. Biomed. Res.* (in press).

Howe, G.R., J. Lindsay, and A.B. Miller. 1980. "A national system for monitoring occupationally related cancer morbidity and mortality." Paper presented at the American Society of Preventive Oncology, Symposium on Occupation and Cancer, March 1980, Chicago.

Kennedy, J.M., H.B. Newcombe, E.A. Okazaki, and M.E. Smith. 1965. *Computer methods for family linkage of vital and health records.* Publ. No. AECL-2222. Atomic Energy of Canada Ltd., Chalk River, Ontario.

Lynch, B.T. and W.L. Arends. 1977. *Selection of a surname coding procedure for the S.R.S. record linkage system.* Department of Agriculture, Washington, D.C.

Medical Research Council of Canada. 1968. *Health research uses of record linkage in Canada.* MRCC Report No. 3. Montreal Road, Ottawa.

Minister of Supply and Services Canada. 1980a. *Mortality atlas of Canada, vol. 1: Cancer.* Cat. No. H49-6/1-1980. Can. Gov. Publ. Centre, Hull, Québec K1A 0S9.

______. 1980b. *Mortality atlas of Canada, vol. 2: General mortality.* Cat. No. H49-6/2-1980. Can. Gov. Publ. Centre, Hull, Québec K1A 0S9.

Newcombe, H.B. 1967. Record linkage: The design of efficient systems of linking records into individual and family histories. *Am. J. Hum. Genet.* **19**:335.

______. 1974. *A method of monitoring nationally for possible delayed effects of various occupational environments.* Publ. No. NRCC-13686. Environmental Secretariat National Research Council of Canada, Ottawa.

Newcombe, H.B., J.M. Kennedy, S.J. Axford, and A.P. James. 1959. Automatic linkage of vital and health records. *Science* **130**:954.

Rowebottom, L.E. 1979. "Statistics Canada: The legal basis of health record linkage." Paper presented at the Workshop on Computerized Record Linkage in Cancer Epidemiology, August 1979, Statistics Canada, Ottawa.

Science Council of Canada. 1977. *Policies and poisons: The containment of long-term hazards to human health in the environment and in the workplace.* Report No. SCC-28, Ottawa.

Smith, M.E. 1979. Automated medical follow-up and delayed industrial risks. In *First International Conference on Health Effects of Energy Production* (ed. N.E. Gentner and P. Unrau), p. 125. Publ. No. AECL-6958, Atomic Energy of Canada Ltd., Chalk River, Ontario.

———. 1980a. The present state of automated follow-up in Canada. Part 1: Methodology and files. *J. Clinical Computing* **9**:1.

———. 1980b. Value of record linkage studies in identifying populations at genetic risk and relating risk to exposure. A paper presented at the International symposium of Chemical Mutagenesis, Human Population Monitoring, and Genetic Risk Assessment (ed. K.C. Bora), Amsterdam ASP Biological, Medical Press, B.V.

Smith, M.E. and H.B. Newcombe. 1980. Automated follow-up facilities in Canada for monitoring delayed health effects. *Am. J. Public Health* **70**:1261.

Smith, M.E., J. Silins, and J.P. Lindsay. 1980. The present state of automated follow-up in Canada. Part 2: The products. *J. Clinical Computing* **9**:19.

Statistics Act. 1970-71-72, c. 15. An Act respecting statistics of Canada. Minister of Supply and Services, Ottawa.

COMMENTS

ACHESON: Could I congratulate Martha Smith on her remarkable paper and say there is justice in the fact that record linkage on a national scale is coming into its own in the country where the term was first used and the technique was first developed by Dr. Newcombe. Furthermore, computer record linkage is much cheaper than manual linkage by clerks.

SMITH: It can be as little as a few cents per search. For example, the study involving 700,000 work histories was one of the cheapest. I think the production runs cost something like $5000 for the total of 700,000 searches of the Mortality Data Base.

R. PETO: How much does it cost to keep the whole system going, that is, for maintaining all these data. Roughly how much are you spending a year?

SMITH: The maintenance of the facilities is in the order of $100,000. This is for the whole operation and includes dealing with customers and updating the mortality file. I am talking about the marginal additional cost to maintain a follow-up facility, given that a system of national vital statistics exists. It is not like the U.S. National Death Index, where they are charging for getting the death files.

R. PETO: What about the costs for all this data coming in?

SMITH: All our research projects are done on a cost-recovery basis. For example, if a customer came to us with a particular file, like the Eldorado Nuclear nominal roll, he would pay. That is done because of the setup agreed upon in the past for getting national statistics. There were agreements between the provinces and the federal government for this purpose. As part of these agreements, we supply forms, for example. We were getting the death data anyhow.

McELHENY: But the expectation would be that if you added up all the costs in the provinces to collect the information to pass it on to you, so to speak, that might be considerably larger than the $100,000.

SMITH: Data has been collected since 1919, so this system basically is using what is available. It is just a matter of organizing it a slightly different way. We are not exactly sure how much it costs the provinces to maintain their vital statistics systems, but I would guess their costs are $5-10 per record.

UTIDJIAN: I understand that in certain provinces the fact but not the cause of death is entered on the record; the death certificate is in two parts, with a perforation, and the cause of death is removed before it is given to most interested parties. Which provinces are those?

SMITH: Both Ontario and Alberta have two-part forms consisting of the death registration form and then a medical certificate. These two provinces have two-part forms for administrative convenience only and this has nothing to do with the confidentiality of the cause of death.

McELHENY: Do any of the other provinces have those limitations?

SMITH: The cause of death is always considered, in all provinces to be confidential information and not generally released for individual deaths.

In almost all the projects that we do, we consider the province to be the owner of the record, and we are the custodian. Very often, when we are doing a study, the mechanics are much easier at a national level. We, however, consult very often the provincial government about doing it. There is a Vital Statistics Council meeting once a year, and the provincial registrars and Statistics Canada review new developments.

Needs for the Future: A Concluding Discussion

RAPPORTEUR: VICTOR K. McELHENY
Banbury Center
Cold Spring Harbor Laboratory

Participants in the occupational cancer conference who were able to remain until the final morning, 2 April 1981, were invited to take part in a general discussion of points where views converged or continued to diverge. The discussion was led by Marvin Schneiderman, one of the organizers of the conference. It focused first on the type of intervention in the workplace that would be needed to improve protection of workers' health and then turned to methods of increasing the chances that epidemiologic and other research would uncover occupational risks earlier than is now possible.

Schneiderman began the discussion by posting a list of topics needing general consideration. These are listed in Table 1.

In opening a consideration of steps needed to reduce occupational risks, Schneiderman urged that participants not be particularly concerned about the cost of such measures, because this would result in spending "a great deal of time trying to read the entrails rather than trying to cook the chicken."

The heat of controversy over occupational cancer, according to Samuels, could be lowered if the public understood that the establishment of absolute truth or falsity was not in the nature of scientific investigation. He urged attention to the possible need for an internationally agreed code for industrial occupations, to allow more exact comparisons not only between countries but also within countries.

The long internal, sometimes more than a century, between identifying an occupation as hazardous and identifying substances creating the hazard was of concern to Acheson who reported that it was 150 years before the substance causing scrotal cancer in chimney sweeps was identified. To diminish the intervals, Acheson urged multidisciplinary meetings.

In the face of urgent demands to protect workers' health, Samuels said, scientists, industry, and governments may have to control industrial processes even before specific carcinogenic substances can be identified.

Acheson agreed that prevention steps should not wait until the hazardous substance is known, but identification of substances also is important because

Table 1
Topics for Consideration in Roundtable

1. Are there any trends?
2. Occupational factors
   - Are they being controlled for adequately?
   - Old materials, new materials, and new jobs must be considered
3. Suggested consensus
   - What are the percentages of cancer attributed to occupational exposure for the past, present, and future?
   - How much is known?
4. High-risk groups
   - What are the specific hazardous substances or processes that pose occupational risk?
5. Directions for future work
   - Siemiatycki study
   - Richard Peto large-scale, case control study of lung cancer
   - Rosenberg–NCHS program, National Death Index, and record linkage
   - The need for industry-occupation coding
6. Modeling
   - Conceptualizations
   - Mathematical expression
   - Multiple exposures and their relationship to quantification of occupational exposures
7. Policy issues
   - Engineering and technology planning
   - Pre-emptive behavior as a "green" goal
8. Costs of action or inaction
   - Coordination of broad support and broad representation
9. Issues for epidemiologists
   - Retention of employee records
   - Confidentiality
   - Standardization of measurements
10. Discovery systems
    - Toxicology interations
    - Marriage of basic biology with epidemiology

this helps track down other potential risks. An example is provided by an alcohol-soluble flavonol, implicated in digestive-system cancers among furniture workers, that also may play a role in the maturing of alcohol in oak casks. Until a carcinogen is identified, its wider relevance cannot be measured. Acheson urged mutagenicity tests on wood dusts.

The design of industrial processes is much more important in preventing occupational cancer than the outmoded epidemiological and medical approach of identifying risky substances and setting exposure standards for them, according to Siemiatycki. He said, "We must promote the idea that workers should not be exposed to products where toxicity is unknown." He added that the trends described by Hoerger (this volume) indicate that this approach already is being applied in fact. Samuels called such an approach "the screening of technology" and urged that it be made a reality.

Siemiatycki said that an admittedly utopian goal, zero exposure, or "green factories," should be the guiding principle in protecting workers' health. Such proper industrial design would be the first line of defense, short-term testing (if validated) would be the second, and epidemiology the third.

Acheson rejoined, "Only the wealthiest countries can afford to consider protecting men at all stages of manufacturing processes from every type of dust." He agreed with Samuels that rich countries have a moral obligation to people in developing countries to which we ship "our outmoded technologies" and that we cannot follow a policy that says, in effect, "Because they are poorer, we will let them die faster." Nonetheless, Acheson urged that we push for the accurate identification of carcinogens.

To Hoerger, the concept of a green factory was "amorphous." Wood dust, he said, has one meaning for a hobbyist in his basement, another to a carpenter building a house, and a third to a worker in a furniture factory.

There often is great difficulty in fixing a level of control to impose on a substance, according to Julian Peto. In the rubber industry, where evidence of a moderate cancer risk has been found but no exact cause determined, dust levels might be controlled at great expense only to find that uncontrolled volatile fractions were to blame. The size of the cancer risk from asbestos in schools or from components of polluted air is difficult to determine, and yet actions are being decided now. At the moment, J. Peto feels that people seem to decide whether they want the level of control to be all or nothing and then collect scientific arguments to support their position—"There are very plausible mathematical arguments to support either extreme, and both are extremely insecure."

Samuels responded that "We can't sit around and count the bodies before we decide to act. We have to reduce unnecessary risk, at the level of practical reason. At the same time, we need ideals like 'green factories.' "

In reducing unnecessary risks, according to Samuels, "you don't just worry about the dust" but also about fumes and vapors from the solvents. "All we can really do in any plant is close or open a system, that is, either expose humans to some degree or not expose them to another degree."

Julian Peto further indicated that he was worried that emphasis on trivial risks might divert attention from important ones, such as tobacco, and that the question of spending \$1,000 or \$1 million in combating a particular risk was important.

Davis reported that less than 10% of the substances in commerce had been tested for carcinogenic effects. According to Davis, between 1970 and 1980, the Occupational Safety and Health Administration managed to regulate a total of 17 carcinogens. At that rate, it would take 100 years to regulate known occupational hazards.

There was debate about the true cost of creating "green factories," or of other risk-reduction steps. Was the true figure $100 billion, or $10 billion a year—or zero? Davis noted that control of fugitive emissions had improved productivity in vinyl chloride manufacture.

Richard Peto noted that some types of data collection, whose value will increase with time, are very inexpensive. Beebe noted that the cost of operating the new U.S. National Death Index was about $1 million a year. Samuels added that in a $2 trillion economy such sums were not an issue; political desire *is*.

Failure to act can be expensive. Schneiderman said that some of the consequences of the explosive spreading of dioxin over the Italian town of Seveso, costing $100 million, might have been avoided by designing high-temperature relief valves costing a few tens of thousands.

In the hope of focusing the discussion on tasks accomplishable by scientists, Stewart said her main concern was the best methods of studying the epidemiology of cancer rather than discussing "these fantastic sums, and cost-benefit analysis and so on." She said, "We have quite enough on our plate without trying to tell everybody how to alter their factories."

Beaumont regarded the prevention of personnel record destruction an important issue among epidemiologists, since this is occasionally done after an inquiry from a govenment agency. Such records often are the sole means of identifying a worker's precise job (and hence of estimating exposures). Acheson said that in the United Kingdom and Canada, organizations of epidemiologists have expressed concern that destruction of workers' records, and excessively restrictive confidentiality rules were beginning to limit vital epidemiological work on occupational and other health risks.

Beebe noted that the National Death Index is designed primarily to serve investigators conducting cohort studies, not case-control studies. By using the National Death Index, researchers can determine the survival from 1979 (the date the Index began) of a group of workers at a particular factory whose personnel records have been preserved. The National Death Index avoids the necessity of applying to 50 different jurisdictions for death certificates. Beebe said, "It is a very basic tool, a very flexible tool that ministers to a lot of things" mentioned in Table 1. He added, "By itself, it doesn't solve anything, but it is a very sharp tool. I think it would greatly enhance the number and cogency of cohort studies that we could do in this country, not just for occupation but for all kinds of hazardous situations."

In response to a question from Davis, Beebe said it had taken 10 years from the formal recommendation by a committee to establish the National Death Index. He deplored the failure to implement the recommendation to extend the index several years back from 1979. Samuels lamented that legislation designed to clarify ethical and legal issues about linkage of Social

Security and Internal Revenue data to the Index, to improve identification of job categories, barely missed passage through Congress last year.

Responding to Schneiderman's request for comments from overseas participants, Axelson said that at least 20% of the reported increase in cancer incidence in Sweden since 1959 represented "a real excess." He expressed surprise at the suggestion by Richard Peto (this volume) that there was no evidence for a generalized increase in cancer rates in the United States other than those due to tobacco. Record linkage, Axelson said, appears overrated from the Swedish experience. "I think it has taken away a lot of thinking and money from regular epidemiology, and in my view we have gained nothing so far." All record-linkage has done, Axelson said, is rediscover the high risk for miners, painters, and chimney sweeps.

McMichael emphasized the need for the best possible epidemiological surveillance to minimize the chances of exposures sneaking up on people dwelling in an ever-changing society, with people constantly changing jobs, eating habits, recreations, reproductive and sexual behavior and so on.

The dominant impression of studies of occupational risk, McMichael said, is of people working "in a lamentably piecemeal fashion, doing little studies dotted all over the place with no adequate standardization of measurements and no good ability to pool data or make satisfactory conclusions." The need, he said, is for "some central work, properly coordinated and widely supported." Such coordination, Schneiderman suggested, might be provided by the International Agency for Research on Cancer in Lyon.

Brochard commented that although a French occupational health organization has existed since World War II and 4,000 doctors have been placed in factories, occupational epidemiology is virtually impossible. Death certificates cannot be obtained for cohort studies but an international organization might be able to alleviate this situation, Brochard added.

According to Paddle, the Chemical Industries Association in Britain, after many years of opposition from many companies on grounds of expense, is working on proposals for collecting four pieces of data on all chemical workers: name, National Health Service number, date of birth, and address. Paddle said that epidemiologists as a group should lobby for pressing ahead with such data collection.

Julian Peto expressed regret that the meeting had devoted so little time to examining the implications of recent advances in molecular understanding epitomized by Legator's ideas (this volume) for monitoring various aspects of potential carcinogenicity. A case can be made now, he said, for large-scale collection of blood and urine samples for current analysis of chromosome abnormalities and storage against the day—less than 10 years off—when DNA sequencing will be far easier and cheaper than now.

Such techniques, he said, would certainly disclose immediate effects from certain exposures, "and thus largely avoid the appalling latency-period problem." People identified as having chromosome abnormalities might then be used in cohort studies that would identify large risks. Up to now, Peto said, "the risks are diluted incredibly. We don't expect to see a five-fold increase in cancer risk in the chemical industry. We would be very surprised if we saw a 2% or 3% increase."

Cairns followed this up with a comment concerning the notion that coffee drinking is a major determinant of pancreatic cancer. "If this is true," he said, "and the epidemiologists' estimates of the extent of the risk are correct, then we are talking of 10,000 cancer deaths a year in the United States."

"It is not certain that the epidemiologists' retrospective studies are correct," Cairns continued. "However, if dietary histories had been taken from some large number of people, and if, say, urine samples had been frozen down, it would now be a simple matter, as Richard Peto pointed out, to pick those who died of pancreatic cancer, plus a group of appropriate controls, and then test the urine samples for whatever one finds to be characteristic of coffee drinkers. In this way, you would find out in 2 months whether the association with coffee held up in a prospective study of this kind."

Afterword

RICHARD PETO
Oxford University
Oxford OX2 6HE, England

MARVIN SCHNEIDERMAN
Clement Associates, Inc.
Washington, D.C. 20007

INTRODUCTION

In concluding a meeting on the quantification of occupational cancer, it is reasonable to ask what new information (or new consensuses) emerged about quantitative matters, and what studies are practicable that might narrow the range of the estimates of the contributions of occupation to cancer in general or to particular cancers. Some of what follows reflects our understanding of areas of agreement among all the views expressed at the meeting.

About 20 substances or processes have been firmly established as causes of cancer among workers exposed to them, 100 or 200 substances that workers are exposed to have been found to be capable of causing cancer in laboratory animals, and several thousand substances that various numbers of workers are exposed to in various degrees have not been tested for cancer in laboratory animals. For a variety of reasons no reliable epidemiological studies of most of these substances have been or will be undertaken (see Karstadt, this volume), therefore the scope for reasonable uncertainty seems large.

Perhaps because of this, divergent views have been expressed as to whether occupational factors are likely to account for a "small" percentage (e.g. 2-4%) or a "large" percentage (e.g. 20-40%) of all U.S. cancer. Both of these, it should be noted, represent large enough absolute numbers of deaths (or new cases) to justify both intensive research and political action, for a mere 2.5% of all U.S. cancer deaths would represent some 10,000 deaths per year. Moreover, the identification of occupational hazards should have a larger place in a national policy for cancer control than might be suggested by whatever may be their relative importance in comparison with other ways of avoiding cancer, for once occupational hazards have been detected their reduction or elimination is likely to be practicable. Nevertheless, quantification remains a worthwhile objective, and whether or not it is currently possible, the process most conducive to it is likely to be a critical examination of the main arguments currently being used for the percentage being "large" and of those currently being used for it being "small," and the establishment of studies that will gather evidence that further limits the range of reasonable uncertainty.

There was considerable discussion at this meeting of a document entitled "Estimates of the fraction of cancer in the U.S. associated with occupational factors" that was prepared in 1978 in connection with the OSHA hearings (see Appendix, this volume). The 1978 document applied the excess risks of cancer that were observed by epidemiologists among small populations of heavily exposed workers to the larger populations of U.S. workers possibly exposed to those agents. It now appears that the 1978 report took insufficient account of intensity and duration of exposure to the agents that were studied. Any study neglecting this kind of exposure information will be inappropriate. There were, however, many occupational factors not considered in the 1978 report, and there was a wide spectrum of opinions among participants at this meeting as to what the current net effect of past occupational exposures is likely to be.

Moreover, no matter what the current effects of past exposures may be, there is no guarantee that the future effects of current exposures will not exceed them, for the increases over recent decades in the production of various chemicals have been enormous (Davis et al., this volume). Due to the long time that commonly elapses between first exposure to a carcinogen and the development of a pathological cancer, as Selikoff (this volume) and others have noted, health effects that are at present difficult to detect may eventually become very large.

One procedure that may help narrow the range of estimates made by different people of the total numbers of today's cancers that are associated with occupational factors is for anyone who is proposing such estimates to do so in the form of a table of numbers of cancers by site and sex. Each entry in the table would contain the suggested number of such tumors being ascribed to occupational factors, and a note of what percentage of all such tumors this represents. Some of the major sites which are related to industrial exposures are also related to nonindustrial exposures (e.g. lung cancer, bladder cancer) which makes ascribing specific cancers to single causes an impossible task.

At this meeting, it was noteworthy that the range of estimates for the likely effects of asbestos was much narrower than previously reported. Another important area of consensus that emerged was that the data on radiation-exposed workers should be analyzed by life-table methods, which should eventually lead to convergence of the interpretation of the Hanford data.

TRENDS

There was not agreement as to the most plausible interpretation of the trends in recorded incidence and in death certification rates. Respiratory cancer mortality and incidence are clearly increasing since the changes are far bigger than could plausibly be ascribed to any form of bias in the data. The national data contain some increases due to introduction or increased use of some occupational carcinogens (e.g. asbestos, radiation, new synthetic chemicals) and, at least in some age groups, possible decreases due to control of others.

On a site-specific basis, the greatest increases have been in the respiratory cancers. On an age-specific basis, most of the reported increases have come in persons 65 or over in the United States. Substantial decreases in mortality (and smaller decreases in incidence) have occurred in persons under 45. The decreases in young women have been greater than the decreases in young men. It is possible that a limited number of major environment pressures are in operation, reinforcing each other, or a set of coincidences has occurred in which many different factors operating on different diseases have been added up to a consistent general trend. Although the major concern at this meeting was with incidence of new diseases it was recognized that substantial improvements in treatment have occurred mostly in those forms of cancer that affect young people—acute lymphocytic leukemia in children, Hodgkin's disease, embryomal tumors, and perhaps breast disease in premenopausal women.

FUTURE EPIDEMIOLOGICAL RESEARCH INTO OCCUPATIONAL FACTORS

At the final session, various future directions for epidemiological research were discussed, and two main recommendations emerged. Martha Smith described the system of national records of disease and death that are available in Canada to occupational epidemiologists, and Gilbert Beebe described various inexpensive and practical ways in which certain substantial defects in the currently available U.S. national records of disease, death, and occupation could be rectified.

The first recommendation that emerged was that the principal suggestions in Dr. Beebe's paper be implemented: they have been clearly thought out and would greatly aid the epidemiological study of occupational factors. (One of them, which was merely that no matter what budgetary pressures might exist, the newly established U.S. National Death Index should survive, is also of great importance in a far wider range of epidemiological and clinical research.)

The second main recommendation was that a large case-control study of at least 10,000 lung cancer cases should be established in relation to occupation, tobacco, diet, and history of residence. The methodology and unit costs might be similar to those of the recent National Bladder Cancer Survey, and the questionnaire and methods to be used might be adapted from those currently being used by the NCI group in New Jersey and Dr. Siemiatycki's group in Montreal. A suggestion was made that certain less common types of cancer (e.g. pleura, lymphomas, scrotum, peritoneum, liver, kidney, nasal sinuses, larynx, and trachea) should also be included, so as to exploit the availability of the large control series for the study of the role of occupational and other factors in these diseases.

APPENDIX

Appendix

The following document which was submitted following the OSHA hearings in 1978 has been the subject of considerable disucssion and therefore is being reproduced in full in order to make it more easily available. The reproduction of this document does not necessarily imply endorsement by participants at this meeting or any of those listed contributors. For the convenience of saving typesetting space the original 52 page document has been condensed to 38 pages.

ESTIMATES OF THE FRACTION OF CANCER IN THE UNITED STATES RELATED TO OCCUPATIONAL FACTORS

Prepared by:

National Cancer Institute
National Institute of Environmental Health Sciences
National Institute for Occupational Safety and Health

Contributors (alphabetical order):

Kenneth Bridbord, M.D., NIOSH
Pierre Decoufle, Sc. D., NCI
Joseph F. Fraumeni, Jr., M.D., NCI
David G. Hoel, Ph. D., NIEHS
Robert N. Hoover, M.D., Sc.D., NCI
David P. Rall, M.D., Ph.D., NIEHS, Director
Umberto Saffiotti, M.D., NCI
Marvin A. Schneiderman, Ph. D., NCI
Aurthur C. Upton, M.D., NCI, Director

Contributor to the Appendix

Nicholas Day, Ph.D., NCI, IARC

September 15, 1978

This statement addresses the question: "What is the best estimate of the fraction of cancer incidence (or deaths) in the United States that is reasonable to attribute to occupational exposure in the present, and in the forseeable future?" Previously published estimates of this fraction have been as low as 1% to 5% for past data [reviews by Higgenson (1-3), Wynder and Gori (4), and Doll (5)] and as high as 10% to 15% [see the discussion by Cole (6)]. All these estimates are somewhat speculative and several were seriously incomplete or deficient. Most are now out of date. If recent evidence is considered and if the full consequences of occupational exposures in the present and recent past are taken into account, estimates of at least 20% appear much more reasonable, and may even be conservative. These estimates refer to the near term and the future.

Four Pitfalls

Four general problems confound attempts to answer this question.

(a) **Incomplete data.** Few industries have been investigated adequately for evaluating the possible occurrence of occupationally related cancers. Because of the insensitivity of epidemiologic surveys and various difficulties in conducting them (7), only agents and industrial processes which lead to rather large excess incidences have been identified to date. The International Agency for Research of Cancer (IARC) has an ongoing program to review data on chemicals for potential carcinogenic effects. To date, some 368 chemicals and industrial processes have been reviewed. According to a recent summary of the results of this program (8), some 26 chemicals or industrial processes have been identified as associated with increased risk of cancer in man (Table 1). This list includes a number of drugs and chemicals to which there is little or no occupational exposure in the United States. Only 8 or 9 of the 26 substances and processes listed in Table 1 involve exposure to large numbers of workers. By way of contrast, some 221 chemicals or mixtures were identified in the same survey as carcinogenic to one or more animal species. Although there is some occupational exposure to the majority of these 221 substances, epidemiological and case studies were in all cases either lacking, or inadequate to determine whether or not the substances are associated with excess cancer incidence in exposed human populations (8). Thus, adequate data are available for only a very small fraction of the substances and industrial processes which pose potential risks to exposed workers. Although it is possible that all the major hazards have already been identified, there is little reason to believe this without much more extensive epidemiologic investigations. In fact, many new processes and materials have been introduced in recent years. Some of these could be as hazardous or more hazardous than those used in the past.

(b) **The fallacy of "one effect – one cause" explanations.** Wynder and Gori (4) offered a tentative allocation of cancer incidence in the United States attributable to specific environmental factors. Their estimates of the proportions of cancers attributable to diet, tobacco, radiation, occupation, alcohol, and exogenous hormones have been widely quoted. However, a major difficulty with their procedures is they have classified all cancers under single "causes." whereas cancer appears to be a disease of interactions. The initiation and development of cancer is a multi-phased, multi-causal process in which both external and internal factors act, probably at each of several stages, before frank, clinical cancer appears. It is likely that many, if not most, cancers are influenced by two or more different external factors acting simultaneously or sequentially. Thus, alcohol by itself appears to be a minor cause of cancer—but alcohol combined with cigarette smoking leads to risks 15 times higher than those experiences by non-smoking non-drinkers. If a drinker smoker develops cancer of the oral cavity, to which "cause" should it be attributed? Drinking or smoking? If we could correctly identify the proportions of cancer incidence "attributable to" each of the classes of environmental factors considered by Wynder and Gori, the sum of these percentages would be considerably higher than 100. One of the best-studied examples of interaction between exogenous agents is that between asbestos and cigarette smoke in inducing lung cancer (9). Most lung cancers "attributable to" asbestos are probably simultaneously "attributable to" smoking. If current theories of a multi-causal process are correct, it seems likely that a large fraction of cancers which at first appear to be "attributable to" smoking should also be "attributable to" asbestos, radiation, and/or other occupational factors.

(c) **Latent period, age, and duration of exposure.** Most occupational carcinogens are characterized by "latent periods" of 10 to 50 years between the onset of exposure and the clinical appearance of tumors (7). This is consistent with a multi-stage process. When occupationally related cancers are detected, they usually reflect exposures which started one or more decades in the past. Accurate numerical assessment is further complicated by the strong dependence of cancer incidence upon age and upon duration of exposure. Even in cases where an excess **risk** is detected within one or two decades, this dependence on age implies that most of the attributable cancers will not occur until later in the life span of the exposed workers, perhaps as much as 40 or 50 years after the first exposure. It is difficult to trace anyone for so long a time, and those epidemiological studies which do not follow people for a full lifetime are likely to underestimate lifetime risks. Most industrial-epidemiologic studies have not (and probably could not) follow a working population to its extinction. This problem is discussed in more detail in the Appendix, but a numerical example illustrates its importance. For many types of cancer, incidence increases approximately as the fourth or the fifth power of age (1); hence the cumulative number of cancers occurring in a population over a lifetime increases as the fifth or sixth power of age. If exposure to a carcinogen results in a constant multiplicative increase in risk at all ages, then the number of cancers occurring in an exposed group will similarly increase as the fifth or sixth power of age. Thus, for example, the number of attributable cancers occurring by age 50 would be only about one-fifth or one-sixth of that expected by age 70. For this reason epidemiological studies often enumerate only a small fraction of the total excess cancers attributable to an agent. Any overall assessment of the importance of occupational carcinogenesis should take this into account.

(d) **Changes in exposure patterns.** The dependence of cancer risk upon age and duration of exposure is further complicated by changes in patterns of exposure to potential carcinogens. Few, if any, workers are exposed throughout their entire working lives to the same chemical at similar concentrations. American workers change jobs fairly frequently; even within the same job, the chemicals to which a worker is exposed may be changed from time to time. By the time an occupationally related cancer develops, the workers will frequently have been exposed to different chemicals and may well have changed occupations. It is particularly difficult to make estimates of the consequences of present-day exposure, because the chemicals for which we have the best dose-response information are those which are generally recognized as carcinogenic. Several of them have been regulated, so that exposure to these chemicals has been reduced; this leaves other carcinogens that are not well controlled.

Previous Attempts to Estimate the Importance of Occupational Carcinogenisis

In 1969, Higginson (1) tabulated estimates of "the extent to which occupational and cultural cancers have been recognized." He attributed to known occupational factors 1% of mouth cancers, 1-2% of lung cancers, 10% of bladder cancers and 2% of skin cancers. (No detailed development of these estimates was given, however.) Higginson limited his attributions to factors that "have been recognized," and the majority of cancers were assigned to "unknown" factors.

In 1976, Higginson and Muir (2) again estimated the impact of environmental factors in human cancer. They stated, again with few supporting details:

> "Although occupational cancers recognized so far provide some of the most satisfactory data for identifying external agents, the absolute number of cancers due to occupational exposures would appear to be relatively small, probably 1% to 3% of all cancers."

In 1977, Wynder and Gori (4) presented estimates of the "percent of cancer incidence in the United States attributable to specific environmental factors." It would appear from Figure 1 in their paper that their median estimates for the fraction of cancers attributable to occupational factors were 4% for men and 2% for women. Their explanation for these estimates was:

> "The data presently available are, at best, educated estimates of the relationship between specific cancers and specific occupational groups. Cole **et al.** (56) suggested

> that 20% of bladder cancers occurring in males in the Boston area are related to occupational exposure. In certain counties of New Jersey, the increased risk for this cancer appeared to be high among workers in certain chemical industries. Bailar (personal communication) estimated that the occupational contribution to total cancer incidence in males lies between 1 and 5%, and a similar estimate was made by Nelson (personal communication). General estimates of the percentage of all human cancers related to occupational exposure range between 1 and 10%. However, identification of specific high-risk groups, hazardous exposure levels, and related cancer incidence rates is yet to be determined."

In addition to the error of "one-effect, one-cause" thinking pointed out above, their reliance on "educated estimates," "personal communications," and "general estimates" makes the resulting conclusions tenuous. And again, of course, no attempt was made to estimate future consequences of past exposures.

In 1977, Doll (5) published a survey of the importance of environmental factors in human cancer in the U.K. He indicated his belief that occupational factors were of relatively small importance, but did not make a numerical estimate.

In 1977, Cole (6) estimated the fraction of cancer that is occupationally-induced to be less than 15% for men and less than 5% for women. He explained the basis for these estimates as follows:

> "I estimated that the occupationally-induced burden was less than 15% for men and less than 5% for women. The major causes of cancer deaths are cancers of the lung, the breast and the colon; and these are largely or totally non-occupationally induced. Lung cancer is 90% cigarette-smoking-induced; breast cancer is probably not at all occupationally induced; there may be some, probably small, ocupational component in cancer of the rectum. Other sites such as cervix or ovary have a negligible occupational component, if any. The above listed sites account for about half of the cancer deaths. For other sites, it is difficult to assess the occupational component. However, even an 'occupationally-related' cancer like bladder cancer can be attributed directly to occupational exposures only about 25% of the time. With half the cancer essentially non-occupationally induced, and half the cancers occupationally-induced less than 25% of the time, a reasonable estimate seemed to be 15% for males."

This argument also assumes that a cancer which is related to a non-occupational factor cannot also be occupationally related. Cole's statement of the basis for his estimates makes it obvious that all these estimates contain a large element of uncertainty.

We conclude that the statement that no more than 1% to 5% of cancers in the United States are attributable to occupational factors is based on partial use of current knowledge, relfects the one-cause one-effect fallacy—and is not particularly useful for estimating future risks. It is not even a correct reflection of the published estimates, which range up to 10% (4) or 15% (6).

Re-formulating the Question

Another defect of the studies summarized above is that they may deal with an inappropriate question. Most appear to have been attempting to provide estimates of the fraction of **present-day** cancer incidence that is attributable to occupational exposures **in the past,** to agents that have already been demonstrated to be carcinogenic. However, such a question is of limited interest because the most important consequences of exposure in the recent past will be manifested until some time in the future. The question that needs to be addressed is "What is the likely contribution of **present-day** occupational exposures to future cancer incidence?" An answer to this question must be somewhat speculative, because we do not know which of the chemicals in the present-day workplace will be identified sometime in the future as causing cancer. Accordingly, to provide a basis for making appropriate estimates, we will first attempt to estimate the contribution of occupational exposures to known carcinogens in the recent past to present and future cancer incidence. It is not particularly helpful merely to speculate about the possible existence of hazardous chemicals in present-day workplaces.

Asbestos as a Well-Studied Example

The consequences of occupational exposure to asbestos in the United States have only begun to be recognized in the recent past (12-14). It has been estimated* (11) that between 8 and 11 million workers have been exposed to asbestos in the U.S. since the beginning of World War II. Of that total, approximately 1.5 to 2.5 million are presently employed. Probably a million have already died, while the remainder—between 5.5 and 7.5 million workers—were formerly employed in environments with significant asbestos exposure, including the survivors among the 4.5 million who worked in shipyards during the 1940's. Of these and other asbestos workers, approximately 4 million are believed to have had heavy exposure to asbestos (11). Epidemiological studies of workers (13-15) have indicated that, of heavily exposed workers who have already died, 20-25 percent have died of lung cancer, 7-10 percent of pleural or peritoneal mesothelioma, and 8-9 percent of gastro-intestinal cancers, adding up to a total of 35-44%. These figures may be underestimates of lifetime cancer risks, because most of these workers have not been followed to the end of their life span.

Of the 4 million heavily exposed workers, at least 1.6 million are thus expected to die of the asbestos-related cancers listed above. [In the absence of exposure to asbestos, about 0.35 million (8-9 percent) would have been expected to die of cancers at these sites.] Assuming that the excess risk to the remaining less heavily exposed workers in one-quarter of that to the heavily exposed workers (an assumption suggested by the data in ref. 16), the total number of cancers attributable to asbestos in the less-heavily exposed group would be expected to be in the range 0.4 to 0.7 million, raising the total to 2.0 to 2.3 million. Since most of these cancers will be manifested over a period of 30-35 years, the expected average number of cancer deaths associated with asbestos per year in that period will be between 58,000 to 75,000.** Such numbers would comprise 13-18% of all cancer deaths expected in the United States in the forseeable future (assuming that total cancer deaths increase to 400,000 to 450,000 per year).

Three features of these estimates deserve emphasis:

1. Although most of the exposure to asbestos has been in the past, most of the predicted effects are expected to be in the future. An estimate of the **present-day** numbers of cancers attributable to asbestos would undoubtedly be smaller.

2. A large fraction of the asbestos-related cancers are also related to smoking (lung and esophagus) or are in the gastro-intestinal tract (esophagus, stomach, and colon), where cancers are usually assumed to be not occupationally related (1, 4, 5, 6). Hence, if the old one-effect, one-cause approach were used, the occupational origin of most of the asbestos-related cancers would be overlooked and they might be attributed to other or "unknown" factors.

3. Although the frequency of asbestos-related cancers is already substantial and is probably increasing rapidly, it has not yet been detected by examination of gross trends in cancer incidence (or mortality) in the general population. There are several reasons for this:

(a) two of the major types of asbestos-related cancer, pleural and peritoneal mesothelioma, are not classifed as such in the national health statistics, but are usually listed as lung cancers or as various abdominal cancers, respectively;

(b) most asbestos-related lung cancers are also smoking-related, so that if one thinks one has the full explanation for the rise in lung cancer incidence in smoking, it is likely that no other causes will be looked for;

(c) any increase in asbestos-related cancers of the stomach and colon would be masked by the other long-term trends in cancer incidence at these sites (down in the stomach, probably up in the colon); these long-term trends are usually attributed to dietary or unknown factors.

* Several authors of this report were responsible for preparing these estimates

** Selikoff (15) made an estimate of 50,000 per year, exclusive of the added cases that would come among the less heavily exposed group.

Perhaps the most important lesson to be learned from the asbestos story is that a major public health disaster can develop while its early manifestations are lost by being attributed to other factors. This would support the argument that the earlier estimates for industrially related cancers may be deceptively low—having left out such information as the asbestos situation has now brought to our attention.

Comparison of Risks due to Asbestos with those due to Five Other High-Expsoure Substances

In Table 2 we have tabulated data on carcinogenic risks associated with exposure to five other substances to which there is large-scale occupational exposure, for comparison with corresponding data on asbestos. The tabulation is similar to that presented in ref. 17, but incorporates more recent data where available, and is limited to the substances and cancer sites for which the best data are available on both exposure and relative risks.

The first three columns in Table 2 list the agent, the affected organs, and the observed risk ratios (R) (from Table1 in ref. 7). The fourth column lists the age-adjusted incidence (I) of cancer at the sites in question in U.S. males (from data presented in the Third National Cancer Survey, ref. 19). The figures tabulated are the age-adjusted incidences in males over 20 years of age, because most occupational exposure starts at around that age. The fifth column lists the estimated number of workers (N) exposed to the chemical in 1972-74 (from ref. 18, derived from the National Occupational Hazard Survey, ref. 10). The notes to Table 2 give further information about each chemical, including summaries of data from the most definitive studies of each, and references to excess cancers at sites other than those listed in the Table.

The last column in Table 2 lists values of the quantity (R−1)NI. This is the average number of excess cancers that would be expected to occur in a population of size N, subject to a site-specific risk R times that in the general population. Although these figures are crude projections of the numbers of excess cancers to be expected in the exposed workers, they are unlikely to be precise estimates of future cancer mortality, for several reasons.

Perhaps the most important reason is that they are projections of the numbers of excess cancers in only one cohort of N workers. Because of turnovers in the workforce, the number of exposed workers and ex-workers subject to excess cancers ay any one time will be several times larger than N. If, for example, the total number of workers who have ever been exposed to a substance is, say, 5 times the number currently exposed, then the figures in Table 2 would underestimate the potential effects by a factor of 5.

It is primarily for this reason that the data for asbestos in Table 2 underestimate the expected future mortality from asbestos-related cancers by a factor of 4-5. Because the data for the other substances in Table 2 were derived in the same way as those for asbestos, they may likewise underestimate the number of cancers attributable to these substances.

The other major assumption that is necessary before the figures in Table 2 can be used as predictions of future cancer mortality is that the relative risks R would remain the same as those reported in the published studies throughout the workers' lives, even if exposures ceased. The basis for this assumption is discussed in Appendix A, where both observational and theoretical reasons for assuming constancey of R are put forward. In any case several of the studies from which the figures in Table 2 are derived reported average risks over a substantial fraction of the workers' lives.

Several other factors complicate the interpretation of the figures in Table 2, including the potential consequences of simultaneous or sequential exposure to other carcinogens or modifying factors. One reason why Table 2 may overestimate numbers of tumor cancers is that some of the workers presently exposed may have less exposure than the workers from whom the risk ratios R were originally derived. For these reasons, the figures should not be interpreted as precise estimates of future cancers, but it is reasonable to compare them with the data derived by the same method for asbestos related cancers. At the least, the data summarized in Table 2 show that the five other agents together pose hazards similar to or greater than those posed by asbestos. The sum of the best projections (see notes to Table 2) for the five compounds is about 33,000 cancers per year, versus 13,900 for asbestos. In presenting this comparison, it should be emphasized that the former figure includes only the primary sites of action. Inclusion of expected excess cancers at other sites would increase the estimates substantially.

It should be re-emphasized that many of the cancers considered here as attributable to occupational exposure would simultaneously be attributable to other factors, especially smoking. They are "attributable to" occupational exposure in the sense that most of them would not have occurred in the absence of exposure, so that they could have been prevented by prevention of occupational exposure.

Other Known and Potential Risks

In addition to the five major agents listed in Table 2, a number of other agents and industrial processes are known or suspected to pose carcinogenic risks to be exposed workers.

We omitted from Table 2 several agents listed as occupational carcinogens in refs. 7, 8 and 17, because we had difficulty matching data on relative risks to data on the number of workers exposed. These agents include cadmium, coal tar pitch volatiles, hematite, and vinyl chloride. The data we used on the number of workers exposed to carcinogenic petroleum fractions are probably conservative. The IARC (8) has already reviewed 221 agents identified as capable of inducing cancer in experimental animals. Although some occupational exposure is known to occur for most of these chemicals, epidemiological and case studies of their possible association with cancer in humans were lacking or were judged to be "inconclusive." Other carcinogens have been reported in the literature. To date only a very small proportion of all the chemicals in use have been tested for carcinogenicity.

Table 3 lists a number of occupational groups that have been shown to be at increased risk of cancer at specific sites, without specific causative agents having been identified. Although risk ratios are available in most of these cases, the imprecision of information on the numbers of workers in the jobs concerned prevented us from making estimates about the number of cancers to be anticipated.

In addition to chemcial carcinogens, occupational exposure to radiation in known to be a significant cause of cancer in U.S. workers. Groups at risk include radiologists, uranium miners, workers in the nuclear industry, military personnel exposed to radiation from nuclear explosions and to nuclear weapons, aircrews, and persons working at high altitudes. Persons working outdoors such as farm workers and fishermen are subject to increased risks of skin cancer associated with solar radiation. We have not attempted to make numerical estimates of expected cancer incidence in these occupations although many millions of workers are at presumptive risk.

Consequences of Present-Day Exposures

The estimates of potential excess cancer mortality that are listed in Table 2 are projections of the **future** consequences of **past** exposures. The estimates of risk ratios listed in Table 2 are derived from studies published between 1947 and 1978, mostly since 1966 (7). The estimated numbers of workers exposed are derived from a survey in 1972-74 (20). The anticipated excess cancer incidences are those expected to be observed in the next three decades, and could exceed those currently occurring and attributable to the agents in question.

There is evidence that occupational exposure to several of these agents has been reduced since the studies developing the risk estimates were published. Exposure to asbestos, benzene, coke oven emissions and vinyl chloride has been limited (although not eliminated) by recent OSHA regulations.

There is also evidence, however, that not all the major occupational carcinogens have been eliminated. Of the agents in Table 2, there is today widespread exposure to arsenic, chromium, nickel, and many petroleum products. Most of the excess risks referenced in Table 3 remain uncontrolled because the causative agents have not been identified. A number of important occupational groups (such as agricultural field workers) have not been adequately surveyed for excess cancer risks. Only a handful of the 221 chemicals found positive in experimental animals and reviewed by the IARC (8) have been regulated as carcinigens in the U.S. workplace. Among those not regulated are a number of synthetic organic chemicals to which there is widespread occupational exposure, but which have not been in production for long enough periods for excess risks to have been identified by epidemiological studies.

For public policy purposes, it would be very desirable to make numerical estimates of the potential consequences of present-day exposure to carcinogens in the workplace. Such estimates would, however, require numerical data on the extent and intensity of exposure, and on dose-response relationships in experimental animals. If sufficient data were available, prediction of future consequences would require quantitative extrapolation from animal responses to man. In our view, existing methods for such extrapolation leave enough questions open concerning their precision so as to make us unwilling to attempt large scale estimates — particularly in the absence of exposure data. Hence, we can say nothing firm about the magnitude of future risks attributable to the unquantified present-day exposures.

There is no evidence, however, that these risks are substantially less than the risks resulting from exposures in the recent past. Although several of the most important known carcinogens have been controlled, others have not; many carcinogenic and potentially carcinogenic chemicals are still present in U.S. workplaces; the total volume of synthetic organic chemicals produced in the U.S. continues to increase rapidly. **If only one of the thousands of chemicals introduced into commerce in the past 30 years proves to be as hazardous as asbestos, this could suffice to maintain comparable rates of occupationally-related cancer for decades into the future.** In our view, any complacency about the future consequences of present-day exposure to uncharacterized chemicals would be unjustified.

Two Alternative Approaches

Other ways can be used to estimate the possible contribution of occupational exposures to human cancer incidence. Although none, to our knowledge, has been used formally and quantitatively, at least two have been used informally to argue that occupationally-related cancers cannot be numerically important.

The first approach is to analyze trends in total cancer incidence (or mortality) in the U.S. population. The argument is made that if occupational factors were important causes of cancer, then total cancer incidence would be increasing rapidly, reflecting the rapid increase in the number and amount of synthetic organic chemicals produced in recent decades. In fact (the argument runs), the continued increase in cancer incidence and mortality is almost solely due to increases in lung cancer and other smoking-related cancers. If the "smoking-related" cancers are subtracted from the total, the argument is that the overall trend is constant or even slightly decreasing.

There are several fallacies in this argument:

1. Most of the increase in production of synthetic organic chemicals is too recent to be reflected in current cancer statistics.

2. The increase in production of synthetics (some of which are potential carcinogens) in the period 1940-1960 may well have been offset by reductions in the intensity of exposure to other chemicals, resulting from improvements in industrial controls stimulated, in part, by government regulation. Exposure to several major carcinogens has been reduced substantially in recent years. Exposure to other potential carcinogens (such as carbon tetrachloride) was reduced earlier, to reduce other types of toxic hazard. The predicted consequence of reduction in exposure to "old" carcinogens and increase in exposure to "new" carcinogens is consistent with what is observed: an increase in cancer at some sites and a decrease at others.

3. To subtract all the "smoking-related" cancers from the total is sophistry, because at least two of the sites in question are precisely those in which "occupationally-related" cancers are best recognized. Many of the smoking-related cancers should be simultaneously attributable to occupational factors. On a per-capita basis smoking among adults is declining and this should result in a decline in the smoking-related cancers — but none of this is factored in when all "smoking-related" cancers are removed from the total. If the smoking-related cancers are not subtracted, total age-adjusted cancer incidence in the U.S. is increasing at more than 1% per annum (37).

4. Not all of the smoking-related cancers, i.e. those in the lung, pancreas, and bladder, are attributable to smoking. Even if a liberal figure is used for attributable risk, the fraction of lung cancer incidence not attributable to smoking is increasing and total cancers possibly industrially related have been increasing more rapidly in the last several years than in the two decades from 1950 to 1970 (38).

5. As pointed out earlier, the major public health impact of asbestos-related cancer is just beginning to be reflected in overall cancer statistics, despite 37 years of heavy exposure. One should hardly expect more recent additions to have shown a great effect already.

A second approach is to compare cancer incidence in men and women. To the extent that exposure to chemical carcinogens occurred in occupations in which most workers are (or were) male, this should be reflected in differences in overall cancer incidence (and trends in incidence) in the two sexes. This argument would tend to support the concept of industrial risk.

The predicted difference is in fact observed: age-adjusted cancer incidence is greater in males than in females at every common site except the gall bladder and thyroid (19). In particular, incidence is much higher in males than in females in the key occupationally related sites: lung, liver, bladder, kidney, hematopoetic and lymphatic system and perhaps stomach and pancreas (19).

Nonetheless, there are some flaws in this argument, too. Not only male workers have substantial exposure to carcinogens. Although male workers doubtless predominate in chemical manufacturing and heavy industry, women have long been employed in large numbers in light industry where there is substantial exposure to certain carcinogens, e.g. the radium dial painters. The fraction of occupationally related cancers in women may increase in future years due to increased employment of women in jobs where they are exposed to carcinogens. Even housewives have greater occupational exposure to some potential carcinogens than typical working men.*

It would clearly be valuable to make a rigorous comparison between employed and never employed women, but such a study would be difficult to conduct and interpret because of the many confounding variables. In our view, there is nothing in the gross cancer statistics for the U.S. population which is inconsistent with the hypothesis that up to 20-40% of all cancers are (or will be in the next several decades) attributable to occupational factors.

Relation between Occupational and Other Contributing Factors

These estimates do not diminish the importance of other contributing factors to cancer risk such as smoking, diet, and perhaps urban-rural differences. While much of the data on occupational cancer risk considered in this paper does not specifically consider factors such as smoking (except for asbestos) and diet, it is also fair to state that the prevailing body of data linking smoking and diet with cancer risk do not adequately consider the contribution of exposure to occupational carcinogens. This is largely because the available scientific methodologies do not facilitate adequate consideration of all contributing factors in any single study or approach. Until recently most scientists did not take into account the multiple etiologies and the multi-stage nature of cancer. In retrospect, it is likely that cancer risk is a function of multiple interacting factors. Past assessments, unfortunately, generally failed to consider adequately one of the most important, and preventable, risk factor, exposure to carcinogenic agents in the workplace.

Opportunities for Prevention

The estimates of cancer attributable to occupational exposure given here should be viewed as pointing up the opportunities that exist to prevent disease in future generations. The causes of cancer are multiple, with more than one factor contributing to cancer risk. In such a situation, any percentage accounting of contributing causes to cancer well exceeds 100%. To prevent cancer, one must concentrate on causative factors that can be reduced so that we can decrease the burden of disease in future generations. It has been argued that present day asbestos workers are at lower risk than earlier workers. Opportunities to reduce risks and subsequent disease in other occupations are at hand.

Summary and Conclusions

1. The estimates that only 1% to 5% of total cancers in the United States are attributable to occupational factors have not been scientifically documented and have little meaning for estimating even short-term future risks.

* We regard the home as a workpace, even if it does not fall within the jurisdiction of OSHA.

2. Most cancers have multiple causes: it is a reductionist error and not in keeping with current theories of cancer causation to attempt to assign each cancer to an exclusive single cause.

3. Because cancer incidence is strongly dependent on age and upon duration of exposure, and because most cancers occur late in life, many industrial epidemiological studies detect only a small fraction of cancers (i.e. those developing early).

4. Past exposure to asbestos is expected to result in up to 2 million excess cancer deaths in the next three decades: this would correspond to roughly 13–18% of the total cancer mortality expected in that period.

5. Reasonable projections of the future consequences of past exposure to established carcinogens suggests that at least five of them may be comparable in their total effects to asbestos.

6. These projections suggest that occupationally related cancers may comprise as much as 20% or more of total cancer mortality in forthcoming decades. Asbestos alone will probably contribute up to 13–18%, and the data in Table 2 suggest at least 10%–20% more. These data do not include effects of radiation, nor effects of a number of other known chemical carcinogens.

7. Although exposure to some of the more important occupational carcinogens has been reduced in recent years, there are still many unregulated carcinogens in the U.S. workplaces; a number of occupations are characterized by excess cancer risks which have not yet been attributed to specific agents.

8. There is no sound reason to assume that the future consequences of present-day exposure to carcinogens in the workplace will be less than those of exposure in the recent past.

9. Patterns and trends in total cancer incidence (and mortality) in the U.S. are consistent with the hypothesis that occupationally-related cancers comprise a substantial and increasing fraction of total cancer incidence.

10. The conclusion that a substantial fraction of cancers in the United States are occupationally related is not inconsistent with conclusions that substantial fraction of cancers are also associated with other factors, such as cigarette smoking and diet.

11. Occupationally-related cancers offer important opportunities for prevention.

REFERENCES

1. HIGGINSON, J. 1969. Present trends in cancer epidemiology. Proc. Canad. Cancer Congr. 8:40-75.
2. HIGGINSON, J., and MUIR, C.S. 1976. The role of epidemiology in elucidating the importance of environmental factors in human cancer. Cancer Detection and Prevention 1:79-105.
3. HIGGINSON, J. 1976. A hazardous society? Individual versus community responsibility in cancer prevention. Amer. J. Publ. Health 66:359-366.
4. WYNDER, E.L., and GORI, G.B. 1977. Guest Editorial: Contribution of the environment to cancer incidence: an epidemiological exercise. J. Nat. Cancer Inst. 58:825-832.
5. DOLL, R. 1977. Strategy for detection of cancer hazards to man. Nature 265:589-596.
6. COLE, P. 1977. Cancer and Occupation: Status and needs of epidemiologic research. Cancer 39:1788-1791 (Discussion on pp. 1807-1808).
7. COLE, P., and GOLDMAN, M.B. 1975. Occupation. Pp. 167-184 In *Persons at High Risk of Cancer* (J.F. Fraumeni, Jr., ed.) Academic Press, New York.
8. TOMATIS, L., AGTHE, C., BARTSCH, H., HUFF, J., MONTESANO, R., SARACCI, R., WALKER, E., and WILBOURN, J. 1978. Evaluation of the carcinogenicity of chemicals: A review of the IARC Monograph Programme (1971-77). Can. Res. 38:877-885.
9. SELIKOFF, I.J., HAMMOND, E.C., and CHURG, J. 1968. Asbestos exposure, smoking and neoplasma. J. Amer. Med. Assoc. 204:106-112.
10. ARMITAGE, P., and DOLL, R. 1961. Stochastic models for carcinogenesis. Proc. 4th Berkeley Symposium on Mathematical Stastics and Probability, Vol. 4:19-38. University of California Press, Berkeley.
11. U.S. DEPARTMENT OF HEALTH, EDUCATION AND WELFARE. 1978. Statemene of Secretary Joseph A. Califano, Jr. April 26, 1978.
12. INTERNATIONAL AGENCY FOR RESEARCH ON CANCER. 1977. Monographs on the Assessment of Carcinogenic Risks of Chemicals to Man. Vol. 14, Asbestos. (Appendix A, pp. 82-84). Lyon, France.
13. SELIKOFF, I.J. 1978. Paper presented at meeting of the New York Academy of Science, June 1978.
14. SELIKOFF, I.J. 1978. Oral testimony at public hearings on OSHA generic cancer policy, June 1, 1978.
15. SELIKOFF, I.J., and HAMMOND, E.C, 1978. Asbestos-associated disease in United States shipyards. CA 28:67-99.
16. MENCK, H., and HENDERSON, B.E. 1976. Occupational differences in rates of lung cancer. J. Occup. Med. 18:797-801.
17. LASSITER, D.V. 1976. In *Occupational Carcinogenesis* (eds. U. Saffiotti and J. Wagoner). Ann. N.Y. Acad. Sci. 271:40-48.
18. BRIDBORD, K. 1978. New Horizons in occupational medicine. National Institute of Occupational Safety and Health, Rockville, Maryland.
19. NATIONAL CANCER INSTITUTE. 1975. Third National Cancer Survey: Incidence data. Nat. Cancer Inst. Monogr. 41:1-454. (S.J. Cutler and J.L. Young, Jr., eds.).
20. NATIONAL INSTITUTE FOR OCCUPATIONAL SAFETY AND HEALTH. 1977. National Occupational Hazard Survey. Vol. III. Survey Analysis and Supplemental Tables. DHEW (NIOSH) Publication No. 78-114. Cincinnati, Ohio.
21. LEE, A.M. and FRAUMENI, J.F., JR. 1969. Arsenic and respiratory cancer in men: An occupational study. J. Nat. Cancer Inst. 42:1046-1052.
22. INFANTE, P.F., RINSKY, R.A., WAGONER, J.V., and YOUNG, R.J. 1977. Leukemia in benzene workers. Lancet:76-78, July 9, 1977.
23. ROCKETTE, H.E. 1977. Cause Specific Mortality of Coal Miners. J. Occup. Med. 19:795-801.

24. LI, F.P., FRAUMENI, J.F., JR., MANTEL, N. and MILLER, R.W. 1969. Cancer mortality among chemists. J. Nat. Cancer Inst. 43:1159-1164.
25. KOSKELA, RIITA-SISKO, HERNBERG, S., KARAVA, R., JARVINEN, E. and NURINEN, M. 1976. A mortality study of foundry workers. Scan. J. Work Environ. Health 2:suppl. 1, 73-89.
26. GIBSON, E.S., MARTIN, R.H., and LOCKINGTON, J.N. 1977. Lung cancer mortality in a steel foundry. J. Occup. Med. 19:807-812.
27. MOSS, E. and LEE, W.R. 1974. Occurrence of oral and pharyngeal cancers in textile workers. Brit. J. Ind. Med. 31:224-232.
28. LLOYD, J.W., DECOUFLE, P., and SALVIN, L.G. 1977. Unusual mortality experience of printing pressmen. J. Occup. Med. 19:543-550.
29. WAGONER, J.K., MILLER, R.W., LUNDIN, F.E., Jr., FRAUMENI, J.F., JR., and HAIJ, M.E. 1963. Unusual cancer mortility among a group of underground metal miners. New Engl. J. Med. 269:284-289.
30. REDMOND, C.K., STROBINO, B.R. and CYPESS, R.H. 1976. Cancer experience among coke by-product workers. In *Occupational Carcinogenesis.* (Eds. U. Safiotti and J. Wagoner) Ann. N.Y. Acad. Sci. 271:102-115.
31. LEMON, R.A., LEE, J.S., WAGONER, J.K. and BLEJER, H.P. 1976. Cancer mortality among cadmium production workers. In *Occupational Carcinogenesis.* (Eds. U. Saffiotti and J. Wagoner.) Ann. N.Y. Acad. Sci. 271:274-279.
32. COOPER, W.C. 1976. Cancer mortality patterns in the lead industry. In *Occupational Carcinogenesis.* (Eds. U. Saffiotti and J. Wagoner.) Ann N.Y. Acad. Sci. 271:250-259.
33. MONSON, R.R., and NAKANO, K.K. 1976. Mortality among rubber workers; I. White male union employees in Akron, Ohio. Amer. J. Epidemiol. 103:284-296.
34. PEDERSEN, E., HOGETVEIT, A.C., and ANDERSEN, A. 1973. Cancer of respiratory organs among workers at a nickel refinery in Norway. Int. J. Cancer 12: 32-41.
35. DOLL, R., MORGAN, L.G., and SPEISER, F.E. 1970. Cancers of the lung and nasal sinuses in nickel workers. Brit. J. Cancer 24:623-632.
36. ENTERLINE, P.E. 1974. Respiratory cancer among chromate workers. J. Occup. Med. 16:523-526.
37. SCHNEIDERMAN, M. 1978. Statement prepared for OSHA hearings.
38. SCHNEIDERMAN, M. 1978. Supplementary statement prepared for OSHA hearings.
39. ACHESON, E.D. 1976. Nasal cancer in the furniture and boot and shoe manufacturing industries. Prev. Med. 5:295-315.
40. BRINTON, L.A. 1977. A death certificate analysis of nasal cancer among furniture workers in North Carolina. Cancer Res. 37:3473-3474.
41. AKSOY, M. et al. 1974. Leukemia in shoe workers chronically exposed to benzene. Blood 44:837-841.
42. NATIONAL INSTITUTE FOR OCCUPATIONAL SAFETY AND HEALTH. 1975. Criteria for a recommended standard: occupational exposure to inorganic arsenic. National Institute for Occupational Safety and Health. HEW Publication No. (NIOSH) 75-149. Rockville, Maryland.

TABLE 1. CHEMICALS OR INDUSTRIAL PROCESSES ASSOCIATED WITH CANCER INDUCTION IN MAN

Derived from Ref. 8, with addition of data on worker exposure from Ref. 19; see also footnotes to Table 3.

Chemical or Industrial Process	Main Type of Exposure	Target Organs in Man	Main Route of Exposure[b]	Estimated No. of Workers Exposed in U.S.
Aflatoxins	E, O	Liver	Oral, inhalation	______[d]
4-amino biphenyl	O	Bladder	Inhalation, skin, oral	100
Arsenic compounds	O, M, E	Skin, lung liver[c]	Inhalation, skin, oral	1,500,000[g]
Asbestos	O	Lung, pleural cavity, g.i. tract	Inhalation, oral	1,600,000
Auramine (manufacture)	O	Bladder	Inhalation, skin, oral	______[d]
Benzene	O	Hemato-poietic system	Inhalation, skin	1,900,000
Benzidine	O	Bladder	Inhalation, skin, oral	2,200
Bis(chloromethyl) ether	O	Lung	Inhalation	______[d]
Cadmium-using industries (? cadmium oxide)	O	Prostate, Lung	Inhalation, oral	1,400,000
Chloramphenicol	M	Hemato-poietic system	Oral, injection	______[d]
Chloromethyl methyl ether	O	Lung	Inhalation	______[d]
Chromium (chromate producing industries)	O	Lung, nasal cavities[c]	Inhalation	1,500,0C (chromium oxides)

O=Occupational; E=environmental; M=Medicinal.

[a]The main types of exposure mentioned are those by which the association has been demonstrated.

[b]The main routes of exposure given may not be the only ones by which such effects could occur.

[c]Denotes indicative evidence

Chemical or Industrial Process	Main Type of Exposure[a]	Target Organs in Man	Main Route of Exposure[b]	Estimated No. of Workers Exposed in U.S.
Cyclophosphamide	M	Bladder	Oral, injection	________[d]
Diethylstilbestrol	M	Uterus, vagina	Oral	________[d]
Haematite mining	O	Lung	Inhalation	19,000
Isopropyl Oil	O	Nasal cavity, larynx	Inhalation	________[d]
Melphalan	M	Hemato-poietic system	Oral, injection	________[d]
Mustard gas	O	Lung, larnyx	Inhalation	________[d]
2-Naphthylamine	O	Bladder	Inhalation, skin, oral	1,000
Nickel (oxides)	O	Nasal cavity, lung	Inhalation	1,400,000[e]
Chlornaphazine	M	Bladder	Oral	________[d]
Oxymetholone	M	Liver	Oral	________[d]
Phenacetin	M	Kidney	Oral	________[d]
Phenytoin	M	Lymphoreticular tissues	Oral, injection	________[d]
Soot, tars and oils	O, E	Lung, skin, scrotum	Inhalation, skin	________[f]
Vinyl chloride	O	Liver, brain[c] lung[c]	Inhalation, skin	2,200,000

[d]Not recorded in the survey: exposure very small in all cases except aflatoxins.
[e]No. of workers exposed to nickel oxide: only about 230 workers exposed to nickel carbonyl
[f]Exposure very large but not characterized numerically

TABLE 2. REPORTED RISKS ASSOCIATED WITH OCCUPATIONAL EXPOSURE: COMPARISON BETWEEN ASBESTOS AND FIVE OTHER HIGH-EXPOSURE SUBSTANCES

Chemical Substance	Affected Organs	Risk Ratio (R)[a]	Age-Adjusted Incidence Per 100,000 Males Over 20 Years (I)[b]	Estimated No. of Workers Currently Exposed (N)[c]	(R-1) NI
Asbestos	Lung, pleural & peritoneal mesothelia	1.5-12	116	1,600,000	900-19,000
Asbestos	Lung, pleural & peritoneal mesothelia	6.6[d]	116	1,600,000	10,400
Asbestos	Esophagus	2.7[d]	9.4	1,600,000	250
Asbestos	Stomach	1.7[d]	26.2	1,600,000	400
Asbestos	Colon/Rectum	1.6[d]	85	1,600,000	800
Arsenic	Respiratory tract	3-8	131	1,500,000[g]	3,900-14,000
Benzene	Leukemia	2-5[e]	17.9	2,000,000	350-1,400
Chromium	Respiratory tract	5-9	131	1,500,000	7,900-16,000
Nickel (oxides)	Respiratory tract	5-10	131	1,400,000	7,300-16,500
Petroleum fractions (including aromatics)	Lung	3 (2-33)[f]	116	3,900,000[f]	9,100

[a] From ref. 7 unless otherwise stated: see also detailed notes
[b] From ref. 18
[c] From ref. 17, derived from ref. 19
[d] From Table 3 in ref. 15
[e] From ref. 21
[f] From ref. 16: see detailed notes
[g] From ref. 42

The figures for risk ratios listed in the table are drawn from the tabulation by Cole and Goldman (ref. 7). The notes below provide further data drawn from the principal published references for each substance.

ASBESTOS

Number of workers potentially exposed: About 1,600,000
Risk Ratios: 1.5 – 12 for lung, pleural and peritoneal mesothelia
Projected number of excess cancers per year: 13,900

From the studies of Selikoff (ref. 15) the relative risk for lung cancer among asbestos-insulation workers in the U.S. is about 6.6, which accounts for about 20% of their deaths. A further 7% of cases are due to mesotheliomas which otherwise occur rarely. Applying the 6.6-fold increase in lung cancer to 1.6 million exposed workers yeilds 10,400 excess cases with roughly another one third or 3,500 due to mesothelioma for a total of 13,900 cases per year. Provisional projections for excess cancers in the respiratory tract, based upon the observed relative risks in Selikoff's study (15) are given in Table 2.

ARSENIC

Number of workers potentially exposed: about 1,500,000
Risk Ratios: 3-8 for respiratory tract cancers
Projected number of excess cancers per year: 7,300

In 1969 Lee and Fraumeni (ref. 21) evaluated the mortality experience of 8,047 white male smelter workers exposed to arsenic trioxide during 1938 to 1963. Smelter workers were found to have a three-fold excess in mortality from all respiratory cancer compared to a statewide population control group. About half of those in the study population were exposed to arsenic less than 10 years. Of those exposed for at least 15 years and followed another 25 years, the relative risk for respiratory cancer was 4.7. If this excess can be applied to the approximately 1,500,000 workers exposed to arsenic, it is projected that about 7,300 excess lung cancers each year may occur. It should be noted that the cancer risk from exposure to arsenic may be influenced by exposures to other occupational chemicals, such as sulfur dioxide.

Exposure to arsenic has also been associated with excess cancers of the skin and liver (7): these sites are not considered here.

BENZENE

Number of workers potentially exposed: about 2,000,000
Risk Ratios: About 5 for leukemia
Projected number of excess cancers per year: 1,400

A study by Infante, Rinsky, Wagoner and Young (ref. 22) examined the mortality experience of workers exposed to benzene from 1940 to 1949. A significant 5-fold excess risk of death from all leukemias was observed compared to controls (7 observed vs. about 1.4 expected). This study represents an understatement of risk since the 25% lost to follow-up in the study population were regarded as alive in the statistical analysis. These data are consistent with numerous case reports of leukemia deaths among workers exposed to benzene. Based on these figures and an estimated occupationally-exposed population of about 2 million, it is projected that about 1,400 excess leukemia cases may occur due to benzene exposure on the job.

CHROMIUM (Trioxide and other hexavalent chromium compounds)

Number of workers potentially exposed: about 1,500,000
Risk Ratios: 3-40 for nasal cavity and sinus, lung and larynx
Projected number of excess cancers per year: 7,900

Enterline (36) noted that the overall SMR for respiratory cancer in a group of 1,200 chromate workers, ages 20-64, who were working some time between January 1, 1937 and December 31, 1940 and who were born after 1889 was 942.6. SMRs decreased steadily over the observational period from a high of 2902.1 in the interval from 1941-45 to a low of 474.7 in 1956-60. From the above, it would seem that a reasonable estimate of the risk ratio for all respiratory cancers among workers exposed to chromium would be at least 5 and perhaps as high as 9. Assuming that an overall risk of 5 can be applied to the approximately 1.5 million exposed workers, it is estimated that about 7,900 excess cancer cases might occur each year.

NICKEL (Oxides)

Number of workers potentially exposed: about 1,400,000
Risk ratio: 5-10 for respiratory tract
Projected number of excess cancers per year: 7,300

A Norwegian study by Pedersen **et al.** in 1973 (34) observed an overall excess respiratory cancer increase of 5.6 fold among nearly 2,000 men exposed to nickel. The highest risk (risk ratio of 14.0) was observed in men first employed before 1930 and followed for at least 40 years. Assuming that an overall risk ratio of about 5 for all respiratory cancers can be applied to the approximately 1,400,000 workers estimated exposed to nickel, it is projected that about 7,300 excess respiratory cancers, excluding nasal cancer, will occur each year. Studies by Doll (35) document the dramatic decrease in risk from respiratory cancer when positive action has been taken to reduce occupational exposure to nickel. Exposure to nickel compounds is also associated with excess cancers of the nasal sinuses (7): these cancers are not considered here.

PETROLEUM PRODUCTS, INCLUDING AROMATIC HYDROCARBONS

Number of workers potentially exposed: about 3,900,000
Risk ratios: 2-33 for lung cancer
Projected number of excess cancers per year: 9,100

The carcinogenic properties of petroleum products, especially polynuclear aromatic hydrocarbons (PNHs) have been well studied. Lung cancer risk ratios in the range of 2 to 33 have been observed for coke oven and gas workers in the U.S., England, and Japan exposed to PNHs which are contained in petroleum products (Doll, Lloyd, Kawai, Kalzumdar, Redmond). Excess lung cancer risk rates have also been observed for roofers in the U.S. (Hammond). Less well appreciated is the fact that many other occupational groups are exposed to aromatic hydrocarbons, including polynuclear aromatics; these groups include mechanics, electricians, and workers in the printing industry. (Menck and Henderson ref. 16). The risk ratios for lung cancer in these groups range from about 2 to 4. The number of workers estimated to be exposed to aromatic hydrocarbons, including polynuclear aromatics, is about 3,900,000. Assuming that an overall lung cancer risk ratio of 3 can be applied to these workers, it is estimated that about 9,100 excess lung cancer deaths each year might occur in this group.

TABLE 3. OCCUPATIONAL GROUPS IN WHICH EXCESS CANCER INCIDENCE HAS BEEN REPORTED WITHOUT IDENTIFICATION OF A SPECIFIC ETIOLOGIC AGENT

Occupational Groups	Cancer Site(s)	% Excess Reported	Reference
Coal Miners	Stomach	40	23
Chemists	Pancreas, lymphomas	64 79	24
Foundry Workers	Lung	50-150	25,26
Textile Workers	Mouth & Pharynx	77	27
Printing Pressmen (newspaper)	Mouth & Pharynx	125	28
Metal Miners	Lung	200	29
Coke By-Product Workers	Large intestine, Pancreas	181 312	30
Cadmium Production Workers	Lung, Prostate	135 248	31
Rubber Industry			
Processing	Stomach, leukemia	80 140	33
Tire Building	Bladder, Brain	88 90	33
Tire Curing	Lung	61	33
Furniture Workers	Nasal cavity & Sinuses	300-400	39
Shoe Workers	Nasal cavity & Sinuses, leukemia	700 100	39,40 41
Leather Workers	Bladder	150	7

Note: With the possible exception of the lung cancers and leukemias, there is no overlap between the excess cancers listed in this table and Table 2.

ESTIMATION OF LIFETIME RISKS FOLLOWING OCCUPATIONAL EXPOSURE

A major part of the preceding paper concerns the prediction of lifetime risk following occupational exposure to carcinogens during all or part of a working life. The estimates were derived assuming that relative risks remain constant for the rest of the lifetime, the estimated values for the relative risks being derived from cohorts with their own particular distributions of age, and both age at, and duration since first exposure. The purpose of this Appendix is to show that the assumption of constancy of relative risk has a reasonable basis. Both relevant epidemiological data and the predictions of mathematical models of carcinogenesis will be considered.

Epidemiological data from four types of exposure are discussed: asbestos, nickel, radiation, and cigarette smoking. The latter two are not primarily occupational exposures, but they provide the two examples best studies with regard to evolution of risk after exposure.

For cigarette smoking, the incidence of lung cancer increases with the daily amount smoked (either linearly or perhaps quadratically) and with the fourth power of duration of smoking, for current smokers. On stopping smoking the incidence does not further increase, but remains approximately constant with age until it approaches that of non-smokers after some 20 years (Doll and Peto 1976). The relative risk therefore falls within five years of stopping smoking, as shown in Figure 1a.

For radiation, leukemia behaves differently from tumors of epithelial origin. Following a single course of radiation treatment for ankylosing spondylitis (Smith and Doll 1978), the relative risk for leukemia rises rapidly, reaching a peak within 3-5 years, then decreases to become inappreciable some 12-15 years after exposure (Figure 1b). The relative risks for epithelial tumors of heavily exposed organs, however, remain low until 10 years after exposure, then rise and remain on a plateau for the remainder of the observation period (Figure 1c).

Other epidemiological data on risks from irradiation show similar behavior for leukemia (A-bomb survivors) and for breast cancer (A-bomb survivors, women given radiation treatment for tuberculosis or post-partum mastitis).

The two examples just given provide the two extreme possibilities, continually elevated risk following exposure of very limited duration, or a rapid fall in risk following cessation of a long lasting exposure.

Asbestos and nickel provide two examples of occupational exposures where cohorts have been followed over an extended period of time. Asbestos causes lung cancer, cancer of the gastrointestinal tract, and mesotheliomas (Selikoff and Hammond 1978). Among a cohort more than two thirds of whom had been exposed for less than two years (Newhouse and Berry), the incidence of mesotheliomas increased with increasing rapidity until the limit of the observation period, 35 years after first exposure (Figure 1d). Conversion of these incidence figures into corresponding values for relative risk is not helpful due to the rarity of the non-occupationally related disease. However, the absolute risk, as given by the incidence figure, shows no sign of leveling off even thirty years after cessation of external exposure. Extrapolation of the incidence curve to higher age groups would seem justified, to give an estimate of 8-10% of deaths due to mesothelioma predicted in the group under study (Newhouse and Berry 1976).

For cancer of the lung the data have not been presented in such clear fashion but all studies indicate an increase in relative risk for the period more than twenty years after start of exposure compared to 10-19 years after start of exposure. Assumption of a constant relative risk would appear to be conservative (Selikoff and Hammond 1978; Peto et al. 1977; Newhouse and Berry 1976; Knox et al. 1968).

For nickel, the main carcinogenic hazard for the cohort from Wales appears to have been removed from the environment around 1930 (Doll, Matthews and Morgan 1977). Nevertheless, there has been no indication that the relative risk for either lung cancer or for cancer of the nasal sinuses has fallen over the decades following the reduction in hazard (Doll et al. 1970, 1977) up to the most recently reported follow-up ending 1971. Similarly in the Norwegian study (Pedersen 1973), the great reduction in exposure to dust and fumes since 1950 is not reflected in any reduction in relative risk. Interestingly, the values for the relative risk (average over follow-up to 1971 in both cases) for the Welsh cohorts exposed before 1930 and the Norweigian cohort exposed before 1950 were similar, approximately 10-fold.

One would conclude from these two examples of occupational exposure that the epithelial tumors induced behave more like epithelial tumors related to radiation than to those related to cigarette smoking. Exposure to the aromatic amines would seem similar with risk among the exposed not falling two decased after removal from the workplace of the known carcinogens but in this situation the replacements for the carcinogens may themselves have been carcinogenic (Fox and Collier 1976).

The different types of behavior described above can be devised from the widely accepted multi-stage theory of carcinogenesis, where a cancer is assumed to arise from a single cell which then passes through a series of stages, the last of which leads irreversibly to a clinically apparent tumor. With k stages, and with probabilities of transition constant over age, one would predict the age-specific incidence to increase with age to be (k-1) power, as is observed for most epithelial tumors with k = 5 or 6 (Whittemore 1977; Cook, Doll and Fellingham 1969).

Now suppose that an external carcinogen, as in an industrial exposure, begins to operate at time t_1, and then is removed at time t_2. If cancer is a multi-stage process, then the effect on the incidence on which stage in the process is primarily effected. If the initial stage is affected then we expect the relative risk at time t $(t>t_2)$ to be of the form:

$$R(t) = 1 + c\,[(1 - t_1/t)^{k-1} + (1 - t_2/t)^{k-1}]$$

where c is proportional to the dose. R(t) is shown graphically for various values of t_1 and t_2 in Figure 2a. The approximate constancy of the relative risk over time for a range of values of t_1 and t_2 is apparent, similar to the behavior for epithelial tumors after irradiation, and probably similar to the effects of asbestos and nickel.

If the penultimate stage is affected, the behavior is different, the relative risk at time t $(t > t_2)$ being given by $1 + (t_2/t)^{k-1} - (t_1/t)^{k-1}$, i.e. decreasing rapidly after cessation of exposure, as in Figure 2b.

Cigarette smoking related lung cancer gives an example of this type of behavior.

For mesotheliomas where because of the low spontaneous incidence relative risk calculations are of little value a multi stage model (with K = 3) has been successfully fitted to both animal data and data from 35 years of follow-up of a cohort (Newhouse and Berry 1976).

The multi-stage model appears to give a coherent picture of the evolution of risk after exposure during a limited interval which is consistent with available epidemiological data, at least for epithelial tumors which comprise the great majority of occupationally related cancers. These data taken together with the implication of the model, give support to the assumption on which many of the numerical estimates of the paper are based, and justify extrapolation of relative risk values obtained from industrially exposed cohorts to the remaining lifetime of the cohort.

REFERENCES

COOK, P.J., DOLL, R., and FELLINGHAM, S.A. 1969. A mathematical model for the age distribution of cancer in man. Int. J. Can. 4:93-112

DOLL, R., MORGAN, L.G., and SPEIZER, F. 1970. Cancers of the lung and nasal sinuses in nickel workers. Brit. J. Can. 24:623-632

DOLL, R., and PETO, R. 1976. Mortality in relation to smoking: 20 years' observation on male British doctors. Brit. Med. J. 2:1525-1536

DOLL, R., MATHEWS, J.D., and MORGAN, L.G. 1977. Cancers of the lung and nasal sinuses in nickel workers: A reassessment of the period of riks. Brit. J. Indust. Med. 34:102-105

FOX, A.J., and COLLIER, P.F. 1976. A survey of occupational cancer in the rubber and cablemaking industries: Analysis of deaths occurring in 1972-74. Brit. J. Indust. Med. 33:249-264

KNOX, J.F., HOLMES, S., DOLL, R., and HILL, I.D. 1968. Mortality from lung cancer and outher causes among workers in an asbestos textile factory. Brit J. Indust. Med. 25:293-303

NEWHOUSE, M.L., and BERRY, G. 1976. Predictions of mortality from mesothelial tumors in asbestos factory workers. Brit. J. Indust. Med. 33:147-151

PEDERSEN, E., HOGETVEIT, A.C., and ANDERSEN, A. 1973. Cancer of respiratory organs among workers at a Nickel refinery in Norway. Int. J. Can. 12:32-41

PETO, J., DOLL, R., HOWARD, W.V., KINLEN, L.J., and LEWINSHOH, H.C. 1977. A mortality study among workers in an English asbestos factory. Brit. J. Indust. Med. 34:169-173

SELIKOFF, I.J., and HAMMOND, E.C. 1978. Asbestos-associated disease in United States Shipyeard. Can. 28(2):87-99

SMITH, P.G. and DOLL, R. 1978. Age and time dependent changes in the rates of radiation induced cancers in patients with ankylosing spondylitis following a single course of x-ray treatment. Presented at the International Atomic Energy Agency Symposium on Late Biological Effects of Ionizing Radiation, Vienna, March 13-17

WHITTEMORE, A.S. 1977. The age distribution of human cancer for carcinogenic exposures of varying intensity. Am. J. Epid. 106(5):418-432

FIGURE 1A

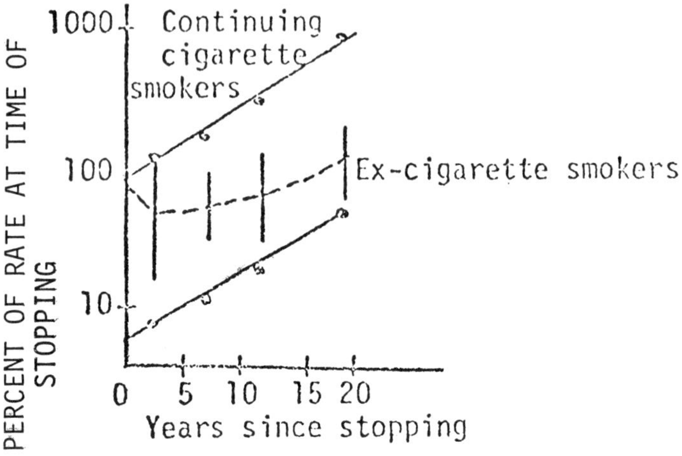

FIGURE 1B

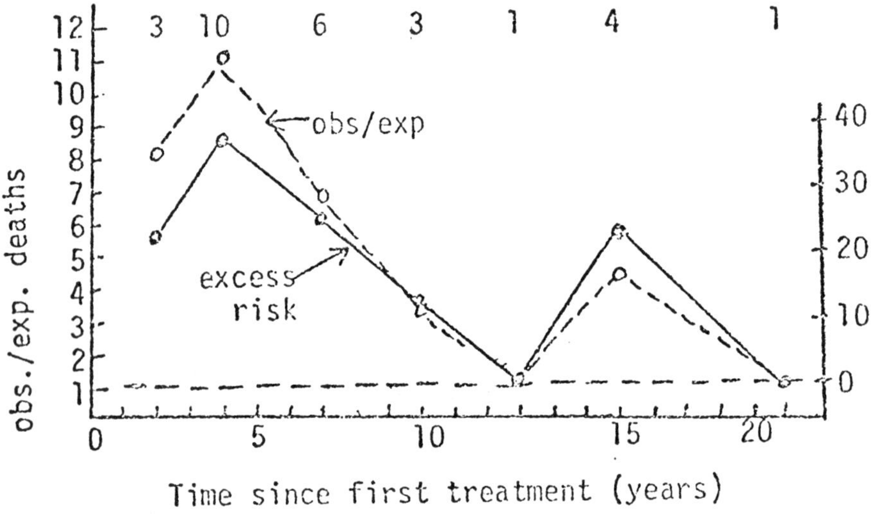

FIGURE 1C

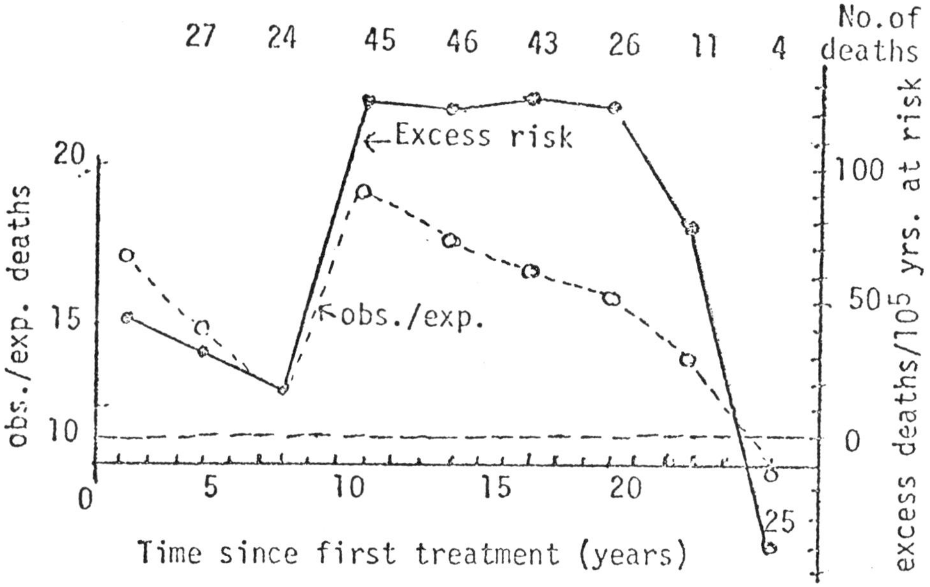

FIGURE 1D

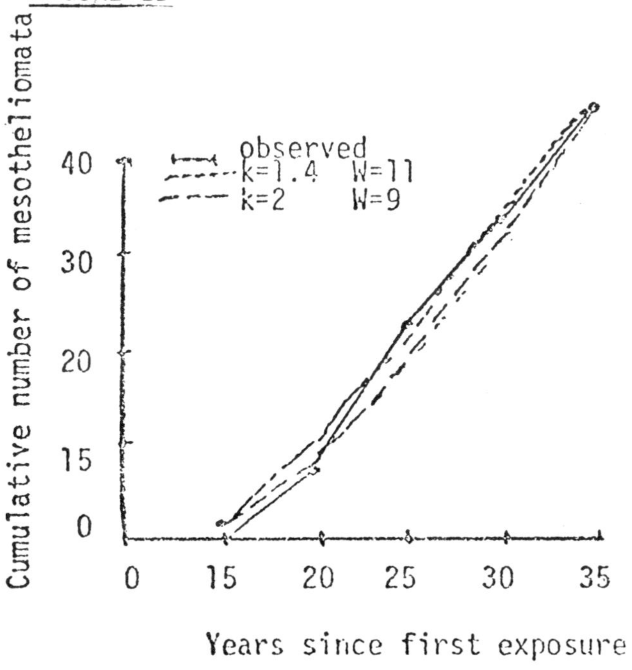

FIGURE 2A

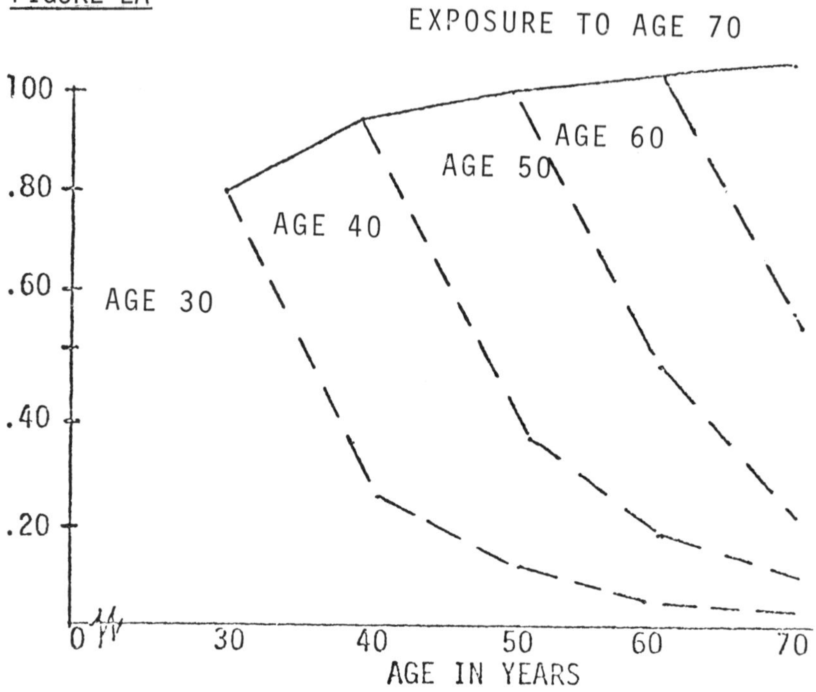

FIRST STAGE EFFECTED EXPOSURE BEGINS AT AGE 20

Evolution of Relative Risk after limited exposure, expressed as percent of Relative Risk associated with exposure through age 70

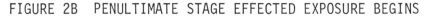

FIGURE 2B PENULTIMATE STAGE EFFECTED EXPOSURE BEGINS AT AGE 20

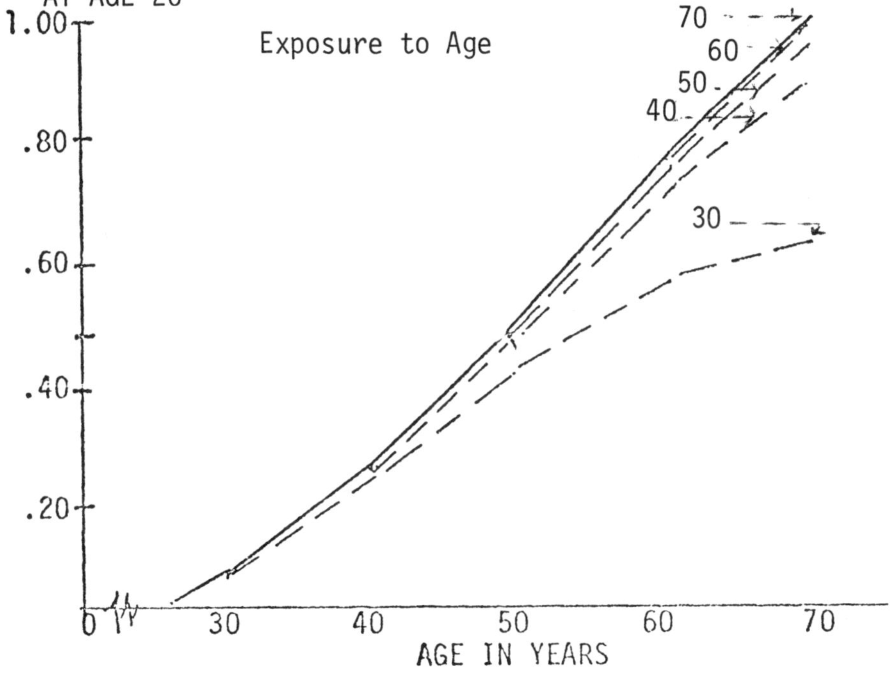

Evolution of Risk After Limited Duration Exposure, Expressed as Percent of Risk Associated with Exposure Through Age 70

LEGENDS FOR FIGURES

1. a. Incidence rate of lung cancer as a percent of rate at time of stopping.

   b. Risk for leukemia following irradiation for ankylosing spondylitis. Left hand vertical axis shows scale for relative risk, right hand vertical axis shows absolute excess number/10^5 population per year.

   c. Risk for tumors of the heavily irradiated sites, following irradiation for ankylosing spondylitis. Vertical axes as in 1b.

   d. Incidence of mesotheliomata, expressed as cumulative number observed, in years since first exposure to asbestos. Expected incidence obtained from Weilbull model with

$$\text{Risk} = c\ (t\text{-}w)^k$$

   where c, w and k are constant (as given in the figure) and t the time since first exposure.

2. Evaluation of risk after exposure of limited duration as predicted by a multi-stage model of carcinogenesis.

   a. First stage effected by the exposure.
   b. Penultimate stage effected by the exposure.

Name Index

Subject Index